An Ultimate Guide to
COMMUNITY MEDICINE

An Ultimate Guide to
COMMUNITY MEDICINE

As per the Competency-based Medical Education Curriculum (NMC)

Fourth Edition

Prithwiraj Maiti

MBBS (RG Kar Medical College)
Postgraduate Trainee
DNB General Medicine
Apollo Multispeciality Hospital
Kolkata, West Bengal, India

Bismoy Mondal

MBBS (RG Kar Medical College) MS (Kolkata)
General Surgery FIAGS (World Laparoscopic Hospital)
MRCS-A (London) MCh (Neurosurgery)
Postdoctoral Trainee
Department of Neurosurgery
Post-Graduate Medical Education and Research
Seth Sukhlal Karnani Memorial Hospital (IPGMER/SSKM)
Kolkata, West Bengal, India

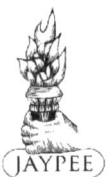

JAYPEE BROTHERS MEDICAL PUBLISHERS
The Health Sciences Publisher
New Delhi | London

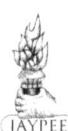

Jaypee Brothers Medical Publishers (P) Ltd.

Headquarters

Jaypee Brothers Medical Publishers (P) Ltd.
EMCA House, 23/23-B
Ansari Road, Daryaganj
New Delhi 110 002, India
Landline: +91-11-23272143, +91-11-23272703
+91-11-23282021, +91-11-23245672
Email: jaypee@jaypeebrothers.com

Overseas Office

J.P. Medical Ltd.
83 Victoria Street, London
SW1H 0HW (UK)
Phone: +44 20 3170 8910
Email: info@jpmedpub.com

Corporate Office

Jaypee Brothers Medical Publishers (P) Ltd.
4838/24, Ansari Road, Daryaganj
New Delhi 110 002, India
Phone: +91-11-43574357
Fax: +91-11-43574314
Email: jaypee@jaypeebrothers.com

EU GPSR Authorised Representative

Logos Europe, 9 rue Nicolas Poussin
17000, La Rochelle, France
Phone: +33 (0) 6 67 93 73 78
E-mail: Contact@logoseurope.eu

Website: www.jaypeebrothers.com
Website: www.jaypeedigital.com

Inquiries for bulk sales may be solicited at: jaypee@jaypeebrothers.com

An Ultimate Guide to Community Medicine

First Edition: 2016
Second Edition: 2017
Third Edition: *2019*
Fourth Edition: **2023**

ISBN: 978-93-5465-340-7

Preface to the Fourth Edition

First of all, we are thankful to the students and readers of our title for their appreciation and blessings throughout these long three years which helped us continue our journey to the 4th edition of *"An Ultimate Guide to Community Medicine".*

In the fourth edition, we have kept the same concise format in order to remain the only student-friendly reference guide of the subject. Yet we have added new contents and updates. All chapters have been thoroughly revised and improvised with the most recent guidelines.

Some of the major updates are as follows:
- Revised National Tuberculosis Control Program guidelines (2022)
- Revised Malaria control guidelines (2022)
- Revised guidelines on initiation of antiretroviral therapy (2022)
- COVID-19 updates (2022)
- New vaccines being introduced in Universal Immunization Program (2017)
- Pradhan Mantri Surakshit Matritva Abhiyan (2016)
- National switch from trivalent OPV to bivalent OPV (2016)
- ESI Act updates (2016)
- New biomedical waste management and handling rules (2016)
- New treatment guidelines on kala-azar (2015)
- Revised IMCI guidelines (2014)
- Swachh Bharat Abhiyan (2014)
- RMNCH+A strategy
- Rashtriya Kishor Swasthya Karyakram
- National Iron Plus Initiative
- Most recent health-related statistics

We would like to express our immense gratitude to our juniors, colleagues, friends, teachers and family because this book is the result of the encouragement, appreciation and guidance from all of them.

Last but not the least, I would like to thank Shri Jitendar P Vij (Group Chairman), Mr Ankit Vij (Managing Director), Mr MS Mani (Group President), Dr Madhu Choudhary (Director-Educational Publishing), Ms Pooja Bhandari (Production Head), Ms Sunita Katla (Executive Assistant to Group Chairman and Publishing Manager), Ms Samina Khan (Executive Assistant to Director–Educational Publishing), Dr Upma Tomar (Development Editor), Mr Rajesh Sharma (Production Coordinator), Ms Seema Dogra (Cover Visualizer), Ms Geeta Barik (Proofreader), Mr Kulwant Singh (Typesetter), Mr Nitin Bhardwaj (Graphic Designer) and the entire team of M/s Jaypee Brothers Medical Publishers (P) Ltd, New Delhi, India, for their meticulous work in publishing this book.

Wishing you all the very best and looking forward for your feedback and valuable suggestions.

Prithwiraj Maiti
Bismoy Mondal

Preface to the First Edition

This book is our first work together with its delicacy, to produce a concise intricate narrative of this vast subject of Community Medicine.

Textbook writing is not a cup of tea for us and since there are innumerable access to tougher textbooks and journals for our colleagues and juniors pursuing this vast career, we never quite got around to writing it. Rather, we have sown the idea of improvising a Standard Students' Guide for this subject, which would glean many new insights, both in theoretical as well as scorers' aspect. So we have given our every strength to it with a dream to revolutionize a subject, which we are sure that many students fail to grow interest in.

This book has been incubating in our heads for the last 2 years since we came across the voluminous syllabi of this subject ourselves and could not have access to a concise form of 'Must know'. There is something distinctly fascinating even about this subject and our idea was to emerge that which precedes through these endeavors.

This whole idea includes itself from the roots of PHC up to WHO in its deliberate and illustrative format, with efficiency of being a handy dealing during examinations. The references and schematic illustrations have been skillfully checked and improvized to avoid echoes of perpetuation and recent values have been updated till date.

We are grateful to many renowned personalities of this subject who were with us being actively involved in the project from its inception. Any kind of mistake is unintended and may kindly be excused; we will surely entertain all the suggestions and rectify them in the subsequent editions.

We are very much hopeful for this title because we have already put our best efforts to ensure the student-friendliness of this book. We hope this book will reduce the pressure of the students during tough times and as well will hold the position of one of the most updated books of the regarding subject in current times. Last but not least, we would be highly elated if this book emphasizes its own potential and accessibility at its best for whom it is written and presented throughout these years.

Prithwiraj Maiti
Bismoy Mondal

Contents

Section 1: Introduction

Chapter 1: History of Medicine   1

Section 2: Guide to Theory Examination

Chapter 2: Long Essay Type Questions   3
- ❖ Concept of Health and Disease   *3*
- ❖ Principles of Epidemiology and Epidemiological Methods   *7*
- ❖ Screening for Disease   *15*
- ❖ Epidemiology of Communicable Diseases   *17*
- ❖ Epidemiology of Chronic Noncommunicable Disease and Conditions   *41*
- ❖ Health Programs in India   *45*
- ❖ Demography and Family Planning   *55*
- ❖ Preventive Medicine in Obstetric, Pediatrics and Geriatrics   *64*
- ❖ Nutrition and Health   *67*
- ❖ Medicine and Social Sciences   *77*
- ❖ Environment and Health   *77*
- ❖ Hospital Waste Management   *78*
- ❖ Occupational Health   *78*
- ❖ Health Information and Basic Biomedical Statistics   *83*
- ❖ Communication for Health Education   *83*
- ❖ Health Planning and Management   *84*
- ❖ Health Care of the Community   *84*
- ❖ International Health   *89*

Chapter 3: Problem Type Questions   90
- ❖ Duties of BMOH in Solving a Problem in his Block   *90*
- ❖ Functions of a BMOH During Investigation of an Epidemic   *91*
- ❖ Format for Writing Duties of a BMOH During a General Outbreak   *92*
- ❖ Duties of a BMOH During Some Important Disease Outbreaks   *96*
- ❖ Duties of BMOH in Solving Different Pediatric, Geriatric and Obstetric Problems   *105*
- ❖ Duties of BMOH During Flood   *120*
- ❖ Duties of BMOH During a Low Immunization Coverage in Block   *124*
- ❖ Duties of BMOH in Solving Problems of Malnutrition in Block   *127*
- ❖ Duties of BMOH in Preventing Low Couple Protection Rate   *132*
- ❖ Duties of BMOH in Preventing Anemia in Pregnant Women   *135*
- ❖ Duties of BMOH in Preventing Incidence of Accidents in a Block   *140*
- ❖ Duties of BMOH in Reducing Popularity of Quacks in a Block   *144*

Chapter 4: Short Notes   147
- ❖ Man and Disease   *147*
- ❖ Concept of Health and Disease   *149*
- ❖ Epidemiology   *158*

- Screening   *167*
- Epidemiology of Communicable Diseases   *168*
- Epidemiology of Noncommunicable Diseases   *178*
- Health Programs in India   *180*
- Demography   *182*
- Preventive Medicine in Obstetrics, Pediatrics and Geriatrics   *185*
- Nutrition and Health   *195*
- Medicine and Social Sciences   *202*
- Environment and Health   *205*
- Hospital Waste Management   *223*
- Disaster Management   *225*
- Occupational Health   *230*
- Genetics and Health   *232*
- Health Information and Basic Biomedical Statistics   *233*
- Communication for Health Education   *241*
- Health Planning and Management   *245*
- Health Care of the Community   *249*
- International Health Organizations   *254*

Chapter 5: Justify/Explain Why   **258**
- Concept of Health and Disease   *258*
- Principles of Epidemiology and Epidemiological Methods   *261*
- Screening for Disease   *266*
- Epidemiology of Communicable Disease   *269*
- Epidemiology of Chronic Noncommunicable Disease and Condition   *288*
- Health Programs in India   *290*
- Demography and Family Planning   *291*
- Preventive Medicine in Obstetrics, Pediatrics and Geriatrics   *292*
- Nutrition and Health   *295*
- Environment and Health   *303*
- Hospital Waste Management   *307*
- Disaster Management   *309*
- Occupational Health   *310*
- Genetics and Health   *313*
- Mental Health   *314*
- Health Information and Basic Biomedical Statistics   *314*
- Communication for Health Education   *316*
- Health Planning and Management   *318*
- Health Care of the Community   *320*

Chapter 6: Differences   **324**
- Community Diagnosis Vs. Clinical Diagnosis   *324*
- Social Medicine Vs. Socialized Medicine   *324*
- Community Diagnosis Vs. Hospital Medicine   *325*
- Disease Control Vs. Disease Elimination Vs. Disease Eradication   *325*
- Impairment Vs. Disability Vs. Handicap   *326*
- Isolation Vs. Quarantine   *327*
- Descriptive Epidemiology Vs. Analytical Epidemiology   *327*
- Cross Infection Vs. Cross Immunity   *327*
- Case Control Study Vs. Cohort Study   *328*
- Longitudinal Studies Vs. Cross-sectional Studies   *328*

* Incubation Period Vs. Generation Time *329*
* Intrinsic Incubation Period Vs. Extrinsic Incubation Period *329*
* Population Pyramid of Developing Country Vs. Developed Country *330*
* Hard Tick Vs. Soft Tick *330*
* Food Fortification Vs. Food Adulteration *331*
* Kwashiorkor Vs. Marasmus *331*
* Growth Monitoring Vs. Nutritional Surveillance *332*
* Old Vs. New ICDS Growth Chart *333*
* Pasteurization Vs. Sterilization *334*
* Preplacement Examination Vs. Periodic Examination *334*
* Social Security Vs. Social Assistance *335*
* Incidence Vs. Prevalence *335*
* Screening Test Vs. Diagnostic Test *336*
* Health Education Vs. Health Propaganda *336*
* Shallow Well Vs. Deep Well *336*
* Slow Sand Filter Vs. Rapid Sand Filter *337*
* Panel Discussion Vs. Group Discussion *338*
* Supplementary Nutrition Vs. Therapeutic Nutrition *338*
* Objective Vs. Target Vs. Goal *338*
* Cost-Effective Analysis Vs. Cost Benefit Analysis *338*
* Family Planning Concept Vs. Family Welfare Concept *339*
* Child Survival and Safe Motherhood (CSSM) Vs. Reproductive and Child Health (RCH) *339*
* Administration Vs. Management *339*

Section 3: Viva Voce

Chapter 7: Immunization **340**
* Immunization *340*
* Types *340*
* Toxoid, Subunit Vaccine, Combined Vaccine and Experimental Vaccine *344*
* Some Other Definitions *345*
* Adverse Events Following Immunization (AEFI) *346*
* Sites of Administration of Different Vaccines *351*
* DPT Vaccine *355*
* Recent Updates: Pentavalent Vaccine *358*
* Oral Polio Vaccine *359*
* Inactivated Polio Vaccine *362*
* Measles Vaccine *364*
* Tetanus Toxoid *366*
* Hepatitis B Vaccine *368*
* Vitamin A in Oil *370*
* Maximum Age of Vaccination *372*
* Delayed Immunization *373*
* Vaccine Vial Monitor *374*
* AD Syringe *375*
* Cold Chain *375*
* Storage of Vaccine at Different Levels *376*
* Vaccine Storage and Transportation Equipment *376*
* Open Vial Policy (2015) *380*

Chapter 8: Family Planning   **381**

    ❖ Conventional Contraceptives   *385*
    ❖ Intrauterine Devices (IUDs)   *389*
    ❖ Hormonal Methods   *395*
    ❖ The Medical Termination of Pregnancy (MTP) Act, 1971   *403*
    ❖ Natural Family Planning Methods   *405*
    ❖ Other Methods of Contraception   *406*
    ❖ Problem-based Questions   *415*

Chapter 9: Specimens   **420**

    ❖ Iron and Folic Acid Tablets   *420*
    ❖ Disposable Delivery Kit   *422*
    ❖ ORS   *423*

Chapter 10: Definitions   **428**

    ❖ Concept of Health and Disease   *428*
    ❖ Epidemiology   *431*
    ❖ Screening   *432*
    ❖ Communicable Diseases   *433*
    ❖ Noncommunicable Diseases   *435*
    ❖ Demography and Family Planning   *436*
    ❖ Preventive Medicine in Obstetrics, Gynecology and Pediatrics   *437*
    ❖ Nutrition   *438*
    ❖ Hospital Waste Management   *439*
    ❖ Disaster Management   *439*
    ❖ Occupational Health   *439*
    ❖ Health Statistics   *440*
    ❖ Other Important Definitions   *440*

Section 4: Guide to Practical Examination

Chapter 11: Statistical and Epidemiological Exercises   **441**

    Numerical Problems   441
    ❖ Mortality Rates   *441*
    ❖ Morbidity and Fertility Indicators   *442*
    ❖ Neonatal, Postnatal and Infant Mortality Rates   *444*
    ❖ Perinatal, Under Five and Child Mortality Rates   *446*
    ❖ Maternal Mortality Ratio   *449*
    ❖ Risk Assessment   *452*
    ❖ Sensitivity, Specificity, Positive and Negative Predictive Value   *454*
    ❖ Relevant Questions   *455*
    ❖ Medical Statistics   *457*
    ❖ Relevant Questions   *461*

Chapter 12: Family   **464**

Chapter 13: Project   **472**

    ❖ Variable   *472*
    ❖ Types   *472*
    ❖ Difference between Project and Program   *472*
    ❖ Census   *472*
    ❖ Data   *473*

Chapter 14: Problem Cards   **475**
- Disease Related   *475*
- Integrated Management of Childhood Illness (IMCI) Related   *484*
- Obstetric Care Related   *485*
- Immunization Related   *489*
- Family Planning Related   *493*
- Growth Chart Related   *494*

Section 5: Special Topics

Chapter 15: COVID-19   **499**
- Nasal Swab Collection   *507*
- Oropharyngeal Swab Collection   *507*
- Covishield   *513*
- Covaxin   *514*

Chapter 16: IMCI Guidelines (WHO, 2014)   **518**
- Follow-up   *526*

Chapter 17: Acute Flaccid Paralysis Surveillance   **533**
- Definition Associated with Surveillance   *533*
- Definition of an AFP Case   *533*
- Background Rate of AFP   *533*
- Purpose of AFP Surveillance   *534*
- Reasons for AFP Surveillance Instead of Polio Surveillance   *534*
- Selection of AFP Cases for Investigation   *534*
- Surveillance at Local/District/State/National Levels   *534*
- AFP Surveillance after Attaining a Zero Polio Status   *535*
- Case Notification   *535*
- Case Verification   *536*
- Case Investigation   *536*
- Collection, Transport and Reporting Results of Stool Specimen   *537*
- Sixty Days Follow-up Examination   *539*
- Outbreak Response Immunization   *539*

Chapter 18: Tuberculosis and RNTCP Guidelines (2022)   **540**
- Tuberculosis and Global Challenges   *540*
- Burden of Tuberculosis   *540*
- Millennium Development Goal and Tuberculosis   *540*
- Revised National Tuberculosis Control Program   *541*
- Drug Sensitive-Tuberculosis Treatment as per NTEP (2022)   *548*
- Special Considerations for Different Manifestations of Tuberculosis (2022)   *549*

Chapter 19: Reproductive, Child and Adolescent Health   **559**
- Basic Concept Behind the Special Attention of Mother and Child   *559*
- Reproductive and Child Health Program   *565*
- Reproductive and Child Health Program–Phase II   *568*
- Adolescent Health   *574*

Chapter 20: Diagnosis and Treatment for Malaria *(According to New NVBDCP Operational Guidelines, 2022)* **576**
- ❖ Treatment of *P. Vivax* Malaria *579*
- ❖ Treatment of *P. Falciparum* Malaria *580*
- ❖ Treatment of Uncomplicated *P. Falciparum* Cases in Pregnancy *581*
- ❖ Mixed Infections *581*
- ❖ Severe and Complicated Malaria *582*
- ❖ Short-term Chemoprophylaxis (Up to 6 Weeks) *583*
- ❖ Chemoprophylaxis for Longer Stay (More than 6 Weeks) *583*
- ❖ Integrated Vector Management *584*

Chapter 21: Biomedical Waste Management **585**
- ❖ Biomedical Waste (Management and Handling) Rules (2016) *585*

Chapter 22: Incubation and Isolation Period of Some Important Diseases **588**
- ❖ Incubation Period *588*

Chapter 23: National Health Policy and Elimination of Some Diseases **591**
- ❖ National Health Goals for Communicable and Noncommunicable Diseases Under 12th Five-Year Plan of National Health Mission (2012–2017) *591*
- ❖ Smallpox Eradication *591*
- ❖ Poliomyelitis Eradication *591*
- ❖ India has Eliminated Following Diseases *592*

Chapter 24: Current Public Health-related Statistics and Recent Updates **593**
- ❖ Socioeconomic Indicators *593*
- ❖ Gross Domestic Products (GDP) *593*
- ❖ Below Poverty Line (BPL) *593*
- ❖ National Sociodemographic Goals of NPP, 2000 (Achieved by 2010) *594*
- ❖ Sustainable Developmental Goals *594*
- ❖ Health-related Goals *595*
- ❖ Global Strategy for Women's, Children's and Adolescent's Health (2016–2030) *596*
- ❖ Recent Health-related Statistics *597*
- ❖ Recent Updates Regarding Infectious Diseases *597*
- ❖ General Guidance *598*
- ❖ Recent Updates Regarding Noncommunicable Diseases *601*
- ❖ Juvenile Justice Act, 2015 *601*
- ❖ Recent Updates Regarding Blindness and Visual Impairment *601*
- ❖ Recent Mortality Statistics *602*
- ❖ Recent Updates in Nutrition *602*
- ❖ Family Planning Related Updates *603*
- ❖ Miscellaneous Recent Updates *603*
- ❖ Swachh Bharat Abhiyan *603*
- ❖ Ayushman Bharat *604*
- ❖ Important Public Health Days *606*

Annexure-1: Drug of Choice for Some Important Communicable Diseases 607
Annexure-2: Some Most Commons in Community Medicine 609

Index *611*

Competency Table

Number	COMPETENCY The student should be able to	Chapter No.	Page No.
CM1.1	Define and describe the concept of public health	2 10	3–5 428
CM1.2	Define health; describe the concept of holistic health including concept of spiritual health and the relativeness and determinants of health	2 5	3–7 258
CM1.3	Describe the characteristics of agent, host and environmental factors in health and disease and the multi factorial etiology of disease	4	154–155
CM1.4	Describe and discuss the natural history of disease	4 10	156 429
CM1.5	Describe the application of interventions at various levels of prevention	4	157–158
CM1.7	Enumerate and describe health indicators	2	5–7
CM1.9	Demonstrate the role of effective communication skills in health in a simulated environment	5	316–317
CM2.2	Describe the sociocultural factors, family (types), its role in health and disease and demonstrate in a simulated environment the correct assessment of socioeconomic status	2 4 12	5 61–64 203–204 464–466
CM2.5	Describe poverty and social security measures and its relationship to health and disease	2	79

Topic: Environmental Health Problems
 Number of competencies: (8)

Number	COMPETENCY	Chapter No.	Page No.
CM3.1	Describe the health hazards of air, water, noise, radiation and pollution	2 4	78 205–208 214–216 218–219
CM3.2	Describe concepts of safe and wholesome water, sanitary sources of water, water purification processes, water quality standards, concepts of water conservation and rainwater harvesting	4	208–214 216–217 219–223
CM3.3	Describe the aetiology and basis of water borne diseases/jaundice/hepatitis/diarrheal diseases	4	218–220
CM3.4	Describe the concept of solid waste, human excreta and sewage disposal	4	208–214 216–217
CM3.5	Describe the standards of housing and the effect of housing on health	4	217
CM3.6	Describe the role of vectors in the causation of diseases. Also discuss National Vector Borne disease Control Program	3 4	96–102 176–178

Number	COMPETENCY The student should be able to	Chapter No.	Page No.
Topic: Principles of health promotion and education **Number of competencies: (3)**			
CM4.1	Describe various methods of health education with their advantages and limitations	5	318
CM4.2	Describe the methods of organizing health promotion and education and counseling activities at individual family and community settings	10	440
Topic: Nutrition **Number of competencies: (08)**			
CM5.1	Describe the common sources of various nutrients and special nutritional requirements according to age, sex, activity, physiological conditions	4 5 10	195–196 295–296 438
CM5.2	Describe and demonstrate the correct method of performing a nutritional assessment of individuals, families and the community by using the appropriate method	2	74–77
CM5.3	Define and describe common nutrition related health disorders (including macro-PEM, Micro-iron, Zn, iodine, Vit. A), their control and management	2 4 5 9	69–70 196–197 299–303 420, 423
CM5.4	Plan and recommend a suitable diet for the individuals and families based on local availability of foods and economic status, etc., in a simulated environment	9 24	401–422 597–598
CM5.6	Enumerate and discuss the National Nutrition Policy, important national nutritional Programs including the Integrated Child Development Services Scheme (ICDS), etc.,	2 4 5	68–69 191–192 197–202 296–298
Topic: Basic statistics and its applications **Number of competencies: (04)**			
CM6.1	Formulate a research question for a study		
CM6.2	Describe and discuss the principles and demonstrate the methods of collection, classification, analysis, interpretation and presentation of statistical data	4 13	233–235 473–474
CM6.3	Describe, discuss and demonstrate the application of elementary statistical methods including test of significance in various study designs	5	315–316
CM6.4	Enumerate, discuss and demonstrate common sampling techniques, simple statistical methods, frequency distribution, measures of central tendency and dispersion	4	235–241
Topic: Epidemiology **Number of competencies: (09)**			
CM7.1	Define epidemiology and describe and enumerate the principles, concepts and uses	2 5 10	7–8 261 431–432
CM7.2	Enumerate, describe and discuss the modes of transmission and measures for prevention and control of communicable and non-communicable diseases	4 5	168,178 269–290

Number	COMPETENCY The student should be able to	Chapter No.	Page No.
CM7.3	Enumerate, describe and discuss the sources of epidemiological data	10 11	433–435 452–463
CM7.4	Define, calculate and interpret morbidity and mortality indicators based on given set of data	10	441–451
CM7.5	Enumerate, define, describe and discuss epidemiological study designs	5 10	262 454
CM7.6	Enumerate and evaluate the need of screening tests	4 5 10	167–168 266–269 432–433
CM8.1	Describe and discuss the epidemiological and control measures including the use of essential laboratory tests at the primary care level for communicable diseases	2	17–27 37–41
CM8.2	Describe and discuss the epidemiological and control measures including the use of essential laboratory tests at the primary care level for noncommunicable diseases (diabetes, hypertension, stroke, obesity and cancer, etc.)	2 4 5	41–47 178–179 288–290
CM8.3	Enumerate and describe disease specific National Health Programs including their prevention and treatment of a case	2 3 4 5 24	69–70 101 180–182 290 598
CM8.5	Describe and discuss the principles of planning, implementing and evaluating control measures for disease at community level bearing in mind the public health importance of the disease	4	245–247

Topic: Demography and vital statistics
Number of competencies: (07)
Number of procedures that require certification: (NIL)

CM9.1	Define and describe the principles of demography, demographic cycle, vital statistics	4 5 10	182–183 291 436
CM9.2	Define, calculate and interpret demographic indices including birth rate, death rate, fertility rates	4	182
CM9.3	Enumerate and describe the causes of declining sex ratio and its social and health implications	4	183
CM9.4	Enumerate and describe the causes and consequences of population explosion and population dynamics of India	4	184
CM9.5	Describe the methods of population control	4 5	184–185 381–415 417–419

Topic: Reproductive maternal and child health
Number of competensies: (09)
Number of procedures that require certification: (NIL)

CM10.1	Describe the current status of reproductive, maternal, newborn and child health	5 10	292–295 437
CM10.3	Describe local customs and practices during pregnancy, childbirth, lactation and child feeding practices	14	486–497

	COMPETENCY	Chapter	
Number	The student should be able to	No.	Page No.
CM10.4	Describe the reproductive, maternal, newborn and child health (RMCH); child survival and safe motherhood interventions	2 4 7 9 19	64–66 187–189 340–376 422 555–556 561–564
CM10.5	Describe Universal Immunization Program; Integrated Management of Neonatal and Childhood Illness (IMNCI) and other existing programs	19	564–571
CM10.6	Enumerate and describe various family planning methods, their advantages and shortcomings	2 14	55–57 59–60 493

Topic: Occupational health
Number of competencies: (05)
Number of procedures that require certification: (NIL)

| CM11.1 | Enumerate and describe the presenting features of patients with occupational illness including agriculture | 5
10 | 310–312
439 |

Topic: Geriatric services
Number of competencies: (04)
Number of procedures that require certification: (NIL)

| CM12.2 | Describe health problems of aged population | 4 | 194 |

Topic: Disaster management
Number of competencies: (04)
Number of procedures that require certification: (NIL)

| CM13.1 | Define and describe the concept of disaster management | 5
10 | 309–310
439 |
| CM14.1 | Define and classify hospital waste | 4
5 | 223–225
307–308 |

Topic: Mental health
Number of competencies: (03)
Number of procedures that require certification: (NIL)

| CM15.1 | Define and describe the concept of mental health | 5 | 314 |

Topic: Health care of the community
Number of competencies:(05)
Number of procedures that require certification: (NIL)

CM17.1	Define and describe the concept of health care to community	2	84
CM17.3	Describe primary health care, its components and principles	2	87–88
CM17.4	Describe national policies related to health and health planning and millennium development goals	4	245–248

Topic: International Health
Number of competencies: (2)
Number of procedures that require certification (NIL)

Number	COMPETENCY The student should be able to	Chapter No.	Page No.
CM18.1	Define and describe the concept of International health	4	245
CM18.2	Describe roles of various international health agencies	2 4	89 245–257

Topic: Recent advances in community medicine
Number of competencies: (04)
Number of procedures that require certification: (NIL)

CM20.1	List important public health events of last five years	24	592–593
CM20.2	Describe various issues during outbreaks and their prevention	24	593–596
CM 20.3	Describe any event important to health of the community	24	590

Chapter

1

History of Medicine

Father of	Name
Biology, Embryology, Zoology	Aristotle
Bacteriology	Louis Pasteur
Anatomy	Vesalius
Modern Physiology and Experimental Medicine	Claude Bernard
Pathology	Rudolph Virchow
Botany	Theophrastus
Microbiology and Protozoology	Antonie Philips van Leeuwenhoek
Virology	WM Stanley
Psychoanalysis	Sigmund Freud
Medicine	Hippocrates
Hindu God of Medicine	Dhanwantari
Indian Medicine	Charaka
Modern Surgery	Ambroise Pare
Indian Surgery and Plastic Surgery	Sushruta
Homeopathy	Samuel Hahnemann
Immunology	Edward Jenner
Polio Vaccine	Jonas Salk
Public Health	Cholera (by Shoe Leather epidemiology during outbreak in London)
Epidemiology	John Snow
First True Epidemiologist	Hippocrates

Person	Activities
Louis Pasteur	• Disproved theory of spontaneous generation • Discovered vaccine against chickenpox, anthrax and rabies • Advanced "Germ theory of disease" (single cause idea/one-to-one causation)
Pettenkofer of Munich	Proposed theory of multifactorial causation of disease

Contd...

Contd...

Person	Activities
Samuel Hahnemann	• First use the term "Homeopathy" • Treatment of diseases by the small amount of a drug which produces symptoms similar to those of the disease • Single medicine at the time of treatment • Minimum medicine dose to be used
Edward Jenner	• Discovered smallpox vaccine

Robert Koch	• Introduced staining techniques for bacteria
	• Introduced methods of obtaining bacteria in pure culture using solid media
	• First to isolate bacteria (anthrax bacilli) in pure culture
	• Discovered tuberculous (TB) bacilli and cholera vibrio
	• Produced new tuberculin
	• Koch phenomenon: It is a hypersensitivity reaction seen in a guinea pig already infected with TB bacilli when the tubercle bacillus or its protein is injected into it.
	• Koch's postulate: It postulates that a microorganism can be accepted as an infectious agent when they are:
	  i. Constantly associated with the lesions of the disease
	  ii. Possible to isolate in pure culture from the lesions
	  iii. Able to reproduce the lesions of the disease when such pure culture is inoculated into suitable laboratory animals
	  iv. Possible to be reisolated in pure culture from the lesions produced in experimental animals
	• Awarded Nobel Prize for medicine (in 1905) for investigation and discoveries in relation to TB

Ross	Malaria and Anopheles mosquito
CEA Winslow	• Defined public health • Science and art of preventing disease • Prolonging life and promoting health and efficacy through organized community efforts
Paul Ehrlich	Termed "chemotherapy" and "autoimmunity"
John Snow	• Studied epidemiology of cholera in London (1848–1854) • Established causative role of polluted water in spread of cholera • Devised system of methodological observations of natural events or experiments
James Lind	First ever to conduct a clinical trial for his study to find treatment of scurvy
Hippocrates	• First true epidemiologist • Described disease formation due to environmental factors in his book "Air, Water and Places"

Chapter

2

Long Essay Type Questions

Authors' Note

In this chapter, we have given model answers to some of the important long questions asked in the university examinations. Strictly speaking, this chapter cannot be a complete one, because if all probable long questions are given in this chapter, it will be a really huge one. So, we have given the important long questions asked in examinations in a separate "try yourself" section at the end, which you have to read from the standard textbooks. Also, when you will read the next chapters "Short notes" and "Explain why", you will get answers of most of the "try yourself" questions given in this chapter.

CONCEPT OF HEALTH AND DISEASE

1. Enumerate the determinants of health. How do socioeconomic conditions act as one of the determinants of health? (4 + 8)

Determinants of Health

a. Biological determinants (genetic constitution of a man).
b. Behavioral and sociocultural determinants (lifestyle changes):
   - Smoking
   - Alcoholism
   - Personal hygiene
   - Customs
   - Cultural patterns.
c. Environmental determinants (external and internal):
   - Housing
   - Water supply
   - Basic sanitation
   - Family structure
   - Community participation in health services.
d. Socioeconomic conditions:
   - Economic status of the country (per capita GNP)
   - Education
   - Occupation
   - Political commitment.
e. Health services.
f. Aging of the population (it increases the prevalence of chronic diseases).

g. Gender (increased concentration on women's health)

h. Development and utilization of newer technologies.

Socioeconomic Conditions as Determinants of Health

The points which we will discuss are the following:

1. Economic status of the country.
2. Education.
3. Occupation.
4. Political commitment.

Economic Status of the Country

❖ Per capita GNP is most commonly used to determine the general economic performance of a country

❖ The per capita GNP is less in developing countries than the developed countries, which is responsible for:
  – Higher infant mortality rates
  – Higher under 5 mortality rates
  – Higher maternal mortality rates and lower life expectancy at birth
  – Lower doctor-population ratio
  – Lower adult literacy rate
  – Lower percentage of people having access to drinking water and adequate sanitation.

Education

Studies has indicated that a higher proportion of people being educated facilitates utilization of the health resources and health services by common people and this leads finally to a decrease in the morbidity and mortality rates.

Occupation

❖ Unemployed person suffers from loss of income and status, which is often a source of psychological damage

❖ On the other hand, employment in a productive work promotes physical and mental health.

Political Commitment

❖ The percentage of Gross National Product (GNP) spent on the health sector is a qualitative indicator of political commitment

❖ The WHO has stated that every country should expend at least 5% of its GNP in the health sector.

❖ India spends ~2% of its GNP in the health sector.

2. **What do you mean by indicators of health? What are the requisite characteristics of indicators of health? Enumerate different indicators of health. Discuss about the mortality indicators of health.** (2 + 2 + 4 + 4)

Definition of Health Indicator (CDC)

A measurable characteristic that describes:
- ❖ The health of a population
- ❖ Determinants of health
- ❖ Health care access, cost, quality, and use.

Requisite Characteristics of Indicators of Health

An ideal health indicator should be:
1. **Valid**, i.e. they should actually measure what they are supposed to measure
2. **Reliable and objective**, i.e. the answers should be same if measured by different people in similar circumstances
3. **Sensitive**, i.e. they should be sensitive to changes in the situation concerned
4. **Specific**, i.e. they should reflect changes only in the situation concerned
5. **Feasible**, i.e. they should have the ability to obtain data needed
6. **Relevant**, i.e. they should contribute to the understanding of the phenomenon of interest.

Different Indicators of Health

1. Mortality indicators
2. Morbidity indicators
3. Disability rates
4. Nutritional status indicators
5. Health care delivery indicators
6. Utilization rates
7. Indicators of social and mental health
8. Environmental indicators
9. Socioeconomic indicators
10. Health policy indicators
11. Indicators of quality of life.

Important Mortality Indicators of Health

1. Life expectancy:
   Life expectancy refers to the number of years a person is expected to live based on the statistical average. It is a positive mortality indicator.

2. Crude death rate $(CDR) = \dfrac{\text{No. of death}}{\text{Mid - year population}} \times 1000$

   - ❖ Mid-year population (MYP) is calculated on July 1st.
   - ❖ CDR is the simplest indicator of mortality as it is **not** age specific.

Specific Death Rates

3. Age specific death rate:

   $\text{Age specific death rate of 5 – 15 years age group} = \dfrac{\text{No. of death in 5 – 15 years}}{\text{Mid year population in 5 – 15 years}} \times 1000$

   It is used to detect the high risk age group.

4. Disease specific death rate:

$$\text{Disease specific death rate of TB} = \frac{\text{No. of deaths due to TB}}{\text{MYP}} \times 1000$$

5. Proportional mortality rate (PMR):

   It is a proportion expressed in %

   Examples:

   1. Proportional mortality rate due to a disease:

   $$\text{PMR due to tuberculosis} = \frac{\text{No. of deaths due to TB}}{\text{All deaths}} \times 100$$

   2. Proportional mortality rate in a particular age group:

   $$\text{PMR in under 5 age group} = \frac{\text{No. of deaths in under 5 years}}{\text{All deaths}} \times 100$$

   Uses of PMR:
   - To find out the most common cause of death, i.e., relative importance of the specific disease as a cause of death, within the population
   - To calculate proportion of deaths in a particular age group (i.e., under-fives)
   - PMR is used when population data are not available

   Limitation of PMR:
   - It cannot be used for making comparisons between population groups or different time periods
   - It does not indicate the risk of dying/developing a disease.

6. Case fatality rate (CFR):

   It detects:
   a. Virulence of an organism
   b. Killing power of a disease.

   $$\text{Case fatality rate (CFR)} = \frac{\text{No. of deaths}}{\text{No. of cases}} \times 100$$

   CFR is used in acute infections.

   Example:
   a. CFR of Rabies is 100%
   b. CFR of Ebola is 40–50%.

   CFR = 30% means that out of 100 cases, 30 will die.

   Survival rate = (100-CFR) in % = (100-30)% = 70%.

7. Survival rate:

   $$\text{Survival rate} = \frac{\text{No. of survivors}}{\text{No. of cases}} \times 100$$

   Example:

   5 years survival rate is used in cancer studies. It implies:
   a. Prognosis of a disease
   b. Standards/ effectiveness of therapy.

Try Yourself

1. Describe the concept of "natural history of disease".

   See in Short Notes (Chapter 4).

2. Using the levels of prevention, describe a plan of action for prevention of following diseases:
   – Tuberculosis
   – Leprosy
   – Polio
   – Coronary heart disease
   – Protein-energy malnutrition (PEM).

   This format of writing this type of questions is same. You can have a look to Page Nos. 17, 24 and 67, where we have written it for leprosy, polio and protein-energy malnutrition, respectively. You can apply the same format to the other diseases to write a complete answer regarding "plan of action for prevention using level of prevention" questions.

PRINCIPLES OF EPIDEMIOLOGY AND EPIDEMIOLOGICAL METHODS

1. **Define epidemiology. Classify epidemiological studies. Mention briefly the important differences between case control and cohort studies.**

   (2 + 4 + 6)

Definition of Epidemiology

Epidemiology is defined as the study of distribution and determinants of health-related states or events in specified population and the application of the study to the control of health problems.

—John M Last (1988)

Classification of Epidemiological Studies

1. Observational studies:
   The investigator only observes natural course of an event but does not intervene.
   a. Descriptive studies:
      The investigator describes pattern of disease occurrence in a population.
   b. Analytical studies:
      The investigator analyzes relationship between health status and other variables in a population. It is of following types:
      - Ecological studies.
      - Cross-sectional studies.
      - Case control studies.
      - Cohort studies.
2. Experimental studies:
   The investigator actively interrupts and intervenes into the natural course of a disease.
   a. Randomized controlled trials (RCTs).
   b. Field studies.
   c. Community trials.

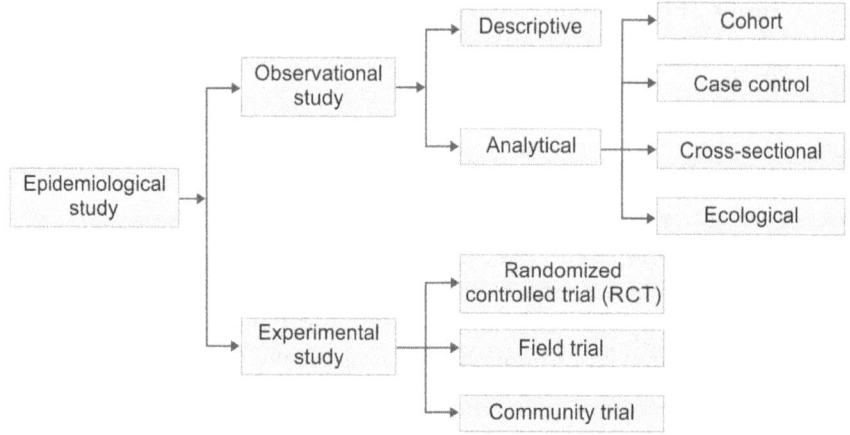

Unit of study in epidemiological studies

Study	Unit of study
Ecological study	Population
Cross-sectional study Case control study Cohort study	Individuals
RCT	Patients
Field trial	Healthy people
Community study	Community

Differences between case control and cohort studies

Features	Case control study	Cohort study
Purpose of the study	It is the first approach to test a hypothesis	It is the approach to test a precisely formulated hypothesis
Direction	Effect to cause	Cause to effect
Starts with	The disease	Exposure
Number of subjects	Fewer	Large
Time needed	Quick results are obtained	Long follow-up results in delayed results
Expense yields	Inexpensive	Very much expensive
Calculates	Calculates odds ratio, which is an indirect measure of relative risk	Relative risk as well as attributable risk and dose response ratio
Study of rare diseases	Possible	Inappropriate
Can evaluate	Multiple exposures	Multiple outcomes
Attrition	Attrition is not a problem due to the short duration of study	Attrition is a common problem due to the long follow-up time
Ethical issue	Minimum	Ethical issue is there because when we accumulate evidence about an etiological factor, we become obliged to intervene and eliminate the factor as a doctor
Bias	• Selection bias • Recall bias	• Loss to follow up bias • Analytic bias

2. **Discuss briefly about the different time trends in disease occurrence and mention their significance.** (6 + 6)

Time Trends in Disease Occurrence

Epidemiologists have identified three types of time trends in disease occurrence:
1. Short-term fluctuations
2. Periodic fluctuations
3. Long-term or secular trends.

Short-term Fluctuations

❖ The best-known short-term fluctuation in the occurrence of a disease is an epidemic.
❖ An epidemic is defined as "the occurrence of cases of an illness or other health-related events in a community or region clearly in excess of normal expectancy".

Types of Short-term fluctuations

1. Common source epidemics:
   a. Single exposure: Bhopal gas tragedy
   b. Multiple Exposure: A contaminated drinking water reservoir may cause periodic epidemics of diarrhea/cholera.
2. Propagated epidemics:
   a. Person to person: COVID-19
   b. Arthropod vector: Dengue
   c. Animal reservoir: Plague

Periodic Fluctuations

a. Seasonal trend:
   – Measles is usually at its height in early spring
   – Upper respiratory tract infections (URTI) frequently show a seasonal rise during winter months
   – Bacterial gastrointestinal infections are prominent in summer months because of warm weather and rapid multiplication of flies.
b. Cyclic trends:
   – Cyclic trend is seen due to variations in herd immunity
   – Measles in pre-vaccination era: Every 2–3 years
   – Rubella in pre-vaccination era: Every 6–9 years
   – Influenza pandemics (due to antigenic shift): 10–15 yearly.

Long Term/Secular Trends

❖ Incidence of communicable diseases is getting reduced gradually due to universal vaccination but incidence of noncommunicable diseases (diabetes/hypertension/coronary artery disease, etc.) is being increased due to sedentary lifestyle and changing food habits. This trend is known as "Epidemiological transition".

3. **What is case control study? Discuss steps of conducting a case control study. What are the advantages and disadvantages of case control study?**

$$(2 + 5 + 5)$$

Definition of Case Control Study

A study that compares patients who have a disease or outcome of interest (*cases*) with patients who do not have the disease or outcome (*controls*), and looks back **retrospectively** to compare how frequently the exposure to a risk factor is present in each group *to determine the relationship between the risk factor and the disease.*

Steps of Conducting a Case Control Study

1. Selection of cases
   Example: Lung cancer patients from hospitals
2. Selection of controls
   Two types of selection:
   a. From general population
      - *Example*: Neighborhood controls
      - Ideal way of selecting controls.
   b. Hospital controls:
      - Hospital controls are different from general population—It gives rise to **selection bias/Berksonian bias**.
3. Matching:
   Process of selecting controls similar to cases in certain characteristics, i.e. age, sex, etc. These characteristics are called "confounders".
   So, *matching is done to eliminate confounding factors.*
   Matching is of two types:
   a. **Group matching/frequency matching**:
      Example: Among cases, we have 30% females. So, among controls, we should have 30% females.
   b. **Individual/pair matching**:
      Example: If we have 45-year-old white females among cases, we should also have 45-year-old white females among controls.
4. Retrospective assessment of exposure:
   This assessment is done using:

Assessment	Bias	Solution
Interview	Interviewer bias	1. Blinding 2. Self-administered questionnaire
Asking history of exposure	Recall bias • Cases will recall the exposure more compared to controls • Recall bias can over-estimate Odd's ratio.	1. Do prospective study 2. Give more time to the controls for recalling the exposure

5. Calculation of Odd's ratio:
   - Odd's ratio: Strength of association in a case-control study
   - Odd's ratio = 1—No association
   - Odd's ratio >1—Positive association
   - Odd's ratio <1—Negative association.

Example:

	Disease	
	Yes	No
Smokers (exposed)	33 (a)	55 (b)
Nonsmokers (nonexposed)	2 (c)	27 (d)
	35	82
	Cases	Controls

- Odds of exposure in cases = Cases (exposed)/ Cases (nonexposed) = a/c = 33/2
  - Odds of exposure in controls = Controls (exposed)/ Controls (nonexposed) = b/d = 55/27
  - Odd's ratio $= \dfrac{\text{Odds in cases}}{\text{Odds in controls}} = \dfrac{33/2}{55/27} = 8.1$

→ It implies that, smoking is 8.1 times more common among cases compared to controls.

Advantages of Case-control Study

❖ Fewer number of subjects required
❖ Results are obtained quickly – less time needed
❖ Attrition(drop-out) is not a problem due to shorter duration of study
❖ Inexpensive
❖ Study of rare diseases possible
❖ Minimum ethical issues as outcome has already occurred and no intervention is to be taken.

Disadvantages of Case-control Study

❖ Only relative risk is calculated in the form of Odd's ratio, incidence cannot be calculated
❖ Cannot yield information about more than 1 disease/outcome.

4. **Define epidemic. Write down the different types of epidemics. Enumerate the steps in the investigation of an epidemic.** (2 + 4 + 6)

Definition of Epidemic

An epidemic is defined as, "the occurrence of cases of an illness or other health-related events in a community or region clearly in excess of normal expectancy". When the occurrence of cases of a disease is more than 2 standard errors from the endemic occurrence, we consider it to be an epidemic.

Types of Epidemics

1. Common source epidemic:
   - Single exposure/point source
   - Continuous exposure/multiple exposure/intermittent source
2. Propagated epidemic
3. Slow epidemic.

Common Source Epidemic

Single exposure epidemic:
❖ Sharp rise, sharp fall
❖ Clustering of cases
❖ All cases develop within 1 incubation period
  Example:
  – Food poisoning
  – Bhopal Gas tragedy.

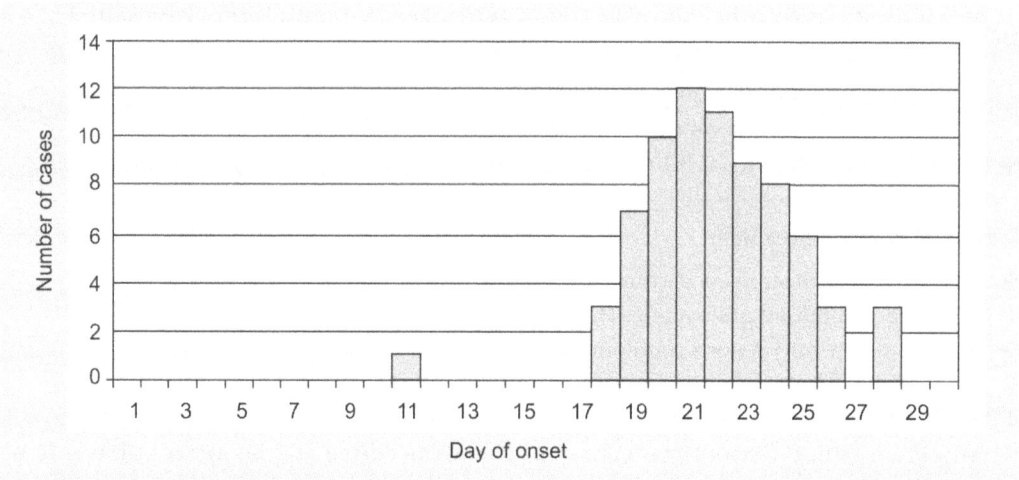

Continuous exposure epidemic:
❖ Secondary waves can be seen
❖ Duration more than one incubation period
  Example:
  – Contaminated well
  – Prostitutes in gonorrhea epidemic
  – Legionnaire's disease outbreak in Philadelphia, etc.

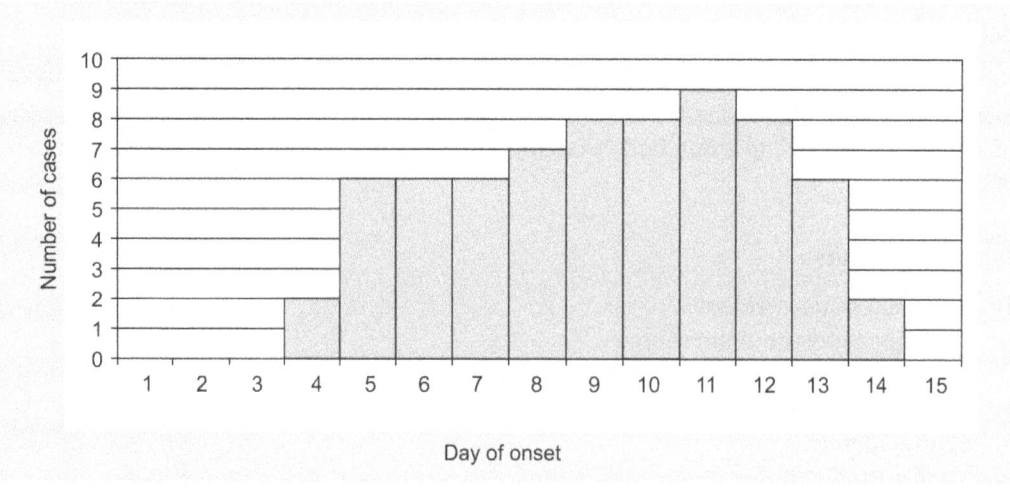

Propagated Epidemic

❖ Gradual rise and gradual fall of cases
❖ Curve has a plateau (horizontal line)
❖ Cases can develop after one incubation period
  Example: Hepatitis A, polio.

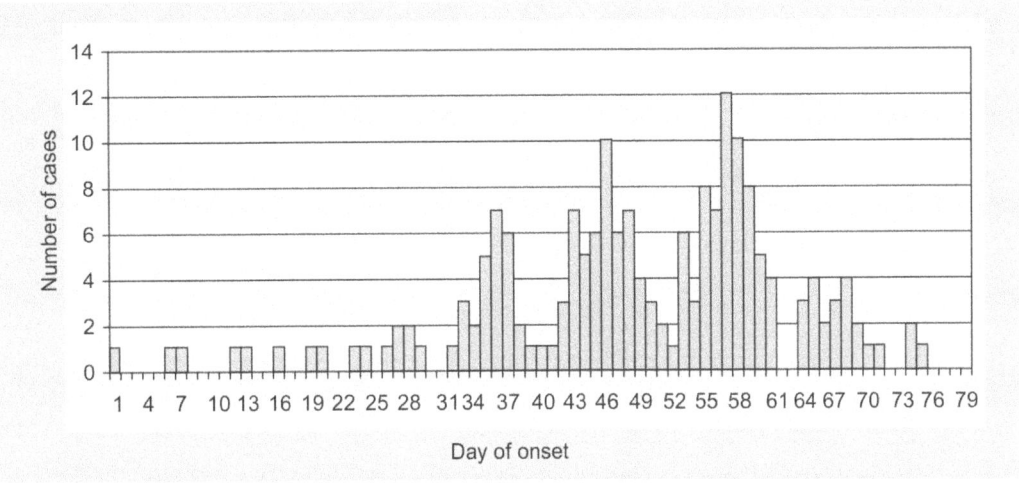

Slow Epidemic

❖ Time scale of the epidemic is shifted from days or weeks to years
  Example: Noncommunicable diseases (diabetes, hypertension, etc.).

Steps in the Investigation of an Epidemic

1. **Verification of diagnosis:**
   By clinical examination ± laboratory investigations
2. **Confirmation of existence of an epidemic:**
   Epidemic frequency ≥ (Endemic Frequency + 2 Standard Errors)
3. **Defining the population at risk:**
   a. Obtaining a map of the area
   b. Counting the population: For this purpose, lay health workers in sufficient numbers should be employed.
4. **Rapid search for all cases and their characteristics:**
   a. Medical survey
   b. Epidemiological case sheet:
      The epidemiological case sheet or "case interview form" should be carefully designed to collect relevant information including: name, age, sex, occupation, history of previous exposure, time of onset of disease, signs and symptoms of illness, personal contacts at home, sources of food and water consumption, etc.
   c. Searching for more cases.
5. **Data analysis:**
   a. **Time distribution:** Time data are usually displayed with a two-dimensional graph. The vertical or y-axis usually shows the number or rate of cases; the horizontal or x-axis shows the time periods such as years, months, or days. The number or rate of cases is

plotted over time. Displaying the patterns of disease occurrence by time is critical for monitoring disease occurrence in the community and for assessing whether the public health interventions made a difference.

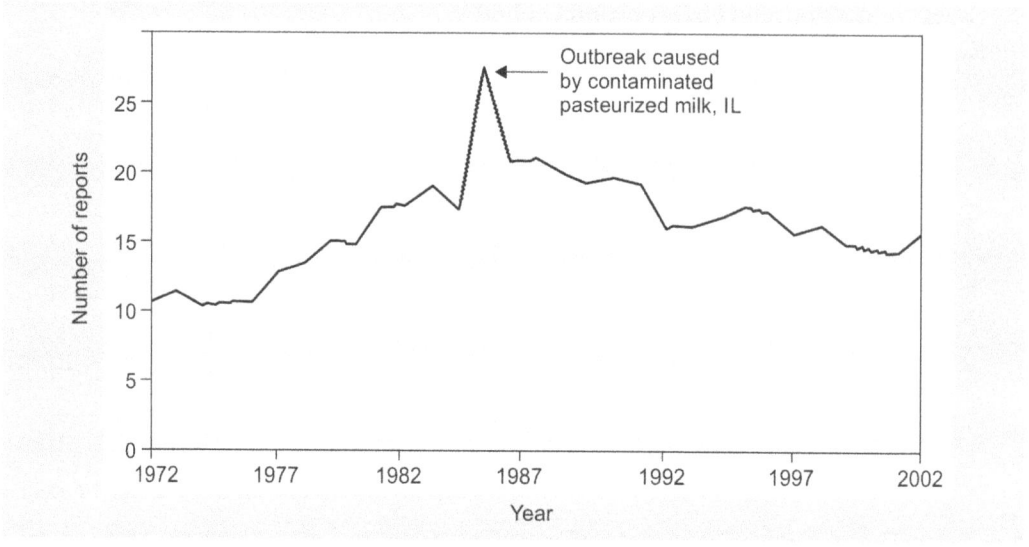

Reported Cases of Salmonellosis per 100,000 Population, by Year: United States, **1972–2002;** *Source:* CDC, USA.

b. **Place distribution:** Describing the occurrence of disease by place provides insight into the geographic extent of the problem.

   A type of map for place data is a spot map. Spot maps are generally used for clusters or outbreaks with a limited number of cases. A dot or X is placed on the location that is most relevant to the disease of interest, usually where each victim lived or worked.

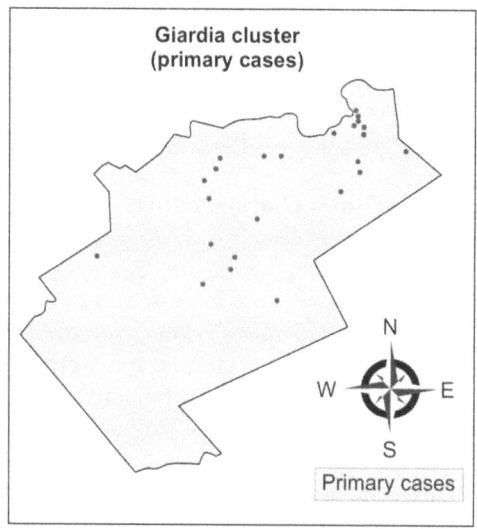

Spot Map of Giardia Cases; *Source:* **CDC, USA.**

c. **Person distribution:** Analyze the data by risk factors, i.e., age, sex, race and socioeconomic status. Age is the single most important "person" attribute, because almost every health-related event varies with age.

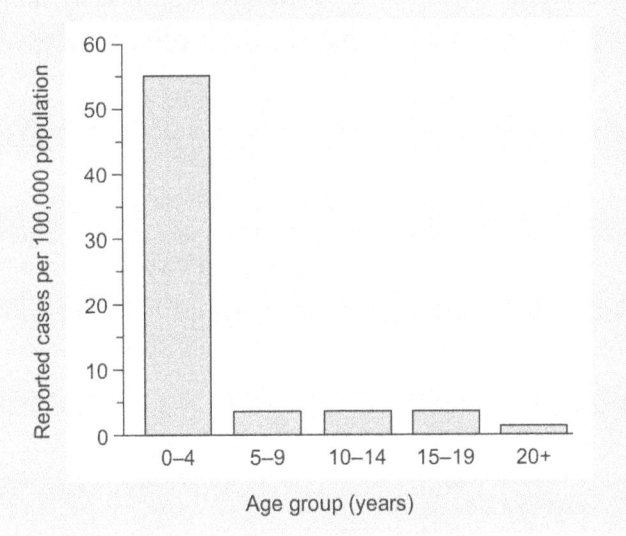

Occurrence of Pertussis by 5-Year Age Groups; *Source:* CDC, USA.

6. **Formulation of hypothesis:**
On the basis of time, place and person distribution, formulate hypotheses to explain the epidemic in terms of:
a. Possible source
b. Causative agent
c. Possible modes of spread
d. The environmental factors which enabled the epidemic to happen.

7. **Testing of hypothesis:**
It is done by comparing the attack rates among those exposed vs nonexposed to each suspected factor.

8. **Evaluation of ecological factors:**
Role of environmental factors in the epidemic is established (*Example*: sanitary conditions) to ensure appropriate measures to prevent further transmission of the disease.

9. **Further investigation of population at risk.**

10. **Writing the final report.**

Try Yourself

1. What are the aim and objectives of epidemiology? Describe uses of epidemiology.
2. Discuss the steps involved in conducting cohort study. Mention the merits and demerits of cohort study and case control study.

SCREENING FOR DISEASE

1. **Define screening. How does it differ from diagnostic tests? Describe the criteria of screening.**

(2 + 4 + 6)

Definition of Screening

Screening is defined as, "the search for unrecognized disease or defect by means of rapidly applied tests, examinations or other procedures in apparently healthy individuals".

Difference between screening and diagnostic tests

Features	Screening tests	Diagnostic tests
Subjects	Apparently healthy individuals	Sick individuals/persons at risk of a particular disease/defect
Application	Applied to groups	Applied to single patient
Based on	One criterion/cut off point	Based on evaluation of a number of criteria (consisting of signs/symptoms/laboratory findings)
Nature of test results	Arbitrary and final	Diagnosis is not final but it is confirmed by summing all the evidences
Accuracy	Less	More
Expense	Less	More
Basis for treatment?	No	Yes
Initiative starts from	From a health agency/healthcare provider	Initiative comes from a patient with a complaint

Criteria of Screening

The criteria for screening includes two components:
  a. Disease to be screened.
  b. Screening test to be applied.

Criteria of a Disease to be Screened

1. The disease should be an important public health problem.
2. There should be a recognizable and well documented early asymptomatic stage.
3. There should be a good body of evidences that early detection and treatment reduces mortality and morbidity associated with the condition.
4. The natural history of the disease (especially the "point of no return") should be completely understood.
5. There should be an established test that can detect the disease prior to the onset of signs and symptoms. There should also be an established test that can confirm the diagnosis.
6. There should be an effective treatment available.
7. There should be a widely-accepted policy determining at which border/cut-off value the person will be considered as patient and treated successively.
8. The expected benefits should always exceed the risks associated with the test.

Criteria of a Screening Test to be Applied

1. *Acceptability*: Tests should be acceptable to the population for whom it will be applied. Painful/irritating/socially unacceptable tests cannot be an effective screening test in a long run.
2. *Repeatability*: The test should give consistent results when repeated more than 1 time on the same individual and under the same conditions. It depends upon three major factors,

which may prevent a screening test from being a repeatable one. All these variations have to be minimized to build a highly specialized screening test.

  a. Observer variation:
    - Intraobserver variation
    - Interobserver variation.
  b. Subject variation:
    - Changes in the parameters to be tested
    - Recall error
    - Regression to the mean value: It is defined as a tendency of the extreme values of a distribution to regress towards the mean value on repeat measurements.
  c. Errors relating to technical methods:
    - Defective instruments.
    - Poor quality reagents.
    - Inborn errors within the test method.
3. *Validity/accuracy of the test*: It refers to the ability of the test to differentiate between diseased and nondiseased persons. Validity has two components:
  a. Sensitivity: It is defined as the ability of a test to detect correctly all those who have the disease (true positive).
  b. Specificity: It is defined as the ability of a test to detect correctly all those who does not have the disease (true negative).

An ideal screening test should have a sensitivity and specificity of 100%. In reality, it remains only a goal of developing a perfect screening test.

Try Yourself

1. What is lead time in screening test? Discuss about sensitivity and specificity of a screening test.
  See in "Short Notes" chapter for the concept of lead time (Chapter 4) Concept of lead time is on page no. 167.
  See in "Statistical and Epidemiological Exercises" Chapter 11.

EPIDEMIOLOGY OF COMMUNICABLE DISEASES

1. **Enumerate different modes of intervention under levels of prevention. Discuss, in brief, the levels of prevention in relation to leprosy.** (4 + 8)

Different modes of intervention under levels of prevention

Level of prevention	Description	Target	Modes of intervention	Actions
Primordial	It is prevention of development of risk factors in populations where it has yet not emerged	Total population/ selected groups	Health education (mass and individual)	

Contd...

Contd...

Level of prevention	Description	Target	Modes of intervention	Actions
Primary	Actions taken prior to the onset of disease (when risk factors are present but disease has not occurred)	Total population/ selected groups/ high risk individuals	Health promotion	Lifestyle modifications to prevent non-communicable diseases (i.e., type II diabetes mellitus, hypertension, dyslipidemia)
			Specific protection	Immunization with vaccines to prevent specific diseases (communicable diseases: OPV for polio, BCG for TB and cancers: HPV vaccine for prevention of cervical cancer)
Secondary	It halts the progression of disease at its early stages and prevents complications	Individuals with established disease	Early diagnosis and early treatment	Screening for cancers, early diagnosis and treatment of communicable diseases
Tertiary	It aims to reduce impairments and dis-abilities when disease has advanced beyond its early stages	Diseased patients	Disability limitation and rehabilitation	Reconstructive surgery in Leprosy, artificial prosthesis and limbs in polio patients

Basic concept of different modes of intervention under levels of prevention

Level of prevention	Risk factor	Disease of onset	Early complication	Late complication	Prevention	Example
Primordial	–	–	–	–	Health education (mass and individual)	• Preventing obesity (Primordial prevention) → Weight reduction (Primary prevention) • Counseling a child not to smoke (Primordial prevention) → Counseling a smoker to quit smoking (Primary prevention)
Primary	+	–	–	–	Health promotion	• Lifestyle modification • Nutritional modification • Food fortification (e.g. addition of vitamin A and D in Vanaspati oil) • Source reduction by spraying insecticidal spray.

Contd...

Contd...

Level of prevention	Risk factor	Disease of onset	Early complication	Late complication	Prevention	Example
					Specific protection	• **N**utritional supplements (e.g. iodination of salts, vitamin A prophylaxis) • **V**accination • **B**ed nets for protection from malaria • **D**e-fluorination of water • **C**hemoprophylaxis/ condoms • **P**ersonal protection (e.g. use of seatbelt and helmets while driving)
Secondary	+	+	–	–	Early diagnosis and early treatment	• Sputum smear for AFB • National health programs
Tertiary	+	+	+	–	Disability limitation	• Physiotherapy in a case of polio
					Rehabilitation	*Types* — *Examples* Physical — Crutch Psychological — Counseling Social — Integration of patient in social activities Vocational — Skill develop-ment

Levels of Prevention in Relation to Leprosy

Primary Prevention

❖ The mainstay of primary prevention in leprosy remains health education.
❖ Health education should be directed towards both:
   a. *Patient and his family*: To prevent dropouts from treatment, the patient and his family should be properly educated about:
      - Need of regular treatment.
      - The infectious nature of the disease and need for periodic medical check-up of contacts of the patients.
      - Self-care for prevention of disabilities resulting from leprosy.
   b. *Common people*: There is a bad social stigma associated with leprosy, especially in India. For this particular reason, health education to common people is of utmost importance to eradicate leprosy from India. People are to be educated that:
      - Leprosy is not a hereditary disease.
      - It is bacterial disease like TB.
      - Not all patients are infectious.
      - Leprosy is a completely curable disease.
      - Regular treatment is essential to achieve a complete cure from leprosy.

- The patients can live a healthy and productive life, but it needs active support from the society.

Specific protection

The mainstay of specific protection from Leprosy are chemoprophylaxis and immunoprophylaxis.

Chemoprophylaxis

It is a well-known fact that immediate contacts of a case of leprosy (especially multibacillary ones) are at higher risk of acquiring leprosy. Trials with Rifampicin as Chemoprophylaxis have been shown to be effective among contacts of Leprosy patients, giving as much as 60% protection.

Immunoprophylaxis

There is currently no vaccine available for leprosy, but it has been shown that a high **BCG coverage in a community has an important contribution on reducing the disease prevalence of leprosy** in the area. So, BCG vaccination should be emphasized and uplifted in a leprosy endemic population.

Secondary Prevention

❖ The mainstay of secondary prevention in leprosy is early diagnosis and treatment of a case of leprosy.
❖ A case of leprosy is defined as, "a person showing clinical signs of leprosy; with or without bacteriological confirmation of the diagnosis and those who has not yet completed a full course of treatment with multidrug therapy".
❖ For the purpose of ease in diagnosis by even a peripheral health worker and as a basis of early treatment, a simple diagnostic protocol has been established.

Diagnostic protocol of leprosy

A case of leprosy is diagnosed by eliciting cardinal signs of leprosy through systematic clinical (and wherever required bacteriological) examination. At least one of the following signs must be present to diagnose leprosy:
1. Hypopigmented or reddish skin lesion(s) with definite sensory deficit
2. Involvement of the peripheral nerves, as demonstrated by definite thickening with loss of sensation and weakness/paralysis of the corresponding muscles of the hands, feet or eyes
3. Demonstration of *Mycobacterium leprae in the lesions.*

The first two cardinal signs can be identified by clinical examination alone, while the third can be identified by examination of the slit skin smear.

Leprosy is classified as paucibacillary or multibacillary, based on the number of skin lesions, presence of nerve involvement and identification of bacilli on slit-skin smear.
❖ **Paucibacillary leprosy (PBL):** A case of leprosy with 1–5 skin lesions, without demonstrated presence of bacilli in a skin smear
❖ **Multibacillary leprosy (MBL):** A case of leprosy with >5 skin lesions *or* with nerve involvement *or with the demonstrated presence of bacilli in a slit-skin smear, irrespective of the number of skin lesions.*

Characteristics	PBL	MBL
Skin lesion	1–5	>5
Peripheral nerve involvement	0–1	>1
Skin smear	Negative at all sites	Positive at any site

Case finding methods

Disease prevalence	Preferred method	Screening applied on
Low (<1 per 1000 population)	Contact survey	Household contacts
Medium (≥1 per 1000 population)	Group survey (skin camps)	Preschool and school children, military recruits, industrial laborers, slum residents
High (≥10 per 1000 population)	Mass survey	Examination of every single person in a community by door to door survey

Management of a Case of Leprosy

Leprosy Case Detection Campaign

In order to detect the hidden leprosy cases, Leprosy Case Detection Campaigns (LCDC), a unique initiative of its kind under National Leprosy Eradication Programme (NLEP), is being implemented in high endemic districts of the country. This involves training of health functionaries. Home visits are conducted by teams comprising of 1 ASHA, 1 male volunteer or field level worker to search for cases. Intensive IEC activities are conducted.

Under ABSULS (ASHA Based Surveillance for Leprosy Suspects), ASHAs bring out cases of leprosy from the villages to the PHC for diagnosis and treatment. Asha workers get ₹ 250/- for early detection of leprosy case without deformity, and ₹ 250/- for a new case with visible deformity of eyes/ hands/feet. They follow up the cases till treatment completion, for which they get ₹ 600/- for MBL, and ₹ 400/- for PBL case.

Multidrug therapy (MDT) for leprosy in adults [NLEP Guidelines, 2019]

Type	Drug	Dosage	Frequency	Duration
PBL	Dapsone	100 mg	Once daily	6 months
	Rifampicin	600 mg	Once monthly	
MBL	Dapsone	100 mg	Once daily	12 months
	Rifampicin	600 mg	Once monthly	
	Clofazimine	50 mg	Once daily	
	Clofazimine	300 mg	Once monthly	

MDT for leprosy in children 10–14 years

Type	Drug	Dosage	Frequency	Duration
PBL	Dapsone	50 mg	Once daily	6 months
	Rifampicin	450 mg	Once monthly	
MBL	Dapsone	50 mg	Once daily	12 months
	Rifampicin	450 mg	Once monthly	
	Clofazimine	50 mg	Once daily	
	Clofazimine	150 mg	Once monthly	

As per the new Leprosy treatment guidelines by WHO (2018)

Age group	Drug	Dosage and frequency	Duration	
			PBL	MBL
Adult	Rifampicin	600 mg once a month	6 months	12 months
	Clofazimine	300 mg once a month and 50 mg daily		
	Dapsone	100 mg daily		
Children (10–14 years)	Rifampicin	450 mg once a month	6 months	12 months
	Clofazimine	150 mg once a month and 50 mg daily		
	Dapsone	50 mg daily		

Tertiary Prevention

The mainstay of tertiary prevention in leprosy remains:
a. Prevention and limitation of disability.
b. Rehabilitation in case of permanent disability.

Disability limitation

❖ Disability is common in untreated/incompletely treated patients; occurring in as much as 25% of cases.
❖ These disabilities can be classified into three groups according to their origin:
  – Disability due to disease progression:
    - Loss of eyebrows and eyelashes (madarosis).
    - Masked facies (a mask-like immobile facial expression).
    - Sagging facies (due to loss of the strength of facial muscles, gravity draws the face downwards).
    - Leonine facies (a face resembling lion).
    - Depressed/perforated nose.
    - Nodules on the ear.
  – Disability due to damage/paralysis of 1 or more peripheral nerve trunks:
    - Inability to close the eyelids completely (Lagophthalmos: Due to damage to the facial nerve).
    - Claw hand (damage to the ulnar nerve).
    - Claw foot (damage to the tibial nerve).
    - Wrist drop (damage to the radial nerve).
    - Foot drop (damage to the peroneal nerve).
  – Disability due to repeated injury/infection of the affected area acquired from loss of sensation:
    - Corneal ulceration and scarring (secondary to exposure keratitis secondary to lagophthalmos).
    - Plantar ulcers.
    - Mutilation of hands and feet.
    - Scar contracture of fingers.
❖ Measures to prevent and limit those disabilities are as follows:
  – Use of protective gloves and footwear to protect denervated body parts from repeated injury.
  – Care of the denervated skin.
  – Healing of wounds/ulcers/cracks in skin.

- Periodic assessment of eyes for acuity of vision/lid gap and any other changes.
- Periodic assessment of nerve function by:
  - Palpation of peripheral nerves for thickening and tenderness (ulnar/median/radial/lateral popliteal/posterior tibial).
  - Sensory testing over palm and sole.
  - Voluntary muscle testing (VMT): Abduction of little finger/abduction of thumb and extension of wrist/dorsiflexion of foot.
- Prevention of joint stiffness in case of paralytic deformities by performing simple exercises.

Rehabilitation

❖ Community-based rehabilitation (CBR) is recognized as the best practice in addressing the needs of people with disabilities, including those affected by leprosy. The definition recognized by the ILO, UNESCO and WHO describes CBR as follows:

   "CBR is a strategy within general community development for the rehabilitation, equalization of opportunities and social inclusion of all people with disabilities".

❖ Since disability is not only about impairments, it follows that the best way to address disability is to **work with the community**.

❖ CBR works to remove all kinds of barriers which block people with disabilities from access to the mainstream of society.

❖ CBR focuses on abilities, not disabilities. It depends on the participation and support of people with disability, family members and local communities.

❖ Rehabilitation services commonly required by people with leprosy-related disability include:

- Physiotherapy
- Orthopedic services
- Occupational therapy
- Reconstructive surgery
- Patient education and awareness programs:
  - Vocational training
  - Integrated education of children affected by leprosy
  - Micro-finance and business creation schemes
  - Provision or improvement of appropriate housing
  - Sensitizing the community to the need to remove barriers to participation
  - Creating awareness of the benefits that might arise from including people with disabilities in the community
  - Encouraging community members to provide appropriate care and support to people with disabilities.

The inter-relationships between prevention of disability, social and economic rehabilitation, and community-oriented activities within CBR

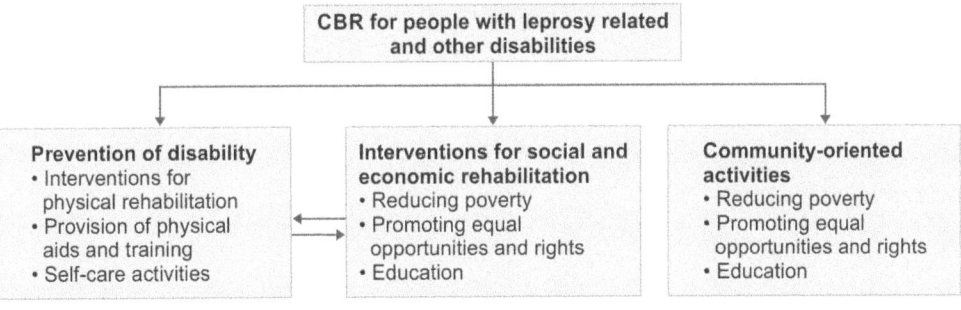

Note:

As a result of the hard work and meticulously planned and executed activities, India achieved elimination of leprosy in December 2005. The goal of elimination of leprosy is defined as less than 1 case per 10,000 population. As on 31st December 2005, prevalence rate recorded in the country was 0.95/10,000 population.

2. **Illustrate how the levels of prevention and the modes of intervention can be applied to poliomyelitis?**   (4 + 8)

Levels of Prevention and Modes of Intervention in Polio

❖ Primary prevention:
  – Health education.
  – Specific protection (vaccination):
    - Oral polio vaccine (OPV)
    - Injectable polio vaccine (IPV).
❖ Secondary prevention:
  – Early diagnosis and supportive treatment.
❖ Tertiary prevention:
  – Disability limitation:
    - Avoidance of factors that potentiate paralysis.
    - Prevention of deformities and contractures.
❖ Rehabilitation:
  – Surgery on contractures and equinus foot.
  – Wheelchair for the disabled.

Primary Prevention

Specific protection

Vaccination is the most effective means of preventing poliomyelitis in the present situation.

Oral polio vaccine

Oral Polio Vaccine (OPV) is a live attenuated vaccine used for active immunization against poliomyelitis, the dreaded childhood disease leading to paralysis of various groups of muscles for under 5 children.

Dosing schedule:

Dose	Age
OPV-0	At birth
OPV-1	6 weeks
OPV-2	10 weeks
OPV-3	14 weeks
OPV-B (booster dose)	16–24 months

Dose: 1 dose = 2 drops = 0.1 mL.

Mode of administration:

Head of the child is tilted backward → mouth is forced to open by gently squeezing the cheeks or pinching the nose → 2 drops are dropped onto the tongue by dropper.

Mother is advised not to administer food, hot liquid, breast milk an hour prior to and after vaccination as these may interact with vaccine viruses.

Recent updates:

❖ Previously trivalent OPV (containing type 1, type 2 and type 3 strains) was administered under UIP.

❖ But from April 25, 2016 onwards, Govt of India started switching from trivalent OPV to bivalent (containing only types 1 and 3) OPV. This date is also called "National switch date".

❖ Rationale of switch/OPV-2 withdrawal:
  – Since 1999, type 2 wild poliovirus has not been detected.
  – The type 2 component of trivalent OPV:
    - Caused >90% of vaccine-derived polioviruses (VDPV)
    - Caused ~40% of vaccine associated paralytic polio (VAPP) cases
    - Interfered with the immune response to poliovirus type 1 and type 3.

Advantages:

❖ Painless, easy to administer

❖ Highly trained staff not required

❖ Induces both humoral and cellular immunity

❖ Quick production of large dose of antibody in single dose only provides herd immunity (*see Short Note on Herd Immunity*)

❖ Useful in controlling epidemics

❖ Even a single dose can produce substantial immunity (except in tropical countries)

❖ Cheaper

❖ Easy to manufacture.

Disadvantages:

❖ Required to be stored and transported in sub-zero temperature (unless stabilized)

❖ Frequent vaccine failure reported

❖ May revert to its wild form and cause neurovirulence.

Injectable polio vaccine

Injectable polio vaccine (IPV) is a type of killed vaccine. It is the first effective polio vaccine was developed in 1952 by Jonas Salk.

Vaccination schedule of IPV

Schedule: Two fractional dose at 6 and 14 weeks of age

Dose: 0.1 mL

Route of administration: Intradermal (right upper arm)

Advantages:

❖ Safe in immunodeficient disorders

❖ Safe in persons with immunosuppressive/corticosteroid therapy

- ❖ Useful >50 years age
- ❖ Safe in pregnancy
- ❖ No risk of VAPP.

Disadvantages:

IPV is unsuitable in epidemics; because:

- ❖ Immunity not achieved immediately by single dose, multiple doses are required
- ❖ Injections can precipitate paralysis during epidemics
- ❖ Costly as its virus content is 10,000 times more than OPV
- ❖ Trained personnel required.

Secondary Prevention

Early diagnosis

- ❖ Polio is mostly diagnosed by means of clinical signs and symptoms.
- ❖ Early symptoms of paralytic polio include:
  - High fever
  - Headache
  - Stiffness in the back and neck
  - Asymmetrical weakness of muscles
  - Sensitivity to touch
  - Difficulty in swallowing
  - Myalgia
  - Loss of superficial and deep reflexes
  - Paresthesia (pins and needles)
  - Irritability
  - Constipation and difficulty passing urine.
- ❖ Paralysis generally develops 1–10 after early symptoms begin, progresses for 2–3 days, and is usually complete by the time the fever breaks.
  - In *children <5 years* of age, *paralysis of one leg* is most common.
  - In *adults*, extensive *paralysis of the chest and abdomen* also affecting all four limbs *(quadriplegia)* is more likely.

Spinal Polio

- ❖ Spinal polio, the most common form of paralytic poliomyelitis, results from viral invasion of the motor neurons of the anterior horn cells, or the ventral gray matter section in the spinal column, which are responsible for movement of the muscles, including those of the trunk, limbs and the intercostal muscles.
- ❖ With the destruction of nerve cells, the muscles no longer receive signals from the brain or spinal cord; without nerve stimulation, the muscles atrophy, becoming weak, floppy and poorly controlled, and finally completely paralyzed *(acute flaccid paralysis)*.
- ❖ Progression to maximum paralysis is *rapid* (2–4 days), and is usually associated with fever and muscle pain.
- ❖ Deep tendon reflexes are also affected, and are usually absent or diminished; *sensation in the paralyzed limbs, however, is not affected.*

Bulbar Polio

❖ Bulbar polio occurs when poliovirus invades and destroys nerves within the bulbar region of the brainstem
❖ The bulbar region is a white matter pathway that connects the cerebral cortex to the brainstem. The destruction of these nerves weakens the muscles supplied by the cranial nerves (especially CN IX, X, XI and XII), producing features of "Bulbar palsy", i.e. difficulty in breathing, speaking, chewing and swallowing.

Bulbospinal Polio

Approximately 19% of all paralytic polio cases have both bulbar and spinal symptoms; this subtype is called respiratory or bulbospinal polio.

Early Supportive Treatment

Because no cure for polio exists, the focus is on increasing comfort, speeding recovery and preventing complications. Supportive treatments include:
❖ Bed rest.
❖ Antibiotics for secondary infections (none for poliovirus).
❖ Analgesics for pain.
❖ Portable ventilators to assist breathing: Portable ventilators may be required to support breathing. Today, many polio survivors with permanent respiratory paralysis use *modern jacket-type negative-pressure ventilators* worn over the chest and abdomen.
❖ Moderate exercise (physical therapy) to prevent deformity and loss of muscle function.
❖ A nutritious diet.

Tertiary Prevention

Disability limitation

❖ Factors that potentiate or facilitate paralytic events should be avoided, e.g.
  – Operations
  – Intramuscular injections
  – Strenuous exercise, etc.
❖ Formation of deformities and contractures should be prevented by moderate exercise and regular follow up.

Rehabilitation

Polio often requires long-term rehabilitation, including:
❖ Occupational therapy.
❖ Physical therapy.
❖ Braces.
❖ Corrective shoes.
❖ Orthopedic surgery.
❖ Electrotherapy.
❖ Massage and passive motion exercises.
❖ Surgical treatments, such as tendon lengthening and nerve grafting.

3. **A 25-year-old man reported medical OPD with high fever, chills, arthralgia and retro-orbital pain. Outline the diagnosis, case management and community intervention as per national guidelines.** **(12)**

Presenting Features

❖ High fever, chills and arthralgia.
❖ Retro-orbital pain.

Diagnosis

According to WHO classification and grading system of dengue infection, this patient is clinically diagnosed as having dengue fever. Fever + Arthralgia + Retro-orbital pain + No objective evidence of plasma leakage (elevated hematocrit/low serum albumin/ascites/pleural effusion/gallbladder edema).

According to WHO classification, dengue fever is diagnosed if fever with any 2/more of the symptoms are seen:

❖ Headache.
❖ Retro-orbital pain.
❖ Myalgia.
❖ Arthralgia.
❖ Rash.
❖ Hemorrhagic manifestations.
❖ No objective evidence of plasma leakage.

Case Management

Management of dengue fever is symptomatic and supportive. According to National Vector Borne Disease Control Programme, the case management of dengue fever is as follows:

❖ Bed rest is advisable during the acute phase
❖ Use cold sponging to keep temperature below 39°C
❖ Antipyretics may be used to lower the body temperature.
   Note: Aspirin/NSAID like Ibuprofen, etc. should be avoided since they may cause gastritis, vomiting, acidosis and platelet dysfunction.
❖ Paracetamol is preferable in the dosages as follows:

Age	Dosage of paracetamol
1–2 years	60–120 mg/dose
3–6 years	120 mg/dose
7–12 years	240 mg/dose
Adult	500 mg/dose

Note: In children the dose is calculated as 10 mg/kg/dose which can be repeated at the interval of 6 hours.

❖ Oral fluid and electrolyte therapy are recommended for patients with excessive sweating or vomiting.
❖ Patients should be monitored in DHF endemic area until they become febrile for one day without the use of antipyretics and after platelet and hematocrit determinations are stable (platelet count is >50,000/cu.mm).

Community Intervention according to National Vector Borne Disease Control Programme (NVBDCP)

1. People should form groups to supplement and reinforce efforts at household level. Such groups can identify commercial activities such as traders dealing in used tyres or small construction projects, etc. which may be creating larval habitats for the vector.
2. The groups should launch awareness campaigns on dengue and seek cooperation for prevention of mosquito breeding and protection from mosquito bites.
3. Community activities against larvae and adult mosquitoes may include:
   - Cleaning and covering water storage containers.
   - Keeping the surroundings clean and improving basic sanitation measures.
   - Burning mosquito coils to kill or repel the mosquitoes/burning neem leaves, coconut shells and husk to repel mosquitoes and eliminating outdoor breeding sites.
   - Aiding in screening houses.
   - Making hand aerosols available for killing mosquitoes.
   - Cleaning weeds and tall grass to reduce available outdoor resting places for adult mosquitoes near houses.
   - Promoting use of mosquito nets to protect infants and small children from mosquito bites during day time and also insecticide treated nets (ITN) and curtains to kill mosquitoes attempting to bite through the nets or resting on nets and curtains.
   - Organizing camps for insecticide treatment of community owned mosquito nets/curtains.
   - In case water containers cannot be emptied, applying Temephos (1 ppm) on weekly basis in coordination with the health authorities.
   - Mobilizing households to cooperate during spraying/fogging.

4. **The BMOH of a block was reported large numbers of cases clinically suspected to be dengue. He also referred 2 cases to district hospital and suspected an outbreak has occurred. As a BMOH, how will you investigate and control the outbreak?** (6 + 6)

Verification of Diagnosis

At first a sample of cases should be examined clinically and laboratory investigation should be done, if possible. There is a reliable classification and grading system of the severity of dengue infection proposed by WHO. It should be applied with accuracy:

Grade	Symptoms/signs	Laboratory findings
DF	Fever + ≥2 of the following: • Headache • Retro-orbital pain • Myalgia • Arthralgia • Rash/hemorrhagic manifestations • No evidence of plasma leakage	• WBC count ≤5,000 cells/cu mm • Platelet count <1,50,000 cells/cu mm • Hematocrit rise up to 5–10% above normal value (Men: 45% and Women: 40%)

Contd...

Contd...

Grade		Symptoms/signs	Laboratory findings
DHF	I	Above criteria for DF: • Hemorrhagic manifestations • Positive tourniquet test (≥20 petechiae/sq.inch) • Evidence of plasma leakage (ascites/pleural effusion/gallbladder edema)	• Platelet count <1,00,000 cells/cu mm • Hematocrit rise of ≥20%
DHF	II	Criteria for DHF grade I: • Evidence of spontaneous bleeding (bleeding from gums/epistaxis/black stools)	
DHF	III	Criteria for DHF grade II: • Circulatory failure (weak rapid pulse/pulse pressure ≤20 mm Hg/ high diastolic pressure/cold skin/restlessness)	
DHF	IV	Criteria for DHF grade III: • Profound shock (undetectable pulse/BP)	

Confirmation of Existence of an Epidemic

An epidemic is confirmed when the occurrence of disease exceeds the usual endemic occurrence by 2 standard deviation. So, the endemic frequency is determined from the existent past records and it is to be compared with the present occurrence.

Epidemic frequency ≥ (Endemic Frequency + 2 Standard Errors)

Defining population at risk:
1. *Obtaining a map of the area*: The map is a prerequisite of starting the investigation of the epidemic. The map should contain information about all the important landmarks, with the help of which one can quickly locate a focus of infection.
2. *Counting the population*: The only importance of counting the population in the locality is that it gives us the much important denominator of attack rates. Through which we can proceed to estimation of the attack rates. As it is a hard work, peripheral health workers (Village health guides/ASHA/Anganwadi workers) may be engaged in this work.

Rapid search for all cases and their characteristics:

This is done by the following methods:
❖ *Medical survey*: This is done to identify all the suspected cases and population at risk. All members of the population should be screened for the disease ideally. But if it is not feasible in reality, the cases and their contacts must be screened.
❖ *Epidemiological case sheet*: The BMOH should prepare an "epidemiological case sheet" which will include all the data relevant to the disease under study:
  – Patient particulars: Name/age/sex/occupation/address of the patient
  – Time of onset of disease/presenting symptoms and signs
  – Socioeconomic history/sanitary condition of the house of the patient, especially the collection of water in and around the house
  – Household contacts with their name, age and sex
  – Previous history of malaria or other mosquito-borne disease.
❖ *Searching for more cases*: The search for new cases and secondary cases should be continued till 2 incubation period passes after occurrence of the last case. It will include all the cases admitted into local hospitals (Government and Private).

Data analysis:

The data collected should be analyzed according to time, place and person.

❖ *Time*: The BMOH has to prepare an "epidemic curve" which should include:
  – A time relationship with exposure.
  – A clear-cut indication of the type of the epidemic: Common source/propagated epidemic.
  – The pattern of the epidemic: Seasonal/cyclic pattern.
❖ *Place*: The BMOH has to prepare a "Spot map" which should properly show the geographical distribution of cases
❖ *Person*: The BMOH has to calculate the attack rates and case fatality rates in exposed and nonexposed individuals.

Formulation of hypothesis:

The BMOH should formulate a proper hypothesis which will include:

❖ Possible source: Asymptomatic cases.
❖ Causative agent: Dengue virus.
❖ Possible mode of transmission: Bite of female *Aedes aegypti* mosquito.
❖ Environmental factors which enabled the epidemic to occur: Rainfall increases the number of breeding places of Aedes mosquito (e.g. flower vase/left out pots/fences, etc.), which can *cause* an epidemic.

Evaluation of entomological factors:

Investigate and comment about the following points:

❖ Agent factors:
  – Species of vector involved.
  – Breeding habits (artificial collection of water).
  – Residing habit of mosquito.
  – Flight range of mosquito.
  – Resistance to insecticides.
❖ Environmental factors:
  – Mosquito breeding places.
  – Drainage system and sanitary condition of the area.
  – Rainfall and its association with prevalence of dengue.
  – If overcrowding is acting as an associated factor in the emergence of epidemic or not.

Further investigation of population at risk:

Active and passive surveillance is done at regular intervals to identify any new cases and reports are sent to the higher authority.

Report writing:

A complete report with all necessary information is to be sent to the higher authority.

5. **Give a brief account of epidemiology of kala-azar. Outline the strategies of control of kala-azar. Enumerate the causes of resurgences of kala-azar.** (5 + 4 + 3)

Epidemiology of Kala-azar

At first it should be told that epidemiological triad consists of three main components:

  1. Agent

2. Host
3. Environment.

For their effective coordination, a critical mode of transmission is also of utmost importance.

Agent Factors

❖ Agent: *Leishmania donovani* is the causative agent of kala-azar. It has two forms in its lifecycle:
  – *Amastigote form*: Nonflagellated, found in man.
  – *Promastigote form*: Flagellated, found in sandfly.
❖ Reservoir of infection: Human.

Host Factors

❖ *Age*: In India, the peak age of kala-azar is 5–9 years.
❖ *Sex*: Males are affected 2 times more than female.
❖ *Socioeconomic status*: Kala-azar usually attacks the people with very low socioeconomic status.
❖ *Occupation*: The following occupations are especially vulnerable to be bitten by sandfly and having kala-azar:
  – Farming
  – Forestry
  – Mining industry
  – Fishing.
❖ *Population movement*: When large numbers of people move from endemic to non-endemic areas, there are greater chances of having the infection spread. So, the following groups are more vulnerable:
  – Tourists
  – Laborers
  – Migrants.
❖ *Immunity*: One attack gives long lasting immunity.

Environmental Factors

❖ *Vectors*: In India, *Phlebotomus argentipes* is the vector of kala-azar.
❖ *Season*: In India, a high prevalence of kala-azar is seen during and after rainy season.
❖ *Altitude*: Kala-azar is most commonly confined to the plains areas. It is not usually seen at a height >600 meters.

Mode of Transmission

❖ In India, kala-azar is transmitted from person to person by the bites of female *Phlebotomus (P. argentipes)* sandfly.
❖ *Extrinsic incubation period* (time required for the development of parasite within sandfly): 6–9 days.
❖ *Incubation period within human*: 1–4 months.
❖ Factors facilitating the transmission:
  – Overcrowding.

- Ill ventilation.
- Accumulation of organic waste materials around houses.

Strategies to Control Kala-azar

Diagnosis

❖ Diagnosis of kala-azar cases is done by using rapid diagnosis test kits in the field. The results can be read in 10 minutes. These kits show >90% specificity and sensitivity
❖ RD test kits are user friendly
❖ Interpretation of the test is also simple as two red lines indicate a positive result and only a single red line indicates negative result
❖ Parasitological diagnosis includes spleen, bone marrow and lymph node aspiration procedures; however, each of the procedures must be measured against the potential risks and gains for the patients
❖ In PKDL cases confirmation of infection either through PCR or by a slit skin biopsy.

Short-time Control Measures (Operational Guidelines on Kala-azar Elimination in India—2015)

As human is the sole reservoir of kala-azar in India, active and passive case detection and effective treatment is the mainstay of controlling kala-azar in a short time basis.

Special notes:
For treatment, single dose single day treatment with liposomal amphotericin B injection is the first drug of choice followed by capsule miltefosine (28 days) and injection amphotericin B (15 injections on alternate days) as well as combination of miltefosine and paramomycin injection.

Liposomal Amphotericin B

❖ It is the first drug of choice
❖ The single infusion treatment with liposomal amphotericin B requires a total quantity of 10 mg/kg for all ages including pregnant, pediatric and elderly patients.

Miltefosine
Miltefosine is a relatively safe oral drug for the treatment of kala-azar.

Mode of Treatment:
The treatment is provided as directly observed treatment (DOT).

Dosing schedule:

Age	Weight	Dosing (Given for 28 days)
Children (2–11 years)	—	2.5 mg/kg OD PC
Adult	<25 kg	50 mg OD PC
	>25 kg	50 mg BD PC

Amphotericin B
Amphotericin B deoxycholate injection intravenously at a dose of 1 mg/kg on alternate days × 15 doses.

Long-term Control Measures

Sandfly Control

❖ The mainstay of sandfly control remains the use of insecticides
❖ The insecticide of choice is **DDT** because the vector of kala-azar, *P. argentipes* is susceptible to DDT. The optimum dose is 1–2 g/sq mt sprayed in 2 rounds
❖ It should be sprayed inside and around the houses, animal shades and all other possible resting places of sandfly up to a height of 2 meters from the floor level
❖ In case of any suspected resistance, hexachlorobenzene (BHC) should be used as the insecticide of second choice.

Sanitation Measures

It should be kept in mind that insecticide spraying becomes optimally effective when it is conjugated with sanitation measures, which includes:

a. Repairing and blocking all cracks and crevices in the wall of the houses (which may be a potential breeding place for sandfly).
b. Removal of firewood and rubbish around houses.
c. Clearance of rodent burrows.
d. Maintenance of a good hygiene at cattle sheds and poultry.

Personal Prophylaxis

Last but not the least, personal prophylaxis adds more potential to the prevention of kala-azar. The following measures can be taken:

a. Avoiding sleeping on the floor
b. Use of fine mesh mosquito nets
c. Use of repellents like lotion/cream, etc.

Causes of Resurgence of Kala-azar

❖ The prevalence of kala-azar was declined due to adoption of insecticidal spraying (DDT) under National Malaria Eradication Programme (NMEP), as sandfly is sensitive to DDT. It had leaded to a substantial reduction in vector density
❖ But withdrawal of spraying resulted in gradual build-up of vector population in 1970s, especially in Bihar, West Bengal and East Uttar Pradesh
❖ At the same time, the following factors made things worse:
 – Presence and expansion of population base of the asymptomatic cases
 – Increased prevalence of post kala-azar dermal leishmaniasis
 – Undernutrition problem of the country
 – Increased prevalence of HIV/AIDS.
❖ At the present times, the most important factor for resurgence of kala-azar remains the population movement and migration (labor/tourists, etc.) from endemic to nonendemic areas, which is facilitating infection throughout the country
❖ Development of drug resistance, especially against SSG (sodium stibogluconate) and non-compliance to drugs also helping in resurgence of kala-azar
❖ Now three strategies have been adopted to prevent resurgence of kala-azar:
 1. Intensified vector control.
 2. Parasite elimination by proper treatment.
 3. Promotion of insecticide treated bed nets (ITBN).

6. **A 10-year-old child reported with dog bite on calf region, in casualty OPD within 2 hours of bite. As SMO suggest measures to prevent rabies in this child.** (12)

The aim of postexposure prophylaxis is to *neutralize the inoculated virus before it can enter the CNS*. Every case of human exposure should be treated as medical emergency. The measures to be taken as SMO are enlisted below:

Postexposure Prophylaxis

The type of postexposure prophylaxis depends on the type/degree of contact, which has been classified into three categories. They are as follows:

Category of contact with rabid animal	Postexposure prophylaxis
Category 1: Touching/feeding animals, licks on intact skin	Local treatment only
Category 2: Minor scratches/abrasions without bleeding, penetration of uncovered skin	Local treatment of the wound + Immediate vaccination
Category 3: Single/multiple transdermal bites/scratches, licks on broken skin, contamination of mucous membrane with saliva from licks, contact with bats	Local treatment of the wound + Immediate vaccination + Administration of rabies immunoglobulin

As the child is presenting with single transdermal bite on the calf region, he should be placed on category 3 of postexposure prophylaxis and given: Local treatment of the wound + Immediate vaccination + Rabies immunoglobulin administration.

Local Treatment of Wound

❖ The purpose of local treatment is to remove as much virus as possible from the site of inoculation before it can be absorbed on nerve endings
❖ It should never be neglected and should be done in every case
❖ Local treatment comprises of the following processes:
  – Cleansing:
    - Immediately flush and wash the wound(s), scratches and adjoining areas with plenty of soap and water, preferable under a running tap, for at least 15 minutes
    - If soap is not available, simply flush the wound with plenty of water
    - In case of punctured wounds, use catheters to irrigate the wound.
  – Chemical treatment:
    The residual virus remaining in the wound should be inactivated by:
    - Alcohol
    - Tincture iodine
    - Povidone iodine.
  – Suturing:
    - Bite wounds should not be immediately sutured to prevent additional trauma which may help spread the virus into deeper tissues
    - If suturing is necessary, it should be done 48–72 hours later, applying minimum possible stitches under the cover of rabies immunoglobulin locally
  – Antibiotic and anti-tetanus measure:
    - It should follow the local treatment mentioned above when indicated.

Postexposure Vaccination

The dose schedules are as follows:

Route	Site of administration	Dosage	Days
Intramuscular	Deltoid muscle in adults/ anterolateral aspect of thigh in children <2 years Multisite regimen	1.0 mL/0.5 mL	5 dose regimen: 1 dose each on day 0, 3, 7, 14, 28 4 dose regimen: 2 doses on day 0 (1 in each deltoid/ thigh), 1 dose each on day 7 and 21
Intradermal	2 sites regimen (deltoid/thigh)	0.1 mL	Injection is given at 2 sites on each visits on day 0, 3, 7, 28

Human rabies immunoglobulin and rabies vaccine administration sites

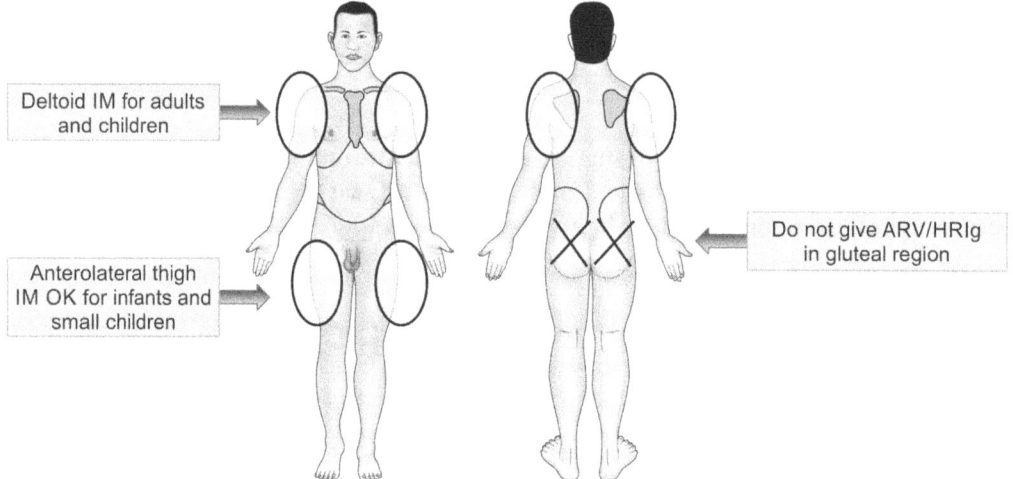

Deltoid IM for adults and children

Anterolateral thigh IM OK for infants and small children

Do not give ARV/HRIg in gluteal region

Note: Postexposure vaccination for previously vaccinated individuals: 1 dose of cell cultured and embryonated egg-based vaccine (CCEEV) delivered IM on day 0 and day 3 is sufficient. Rabies immunoglobulin is not indicated in such cases.

Postexposure Passive Immunization

❖ Rabies immunoglobulin is used for passive immunization as soon as possible after the initiation of postexposure vaccination
❖ It should be mentioned that after 7 days of first dose of vaccine, rabies immunoglobulin is not recommended because an active antibody response to rabies vaccine (CCEEV) is presumed to occur after this period
❖ The schedule of rabies immunoglobulin is as follows:

Dose:
20 IU/kg for human rabies Ig; 40 IU/kg for equine rabies Ig.
Site of administration:
All/as much as possible Ig should be administered into/around the wound.
If any amount remains, it should be administered at a site distant from the site of vaccination.
Caution:
In case of equine Ig, there is a small risk of anaphylaxis due to its heterogenous origin. So the physician should always be ready with a syringe of adrenaline before administering it.

7. **A child bitten by a street dog on hand and fingers was brought to the casualty ward of medical college within an hour of time. As a MO I/C what measures will you suggest to prevent rabies in this case?** (12)

As the child is presenting with multiple transdermal bites on multiple sites, he should be placed on category 3 of postexposure prophylaxis.

So, the child should be given: Local treatment of the wound + Immediate vaccination + Rabies immunoglobulin administration.

8. **A 30-year-old male attended OPD with 6 hypopigmented patches on different parts of the body. Write down the diagnosis. Outline the management of the case as per national program.** (4 + 8)

The patient is diagnosed as a patient of "Multibacillary leprosy".

Diagnosis of Leprosy

Type	No. of skin lesions (hypopigmented patches)
Paucibacillary leprosy	1–5 skin lesions
Multibacillary leprosy	>5 skin lesions

The following portion may be added if it comes as a long question:

Clinical Examination

To diagnose a case of leprosy clinically, a set pattern must be followed. It is called "Case taking", which consists of:

Interrogation

❖ Patient particulars (name, age, sex, place of residence, occupation)
❖ Family history of leprosy
❖ History of contact with leprosy cases
❖ Presenting complaint
❖ Details of previous history of treatment.

Physical Examination

❖ A thorough examination of body surface in good natural light for any evidence of leprosy (characteristic skin lesion: hypopigmented patch)
❖ Palpation of the commonly involved peripheral and cutaneous nerves for detection of *nerve thickening/nerve tenderness*. These include:
  – Ulnar nerve
  – Dorsal branch of radial nerve
  – Greater auricular nerve
  – Lateral popliteal nerve.
❖ Testing for loss of sensation for the following stimulus:
  – Heat
  – Cold

- Pain
- Light touch.
❖ Testing for paresis/paralysis of the muscles of hands and feet.

Bacteriological Examination

Skin smears are useful for diagnosing multibacillary leprosy. As the differentiation of paucibacillary and multibacillary leprosy can be done by detecting only the number of characteristic skin lesions, the bacteriological examination should not be a prerequisite for diagnosis and implementation of multidrug therapy (MDT).

Skin Smear

Skin smear is taken by "Slit and Scrape" method from two sites:
1.   An active lesion.
2.   One of the ear lobe.

Slit and Scrape Method

❖ The skin is cleaned with ether/spirit and allowed to dry
❖ A fold of skin is nipped in between thumb and index finger of the left hand
❖ A sterile knife is held at the right hand
❖ The point of the knife is held vertical to the skin fold
❖ The knife is pushed into the skin to a depth of 2 mm (to reach the dermis)
❖ An incision of about 5 mm is made
❖ Then the blade of the knife is rotated transversely to the line of cut
❖ The point of the knife is then used to scrape first on one side and then on the other side of the incision 2–3 times to obtain a tissue pulp from the dermis.

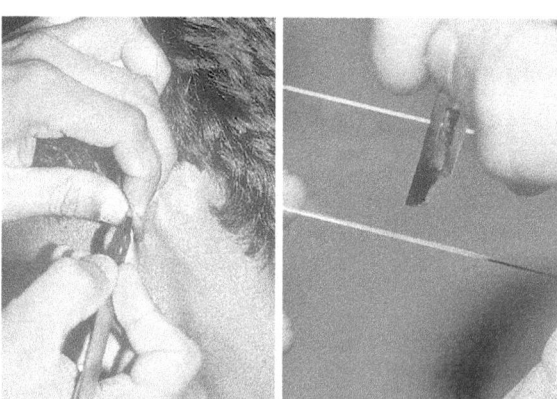

(Courtesy: Margreet Hogeweg)

❖ The scraped material is transferred on a glass slide and spread over an area with a radius of 4 mm.
❖ 6 smears can be made on one microscopic slide.

❖ The sites of the smears should be recorded accurately so that the next sets of smears can be taken from the same sites for assessing the effect of treatment.

❖ The wound is dressed and closed with a tape applied over the site.

Nasal Smear

❖ This is used for assessing the infectivity of the patient.

❖ The procedure should be done in the early morning.

❖ The patient blows his nose into a clean and dry sheet of plastic

❖ The smear should be made and fixed immediately/as soon as possible.

Working Out the Bacteriological and Morphological Index

Bacteriological Index

❖ This index includes both:
  – Live bacilli: Solid staining.
  – Dead bacilli: Fragmented/granular.

❖ The bacteriological index (BI) is calculated by the following way:

Score	No. of bacilli	No. of oil immersion field observed
0	0	100
1+	1–10	100
2+	1–10	10
3+	1–10	1
4+	10–100	1
5+	100–1000	1
6+	>1000	1

BI = (Total no. of plus (+)/Total No. of sites observed)

E.g.: If score from right ear and left ear are 4+ and 2 + accordingly, then the BI is: (4 + 2)/2 = 3.

Note: Before confirming a BI of 1+ and 2 +, at least 100 fields should be examined.

Before confirming a BI of 3 +, 4 +, 5 + and 6 +, at least 25 fields should be examined.

Morphological Index

❖ This index includes only the live bacilli (solid staining bacilli).

❖ The criteria for calling a bacilli "live", the following criteria are looked for:
  – Uniform staining of the entire organism.
  – Rounded ends.
  – Parallel sides.
  – Length = 5 × Width.

❖ The MI is calculated after examining 200 pink stained free (not in clumps) solid bacilli.

Histamine Test

❖ This test is used to detect early stage peripheral nerve damage by leprosy.

❖ Procedure and interpretation of the test:

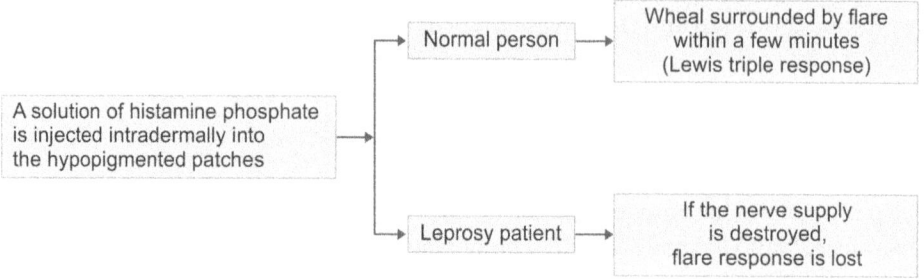

Immunological Test

It is of two types:
1. Tests for detecting cell-mediated immunity (CMI) → Lepromin test.
2. Tests for detecting humoral immunity (HI) → FLA-ABS test.

Lepromin Test

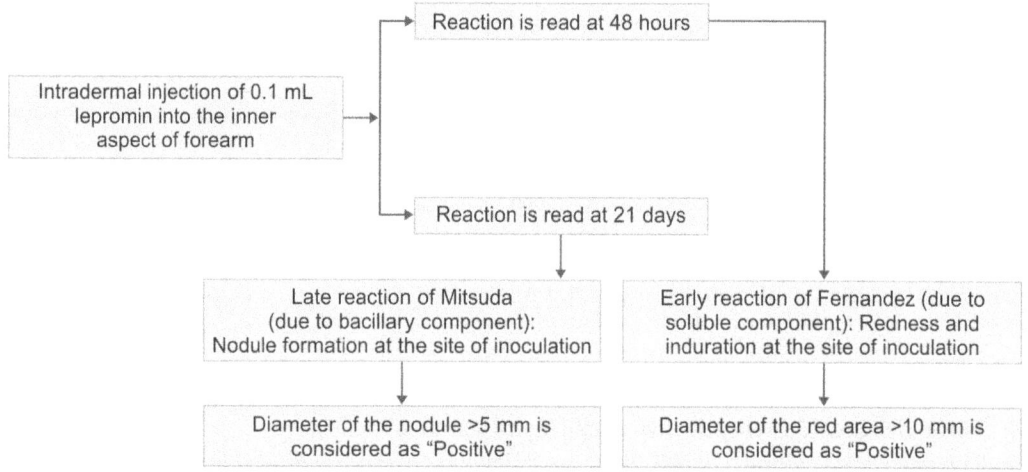

❖ This test is valuable in both:
  – Classification of the disease
  – Estimation of prognosis.
❖ Lepromin –ve individuals are prone to develop multibacillary leprosy later, which have a worse prognosis.
❖ Lepromin +ve individuals show better prognosis as they either develop paucibacillary leprosy/escape from the disease.

FLA-ABS Test (Fluorescent Leprosy Antibody Absorption Test)

❖ This test is now widely used for detection of subclinical cases of leprosy.
❖ This test detects *M. leprae* specific antibodies in the blood of the patient.

Management of a Case of Leprosy

As per the new Leprosy treatment guidelines by WHO (2018):

			Duration	
Age group	Drug	Dosage and frequency	PBL	MBL
Adult	Rifampicin	600 mg once a month	6 months	12 months
	Clofazimine	300 mg once a month and 50 mg daily		
	Dapsone	100 mg daily		
Children (10–14 years)	Rifampicin	450 mg once a month	6 months	12 months
	Clofazimine	150 mg once a month and 50 mg daily		
	Dapsone	50 mg daily		

Try Yourself

1. A 6-month-old patient with ARI had a respiratory rate of 56/min. There was no chest indrawing and danger signs. Classify ARI with justification and discuss the management accordingly.
2. Discuss the reasons behind reappearance of kala-azar in West Bengal. Suggest the measures for its control.
3. What are the diseases covered by National Vector Borne Disease Control Programme (NVBDCP). What are the malariometric indices? Write down the antimalarial drug policy in NVBDCP.
4. Enumerate three different parameters used for measuring malaria problem in a community. Define and explain two important parameters.
5. Outline the role of various epidemiological factors in the causation of measles. Suggest preventive and control measures in case of an outbreak of measles.
6. How will you investigate an outbreak of watery diarrhea in your college hostel? Describe the control and preventive measures to be adopted.
7. Discuss polio eradication in the light of epidemiological factors influencing poliomyelitis.
8. Name vector-borne diseases. Explain epidemiology of one of them.
9. Enumerate the various STDs. Describe the social factors involved in their spread.

EPIDEMIOLOGY OF CHRONIC NONCOMMUNICABLE DISEASE AND CONDITIONS

1. What are the danger signs of cancer? Outline the epidemiology of oral cancer and methods of its prevention in the community.   (3 + 4 + 5)

Danger Signs of Cancer

These are the signs people should be educated about to accelerate early diagnosis and treatment because most of the cancers, when present in an early stage are preventable or curable. Some of the danger signs of cancers are:

❖ An unexplained loss of weight
❖ A lump/hard area in the breast

❖ A change in a wart/mole
❖ A swelling/sore that is not getting better
❖ A persistent cough
❖ A persistent hoarseness of voice
❖ Excess blood loss at times of period/blood loss outside usual dates
❖ A persistent change in digestive/bowel habits.

Epidemiology of Oral Cancer

1. *World scenario*: According to Oral Cancer Foundation, oral cancer is the 11th most common cancer in the world with >300,000 new cases annually. The Indian subcontinent accounts for 1/3rd of the world burden.
2. *Problem in India*: With an annual incidence of 130,000 new cases per year, oral cancer remains an important problem in India. In fact, India alone has reported the highest prevalence of oral cancer globally.
3. *Epidemiological factors*:
   a. Tobacco use (including smoking tobacco in form of biri/cigarette/cigar/hookah as well as smokeless tobacco in form of gutka/quid/snuff/misri) and excessive alcohol consumption are estimated to account for ~90% of all oral cancers.
   b. The most common form of tobacco chewing in India is in the form of **betel quid** (betel leaf+ tobacco+ lime+ spices). Sun-dried tobacco and slaked lime are placed in the palm of hand and rubbed with the thumb. The desired mixture is called *Khaini*. It is placed at mouth and slowly sucked and swallowed at regular intervals.
   c. Studies are suggesting that almost all cases of oral cancers have occurred among tobacco smokers/tobacco chewers and in case of chewing tobacco, cancer has always occurred at that side of the mouth where tobacco quid was kept.
   d. Usually oral cancer is always preceded by some oral lesions like white patches *(leukoplakia)* and red patches *(erythroplakia)*, which are easy to detect due to their long existence of 10-15 years before proceeding to invasive carcinoma. These lesions are reversible at early stages because stopping tobacco use at these stages can completely cure them.

Note: A common cancer of oral cavity at coastal regions of Andhra Pradesh is epidermoid carcinoma of hard palate, which occurs in people who smoke cigar reversely, i.e. smoking with the burning end placed inside the mouth.

Methods of Prevention of Oral Cancer

Primary Prevention

Control of tobacco and alcohol consumption:
❖ As oral cancer is caused by tobacco use (especially smokeless tobacco like gutka/quid/snuff/misri), so intensive public health education is required to change this harmful habit.
❖ Legislative actions are essential in this aspect with proper highlighting on the tobacco products of their harmfulness and their potential to cause cancers and ban/restriction of the sale of tobacco products in selected high prevalence territories/throughout the country like India, which bears above 30% of the oral cancer burden of the world.
❖ Intersectoral coordination is required at this step, as well as engagement of mass media to ensure community participation at the highest level.

Secondary Prevention

Early diagnosis and treatment of precancerous lesions:

❖ It is a well-established fact that after the first appearance of oral lesions like leukoplakia and erythroplakia, the transformation of them into invasive oral cancer is a long-term event, taking not less than 10–15 years

❖ These oral lesions are easily visible and can be cured only by complete cessation of tobacco use

❖ There is also an important concept called "*Field cancerization*", which implicates that multiple individual primary tumors develop independently in the upper digestive tract as a result of years of chronic exposure of the mucosa to carcinogens. The 5-year survival rate for the first primary tumor is considerably better than 50%, but in such individuals, second primary tumors are the most common cause of death

❖ So, early diagnosis is of utmost importance in case of oral cancer

❖ Invasiveness of oral cancers is a matter of concern because the only treatment modalities left at that stage are surgery and radiotherapy, which requires a tertiary care support and highly specialized personnel. It should be kept in mind that in developing countries over 50% cases present at advanced stage

❖ For early diagnosis of oral lesions, an effective way is to involve grass-root level workers like village health guides, ASHA workers, anganwadi workers and multipurpose workers and properly educate them so that they can properly identify early oral lesions and can advise the patients to take preventive measures and can refer oral cancers to district hospitals/tertiary care units at an early stage

❖ For the purpose of mass screening in a high prevalence area, "oral camps" may be strategically planned to detect precancerous oral lesions and oral cancers at the same time

❖ Last but not the least, an effective case detection system is useless without a well-established infrastructure and manpower to treat cancer. So, infrastructure development and manpower training should be uplifted with active collaboration from Government and Private Agencies.

2. A 35-year-old sedentary obese man with smoking habit is found to have a blood pressure of 126/100 mm Hg. How will you classify this blood pressure? Describe the management with special emphasis on diet of the person.

(2 + 10)

ACC/AHA 2017 Hypertension Guidelines

Designation	SBP (mm Hg)		DBP (mm Hg)
Normal BP	<120	AND	<80
Elevated BP	120-129	AND	<80
Stage 1 hypertension	130-139	OR	80–89
Stage 2 hypertension	≥140	OR	≥90

According to the new guidelines, the person is classified to have a stage 2 hypertension.

Management (According to New ACC/AHA Guidelines)

Nonpharmacological interventions

Intervention	Dose
Weight loss	Ideal body weight is best goal but at least 1 kg reduction in body weight for most adults who are overweight
DASH dietary pattern*	Diet rich in fruits, vegetables, whole grains, and low-fat dairy products with reduced content of saturated and trans fat
Reduced intake of dietary sodium	<1,500 mg/day is optimal goal but at least 1,000 mg/day reduction in most adults
Enhanced intake of dietary potassium	3,500–5,000 mg/day, preferably by consumption of a diet rich in potassium
Physical activity	Aerobic physical exercise 90–150 min/wk
Moderation in alcohol intake	In individuals who drink alcohol, reduce alcohol to: • Men: ≤2 drinks daily • Women: 1 drink daily

*DASH: Dietary Approaches to Stop Hypertension.

Recommendations for treatment and follow-up:
1. Normal BP:
   – Promote optimal lifestyle habits
   – Reassess in 1 year.
2. Elevated BP:
   – Nonpharmacological therapy
   – Reassess in 3–6 months.
3. Stage 1 hypertension:
   A. Estimated 10 years cardiovascular disease risk <10%:
      - Nonpharmacological therapy
      - Reassess in 3–6 months.
   B. Estimated 10 years cardiovascular disease risk ≥10%:
      - Nonpharmacological therapy + BP-lowering medications*
      - Reassess in 1 month.
4. Stage 2 hypertension:
      - Nonpharmacological therapy + BP-lowering medications*
      - Consider initiation of pharmacological therapy with 2 antihypertensive agents of different classes
      - Reassess in 1 month.
*If BP goals are met: Reassess in 3–6 months
If BP goals are not met: Consider intensification of therapy.

3. Define diabetes mellitus. What are the diagnostic criteria for diabetes mellitus? Discuss the role of lifestyle modifications including medical nutritional therapy in management of diabetes mellitus. **(2 + 4 + 6)**

Diabetes Mellitus

Diabetes mellitus (DM) refers to a group of common metabolic disorders that share the phenotype of hyperglycemia.

Diagnostic Criteria of DM

❖ Symptoms of diabetes plus random blood glucose concentration ≥200 mg/dL or
❖ Fasting plasma glucose ≥126 mg/dL or
❖ Hemoglobin A1c ≥ 6.5% or
❖ 2-hour plasma glucose ≥200 mg/dL during an oral glucose tolerance test.

Role of Lifestyle Modifications in Management of Diabetes Mellitus

❖ Individuals with prediabetes or increased risk of diabetes should be referred to a structured program to reduce body weight and increase physical activity as well as being screened for cardiovascular disease.
❖ The Diabetes Prevention Program (DPP) demonstrated that intensive changes in lifestyle (diet and exercise for 30 min/day – 5 times/week) in individuals with impaired glucose tolerance (IGT) prevented or delayed the development of type 2 DM by 58%.

Medical Nutrition Therapy (MNT)

❖ MNT is a term used by the ADA to describe the optimal coordination of caloric intake with other aspects of diabetes therapy (insulin, exercise, weight loss).
❖ **Primary** prevention measures of MNT are directed at preventing or delaying the onset of type 2 DM in high-risk individuals (obese or with prediabetes) by promoting *weight reduction.*
❖ **Secondary** prevention measures of MNT are directed at preventing or delaying diabetes-related complications in diabetic individuals by *improving glycemic control.*
❖ **Tertiary** prevention measures of MNT are directed at managing diabetes-related *complications* (cardiovascular disease, nephropathy, etc.) in diabetic individuals.

Nutritional Recommendations for Adults with Diabetes or Prediabetes (ADA)

❖ Hypocaloric diet that is low-carbohydrate
❖ Monitor carbohydrate intake in regard to calories
❖ Minimize intake of sucrose-containing foods
❖ Fructose preferred over sucrose or starch
❖ Minimal trans-fat consumption
❖ Diet rich in monounsaturated fatty acids may be better
❖ Routine supplements of vitamins, antioxidants, or trace elements not advised.

HEALTH PROGRAMS IN INDIA

1. **A 7-day-old baby is brought to your OPD block with excessive cry, refusal of feeds and convulsions. Discuss the diagnosis, case management and preventive strategies as per National Program. (12)**

As the age is 7 days, the baby will fall into the IMCI classification for age up to 2 months.

Symptoms:
1. Refusal of feeds
2. Vomiting
3. Convulsions.

Diagnosis According to IMCI Classification (2014)

Very Severe Disease

Check for general danger signs

Ask:	Look:				
• Is the child able to drink or breastfeed? • Has the child had convulsions?	• See if the child is lethargic or unconscious • Is the child convulsion now?	Urgent attention	• Any general danger sign	Pink: Very severe disease	• Give diazepam if convulsing now • Quickly complete the assessment • Give any pre-referral treatment immediately • Treat to prevent low blood sugar • Keep the child warm • Refer *urgently*

A child with any general danger sign needs *urgent* attention; complete the assessment and any pre-referral treatment immediately so referral is not delayed.

Case management:

❖ Give diazepam if convulsing now

❖ Quickly complete the assessment

❖ Give any pre-referral treatment immediately

❖ Treat to prevent low blood sugar

❖ Keep the child warm

❖ Refer urgently.

Give Diazepam to Stop Convulsions

❖ Turn the child to his/her side and clear the airway. Avoid putting things in the mouth

❖ Give 0.5 mg/kg diazepam injection solution per rectum using a small syringe without a needle (like a tuberculin syringe) or using a catheter

❖ Check for low blood sugar, then treat or prevent

❖ Give oxygen and refer

❖ If convulsions have not stopped after 10 minutes repeat diazepam dose

Age or weight	Diazepam (10 mg/2 mL)
2 months up to 6 months (5–7 kg)	0.5 mL
6 months up to 12 months (7–10 kg)	1.0 mL
12 months up to 3 years (10–14 kg)	1.5 mL
3 years up to 5 years (14–19 kg)	2.0 mL

Treat The Child to Prevent Low Blood Sugar

❖ If the child is able to breastfeed:
  – Ask the mother to breastfeed the child

❖ If the child is not able to breastfeed but is able to swallow:
  – Give expressed breast milk or a breast-milk substitute
  – If neither of these is available, give sugar water*
  – Give 30–50 mL of milk or sugar water* before departure.

❖ If the child is not able to swallow:
  – Give 50 mL of milk or sugar water* by nasogastric tube
  – If no nasogastric tube available, give 1 teaspoon of sugar moistened with 1–2 drops of water sublingually and repeat dose every 20 minutes to prevent relapse.*

* *To make sugar water: Dissolve 4 level teaspoons of sugar (20 grams) in a 200 mL cup of clean water.*

Preventive Strategies under National Program

To prevent very severe disease, the following measures should be taken:
* Immunization of young infants
* Better maternal and child health care
* Improvement of living conditions.

Immunization of Young Infants

Immune the young infants as per national guidelines.

Better Maternal and Child Health Care

* Maternal nutrition:
  Improving prenatal and postnatal nutrition will reduce the low birth weight problem and will improve the quality of breast milk, respectively; both of which has a great impact on childhood infections
* Child nutrition:
  For child nutrition, the following measures should be taken:
  - Promotion of breastfeeding
  - Appropriate weaning practices
  - Supplementary feeding
  - Vitamin A supplementations.

Improvement of Living Conditions

* Health education should be given to the family and community about the impact of general cleanliness and personal hygiene on child health.
* *It should be emphasized that at the time of illness, breastfeeding should never be reduced or discontinued.*
* Families with young children must be educated about the danger signs so that appropriate steps can be taken at right times.
* Immunization coverage of the vulnerable areas should be enhanced to maximum with step-by-step planning and implementation.

2. **A 9-month-old child presented with history of frequent passage of loose stool for 2 days. The child is irritable and skin turgor going back slowly. Classify the condition with proper justification in accordance with national program guidelines. Outline the management of the child. What advices you should give to the mother for prevention of occurrence of such condition in the future?** (4 + 6 + 2)

As the age of the child is 2 months, he will fall under the IMCI classification of 2 months to 5 years.

Presenting signs and symptoms:
1. Frequent passage of loose stool for 2 days
2. Irritability
3. Skin turgor goes back slowly.

IMCI classification placement: Some dehydration.

For proper justification, we are discussing how to classify the dehydration in diarrhea according to IMCI classification.

Does the child have diarrhea?

It yes. ask:	Look, and feel:	for DEHYDRATION Classify DIARRHEA	Signs	Classify	Treatment
• For how long? • Is there blood in the stool?	• Look at the child's general condition in the clinic: – Lethargic or unconscious? – Restless and irritable? • Look for sunken eyes.		Two of the following signs: • Lethargic or unconscious • Sunken eyes • Not able to drink or drinking poorly • Skin pinch goes back very slowly	Pink: Severe dehydration	• If child has no other severe classification: – Give fluid for severe dehydration (Plan C) OR • If child also has no other severe classification: – Refer URGENTLY to hospital with mother giving frequent sips of ORS on the way – Advise the mother to continue breastfeeding • If child is 2 years or older and there is cholera in your area, give antibiotic for cholera
	• Offer the child fluid. Is the child: – Not able to drink or drinking poorly? – Drinking eagerly, thirsty? • Pinch the skin of the abdomen. Does it go back: – Very slowly (longer than 2 seconds)? – Slowly?		Two of the following signs: • Restless, irritable • Sunken eyes • Drink eagerly, thirsty • Skin pinch goes back slowly	Yellow: Some dehydration	• Give fluid, zinc supplements, and food for some dehydration (Plan B) • If child also has a severe classification: – Refer URGENTLY to hospital with mother giving frequent sips of ORS on the way – Advise the mother to continue breastfeeding • Advise mother when to return immediately • Follow-up in 5 days if not improving
			Not enough signs to classify as some or severe dehydration	Green: No dehydration	• Give fluid, zinc supplements, and food to treat diarrhea at home (Plan A) • Advise mother when to return immediately • Follow-up in 5 days if not improved
		and if diarrhea 14 days or more	• Dehydration present	Pink: Severe persistent diarrhea	• Treat dehydration before referral unless the child has another severe classification • Refer to hospital
			• No dehydration	Yellow: Persistent diarrhea	• Advise the mother on feeding a child who has persistent diarrhea • Give multivitamins and minerals (including zinc) for 14 days • Follow-up in 5 days
		and if blood in stool	• Blood if blood in stool	Yellow: Dysentery	• Give ciprofloxacin for 3 days • Follow-up in 3 days

Plan B: Treat Some Dehydration with ORS

In the clinic, give recommended amount of ORS over 4-hour period

❖ Determine amount of ORS to give during first 4 hours

Weight	<6 kg	6 – <10 kg	10 – <12 kg	12–19 kg
Age*	Up to 4 months	4 months up to 12 months	12 months up to 2 years	2 years up to 5 years
In mL	200–450	450–800	800–960	960–1600

    * *Use the child's age only when you do not know the weight. The approximate amount of ORS required (in mL) can also be calculated by multiplying the child's weight (in kg) times 75.*

- – If the child wants more ORS than shown, give more
- – For infants under 6 months who are not breastfed, also give 100–200 mL clear water during this period if you use standard ORS. This is not needed if you use low osmolarity ORS.

❖ Show the mother how to give ORS solution:
- – Give frequent small sips from a cup
- – If the child vomits, wait 10 minutes. Then continue, but more slowly
- – Continue breastfeeding whenever the child wants.

❖ After 4 hours:
- – Reassess the child and classify the child for dehydration
- – Select the appropriate plan to continue treatment
- – Begin feeding the child in clinic.

❖ If the mother must leave before completing treatment:
- – Show her how to prepare ORS solution at home
- – Show her how much ORS to give to finish 4-hour treatment at home
- – Give her enough ORS packets to complete rehydration. Also give her 2 packets as recommended in Plan A
- – Explain the 4 rules of home treatment:
  1. Give extra fluid
  2. Give zinc (age 2 months up to 5 years)
  3. Continue feeding (exclusive breastfeeding if age less than 6 months)
  4. When to return.

❖ If still breastfeeding, give more frequent, longer breastfeeds, day and night.

❖ If taking other milk:
- – Replace with increased breastfeeding, or
- – Replace with fermented milk products, such as yoghurt, or
- – Replace half of the milk with nutrient-rich semisolid food.

❖ For other foods, follow feeding recommendations for the child's age.

Follow-up

After 2 days:

Ask: Has the diarrhea stopped?

Treatment

❖ If the diarrhea has not stopped, assess and treat the young infant for diarrhea (SEE "Does the Young Infant have Diarrhea").

❖ If the diarrhea has stopped, tell the mother to continue exclusive breastfeeding.

Advice to the mother for prevention of occurrence of such condition in future:

❖ If the child is on breastfeeding till now, the mother should be advised to continue it.

❖ The mother should be told to continue supplementary feeding properly and in adequate amounts.

❖ Vitamin A supplementation measures should be taken by the mother. Foods rich in vitamin A like carrot/spinach/amaranth/butter/margarine/green leafy vegetables should be given to the child.

❖ The mother should be advised to upgrade the hygienic condition inside and around the house by:

– Keep the environment as clean as possible.
– Use plenty of water:
  - To wash the hands before preparing food.
  - Before and after eating.
  - Before feeding the child.
  - After defecation.
– Use sanitary latrine for defecation purpose. If there is no sanitary latrine, then the mother should educate all the family members to defecate at a minimum distance of 10 meters from any water source.
– Eat food as soon as possible after preparation because unhygienic storage of food enhances contamination.

3. **A 4-year-old child with difficulty breathing has been brought to the subcenter. On examination, you got a respiratory rate of 45/min along with chest indrawing. How will you assess, classify and manage the case? What advices you should give to the mother?** (8 + 4)

Presenting Signs and Symptoms

1. Fast breathing (respiratory rate >40/min in 12 months to 5 years of age is called "Fast breathing")
2. Chest indrawing.

History: Passage of watery stool every 2–3 hours.

As the age of the child is 4 years, he will fall under the IMCI classification of 2 months to 5 years.

IMCI Classification Placement: Pneumonia

❖ For proper justification, we are discussing how to classify the dehydration in diarrhea according to IMCI classification.

THEN ASK ABOUT MAIN SYMPTOMS:

Does the child have cough or difficult breathing?

Classify cough or Difficult breathing

It yes, ask:	Look, listen, feel:			
• For how long?	• Count the breaths in 1 minute • Look for chest indrawing • Look and listen for stridor • Look and listen for wheezing	Young infant must be calm		

If wheezing with either fast breathing or chest indrawing:
Give a trial of rapid acting inhales bronchodilator for up to three times 15–20 minutes apart. Count the breaths and look for chest indrawing again, and then classify.

If the child is:	Fast breathing is:
2 months up to 12 months	50 breaths per minute or more
12 months up to 5 years	40 breaths per minute or more

Signs	Classification	Treatment
• Any general danger sign or • Stridor in calm child	*Pink:* Severe pneumonia or very severe disease	• Give first dose of an appropriate antibiotic • Refer *urgently* to hospital**
• Chest indrawing or • Fast breathing	*Yellow:* Pneumonia	• Give oral Amoxicillin for 5 days*** • If wheezing (or disappeared after rapidly acting bronchodilator) given an inhaled bronchodilator for 5 days**** • If chest indrawing in HIV exposed/infected give first dose of amoxicillin and refer • Sooth the throat and relieve the cough with safe remedy • If coughing for more than 14 days or recur wheeze, refer for possible TB or asthma assessment • Advise mother when to return immediately • Follow-up in 3 days
• No signs of pneumonia or very severe disease	*Green:* Cough or cold	• If wheezing (or disappeared after rapidly a bronchodilator) give an inhaled bronchodilator 5 days**** • Soothe the throat and relieve the cough with safe remedy • If coughing for more than 14 days or recur wheezing, refer for possible TB or asthma assessment • Advise mother when to return immediately • Follow-up in 5 days if not improving

* If pulse oximeter is available, determine oxygen saturation and refer to hospital if <90%.

** If referral is not possible, manage the child as described in the pneumonia section of the national referral guidelines or as in WHO Pocket Book for hospital care for children

*** Oral amoxicillin for 3 days could be used in patients with fast breathing but no chest indrawing in low HIV settings.

**** In settings where inhaled bronchodilator is not available, oral salbutamol may be tried but not recommended for treatment of severe acute wheeze.

Advices to the Mother

❖ If still breastfeeding give more frequent, longer breastfeeds, day and night
❖ If taking other milk:
  – Replace with increased breastfeeding, or
  – Replace with fermented milk products, such as yoghurt, or
  – Replace half of the milk with nutrient-rich semisolid food.
❖ For other foods, follow feeding recommendations for the child's age.

Follow up:
After 5 days:
Ask:
❖ Has the diarrhea stopped?
❖ How many loose stools is the child having per day?

Treatment

❖ If *the diarrhea has not stopped* (child is still having 3 or more loose stools per day), do a full reassessment of the child. Treat for dehydration if present. Then refer to hospital
❖ It *the diarrhea has stopped* (child having less than 3 loose stools per day), tell the mother to follow the usual feeding recommendations for the child's age.

Return immediately if the child has any of the following signs:

❖ Not able to drink/breastfeed
❖ Becomes sicker
❖ Develops a fever
❖ Blood in stool
❖ Drinking poorly.

4. Enlist major causes of blindness in India. What is the definition of blindness under NPCB? Outline the strategies adopted for controlling of blindness under the National Programme for Control of Blindness (NPCB). (4 + 8)

Major Causes of Blindness in India

❖ Cataract (62.6%)
❖ Refractive error (19.70%)
❖ Glaucoma (5.80%)
❖ Posterior segment disorder (4.70%)
❖ Surgical complication (1.20%)
❖ Posterior capsular opacification (0.90%)
❖ Corneal blindness (0.90%)
❖ Others (4.19%).

Definition of Blindness Under NPCB

Simple Definition

Inability of a person to count fingers from a distance of 6 meters or 20 feet.

Technical Definition

❖ Vision 6/60 or less with the best possible spectacle correction
❖ Diminution of field vision to 20° or less in better eye.

Goals and Objectives of NPCB in the XII Plan

❖ To reduce the backlog of blindness through identification and treatment of blind at primary, secondary and tertiary levels based on assessment of the overall burden of visual impairment in the country
❖ Develop and strengthen the strategy of NPCB for "Eye Health" and prevention of visual impairment; through provision of comprehensive eye care services and quality service delivery
❖ Strengthening and upgradation of Regional Institutes of Ophthalmology (RIOs) to become center of excellence in various sub-specialities of ophthalmology
❖ Strengthening the existing and developing additional human resources and infrastructure facilities for providing high quality comprehensive eye care in all districts of the country
❖ To enhance community awareness on eye care and lay stress on preventive measures
❖ Increase and expand research for prevention of blindness and visual impairment
❖ To secure participation of voluntary organizations/private practitioners in eye care.

Strategies Adopted for Controlling of Blindness under the NPCB

❖ Comprehensive eye care services addressing major blinding causes: cataract, refractive errors and low vision, childhood blindness, corneal blindness, glaucoma, diabetic retinopathy, etc.
❖ Development of eye care services and improvement in quality of eye care by training of personnel, supply of high tech equipment, strengthening follow-up services and monitoring of services
❖ Decentralized implementation of the schemes through state and district health societies
❖ Reduction in backlog of blind persons active screening of population over 50 years, organizing screening camps and transporting operable cases to eye care facilities
❖ Involvement of voluntary organization in various NPCB activities
❖ Participation of community and Panchayati raj institutions in organizing services in the rural area
❖ Screening of school going children for identification and treatment or refractive errors, with special attention to underserved areas
❖ Promoting eye donation, processing and utilization of donated eyes for treatment of corneal blindness
❖ Special focus of illiterate women in rural areas, convergence with ongoing schemes for development of women and children
❖ Free treatment to poor patients through qualified government and nongovernmental organizations
❖ Public awareness about prevention and timely treatment of eye ailments.

Structural Organization of National Programme for Control of Blindness (NPCB)

1. *Central level:* Ophthalmology section, Directorate General of Health Services, Ministry of Health and Family Welfare.
2. *State level:* State Ophthalmic Cell, Directorate of Health Services, State Health Services (State Program Officer at State Level is looking after the program)
3. *District level:* District blindness control society (DBCS) (District Blindness Cell Program Officer at District Level is looking after the program).

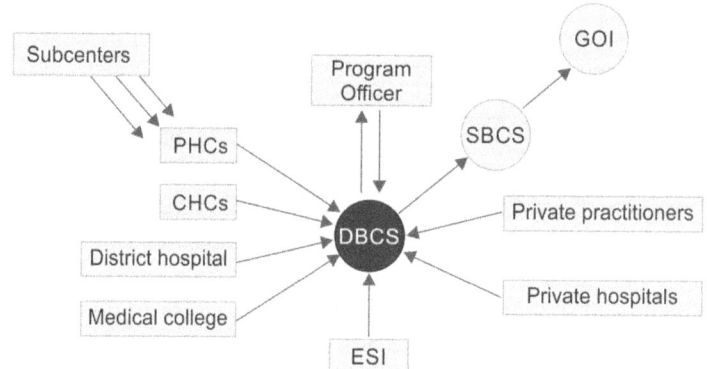

(PHC: Primary Health Center; CHC: Community Health Center; ESI: ESI hospitals; DBCS: District Blindness Control Society; SBCS: State Blindness Control Society; GOI: Government of India)

Detail Insight into the Strategies

Constructional Strategies

1. To shift from eye camp approach to a fixed facility surgical approach.
2. Construction of dedicated eye operation theaters and eye wards at district and subdistrict hospitals.
3. Supply of ophthalmic instruments to the whole country.
4. Setting up 5 centers for excellence for eye care services at tertiary level.

Administrative Strategies

1. Appointment of ophthalmic surgeons and ophthalmic assistants in new district and sub-divisional hospitals.
2. Appointment of ophthalmic assistants in PHCs/vision centers.
3. Appointment of eye donation counsellors on contract basis in eye banks.
4. Promotion of eye donation and eye banking.
5. Involvement of private practitioners.

Cause Prevention Strategies

1. To shift from conventional cataract surgery to intraocular lens (IOL) implantation for better postoperative vision.
2. To improve follow-up services for cataract operated persons.

3. To identify bilateral blind persons, preparation of village-wise blind registers and giving preference to bilateral blind patients for cataract surgery.
4. Grant in aid for NGOs for management of eye diseases other than cataract (including glaucoma, diabetic retinopathy, corneal opacity and corneal ulcer, childhood blindness, etc.).
5. Vitamin A supplementation and MMR vaccination for prevention of childhood blindness through DBCS funding.

Try Yourself

1. Enumerate the various national health programs in India. Write in detail about any one of them.
2. What are the diseases covered under National Vector Borne Disease Control Programme? Describe the program strategy for one of them.
3. What is DOTS? Describe the strategy for the treatment under DOTS.
4. What is the difference between planning and family welfare? Describe the components and strategies under RCH program.

DEMOGRAPHY AND FAMILY PLANNING

1. **A 25-year-old mother with 2 children aged 5 years and 1 year came to the OPD for family planning advices. Discuss different methods of contraception that can be offered to her with merits and demerits.** **(10)**

As the family has been completed as per 2 child norm, the mother should be firmly advised to adopt the permanent sterilization methods (female or male). But if the mother refuses to take it to have another child at future, then she should be advised to adopt any of the following methods:
a. Condoms.
b. Intrauterine contraceptive devices (IUCDs).
c. Oral contraceptive pills (OCPs)
d. DMPA.

Merits and demerits of the proposed methods

Methods	Merits/benefits	Demerits/limitations

Female sterilization/ Tubectomy	• Very effective and simple surgery performed on women under local anesthesia
	• Permanent procedure
	• Effective immediately
	• Nothing to remember, no supplies needed, no repeat clinic visits required after initial follow-up visits on 7th day to remove the stitches
	• Does not interfere with sexual intercourse
	• No effect on breast milk production
		• Short-term discomfort/pain following procedure
		• Uncommon complications of surgery include:
		  – Bleeding from surgical site
		  – Infection
		  – Injury to internal organs
		  – Requires a trained provider and health facility providing the service
		  – Does not protect against STIs and HIV

Contd...

Contd...

Methods	Merits/benefits	Demerits/limitations
	• No known long-term side effects or health risks • Can be performed any time during the menstrual cycle when it is reasonably sure that the woman is not pregnant/within 7 days of delivery/postabortion, after ruling out infection	
Male sterilization/vasectomy	• Very effective, permanent procedure • Not effective immediately after the procedure. The couple needs to use a backup method such as condom for the first 3 months after the procedure for the semen to be sperm free • Does not interfere with sexual intercourse/sexual pleasure • Simple surgery performed under local anesthesia by trained providers • No known long-term side effects • No repeat clinic visits required, no supplies needed, except the use of backup method/condoms for the first 3 months • Easier to perform than female sterilization • No change in sexual function • No effect on hormone production	• Permanent • Delayed effectiveness (requires at least 3 months or 20 ejaculations for procedure to be effective) • Does not protect against STIs and HIV • Scrotal support to be maintained for the initial few days to prevent pain at the operation site
Condoms	• Moderately effective • Effective immediately • Only method that prevents STIs, including HIV/AIDS, as well as pregnancy (dual protection), when used correctly during intercourse • No effect on breast milk production • No hormonal side effects • Can be stopped at any time • Easy to keep stock handy, can be used by men of any age • Can be used without initially seeing a healthcare provider • Enables a man to take responsibility for preventing pregnancy and disease • Condoms are readily available free of cost at the government health facilities or home delivered by ASHA at a nominal cost	• Condoms should not be reused and should be discarded after every act of intercourse • Supplies must be readily available before intercourse begins • Some men or women may feel that it interferes with their sexual pleasure • Latex condoms may cause itching for a few people who are allergic to latex

Contd...

Contd...

Methods	Merits/benefits	Demerits/limitations

Intrauterine contraceptive devices (IUCDs)	• Highly effective, reversible FP method
	• Can be used for spacing or limiting with pregnancy rates of <1%
	• Available free of cost at government health facilities
	• Independent of sexual activity
	• Does not interfere with sexual intercourse
	• Immediately reversible with no delay in return to fertility
	• Does not interfere with breastfeeding
	• No interactions with any medicines
	• Initial follow-up visit required after next periods or 6 weeks of postpartum insertion followed by visits at 3 and 6 months (to ensure retention as this is the period of maximum spontaneous expulsion) then the woman needs to return to the clinic only if she has a problem
	• Women do not need to purchase any supplies
	• Can act as emergency contraceptive method when inserted within 5 days of unprotected sex
		• Possibility of minor side effects which decrease after initial few months:
		  – Longer and heavier menstrual periods
		  – Bleeding or spotting between periods
		  – More cramps or pain during periods
		  – Does not protect against STIs and HIV
		  – Requires a trained healthcare provider to insert and remove the IUD
		  – May be expelled spontaneously, in a few cases

Oral contraceptive pills (OCPs)	• Effective (almost 100%) if used according to directions • Highly effective, reversible, easy to use • Effective within first 2 weeks • Safe for most women • Regulate the menstrual cycle • Reduce menstrual flow (which may be useful to anemic women) • Decrease the risk of ovarian and uterine cancer, benign breast disease, and incidence of acne • Do not interfere with sexual intercourse • Pelvic examination not required before use • Can be provided by trained non-medical staff • Immediate return of fertility on discontinuation	• Must be taken every day • Require regular/dependable supply • Pills may cause side effects in some women, such as nausea/headache/ bleeding between menses or mid-cycle bleeding/weight gain • Do not protect against STIs and HIV • Risk of developing cardiovascular disease in women >35 years of age and who smoke
DMPA (Depo Medroxy Progesterone Acetate) Dose: 150 mg IM every 3 months	• Available free of cost under NHM in the name of 'Antara' • Effective, reversible method • Preferably given within 1–5 days of menstruation but can be given any time after menstruation • Reduces menstrual cramps	• May cause amenorrhea/irregular bleeding • Delayed return of fertility: Fertility returns usually 7–10 months after last injection

2. **Enumerate fertility indicators. What do you mean by NRR = 1? Write in brief: advantages and disadvantages of contraceptive methods which an eligible couple should adopt in different phases of their reproductive life to achieve "small family norm".** (3 + 2 + 7)

Fertility Indicators

Birth Rate

$$\text{Birth rate} = \frac{\text{Number of live births during the year}}{\text{Estimated mid-year population in the same year}} \times 1000$$

General Fertility Rate (GFR)

$$\text{GFR} = \frac{\text{Number of live births during the year}}{\text{Mid-year female population of age 15–44 years in the same year}} \times 1000$$

General Marital Fertility Rate (GMFR)

$$\text{GMFR} = \frac{\text{Number of live births in a year}}{\text{Mid-year married female population in 15–49 years in the same year}} \times 1000$$

Age-specific Fertility Rate (ASFR)

$$\text{ASFR} = \frac{\text{Number of live births in a particular age group}}{\text{Mid-year female population of the same age group}} \times 1000$$

Age-specific Maternal Fertility Rate (ASMFR)

$$\text{ASMFR} = \frac{\text{Number of live births in a particular age group}}{\text{Mid-year married female population of the same age group}} \times 1000$$

Total Fertility Rate (TFR)

$$\text{TFR} = \sum_{15-19}^{45-49} ASFR \div 1000$$

Total Marital Fertility Rate (TMFR)

$$\text{TMFR} = 5 \times \sum_{15-19}^{45-49} ASMFR \div 1000$$

Gross Reproduction Rate (GRR)

$$\text{GRR} = 5 \times \sum_{15-19}^{45-49} ASFR \text{ for female live births} \div 1000$$

Net Reproduction Rate (NRR)

Net reproduction rate is defined as the number of daughters a newborn girl will bear during her lifetime assuming fixed age specific fertility and mortality rates.

❖ An NRR of one means that each generation of mothers is having exactly enough daughters to replace themselves in the population. Assuming an equal sex ratio, it is equivalent is equivalent to attaining approximately the 2 child norm.

❖ If the NRR is less than one, the reproductive performance of the population is below replacement level.

Couple Protection Rate (CPR)

Couple protection rate is defined as the percentage of eligible couple effectively protected against childbirths by one or the other approved methods of family planning (Sterilization/IUD/Condom/Oral pills).

Choice of Contraceptive Methods

Situation	Choice of contraceptive
Delaying the first child	◆ Condoms ◆ Oral contraceptive pills (OCPs) ◆ Intrauterine contraceptive devices (IUCDs)
Healthy spacing between 2 deliveries	◆ Condoms ◆ IUCD ◆ OCP ◆ DMPA
Limiting methods	◆ Female sterilization (tubectomy) ◆ Male sterilization (vasectomy)

Advantages and Disadvantages of Contraceptive Methods

Methods	Advantages	Disadvantages
Condom	◆ Easily available ◆ Safe and inexpensive ◆ Easy to use ◆ Light, compact and disposable ◆ Provides protection against STD	◆ It may slip off/tear during coitus due to incorrect use ◆ It interferes with sex sensation ◆ Many men do not use them regularly/carefully
Diaphragm	◆ Absence of risks ◆ Absence of medical contraindications	◆ Initially a physician/trained person is needed to demonstrate the technique of insertion of the diaphragm into the vagina ◆ Risk of *toxic shock syndrome* if left in the vagina for an extended period ◆ Use of it requires privacy for insertion and facilities for washing and storing it properly
Spermicides	If used along with diaphragm, it is a good contraceptive	◆ They have a high failure rate when used alone ◆ They must be introduced into those regions of vagina where sperms are likely to be deposited ◆ They must be used almost immediately before intercourse ◆ There are risks of burning and irritation

Contd...

Contd...

Methods	Advantages	Disadvantages
Intrauterine devices (IUDs)	• No hospitalization is required in insertion of IUDs and takes few minutes only • Once inserted, IUD stays in place as long as required • Inexpensive • Free from reversible side effects	There are certain side effects like: • Vaginal bleeding (should receive Ferrous sulfate tablets 200 mg 3 times daily) • Risk of iron deficiency anemia if bleeding is severe • Pain (low backache/lower abdominal cramp/pain down the thighs) • Risk of pelvic inflammatory disease (PID: Presenting symptoms are fever, vaginal discharge, pelvic pain and abdominal bleeding) • Risk of uterine perforation and ectopic pregnancy
Hormonal contraceptives	They give protection against at least 6 diseases: • Benign fibrocystic disease and fibroadenoma of breast • Ovarian cysts • PID • Iron deficiency anemia • Ectopic pregnancy • Ovarian cancer	• Cardiovascular risks (AMI/cerebral and venous thrombosis) • Increased risk of cervical cancer • Alteration in the quality of breast milk • Risk of hepatocellular adenoma • Breast tenderness • Weight gain • Aggravation of migraine • Breakthrough bleeding in between menstrual periods
Depot formulations (DMPA and NET-EN)	• Highly effective • Long lasting • Reversible contraceptive (Women continue being pregnant after 5.5 months of discontinuation)	Disruption of normal menstrual cycle (with symptom of unpredictable and excessive bleeding)
Safe period method	—	• If a woman's menstrual cycle is irregular, then it is difficult to predict the safe period • High failure rates • Compulsory abstinence of sexual intercourse for a period of 1 week • Requires a high degree of motivation, cooperation and education • Risk of ectopic pregnancy and embryonic abnormalities
Male sterilization/ Vasectomy	• If properly performed, vasectomies are almost 100% effective • It is a simple, faster and cost effective operation	• Operative complications: Pain/scrotal hematoma/local infection • Sperm granules (caused by accumulation of sperm, symptoms are pain and swelling) • Spontaneous recanalization • Autoimmune response against sperm
Female sterilization/ ligation	• Short operating time • Shorter stay in hospital • High success rate • Small scar after operation	—

3. **Enumerate types of family. Describe the stages of family cycle. Discuss the role of family in health and disease.** (2 + 4 + 6)

Types of Family

- ❖ According to structure of family:
  - – Nuclear family
  - – Joint family
  - – 3 generation family.
- ❖ According to pattern of marriage:
  - – Monogamous
  - – Polygamous
  - – Polyandrous.
- ❖ According to sanction of marriage:
  - – Exogenous family
  - – Endogenous family.
- ❖ According to dependency:
  - – Patriarchal family
  - – Matriarchal family.
- ❖ Abnormal family:
  - – Broken family
  - – Problem family.

(For more details, please read Chapter 12)

Short Description of the Classification of Families According to Structure

Nuclear Family
- ❖ It consists of the married couple and their children (till they are regarded as dependents).
- ❖ In the nuclear family, husband usually plays the dominant role in the household.
- ❖ The absence of any guardians (like grandparents/relatives) places a greater burden in terms of responsibility for child rearing.
- ❖ The husband-wife relationship tends to be more intimate in nuclear family than joint family.

Joint Family
- ❖ It consists of a number of married couples and their children who live together in the same household.
- ❖ All the men are related by blood and all the women are their wives/unmarried girls/widows.
- ❖ All the property is held in common. There is a common family purse where all the family income goes and from where all expenditures are met.
- ❖ The senior most male member is the dominant member. The wife of him shares his power when the women members of the family are concerned.
- ❖ The familial relations get priority over marital relations.

Three Generation Family
- ❖ Here, three generations related to each other (young couples with their children and parents) live together due to unavailability of a separate house.

Stages of Family Cycle

A typical family cycle generally has six stages:

	Stage of family cycle	Events	
Stage No.	Description	Beginning of stage	End of stage
1	Formation	Marriage	Birth of 1st child
2	Extension	Birth of 1st child	Birth of last child
3	Complete extension	Birth of last child	1st child leaves home
4	Contraction	1st child leaves home	Last child leaves home
5	Completed contraction	Last child leaves home	1st spouse dies
6	Dissolution	1st spouse dies	Death of survivor

It should be noted that such a typical model is applicable only to the areas with low mortality and that any exception to this model (like divorce/no child, etc.) has to be taken into account.

Role of Family in Health and Diseases

"The secret of national health lies in the homes of the people."   **—Florence Nightingale**

Family

Family is defined as a group of people living together who are related biologically/by marriage/ by adoption and sharing a common kitchen.

❖ *Biologically*: It shares a pool of genes.

❖ *Culturally*: It reflects the culture of the wider society of which it is a part.

❖ *Socially*: It shares a common physical and social environment.

No scientific practice towards an individual is complete without the knowledge of his/ her family. All of the characteristics of a family are important in initiating diseases as well as promoting health and nutrition of the members like:

❖ Composition and structure of a family,

❖ Cultural and socioeconomic aspects of a family,

❖ Environmental conditions, etc.

There are certain functions of family which are relevant to health and disease:

1. Child rearing.
2. Socialization.
3. Personality formation.
4. Care of dependent adults.
5. Stabilization of adult personality.
6. Familial susceptibility to disease.
7. Broken families.
8. Problem families.

Child Rearing

❖ One of the most important functions of a family is *physical care for their dependent young*, so that they survive in adulthood and continue the family.

❖ It is worthy to note that *patterns of child care* (like feeding/nutrition/personal hygiene/ clothing/discipline, etc.) are passed from one generation to another.

❖ When a community health worker tries to improve the health of the child, he meets several obstacles which arise from traditional ways supported by religions/social customs.

Socialization

❖ It refers to the *process whereby individuals develop qualities essential for functioning effectively in the society*
❖ Family teaches the young the following things to make them fit for membership in the wider society:
  – Value of society
  – Culture
  – Beliefs
  – Code of conduct.
❖ Organizations such as school and religious places also take an important role in the socialization process.

Personality Formation

❖ The word "Personality" implies *certain physical and mental traits, which are characteristic of a given individual and which, to some extent, determine the behavior or adjustment of the individual to his surroundings*
❖ The personality of an individual is largely determined by his early experience in the family; especially with his father, mother and siblings *who provide the earliest and most immediate component of the child's external environment*
❖ So here the family acts like a **"Placenta"** by excluding/modifying/giving influences; leading to the foundation of physical, mental and social health of the child.

Care of Dependent Adults

❖ The family is expected to provide the front line care to:
  – Women during pregnancy and child birth
  – Aged and handicapped
  – Sick and injured.
❖ Without the support of family, no amount of medical care can succeed because family does more nursing than the hospital. In India, joint family provides such support.

Stabilization of Adult Personalities

❖ The family acts like a *"Shock absorber"* to the stress and strains of life by meeting the emotional needs of both adults and children
❖ These stress and strains include:
  – Injury
  – Illness
  – Births and deaths
  – Tension
  – Emotional upsets
  – Anxiety
  – Economic insecurity, etc.
❖ Certain chronic diseases have been accepted as *"Stress diseases"*, because they have a prominent emotional component in their development.
  – Peptic ulcer
  – Hypertension

- Rheumatism
- Colitis, etc.

Broken Family

❖ A broken family is one where the *parents have separated/where death of one/both of the parents has occurred.*
❖ This separation may be of two types:
  1. *Paternal separation*: Separation of the child from its father.
  2. *Dual parental separation*: Separation of the child from both of the parents.
❖ *Mental deprivation is one of the most dangerous factors in the psychological development of the children who are victims of broken families and these children frequently get involved in crime/prostitution/vagrancy in near future.*

Problem Families

❖ Problem families are those which *lag behind the rest of the community, where the standards of life are far below the accepted minimum and where parents are unable to meet the physical and emotional needs of their children.*
❖ The underlying factors in problem families are:
  - Poverty
  - Backwardness
  - Illness
  - Mental and emotional instability
  - Character defects
  - Marital disharmony, etc.

Note: Children who belong to problem families are frequent victims of crime/prostitution/vagrancy. So the health services delivery system should focus on broken families and problem families for rehabilitating them in the community.

Try Yourself

1. Define population explosion. What are the demographic trends in India? What measures do you suggest for the control of population explosion?

PREVENTIVE MEDICINE IN OBSTETRIC, PEDIATRICS AND GERIATRICS

1. **How RCH (Reproductive and Child Health) program differs from CSSM (Child Survival and Safe Motherhood) program? Describe briefly the strategies of RCH program.**   (4 + 8)

Please see the difference between RCH and CSSM in Chapter 6 on page no, 339.

Strategies of RCH Program

The major strategies under the second phase of RCH are:
❖ Essential obstetric care:
  - Institutional delivery
  - Skilled attendance at delivery
  - The policy decisions
❖ Emergency obstetric care:
  - Operationalising first referral units (FRUs)

- Operationalising PHCs and CHCs for round the clock delivery services
- Setting up of blood storage centers (BSC) at FRUs
❖ Strengthening referral system.

Essential Obstetric Care

Institutional Delivery

❖ To promote institutional delivery in RCH Phase II it is envisaged that 50% of the PHCs and 100% of the CHCs would be made operational as 24-hour delivery centers, in a phased manner, by the year 2010
❖ These centers would be responsible for providing the following services round the clock:
- Basic emergency obstetric care
- Essential newborn care
- Basic newborn resuscitation service.

Skilled Attendance at Delivery

The WHO has emphasized that skilled attendance at every birth is essential to reduce the maternal mortality in any country. A guideline for normal delivery and management of obstetric complications at PHCs/CHC for MOs and for ANC and skilled attendance at birth for ANM (auxiliary nurse midwife)/LHVs (lady health visitors) have been formulated and disseminated to the states.

The Policy Decisions

ANMs/LHVs/SNs have now been permitted to use drugs in specific emergency situations to reduce maternal mortality. They have also been permitted to carry out certain emergency interventions when the life of the mother is at stake.

Emergency Obstetric Care (EmOC)

❖ Operationalization of FRUs and skilled attendance at birth are the two activities which go hand in hand. In view of this, simultaneous steps have been taken to ensure tackling obstetric emergencies
❖ It has been decided that all the FRUs will be made operational for providing emergency and essential obstetric care during the second phase of RCH. Some of the steps taken are:
- *Training of MBBS doctors in life-saving anesthetic skills for EmOC*
- *Establishing blood storage at FRUs*
- *Preparing guidelines for operationalization of the FRUs*
- *Training of MBBS doctors for management of obstetric cases including cesarean section, etc. with the help of professional organizations such as FOGSI* (Federation of Obstetric and Gynaecological Societies of India).

Training of MBBS Doctors in Life-saving Anesthetic Skills for EmOC

Provision of adequate and timely emergency obstetric care (EmOC) has been recognized globally as the most important intervention for saving lives of pregnant women who may develop complications during pregnancy or childbirth.

Operationalization of FRUs

❖ *The operationalization of FRUs at subdistrict/CHC level for providing EmOC to pregnant women is a crucial strategy of RCH-II*

❖ It has not been possible to operationalize these FRUs till now due to shortage of specialist manpower, i.e. gynecologist and anesthetist, particularly at district and subdistrict level
❖ In view of this, for effective and better management of emergency obstetric needs at the grassroot level, it was felt to institute a training programme of appropriate duration to train MBBS doctors in life-saving anesthetic skills for emergency obstetric care
❖ Accordingly, the experts in field formulated an *18 weeks program for training of MBBS doctors in anesthetic skills*
❖ It should be remembered that in no way, it is the replacement of the specialist anesthetists who are working after pursuing degree/diploma in the subject.

Setting up of Blood Storage Centers (BSCs) at FRUs

❖ Timely treatment for complications associated with pregnancy is sometimes hampered due to nonavailability of blood transfusion services at FRUs
❖ The Drugs and Cosmetics Act has been amended to facilitate establishment of blood storage centers at such FRUs
❖ Guidelines for these blood storage centers (BSCs) have been prepared and disseminated to the States.

Strengthening Referral System

❖ During RCH Phase-I, funds were given to the Panchayat for providing assistance to poor people in the case of obstetric emergencies
❖ Feedbacks from the states indicate that there was no active involvement of Panchayats in running the scheme
❖ Based on these experiences, some modes of referral linkage in RCH Phase II have been proposed:
 – Involve local self-help groups, NGOs and women groups
 – Outsourcing.

Try Yourself

1. What is MCH? Discuss briefly the MCH activities at primary health center level. How will you evaluate the same?
 Please read the Chapter 19, "Reproductive, Child and Adolescent Health".

2. Definition, causes, prevention and controlling measures to the following:
 – IMR
 – MMR
 – PMR
 – U5MR
 Please read the Chapter 11, "Statistical and Epidemiological Exercises", and Chapter 3, "Problem Type Questions".

3. What are the importance and objectives of school health program? Mention various aspects of school health services which are to be provided.
 Please read the Chapter 4, "Short Notes" on page no. 189.

4. Discuss the various functions and organizational aspects of ICDS scheme.
 Please read the Chapter 4, "Short Notes" on page no.68 of this chapter, also on page no. 197.

NUTRITION AND HEALTH

1. Large number of malnutrition (Protein-energy malnutrition-PEM) cases among under 5 have been identified in your block. What social factors are responsible for it? Name the nutritional programs currently available in India. Describe briefly any one of them.   (3 + 3 + 4)

Social Factors Responsible for High Prevalence of PEM in a Block

We can divide the time period in three categories to describe the social factors responsible for malnutrition:

1. Antenatal factors.
2. Intranatal factors.
3. Postnatal factors.

Antenatal Factors

Some foods are restricted in the time of pregnancy in some parts of India. Restriction of nutritious foods like eggs/fish/meat/milk/green leafy vegetables has a negative effect on the health of the mother and at the same time, on the developing fetus.

Intranatal Factors

In most of the underdeveloped rural areas of India, deliveries are conducted by completely untrained dais and birth attendants, who are not aware of the concept of aseptic delivery and about the life-threatening dangers of sepsis resulting from uncleanliness at the time of delivery. But the villagers have great faith in them, which prevents them from coming to the nearby health care facilities.

Postnatal Factors

In some parts of India, there is a widespread belief that colostrum is harmful for the baby, for which they restrict any type of contact between mother and child for the first 3 days after delivery, instead the baby is given water, sugar solution, etc., which has definitely a negative impact on the health of the baby.

❖ In almost all parts of the country there is a custom among Hindu communities of giving honey to the baby at a time within the exclusive breastfeeding period (first 6 months after birth). This practice of prelacteal feeding is proven danger to the health of the baby

❖ Other harmful practices that pushes the baby towards the danger of malnutrition are:
  - Branding of the skin of the baby
  - Administration of opium and purgative to the baby.

Nutritional Programs Currently Available in India

The various nutritional programs currently available and running in India and their respective controlling and funding ministry are as follows:

Program	Ministry	Current status
Vitamin A prophylaxis program		
Prophylaxis against nutritional anemia	Ministry of Health and Family Welfare	Running
Iodine deficiency disorder control program		
Special nutrition program	Ministry of Social Welfare	These two programmes are gradually being phased out because of universalization of ICDS
Balwadi nutrition program		
ICDS program		Running
Mid-day meal program	Ministry of Education	Running
Mid-day meal scheme	Ministry of Human Resource Development	Running

Overview of Nutritional Programs Currently Running in India

1. Integrated Child Development Scheme (ICDS)

ICDS is the country's most comprehensive and multidimensional program. It is a 100% centrally sponsored scheme of the Ministry of Women and Child Development.

Objectives

❖ Lay foundation for the proper psychological, physical and social development of the child
❖ Improve nutritional and health status of children below six years
❖ Reduce incidence of mortality, morbidity, malnutrition and school dropouts
❖ Achieve effective coordination of policy and implementation amongst various departments
❖ Enhance the capabilities of the mother to look after the normal health and nutritional needs of child through proper nutrition and health education.

Focal Point to Deliver all the Services under ICDS

Anganwadi center (1 for 1,000 population).

Beneficiaries and services provided

Beneficiaries	Services provided
Children <3 years	♦ Supplementary nutrition ♦ Growth monitoring ♦ Immunization ♦ Health checkup ♦ Referral services
Children 3–6 years	♦ Nonformal preschool education ♦ Supplementary nutrition ♦ Growth monitoring ♦ Immunization ♦ Health checkup ♦ Referral services
Expectant and nursing mothers	♦ Health checkup ♦ Tetanus toxoid immunization to pregnant women ♦ Supplementary nutrition ♦ Nutrition and health education
Other women of 15–45 years	♦ Nutrition and health education

Contd...

Contd...

Beneficiaries	Services provided
Adolescent girls of 11–18 years	• IFA supplementation and de-worming intervention • Nonformal education • Home-based skill training and vocational training • Supplementary nutrition

Integrated packages of services under ICDS scheme

Packages	Services
Nutrition	• Supplementary nutrition • Growth monitoring • Nutrition and health education
Health	• Health checkup • Immunization • Identification and treatment of common childhood illnesses • Referral services
Supportive services and convergence	• Safe drinking water • Environmental sanitation • Women's empowerment programs • Adult literacy
Early childhood care and preschool education	• Early care and stimulation of children under 3 years • Preschool education to children in the 3–6 years age group

Special Note: Supplementary Nutrition

Age	Nutrition provided
Normal children (6 months to 6 years)	500 KCal and 12–15 g protein
Severely malnourished children (6 months–6 years)	800 KCal and 20–25 g protein
Pregnant and lactating mothers	600 KCal and 18–20 g protein

2. National Programme for Prevention of Nutritional Blindness due to Vitamin A Deficiency

Objective

The specific objective of the program is to reduce the prevalence of diseases due to vitamin A deficiency.

Activities

❖ A massive dose of vitamin A is given every 6 months to children between 6 months and 5 years
❖ The recommended schedule for the mega-dose administration is:
  – *6–11 months*: 1 dose of vitamin A of 1,00,000 IU.
  – *1–5 years*: A total of 8 doses of vitamin A of 200,000 IU every 6 months.
❖ The long-term strategy emphasizes the improvement of dietary intake of vitamin A through regular consumption of vitamin A rich foods:
  – Green leafy vegetables
  – Yellow fruits
  – Dairy products and promotion of breastfeeding.

3. Intensified National Iron Plus Initiative (I-NIPI)

Intensified National Iron Plus Initiative (I-NIPI) of the Anemia Mukt Bharat campaign is a recently launched program by Ministry of Health and Family Welfare, Government of

India in April, 2018 under POSHAN (PM's Overarching scheme for holistic nourishment) abhiyaan.

Hemoglobin levels to diagnose anemia (g/dL):

Age groups	No anemia	Mild	Moderate	Severe
Children 6–59 months of age	≥11	10–10.9	7–9.9	<7
Children 5–11 years of age	≥11.5	11–11.4	8–10.9	<8
Children 12–14 years of age	≥12	11–11.9	8–10.9	<8
Nonpregnant women (15 years of age and above)	≥12	11–11.9	8–10.9	<8
Pregnant women	≥11	10–10.9	7–9.9	<7
Men	≥13	11–12.9	8–10.9	<8

Source: Hemoglobin concentration for the diagnosis of anemia and assessment of severity, WHO

Beneficiaries	Intervention/dose	Regime
Children of 6–59 months	1 mL of IFA syrup containing 20 mg of elemental iron and 100 µg of folic acid	Biweekly throughout the period 6–60 months of age and deworming for children 12 months and above
School children 5–9 years	Tablets of 45 mg elemental iron and 400 µg of folic acid	Weekly throughout the period 5–10 years of age and biannual deworming
Adolescents of 10–19 years	60 mg elemental iron and 500 µg of folic acid	Weekly throughout the period 10–19 years of age and biannual deworming
Pregnant and lactating women	60 mg elemental iron and 500 µg of folic acid	1 tablet daily, starting from 14th week of gestation, continued throughout pregnancy (minimum 180 days during pregnancy) and to be continued 180 days postpartum: a total of 1 year
Women in reproductive age group	60 mg elemental iron and 500 µg of folic acid	Weekly throughout the reproductive period

4. National Iodine Deficiency Disorder Control Programme

India commenced the National Goiter Control Programme in 1962, which was intensified into a greater national program called National IDD Control Programme.

Components
a. Use of iodized salt in place of common salt.
b. Monitoring and surveillance.
c. Manpower training.
d. Mass communication.

Use of iodized salt in place of common salt
❖ The daily requirement of iodine for adults is 150 µg
❖ According to this assumption, the Prevention of Food Adulteration Act in India has fixed the iodization level to at least 30 ppm at the production point and at least 15 ppm at the consumer level
❖ Iodization of common salt is the most effective way towards mass prophylaxis in an IDD prevalent zone

❖ Another effective way to control IDDs in the country is the use of intramuscular injection of iodized oil. Beside the advantage that it can be applied on a large scale basis, the cost is higher than that of iodized salt.

Monitoring and surveillance

The following indicators are most commonly used to monitor the efficacy of the control program:
❖ Prevalence of neonatal hypothyroidism: It is the most sensitive indicator
❖ Measurement of urinary iodine excretion
❖ Prevalence of goiter and cretinism in a community
❖ Measurement of iodine levels in food, water and salt.

Manpower training and mass communication

They are also important components of National IDD Control Programme, which include proper training of healthcare providers and peripheral health workers and at the same time, creating public awareness by collaboration with mass media to achieve effective IDD control at the fullest extent.

5. Mid-day Meal Scheme

Objectives

The objectives of the mid-day meal scheme are:
❖ Improving the nutritional status of children in classes I–VIII in government, local body and Government aided schools, and EGS and AIE centers
❖ Encouraging poor children, belonging to disadvantaged sections, to attend school more regularly and help them concentrate on classroom activities
❖ Providing nutritional support to children of primary stage in drought-affected areas during summer vacation.

Nutritional content: Calorific and nutrition value and food norm per child per day.

To achieve the above objectives a cooked mid-day meal with the following nutritional content is provided to all eligible children.

Items	Primary	Upper primary
Calorie	450	700
Protein	12 grams	20 grams
Rice/wheat	100 grams	150 grams
Dal	20 grams	30 grams
Vegetables	50 grams	75 grams
Oil and fat	5 grams	7.5 grams
Micronutrients and de-worming medicines	In convergence with school health program of NRHM	

Rationale of Mid-day Meal Scheme

❖ *Promoting school participation*: Mid-day meals have great effects on school participation, not just in terms of getting more children enrolled in the registers but also in terms of regular attendance on a daily basis

❖ *Preventing classroom hunger*: Many children reach school on an empty stomach. Even children who have a meal before they leave for school get hungry by the afternoon and are not able to concentrate—especially children from families who cannot give them a lunch box or are staying a long distance away from the school. Mid-day meal can help to overcome this problem by *preventing "classroom hunger"*

❖ *Facilitating the healthy growth of children*: Mid-day meal can also act as a regular source of "supplementary nutrition" for children, and facilitate their healthy growth

❖ *Intrinsic educational value*: A well-organized mid-day meal can be used as an opportunity to impart various good habits to children (such as washing one's hands before and after eating), and to educate them about the importance of clean water, good hygiene and other related matters

❖ *Fostering social equality*: Mid-day meal can help break the barriers of caste and class among the students

❖ *Enhancing gender equity*: The gender gap in school participation tends to narrow, as the Mid-day Meal Scheme helps erode the barriers that prevent girls from going to school. Mid-day Meal Scheme also provide a useful source of employment for women, and helps liberate working women from the burden of cooking at home during the day. In these and other ways, women and girl children have a special role in Mid-day Meal Scheme

❖ *Psychological benefits*: Physiological deprivation leads to low self-esteem, consequent insecurity, anxiety and stress. The Mid-day Meal Scheme can help address this and facilitate cognitive, emotional and social development.

2. **Enumerate different types of food intoxicants. Suggest measures to control epidemic dropsy in your area.** (4 + 8)

Different Types of Food Intoxicants

Original food	Toxicants	Disease caused
Seeds of Lathirus sativus	Beta oxalyl amino alanine (BOAA)	Neurolathyrism
Bajra/rye/sorghum/wheat	Ergot	Nausea, repeated vomiting, giddiness drowsiness, cramps, gangrene of limbs
Mustard oil	Argemone oil	Epidemic dropsy
Gondhi (a millet)	Seeds of Jhunjhunia	Endemic ascites

Measures to Control Epidemic Dropsy

Source Reduction

As crops of argemone grow wild with mustard in the time of March in India, accidental contamination of mustard seeds can be prevented by *removing argemone weeds growing among mustard crops.*

Tests for Detection of Argemone Oil in Mustard Oil

❖ *Nitric acid test*: Add nitric acid in a sample of oil and shake the tube; a color change from brown to orange red shows the presence of argemone oil

❖ *Paper chromatography test*: This is the most sensitive test.

Legal Restriction

Unscrupulous dealers can be dealt with by strict enforcement of Prevention of Food Adulteration Act, 1954, which states that, "A minimum imprisonment of 6 months with a minimum fine of ₹ 1000/- is envisaged under the act for cases of proven adulteration; whereas for the cases of adulteration which may render the food injurious to cause death/such harm which may account to grievous hurt, the punishment may go up to life imprisonment and a fine which shall not be less than ₹ 5000/-."

Educating the People

People should be educated about the danger signs of the disease and they should be told to immediately bring such cases to the nearby health facility if they find so:

❖ Sudden noninflammatory bilateral swelling of legs
❖ Diarrhea
❖ Dyspnea
❖ Cardiac failure
❖ Sudden worsening of vision (due to glaucoma).

3. **What is malnutrition? Discuss its prevention strategies in terms of different levels of prevention.**

(4 + 8)

Definition of Malnutrition (UNICEF, 2006)

❖ Malnutrition is a broad term used as an alternative to undernutrition but technically it also refers to overnutrition
❖ People are malnourished if their diet does not provide adequate calories and protein for growth and maintenance/they are unable to fully utilize the food they eat due to illness (undernutrition)
❖ People are also malnourished if they consume too much calories (overnutrition).

Preventive Strategies

Level of prevention	Components	Preventive measures
Primary prevention	Health promotion	• Supplemental nutrition to pregnant and lactating women • Promotion of breastfeeding • Development of low cost weaning foods • Improve family diet • Family planning • Nutrition education
	Specific protection	• Child's diet must contain protein and energy rich foods (milk/egg/fruits) • Immunization • Food fortification
Secondary prevention	Early diagnosis and treatment	• Early diagnosis of any lag in growth (maintenance of growth charts) • Early diagnosis and treatment of infections and diarrhea • Supplementary feeding programs during epidemics • Deworming
Tertiary prevention	Rehabilitation	• Nutritional rehabilitation services • Hospital treatment • Follow-up services

4. Describe the methods of assessment of nutritional status of a community.

$(6 + 6)$

(Remember: The terms "Nutritional survey" and "Nutritional surveillance" are not same.)

Nutritional survey	Nutritional surveillance
Method of assessment of nutritional status of a group of people/a community.	Method of assessment of nutritional status of a group of people/a community *as well as periodical monitoring* of the success of a nutritional program.

Objectives

To determine the extent of nutritional problems/diseases in a community and their contributing factors for prevention and control of nutritional diseases.

Methods

❖ Clinical examination
❖ Anthropometric examination
❖ Laboratory and biochemical examination
❖ Biophysical examination
❖ Functional examination
❖ Assessment of ecological factors
❖ Vital statistics
❖ Diet survey.

Clinical Examination

It involves head to toe examination for changes believed to be related to consumption of food.

Sites to be examined:
Superficial tissues like, hairs, eyes, skin, buccal mucosa, tongue, ears, nose, lips, teeth, gums, glands, nails, chest, abdomen and edema.

Categorization of signs according to WHO expert committee:

Not related to nutrition	Alopecia, pyorrhea, pterygium
Needs further investigations	Malar pigmentation, corneal vascularization, geographic tongue
Known to be of value	Angular stomatitis, Bitot's spots, calf tenderness, absence of knee or ankle jerks, enlargement of thyroid, etc.

Anthropometric Examination

Though genetically determined, profoundly determined by nutritional status.
a. **Weight:**
   – Weight for age helps in assessing nutritional status
   – Periodical assessment among children plotted in "Road to Health" card.
   – Describes severity of malnutrition.

Methods:

In children	In adult
Current weight (in kg) of child is compared with the expected standard weight and the deficiency in percentage is expressed in terms of degrees of malnutrition	Nutritional status measured in terms of BMI $BMI = Weight\ in\ kg/(Height\ in\ meter)^2$ Interpretation of BMI (WHO standards for Asian population):

Value	Interpretation
<18.5	Underweight
18.5–23	Normal weight
23–27.5	Overweight
≥27.5	Obese

b. **Height:**
   - Measurement of linear dimension
   - Measurement of skeletal elongation
   - Height for age: It indicates duration of malnutrition (perhaps best parameter of malnutrition).

c. **Circumference of chest to head ratio:**

Normal	In PEM
Chest to head circumference ratio <1 → at birth =1 → at 1 year of age >1 → after 1 year	Chest to head circumference ratio <1 in pre-school children

d. **Circumference of mid-arm:**
   Gives information about muscle mass (as muscle wasting is a cardinal feature of PEM) especially in early childhood.

Mid-arm circumference (in cm)	Interpretation
>12.5 (Green)	Well nourished
11.5–12.5 (Yellow)	Mild – moderately nourishment
<11.5 (Red)	Severe malnutrition

   - Tape used: Shakir's tape
   - Child between 1–4 years of age will have almost the constant measurement.

e. **Skin fold thickness:**
   - Gives information about subcutaneous reserve of calories
   - Instrument used: Herpenden's callipers
   - Site: Over triceps of left arm or infrascapular region
   - For preschool children cut-off point: 10 mm.

Laboratory and Biochemical Examination

a. **Laboratory tests**

Examples:
- Hemoglobin estimation and serum transferrin
- Stools → for intestinal parasites
- Urine → for albumin, sugar and urinary nitrogen.

b. **Biochemical tests**

Assessment of different direct and indirect indicators of vitamin levels of blood.

Biophysical indicators
- Cytological examination of buccal mucosa is done to study the cornified cells
- % of cornified cells increases with degree of malnutrition
- Normal level in children: 30–40%.

Functional indicators

For example, testing the functional integrity of coagulation cascade by measuring prothrombin time (which is extremely sensitive to the vitamin-K dependent clotting factors). So PT helps in determining deficient vitamin-K level indirectly.

Assessment of ecological factors

Influential ecological factors that may be responsible for malnutrition are as follows:
- Conditioning infections and infestations
- Cultural factors
- Socioeconomic factors
- Food production
- Food consumption
- Availability of health services.

Vital statistics

Malnutrition influences following indicators of vital statistics:
- Age-specific death rate among 1–4 years
- Cause specific (due to PEM) death rate among under-fives
- Proportional mortality rate among under-fives due to PEM.

Diet Survey/Assessment of Dietary Intake

(May come as an individual short note)
It is the study of food consumption pattern in a group of individuals.
Here the investigator makes home visits daily for 7 days, i.e. dietary cycle.

Methods of diet survey

Diet survey technique	Methodology	Advantages	Disadvantages
Weighing raw food	Investigator visits households and weighs all food which is going to be cooked and eaten as well	• Practicable, hence widely used • Fairly accurate if carried properly	• Weighs food that has to be discarded • Takes longer duration • Value obtain for whole family

Contd...

Contd...

Diet survey technique	Methodology	Advantages	Disadvantages
Weighing cooked food (Recipe method)	Investigator visits the household and weighs all cooked food which is going to be consumed	• Most accurate method	• Not easily acceptable • Difficult • Plate wastes are included
Questionnaire method	Person asked about previous 24–48 hours (recall method) or a literate person is asked to keep record of his diet for next 24–48 hours (record method)	• Useful for large population • Easy and less time consuming	• Less accurate (especially the recall method)
Food inventory/Log book method	• Here quantity of food present in the house at the beginning of the survey is weighted and recorded • An account of food items purchased during 1 week of study period should be kept by the head of the family • Food items remaining unused is also weighted and recorded	• Easy, simple • Acceptable	• Requires cooperation of the family • Value obtained for whole family
Food list method	Investigator will have question-naire containing a list of foods consumed by the family and the quantity of the food stated by the housewife are entered	• Easy and simple	• Have to rely on housewives
Analysis of cooked food	Involves actual analysis of composite sample of each cooked food item for presence of various nutrients	• Most reliable and accurate • Provides value for individual	• Time consuming • Expensive

Try Yourself

1. Enumerate the nutritional problems in public health. Describe in detail protein-energy malnutrition with respect to its symptoms and preventive measures.

MEDICINE AND SOCIAL SCIENCES

Try Yourself

1. Define family. Explain the types of families. Briefly explain functions of families. Discuss how social and cultural factors influencing health and disease.

Please see Chapter 2, "Long Essay Type Questions", and Chapter 12, "Family" on page no. 61.

ENVIRONMENT AND HEALTH

Try Yourself

1. What are the methods of disposal of refuse? Describe a method that you consider suitable for rural community.
2. Discuss the role of environmental sanitation in controlling communicable diseases with emphasis on safe water supply and disposal of wastage.
3. What are the measures for prevention and control of air pollution?

HOSPITAL WASTE MANAGEMENT

Try Yourself

1. What are the health hazards caused by healthcare waste? What are the different categories of biomedical waste in India? Describe the mode of treatment and disposal.

(*Please see Chapter 21, "Biomedical Waste Management"*).

OCCUPATIONAL HEALTH

1. **What is pneumoconiosis? Enumerate its different types with causative factors. Enumerate the benefits provided under ESI Act and describe any one of them which is relevant to pneumoconiosis.** (2 + 3 + 3 + 4)

Pneumoconiosis

It is a respiratory disease caused by prolonged exposure to dusts within the range of *0.5–3.0 µM* size, which can reduce one's working capacity due to pulmonary fibrosis.

The reason behind the fact that only dust particles in the range 0.5–3.0 µM can deposit in the lungs and cause pneumoconiosis is that particles <0.5 µM are not deposited in the lungs due to their property of "Brownian movement", where particles of >3.0 µM size are usually cleared instantly by combined action of cilia and mucus of respiratory tract.

Different types of pneumoconiosis and their causative factors

Type	Causative factor	Industry
Silicosis	Inhalation of dust containing free silica/silicon dioxide	• Mining industry • Pottery • Ceramic industry • Sand blasting • Construction work • Steel industry
Anthracosis	Inhalation of coal dust	• Coal miners
Byssinosis	Inhalation of cotton fiber dust	• Textile industry
Bagassosis	Inhalation of sugar cane dust	• Cane-sugar industry
Asbestosis	Inhalation of fine particles of asbestos	• Cement industry • Textile industry • Construction work
Farmer's lung	Inhalation of spores from moldy hay	• Farming

Benefits given Under the ESI Act Relevant to Pneumoconiosis

Benefit to Employees

1. Medical benefit.
2. Sickness benefit.
3. Maternity benefit.
4. Disablement benefit.

5. Dependant's benefit.
6. Funeral expenses.
7. Rehabilitation allowance.

Medical Benefit

Medical benefit consists of full medical care including:
- ❖ Hospitalization free of cost in case of sickness, employment injury and maternity
- ❖ Out-patient care and in-patient treatment
- ❖ Supply of drugs and dressings
- ❖ Specialist services
- ❖ Pathological and radiological investigations
- ❖ Domiciliary services
- ❖ Antenatal, intranatal and postnatal services
- ❖ Immunization and family planning services
- ❖ Emergency services
- ❖ Ambulance services
- ❖ Health education
- ❖ Other free services: Spectacles, hearing aids, artificial limbs, hernia belts, spinal braces, surgical boots, jackets, etc.

Medical care is provided in two ways:
1. *Direct pattern*: Through ESI hospitals and dispensaries.
2. *Indirect pattern*: Through a panel of insurance medical practitioners.

2. Define social security. Briefly discuss any one of the social security systems in our country.

$$(2 + 10)$$

Definition of Social Security

Social security is defined as, "security that society furnishes through appropriate organization, against certain risks to which its members are exposed".

The risks that social security covers in most countries are:
- ❖ Sickness
- ❖ Invalidity
- ❖ Maternity
- ❖ Old age
- ❖ Death.

Examples:
- ❖ Workmen's Compensation Act, 1923
- ❖ Employees State Insurance Act, 1948
- ❖ Central Maternity Benefit Act, 1961
- ❖ The Family Pension Scheme, 1971, etc.

Here we are discussing the Employees State Insurance Act, which provides for cash and medical benefits to industrial employees in cases of sickness, maternity and employment injury.

The Employees State Insurance Act (ESI Act), 1948

Introduction

The ESI scheme, introduced by an Act of Parliament in 1948, is a unique piece of social legislation in India. It has introduced for the first time in India the principle of contribution by the employer and employee. The Act provides for medical care in cash and kind, benefits in the contingency of sickness, maternity, employment injury, and pension for dependents on the death of worker because of employment injury.

Administration

The administration of the ESI scheme under the Act is entrusted to an autonomous body called the **ESI Corporation**.

Benefit to Employees

1. Medical benefit.
2. Sickness benefit.
3. Maternity benefit.
4. Disablement benefit.
5. Dependent's benefit.
6. Funeral expenses.
7. Rehabilitation allowance.

Medical Benefit

Full medical care is provided to an insured person and his family members from the day he enters insurable employment. There is no ceiling on expenditure on the treatment of an insured person or his family member. Medical care is also provided to retired and permanently disabled insured persons and their spouses on payment of a token annual premium of ₹ 120/-.

❖ System of treatment
❖ Scale of medical benefit
❖ Benefits to retired ips
❖ Administration of medical benefit in a state
❖ Domiciliary treatment
❖ Specialist consultation
❖ In-patient treatment
❖ Imaging services
❖ Artificial limbs and aids
❖ Special provisions
❖ Reimbursement.

Sickness Benefit

Sickness benefit in the form of cash compensation at the rate of 70% of wages is payable to insured workers during the periods of certified sickness for a *maximum of 91 days in a year. In order to qualify for sickness, benefit the insured worker is required to contribute for 78 days in a contribution period of 6 months.*

❖ **Extended sickness benefit:** Extendable up to 2 years in the case of 34 malignant and long-term diseases at an enhanced rate of 80% of wages.

❖ **Enhanced sickness benefit:** Enhanced sickness benefit equal to full wage is payable to insured persons undergoing sterilization for 7 days/14 days for male and female workers respectively.

Maternity Benefit

Maternity Benefit for confinement/pregnancy is payable for *26 weeks, which is extendable by further one month on medical advice at the rate of full wage subject to contribution for 70 days.*

Disablement Benefit

❖ **Temporary disablement benefit:** From day one of entering insurable employment and irrespective of having paid any contribution in case of employment injury. Temporary disablement benefit at the rate of 90% of wage is payable so long as disability continues.

❖ **Permanent disablement benefit:** The benefit is paid at the rate of 90% of wage in the form of monthly payment depending upon the extent of loss of earning capacity as certified by a Medical Board.

Dependant's Benefit

Dependants Benefit (DB) paid at the rate of 90% of wage in the form of monthly payment to the dependants of a deceased Insured person in cases where death occurs due to employment injury or occupational hazards.

Funeral Expenses

An amount of ₹15,000/- is payable to the dependents or to the person who performs last rites from day one of entering insurable employment.

Confinement Expenses

An insured woman or an insured person in respect of his wife in case confinement occurs at a place where necessary medical facilities under ESI Scheme are not available.

Vocational Rehabilitation

To permanently disabled insured person for undergoing VR training at VRS.

Physical Rehabilitation

In case of physical disablement due to employment injury.

Old age medical care: For insured person retiring on attaining the age of superannuation or under VRS/ERS and person having to leave service due to permanent disability insured person and spouse on payment of ₹ 120/- per annum.

3. **Define ergonomics. Discuss the importance of preplacement examination with suitable examples.**   (2 + 10)

Definition of Ergonomics

Ergon = Work.

Nomos = Laws.

Ergonomics = Fitting the job to the worker.

"Ergonomics is the scientific discipline concerned with the understanding of the interactions among humans and other elements of a system and the profession that applies theoretical principles, data and methods to design in order to optimize human well-being and overall system performance." **—International Ergonomics Association (2000)**

The objective of ergonomics is to achieve the best mutual adjustment of man and his work, for the improvement of human efficiency and well-being.

Importance of Preplacement Examination

❖ The purpose of preplacement examination is *to place the right man in the right job*, so that the worker can perform his duties efficiently, without any detrimental effect to his health

❖ These examinations must be planned in relation to morbidity, age, sex, occupational hazards and other factors

❖ A preplacement examination usually includes the following:
  - Personal history
  - Clinical examination
  - Psychological examination
  - Laboratory tests for blood and urine
  - Chest X-ray
  - ECG
  - Vision testing
  - Blood test for locally endemic diseases

❖ These examinations should not only disclose diseases at an early stage, but they should also decide the limit of the person's working capacity; resulting in placement of workers from a health point of view

❖ Proper placement prevents impairment of health of individual worker/accidents at the workplace.

Rating of Workers Ability

The industrial physician will examine the worker according to his capacity in the following fields:

P: Physical capacity—heavy physical work
F: Feet, lower extremities—standing
N: Nose and throat—dust exposure, risk of lesions in upper respiratory tract
R: Respiration, lung function—dust exposure, risks of pneumoconiosis
S: Skin—risks of occupational dermatoses
V: Vision
I: Intelligence.

The worker's capacity will be rated for each factor in the following way:

1. Excellent
2. Average
3. Moderate
4. Below minimum standards.

The result of an examination may be:

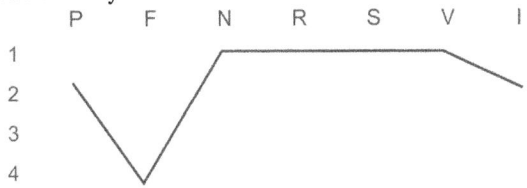

So, the preplacement examinations and periodic clinical examinations according to the demands of particular work and proper placement are the most important procedures in occupational health.

Example:

Occupational hazards	Undesired health problems
Lead	Anemia/hypertension/nephritis
Dye	Asthma/skin disease/bladder and kidney problems
Silica	Chronic lung disease, healed/active TB of lung
Radioactive substances and X-rays	Cancers of blood cells

Try Yourself

1. Classify occupational hazards. As a factory medical officer, what measures will you take to control such problems?
2. How does application of ergonomics help to improve human efficacy and wellbeing? What protection is available for young women under Factory Act?
3. What are the health hazards of coal mines? What are the measures would you take to reduce the hazards?

HEALTH INFORMATION AND BASIC BIOMEDICAL STATISTICS

Try yourself

1. Discuss briefly the advantages and disadvantages of various sources of health information system available in India, describe the three important indicators, which directly access ill health in a community.
   Please see Chapter 4, "Short Notes" on page no. 233.
2. What is sampling? Explain with suitable examples the different methods of sampling.
   Please see Chapter 4, "Short Notes" Sampling is on page no. 235.

COMMUNICATION FOR HEALTH EDUCATION

Try Yourself

1. Define health education. What are the content and principles of health education? Describe the various approaches and application of health education.
2. What is the concept of information, education and communication? Describe in brief the various methods to deliver it.

HEALTH PLANNING AND MANAGEMENT

Try Yourself

1. Define health planning. Describe the steps involved in a planning cycle.
   Please see Chapter 4, "Short Notes" on page no. 245.

HEALTH CARE OF THE COMMUNITY

1. Enumerate the principles of primary health care. How it is delivered in rural areas?   (4 + 8)

Principles of Primary Health Care

Introduction

Primary health care is essential health care made universally accessible to individuals and acceptable to them, through their full participation and at a cost the community and country can afford.

Principles of Primary Health Care

1. Equitable distribution.
2. Community participation.
3. Intersectoral coordination.
4. Appropriate technology.

Equitable distribution

❖ Equitable means something for all, but more for the needy. Example: Mothers and children are a vulnerable group; so priority is given to MCH services, to address the needs of this group.
❖ At present the health services are concentrated in major towns and cities, while urban slums and rural areas are highly deprived of these.
❖ Primary health care aims to eliminate this social injustice by shifting the gravity of health services from urban to rural areas and bring these services as close to the home as possible.

Community participation

❖ The universal coverage of health services cannot be achieved without the involvement of local community.
❖ So, there should be a continuous effect to involve communities in healthcare delivery system with maximum reliance on the local resources (money/material/manpower/knowledge).
❖ The community participation has been achieved in India by a revolutionary approach by recruiting ASHA workers, who are permanent residents, for each village.
❖ By overcoming the cultural and communication barriers, they provide primary health care in a way that is acceptable to the community.

Intersectoral coordination

❖ The components of primary health care cannot be provided by the health sector alone, but there should be coordination among all the health-related sectors like:
  – Agriculture
  – Animal husbandry
  – Food
  – Industry

- Education
- Housing, etc.

Examples are:

1. **National Iodine Deficiency Disorders Control Programme (NIDDCP):**
   Nodal ministry is Ministry of Health and Family Welfare, supported by:
   - Ministry of Industries which produces salt
   - Ministry of Railways, which gives subsidy for freight to transport the salt throughout the country
   - Ministry of Information and broadcasting which helps in generating a demand for iodized salt through health education and publicity.

2. **Integrated Child Development Services (ICDS):**
   Nodal ministry is Ministry of Women and Child Development, supported by:
   - Ministry of Health and Family Welfare
   - Sarva Shikshya Abhiyan of Ministry of Human Resource Development
   - Department of Food and Public Distribution
   - Ministry of Drinking water and Sanitation
   - Ministry of Rural Development.

❖ To achieve this coordination, the following measures can be taken:
   - Introduction of suitable legislation
   - Reviewing the administrative system
   - Reallocation of resources
   - A suitable planning to avoid unnecessary duplication of activities.

Appropriate technology

❖ It is defined as technology that is:
   - Scientifically sound
   - Adaptable to local needs
   - Acceptable to those who apply it and those for whom it is used
   - Can be maintained by the people themselves
   - The cost of the resources used in the technology should be within the limits the community and country can afford.

❖ The term "appropriate" is used because a technology that is appropriate and affordable for a large multi-facility hospital may be totally inappropriate for a rural settings, where the availability of resources are poor.

❖ An example of appropriate technology is **ORS** (Oral rehydration solution) because it is cheaper, scientifically valid, socially acceptable and it can be made by the people who wants to apply it if they have the correct knowledge.

Delivery of Primary Health Care in Rural Areas

Model

A simplest model of healthcare delivery system is as follows:

Inputs	Healthcare services	Healthcare system	Outputs
◆ Health status	◆ Curative	◆ Public	
◆ Health problems	◆ Preventive	◆ Private	Changes in health status
◆ Resources	◆ Promotive	◆ Voluntary	
		◆ Indigenous	

The following schemes are in operation to achieve equitable distribution and universal coverage of health services in the rural areas:

1. ASHA scheme
2. ICDS scheme
3. Training of local dais.

ASHA Scheme

❖ Under the ASHA (Accredited social health activist) scheme, there is an ASHA worker for a population of 1,000.
❖ The guidelines for selection of ASHA worker are:
   - ASHA must be a resident of the village, preferably a woman.
   - She should have a formal education of at least 8th standard.
   - She should be preferably in the age group of 25–45 years.
   - She should have communication skills and leadership qualities.

Note: The general norm of selection is one ASHA for 1,000 population.

Roles and responsibilities of an ASHA worker

Roles	Description
Awareness and information to the community/women of the community about:	• Importance of nutrition/basic sanitation/personal hygiene as determinants of health • Need for utilization of health and family welfare services • Importance of breastfeeding/immunization/complementary feeding/family planning/prevention of STDs
Referral services	ASHA will arrange escort/accompany pregnant women/child requiring referral to the nearest PHC/CHC/FRU
Primary health care for minor illnesses	• Diarrhea • Fever • First aid services
Depot holder and provider of:	• DOTS • ORS • IFA tablets • Chloroquine • Disposable delivery kits • Oral pills • Condoms
Facilitation of utilization of government health services	• Antenatal checkup • Postnatal checkup • Immunization • Supplementary nutrition
Development of a comprehensive village health plan	ASHA will develop it working with: • Village health guides • Anganwadi workers and sanitation committee of Gram Panchayat
Notification services	ASHA will notify nearby PHC/subcenter about: • Birth • Death • Disease outbreaks in the community • Any unusual health problem in the community

ICDS Scheme

❖ Under the ICDS (Integrated child development services) scheme, there is an anganwadi worker (AWW) for a population of 400–800
❖ The anganwadi worker is selected from the community, she undergoes training for 4 months about health/nutrition/child development.
❖ She is a part time worker and is paid a honorarium of ₹ 1,500/- per month for the services she gives to the community:
  – Maintenance of growth charts
  – Immunization
  – Supplementary nutrition
  – Health education
  – Nonformal preschool education
  – Referral services.
❖ The beneficiaries are:
  – Nursing mothers
  – Pregnant women
  – Women of reproductive age group (15–45 years)
  – Children <6 years of age.

2. **Enumerate the functions of primary health care. What are the services provided by a subcenter?**

   (6 + 6)

Functions of Primary Health Care

The Alma-Ata Declaration has outlined 8 essential components of primary health care:
1. Education concerning prevailing health problems and the methods of preventing and controlling them
2. Promotion of food supply and proper nutrition
3. An adequate supply of safe water and basic sanitation
4. Maternal and child health care, including family planning
5. Immunization against major infectious diseases
6. Prevention and control of locally endemic diseases
7. Appropriate treatment of common diseases and injuries
8. Provision of essential drugs.

Services Provided by a Subcenter

1. Maternal health care:
   Antenatal care:
   a. Early registration of pregnancy
   b. Minimum three antenatal check-ups
   c. Recording of general check-up, weight, blood pressure, abdominal examination, hemoglobin, routine urine examination and blood group
   d. Iron and folic acid supplementation
   e. Tetanus toxoid immunization
   f. Identification of high-risk pregnancy and referral.

Intranatal care:
a. Promotion of institutional deliveries
b. Skilled attendance at home deliveries
c. Prompt referral in case of complications.
Postnatal care:
a. Postpartum home visits
b. Initiation of breastfeeding within 1/2 hour of delivery
c. Counseling on diet, hygiene and contraception
d. Provision of facilities of Janani Suraksha Yojana.
2. Child health care:
a. Essential newborn care
b. Promotion of exclusive breastfeeding for 6 months
c. Full immunization of all infants and children against vaccine preventable diseases
d. Vitamin A prophylaxis
e. Prevention and control of childhood diseases.
3. Family planning and contraception:
a. IEC to adopt appropriate family planning method
b. Provision of contraceptives such as condoms, oral pills, emergency contraceptives and IUD insertion
c. Follow up services to the eligible couples adopting permanent methods of tubectomy and vasectomy.
4. Counseling and appropriate referral for safe abortion service (MTP)
5. Adolescent health care
6. Assistance to school health services
7. Water quality monitoring
8. Promotion of sanitation
9. Field visits by appropriate health workers for disease surveillance and family welfare services awareness
10. Community need assessment
11. Curative services for minor ailments
12. Running National Health programmes:
   – National AIDS Control Programme (NACP)
   – National Vector Borne Disease Control Programme (NVBDCP)
   – National Leprosy Eradication Programme (NLEP)
   – Integrated Disease Surveillance Projects (IDSP)
   – Revised National Tuberculosis Control Programme (RNTCP)
   – National Programme for Control of Blindness (NPCB)
   – National Programme for Prevention and Control of Cancer, Diabetes, Cardiovascular Diseases and Stroke (NPCDCS).

Try Yourself

1. Define "Health for all". Describe briefly the primary healthcare delivery in rural India.
2. Discuss briefly the three tier system of healthcare delivery in rural India.
3. Briefly describe the services given by the health functionaries at the village level.
4. List the elements of primary health care. Briefly explain the principles of PHC.

INTERNATIONAL HEALTH

1. **What are the roles of UNICEF in improving child survival in India? What are the functions of WHO?**

   (6 + 6)

Roles of UNICEF in Improving Child Survival in India

Historical Interest

In 1980s, UNICEF proposed 4 techniques to vanquish common infections of early childhood using simple medical technologies, which collectively were referred to as **'GOBI'**:

❖ **'G'** for *growth monitoring* to keep a regular check on child well-being

❖ **'O'** for *oral rehydration therapy* to treat bouts of childhood diarrhea

❖ **'B'** for *breastfeeding* as the perfect nutritional start in life; and

❖ **'I'** for *immunization* against the six vaccine-preventable childhood killers: tuberculosis, diphtheria, whooping cough, tetanus, polio and measles.

UNICEF's Present Cooperation with India

1. **Eliminate open defecation:**

   The Government of India has a target to make India "Open Defecation Free" by 2019 and UNICEF India is a key partner in its flagship programme to achieve this target through the *Swatchh Bharat Mission* (SBM).

2. **Neonatal health:**

   As the lead technical partner in the country for Newborn and Child Health, UNICEF has been involved from the beginning of the Integrated Management of Newborn and Childhood Illness (IMNCI) programme in India.

3. **Infant and young child feeding:**

   UNICEF supports ICDS and NRHM, India's flagship programmes whose goal is to improve nutrition, health and development outcomes in infants and young children.

4. **Immunization:**

   UNICEF was a major partner in drafting the government's Comprehensive Multiyear Plan for immunization 2013-17 (CMYP), which provides a framework to achieve the UIP.

Functions of WHO

The World Health Organization (WHO) is the body of the United Nations (UN) responsible for directing and coordinating health. The organization's 12th General Programme of Work details the **6 core functions** it is focusing on between 2014 and 2019. These functions are:

1. *Providing leadership* on matters critical to health and engaging in partnerships where joint action is needed.

2. Shaping the *research* agenda and stimulating the generation, translation and dissemination of valuable knowledge.

3. *Setting norms and standards* and promoting and monitoring their implementation.

4. Articulating ethical and *evidence-based policy* options.

5. Providing *technical support*, catalyzing change, and building sustainable institutional capacity.

6. Monitoring the health situation and assessing *health trends*.

Chapter

3

Problem Type Questions

Authors' Note

Problem type questions are asked in university examinations all over India as long questions. In WBUHS, it is also known as BMOH questions, as the problems in a community is solved by active leadership of a Block Medical Officer. In other states, it is known as problem type questions where a problem in a community is addressed by a healthcare provider and solved with active community participation and involvement from other health-related sectors. So, the format of answering these type of questions is same. This format should be memorized first while answering these questions as it carries separate marks. In this chapter, we have addressed some of the most common health-related problems in a typical Indian society and a roadmap of how to solve those problems.

DUTIES OF BMOH IN SOLVING A PROBLEM IN HIS BLOCK

Introduction
❖ Full form of BMOH: Block Medical Officer of Health
❖ Introduction: When presented with a problem, the main duty of a BMOH is to assess the problem and device-specific solution using administrative machinery under his jurisdiction through his:
  – Supervisory
  – Administrative
  – General functions.
❖ Thereby tackling the problem, keeping in view the resources and limitations of the system and needs of the area.

Functions of a BMOH
Supervisory Functions
❖ Investigation and assessment of the problem:
  a. Analysis of health situation (planning cycle)
    - Population, age and sex distribution
    - Statistics of mortality and morbidity
    - Epidemiological and geographical distribution of disease
    - Medical facility in the region
    - Training facility
    - Attitude and belief of people towards the problem.
  b. Establishment of objective and goals
  c. Assessment of resources
  d. Fixing priorities

e. Write up of formulated plans
f. Programming and implementation
g. Monitoring
h. Evaluation.
❖ Providing medical care
❖ Training
❖ Information, education and communication (IEC) activities
❖ Supervising and scrutinizing work of staff in implementation of plan.

Administrative Functions

❖ Management of personnel
❖ Financial power
❖ Stores and supplies of essential drugs
❖ Organizing tours
❖ Conducting monthly meeting.

General Functions

❖ Medical care
❖ MCH services and family planning
❖ School health services
❖ Attend OPD
❖ Attend wards
❖ Attend emergency duties
❖ Attend medicolegal issues
❖ Maintenance of vital statistics information.

Intersectoral Coordination

Through involvement of:
❖ Local people
❖ Influential people of the body
❖ Coordination with NGOs and voluntary organization working for the same cause
❖ Involving various mass media.

Writing Reports

FUNCTIONS OF A BMOH DURING INVESTIGATION OF AN EPIDEMIC

1. Verification of diagnosis
2. Confirmation of existence of epidemic
3. Defining population at risk:
   a. Obtaining map of the area
   b. Population of the area.
4. Rapid search of all cases and their characteristics:
   a. Medical survey
   b. Epidemiological case sheet
   c. Searching for more cases.
5. Data analysis
6. Formulation of hypothesis
7. Testing of hypothesis

8. Evolution of ecological factors
9. Further investigation of population at risk
10. Writing report.

FORMAT FOR WRITING DUTIES OF A BMOH DURING A GENERAL OUTBREAK

Situation Analysis

Data Collection

❖ Primary data: By door to door survey
❖ Secondary data: Voluntary agencies, panchayat functionaries.

Data Analysis

On the basis of:
❖ Mortality, morbidity
❖ Healthcare facility available
❖ Community participation.

Assessment of Determinants

❖ Water
❖ Food
❖ Entomological
❖ Ecological.

Verification of Diagnosis

Done by-BMOH or any qualified person must visit the area for:
❖ Clinical diagnosis
❖ Laboratory diagnosis.

Confirmation of Existence of an Epidemic

[Epidemic occurs when there is an excess of occurrence of disease above expected disease frequency (Epidemic frequency ≥ Endemic frequency + 2 Standard errors)]
    Following protocol should be followed: Is it an Epidemic? If yes → What is its Type? → Comparison and interpretation of such epidemic.

Estimation of Magnitude of Problem

❖ Rapid search for all cases with unnoticed cases:
    – Medical survey
    – Epidemiological case sheet
    – Searching for more cases.
❖ Medical survey for the population
❖ Defining population at risk/demographic distribution
❖ Obtaining map of that area/geographic distribution
❖ Availability of health facility of the community
❖ Frequency of reporting.

Resource Analysis

Identification of available resources and whether additional resources are available/needed:

Manpower

A. Based on available internal resources:
  - *Supervisory functions*: Supportive supervision regarding all work done by subordinates (such as BPHN, MO, etc.)

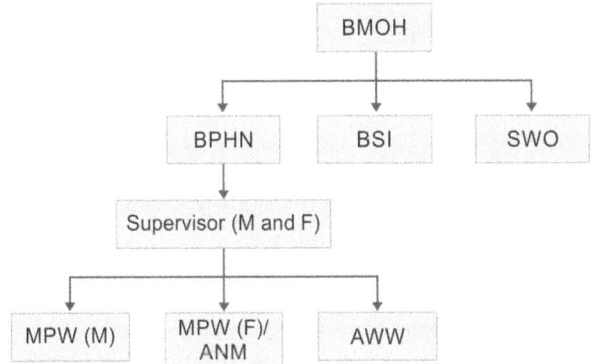

(BMOH: Block medical officer of health; BPHN: Block primary health nurse; BSI: Block sanitary inspector; SWO: Social welfare officer; MPW: Multipurpose worker; M: Male; F: Female; ANM: Auxiliary nurse midwife; AWW: Anganwadi worker)

  - *Administrative functions*: Includes taking decision of number of workers to be appointed, their work division, etc.

B. Additional resources that can be utilized (if required):

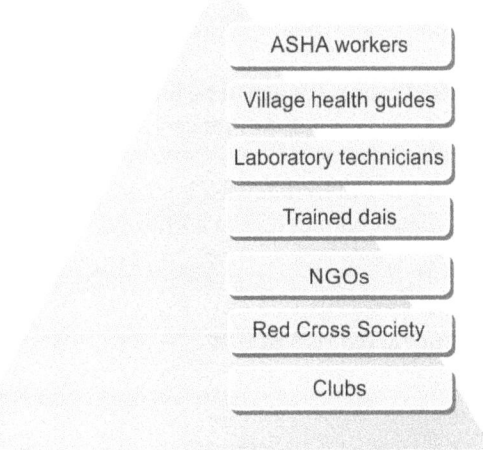

Additional manpower resources
(NGOs: Nongovernmental organizations)

Materials
❖ Equipment
❖ Drugs
❖ Laboratory transports
❖ Other supplies.

Money
An action plan is given to the CMOH for sanctioning a fund.

Writing up the formulated plan
❖ Detailed information about the plan
❖ Detailed information about the resources (needed and available)
❖ Interventions to be taken.

Fixing the Priorities

On the basis of:
❖ Health needs and demands of the community
❖ Financial constrains to mortality and morbidity data.

Establishment of Goal, Target and Objective

❖ Goal: Elimination of _____ from the area (fill in the blanks according to the question)
❖ Target:
 – To provide adequate treatment of affected cases
 – To reduce mortality and morbidity
 – Inhibition of transformation of cases to its complicated form.
❖ Objective: To reduce magnitude of the problem in given population and stated time.

Formulation of Plan

❖ Detailed information of:
 – Resources required
 – Results expected
 – Time and cost required for each stage to be implemented.
❖ Discuss limitation of cost, time, manpower at each step
❖ Intervention to be taken
❖ Allotment of responsibility to different levels (1st/2nd/3rd tier)
❖ Submission of the formulated plan to higher authority.

Mobilization of Resource

Programming and Implementation of Control Measures

Short-term measure:
❖ Control of reservoir:
 – Active surveillance: Usually done by MPW
 – Passive surveillance: Done when the patient comes for treatment in clinics

 – Treatment proper: (according to specific disease in question).

Long-term measure:

- ❖ Control of vector (for vector-borne diseases)
- ❖ Control of transmission
- ❖ Establishment of _____ clinic (fill in the blanks according to the question)
- ❖ IEC activities:
  - – Aim of health education through IEC activities
  - – Activities:
    - - Directly through meeting with patients and community to increase awareness
    - - By slide shows, pamphlets, leaflets, posters, and videos
    - - IEC activities showing danger signs for immediate hospital admission and sign of complications.
- ❖ Engineering measures
- ❖ Completing treatment to prevent relapse
- ❖ Training and supervision of _____ (fill in the blanks according to the question)
- ❖ Socioeconomic improvement
- ❖ Improvement of literacy status.

Monitoring

To detect:
- ❖ If all cases are being adequately identified and treated or not
- ❖ If the program is being implemented in right direction or not.

Evaluation

For assessment of:
- ❖ Achievements in terms mortality and morbidity rates
- ❖ Adequacy, efficacy, success and its acceptance by all parts of the community involved.

Reporting

By BMOH to the higher authorities for proper further actions to be taken.

Just change the following points for writing function of a BMOH during outbreak of a specific disease:

Assessment of Determinants

- ❖ Water
- ❖ Food
- ❖ Entomological
- ❖ Ecological.

Verification of Diagnosis

- ❖ Clinical diagnosis: Write down diagnostic clinical features
- ❖ Laboratory diagnosis: Write down screening tests and confirmatory tests.

Resources

Material: Drugs, insecticides (if required), IEC activities.

Programming and Implementation of Control Measures

Short-term measure:

❖ Control of reservoir:
  – Active surveillance: Usually done by MPW
  – Passive surveillance: Done when the patient comes for treatment in clinics
  – Treatment proper.

Long-term measure:

❖ Control of vector (for vector borne diseases)
❖ Control of transmission
❖ Establishment of _____ clinic (fill in the blanks according to the question)
❖ IEC activities:
  – Aim of health education through IEC activities.
❖ Completing treatment to prevent relapse
❖ Training and supervision of _____ (fill in the blanks according to the question)
❖ Socioeconomic improvement
❖ Improvement of literacy status.

DUTIES OF A BMOH DURING SOME IMPORTANT DISEASE OUTBREAKS

❖ Malaria
❖ Dengue
❖ Kala-azar
❖ Sexually transmitted diseases (STDs)
❖ Acquired immunodeficiency syndrome (AIDS).

Malaria

Assessment of Determinants

a. Host factors:
  – Age incidence
  – Sex incidence
  – Pregnancy
  – Occupation
b. Environmental factors:
  – Season
  – Rainfall
  – Prevalence of breeding places
  – Housing standard
c. Agent factors:
  – Specific agent causing malaria
  – Reservoir of infection

Verification of Diagnosis

❖ Clinical diagnosis:
  – By various clinical presentation carried out by different malaria parasites.

❖ Laboratory diagnosis:
  – Blood smears
  – Malaria testing kits.

Resources

Material:
❖ Insecticide
❖ Mosquito nets
❖ Medicine.

Programming and Implementation of Control Measures

Short-term measure:
❖ Control of reservoir:
  – Active surveillance: Usually done by MPW
  – Passive surveillance: Done when the patient comes for treatment in clinics
  – Treatment proper:
See guideline of NVBDCP 2022, Chapter 20.

Long-term measure:
❖ Control of vector:

Antiadult measures	◆ Use: – Residual spraying, DDT, malathion, parathion – Area where API>2, residual spraying of 2 rounds DDT – Where DDT and malathion both are resistant use *Pyrethroids* ◆ Space application of mist/fog ◆ Individual protection: Repellant, mosquito nets, coils, creams
Antilarval measures	◆ Larvicide: Paris green, temphos ◆ Source reduction/genetic control by *Bacillus thuringiensis* ◆ Larvivorus fish like gambusia

❖ Control of transmission: By chemoprophylaxis, *See Chapter 20.*
❖ Establishment of malaria clinics
❖ IEC activities: Regarding cause, danger signs and complication of malaria
❖ Engineering measures: To be taken by improving drainage system
❖ Completing treatment to prevent relapse/recrudescence
❖ Training and supervision of:
  – MPW (male) and HW (male)
  – Laboratory technician
  – Voluntary workers.
❖ Socioeconomic improvement
❖ Improvement of literacy status.

Dengue

Assessment of Determinants

a. Host factors:
  – Age incidence
  – Sex incidence

- Pregnancy
- Occupation
- Host susceptibility.
b. Environmental factors:
  - Season: Rainy
  - Rainfall: Increases mosquito breeding in flower vase, left out earthen pot, etc.
  - Flood, overcrowding, mosquito breeding places
  - Humidity: 80–85% optimum
  - Prevalence of breeding places
  - Housing standard.
c. Agent factors:
  - Causative agent: Dengue virus—1/2/3/4
  - Possible mode of transmission: By bite of *A. aegypti* mosquito
  - Breeding and feeding habits
  - Reservoir of infection
  - Species of vector involved *A. aegypti, A. albopictus*
  - Density
  - Flight range
  - Resistance to insecticides.

Verification of Diagnosis

❖ Clinical diagnosis:
  - Acute onset of fever (39–40°C) with chills and rigor
  - Headache
  - Muscle and joint pain
  - *Retro-orbital pain*, especially on eye movement, pressure on eye, photophobia.
❖ Other symptoms and signs:
  - Anorexia
  - Abdominal tenderness
  - Dragging pain in inguinal region
  - Abdominal colic and sore throat.
❖ Presentation:
  - 80% cases: Fever undergoes remission for hours to 2 days, which is followed by recurrence.
    - Order of appearance of rash: Chest >Trunk >Extremities.
  - 20% cases: DHF occurs which presents with:
    - Petechiae, purpura, ecchymosis, epistaxis, gum bleeding, hematemesis ± melena, hepatomegaly.
❖ Diagnosis confirmed by:
  - Positive tourniquet test >20 petechiae/sq inch
  - Platelet count ≤1,00,000/cu mm
  - Hematocrit value increases by ≥20% above baseline values
  - Serologically becomes +ve.

Resources

Material: Insecticide, mosquito nets, proper treatment measures.

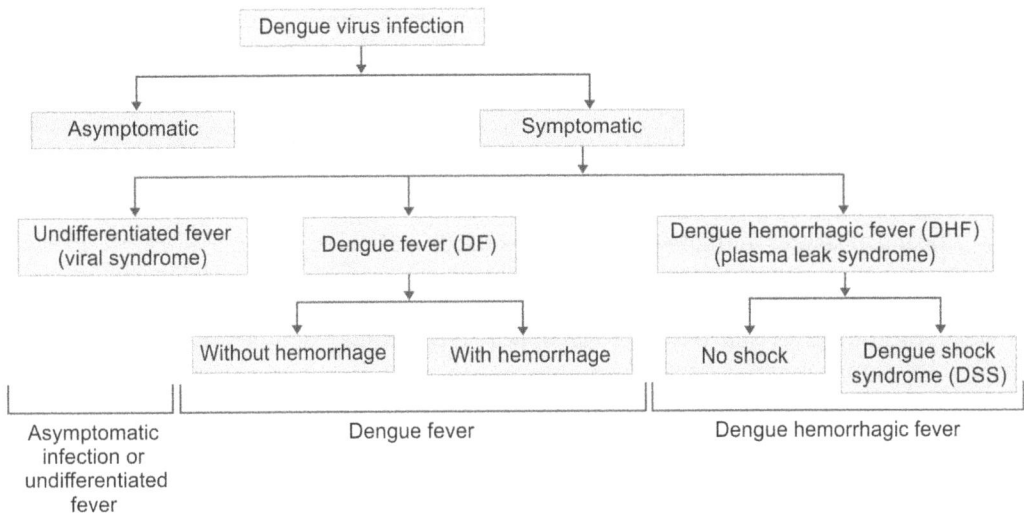

Clinical presentation of dengue

Source: Dengue hemorrhagic fever: Diagnosis, treatment, prevention and control, 2nd edition WHO, Geneva; 1997.

Programming and Implementation of Control Measures

Short-term measure

❖ Control of reservoir:
  – Active surveillance: Usually done by MPWs—
    - Ask family members for clinical symptoms and signs by door-to-door visit
    - Collect blood sample and send to laboratories
    - Perform on spot tourniquet test.
❖ Passive surveillance: Done when the patient comes for treatment in clinic
❖ Treatment proper: As it is a viral disease, there is no specific treatment.

Only symptomatic management

Symptoms	Management
Pyrexia	Paracetamol
Features of dehydration	Oral fluid and electrolyte therapy
Shock	Specific management

Long-term measure

❖ Control of vector:

Antiadult measures	♦ Use:
	  – Residual spraying, DDT, malathion
	  – Space application of mist/fog
	♦ Individual protection: Repellant, mosquito nets, coils, creams

Antilarval measures	♦ Larvicide: Paris green, temphos ♦ Source reduction/genetic control by *Bacillus thuringiensis* ♦ Larvivorus fish like gambusia

❖ Control of transmission: By personal protective measures: repellants, mosquito nets, coils, creams
❖ Establishment of dengue clinic
❖ IEC activities: With emphasis on:
  – Personal protective measures
  – Intake of PCM during fever
  – Strict avoidance of aspirin like drugs
  – Taking measures for removing artificial collection of water.
❖ Engineering measures: For proper drainage of water
❖ Completing treatment to prevent relapse
❖ Training and supervision of—MPW, laboratory technicians, voluntary workers
❖ Socioeconomic improvement
❖ Improvement of literacy status.

Kala-azar

Assessment of Determinants

Agent factors:
❖ Agent: *Leishmania donovani*
❖ Reservoir of infection: Human.

Host factors:
❖ Age: In India, the peak age of kala-azar is 5–9 years
❖ Sex: Male-female prevalence ratio = 2:1
❖ Socioeconomic status: Kala-azar usually attacks the people with very low socioeconomic status
❖ Occupation: The following occupations are especially vulnerable to be bitten by sandfly and having kala-azar:
  a. Farming
  b. Forestry
  c. Mining industry
  d. Fishing.
❖ Population movement: When large numbers of people move from endemic to nonendemic areas, there are greater chances of having the infection spread. So, the following groups are more vulnerable:
  a. Tourists
  b. Laborers
  c. Migrants.
❖ Immunity: One attack gives long-lasting immunity.

Environmental factors:
❖ Vectors: In India, *Phlebotomus argentipes* is the vector of kala-azar
❖ Season: In India, a high prevalence of kala-azar is seen during and after rainy season
❖ Altitude: Kala-azar is most commonly confined to the plains. It is not usually seen at a height >600 meters.

Mode of transmission:
❖ In India, kala-azar is transmitted from person to person by the bites of female *Phlebotomus* (*P. argentipes*) sandfly
❖ Extrinsic incubation period (time required for the development of parasite within sandfly): 6–9 days
❖ Incubation period within human: 1–4 months

❖ Factors facilitating the transmission:
  – Overcrowding
  – Ill ventilation
  – Accumulation of organic waste materials around houses.

Verification of Diagnosis

❖ Clinical diagnosis:
  – Fever
  – Weight loss
  – Mucosal ulcers
  – Fatigue
  – Anemia
  – Substantial swelling of the liver and spleen (in visceral leishmaniasis).
❖ Laboratory diagnosis by:
  – Blood smear
  – Bone marrow aspiration
  – Serology.

Resources

Material: Mosquito nets, proper drugs, etc.

Programming and Implementation of Control Measures

Short time control measures (Operational Guidelines on Kala-Azar Elimination in India, 2015)

As human is the sole reservoir of kala-azar in India, active and passive case detection and effective treatment is the mainstay of controlling kala-azar in a short time basis.

Special notes:

For treatment, single dose single day treatment with liposomal amphotericin B injection is the first drug of choice followed by capsule miltefosine (28 days) and injection amphotericin B (15 injections on alternate days) as well as combination of miltefosine and paramomycin injection.

Liposomal Amphotericin B

It is the first drug of choice. The single infusion treatment with liposomal amphotericin B requires a total quantity of 10 mg/kg for all ages including pregnant, pediatric and elderly patients.

Miltefosine

Miltefosine is a relatively safe oral drug for the treatment of kala-azar.

Mode of treatment:

The treatment is provided as directly observed treatment (DOT).

Dosing schedule:

Age	Weight	Dosing (given for 28 days)
Children (2–11 years)	—	2.5 mg/kg OD PC
Adult	<25 kg	50 mg OD PC
	>25 kg	50 mg BD PC

Amphotericin B

Amphotericin B deoxycholate injection intravenously at a dose of 1 mg/kg on alternate days × 15 doses.

Long-term Control Measures

Sandfly Control

❖ The mainstay of sandfly control remains the use of insecticides
❖ The insecticide of choice is **DDT** because the vector of kala-azar, *P. argentipes* is susceptible to DDT. The optimum dose is 1–2 g/sq mt sprayed in 2 rounds
❖ It should be sprayed inside and around the houses, animal shades and all other possible resting places of sandfly up to a height of 2 meters from the floor level
❖ In case of any suspected resistance, benzene hexachloride (BHC) should be used as the insecticide of second choice.

Sanitation Measures

It should be kept in mind that insecticide spraying becomes optimally effective when it is conjugated with sanitation measures, which includes:

a. Repairing and blocking all cracks and crevices in the wall of the houses (which may be a potential breeding place for sandfly)
b. Removal of firewood and rubbish around houses
c. Clearance of rodent burrows
d. Maintenance of a good hygiene at cattle sheds and poultry.

Personal Prophylaxis

Last but not the least, personal prophylaxis adds more potential to the prevention of kala-azar. The following measures can be taken:

a. Avoid sleeping on the floor
b. Use of fine mesh mosquito nets
c. Use of repellents like lotion/cream, etc.

Sexually Transmitted Infections/Diseases (STI/STD)

Assessment of Determinants

Host factors

❖ Age: 20–30 years
❖ Sex: M>F
❖ Marital status: Single, divorced
❖ Low socioeconomic condition.

Social factors

❖ Prostitution
❖ Broken families
❖ Sexual disharmony
❖ Alcoholism
❖ Emotional immaturity
❖ Social stigma.

Other factors

❖ Unplanned urbanization and industrialization
❖ ↑ No. of bridge population.

Verification of Diagnosis

❖ Clinical diagnosis:
  – According to organism involved
  – Some are asymptomatic (important for screening).
❖ Laboratory diagnosis:
  – Blood tests (for HIV, later stages of syphilis)
  – Urine tests
  – Culture of discharge/other fluids.

Resources

Material: Contraceptives (barrier method)
Example: Condoms, diaphragm, spermicidal jelly.

Programming and Implementation of Control Measures

Short-term measure:
❖ Control of reservoir:
  – *Active surveillance*:
    Usually done by MPW for screening purpose.

Persons to be screened	Screening for which disease
Every one	• In high-risk areas • For high-risk group, e.g. pregnant woman, blood donors, industrial worker, prostitutes
Pregnant women	• For HIV, hepatitis B, chlamydia and syphilis generally takes place at the first prenatal visit for all pregnant women • Gonorrhea and hepatitis C screening tests are recommended at least once during pregnancy for women at high risk of these infections
Women age >21 years	Pap smear for detecting HPV infections
Women age <25 years	Chlamydia, gonorrhea
Males	Homosexuals, male prostitutes should be screened on regular basis
People with HIV	• Increased chance of STD/STIs • Should be screened for: Syphilis, gonorrhea, chlamydia and herpes tests for people with HIV

  – *Passive surveillance*: Done when the patient comes for treatment in clinics.
  – *Treatment proper*:
    - Adequate and complete treatment of patients and their contacts
    - Counseling of the patient
    - Never isolate the patient.
    Syndromic management for:
    - Vaginal discharge
    - Genital ulcers
    - Urethral discharge
    - Scrotal swelling
    - Inguinal swelling
    - Lower abdominal pain in woman.

- *Epidemiological approach*
- *Provision of personal prophylaxis kits*: Such as condom, diaphragm
- *Vaccination*: Against HPV, Hep-B in high-risk areas
- Exposed part should be washed with soap and water as early as possible.

Long-term measure:
❖ Training of health workers for:
- Proper diagnosis of cases and prompt reporting
- Influence and educate people about prevention and control of diseases.
❖ IEC activities:
By—plays, pamphlets, banners, television advertisement, etc.
Addressing:
- De-addiction
- Condom promotion
- Social marketing
- Counseling
- Partner management.
By—involvement of society local people, mass media, etc.
Addressing:
- Coordinate with NGOs and voluntary organization
- Discourage use of used razors, syringes, etc.
- Education regarding safe sexual partners and promoting use of barrier methods like condom
- Promoting monogamous relationship
- HIV + women should be discouraged to become pregnant.
❖ Completing treatment to prevent relapse
❖ Socioeconomic improvement
❖ Improvement of literacy status.

Acquired Immunodeficiency Syndrome (AIDS)

Assessment of Determinants

Almost same as STDs/STIs. *See Chapter 24: Current Public Health-related Statistics and Recent Updates*

Verification of Diagnosis

❖ Clinical diagnosis:
WHO case definition for AIDS surveillance:
For age ≥12 years
At least 2 major + 1 minor criteria should be fulfilled:

Major criteria	Minor criteria
◆ Weight loss ≥10% of BW	◆ Cough >1 month
◆ Chronic diarrhea for >1 month	◆ Generalized pruritic dermatitis
◆ Fever for >1 month	◆ History of herpes zoster
	◆ Oropharyngeal candidiasis
	◆ Chronic progressive/disseminated HSV infection
	◆ Generalized lymphadenopathy

❖ Laboratory diagnosis: By using appropriate screening tests (Detection of anti-HIV antibody usually by EIA) and confirmatory tests (usually by ELISA/Western Blot).

Resources
❖ Material
❖ Funding
❖ Manpower.

Programming and Implementation of Control Measures

Short-term measure

Control of reservoir:
❖ Active surveillance: Usually done by MPW
❖ Passive surveillance: Done when the patient comes for treatment in clinic
❖ Treatment proper: Proper regimen of antiretroviral drugs. *See Chapter 24: Current Public Health-related Statistics and Recent Updates.*

Long-term measure
❖ *Control of vector* (for vector-borne diseases)
❖ *Control of transmission*
❖ Establishment of _____ clinic (fill in the blanks according questions)
❖ IEC activities:
   Aim of health education through IEC activities
❖ Engineering measures
❖ Completing treatment to prevent relapse
❖ Training and supervision of _____ (fill in the blanks according question)
❖ Socioeconomic improvement
❖ Improvement of literacy status.

DUTIES OF BMOH IN SOLVING DIFFERENT PEDIATRIC, GERIATRIC AND OBSTETRIC PROBLEMS

Duties of BMOH Regarding High IMR

1. Infant mortality rate (IMR) is rising in your block area. As BMOH, suggest measures to improve this situation. (12)

Situation Analysis

1. Data collection from:
   - Birth and death records
   - Immunization cards
   - ANC register
   - Maternal and child health (MCH) card
   - Subcenter record
   - House-to-house survey.
2. Analysis of data on the basis of:
   - Geographical distribution of IMR
   - Socioeconomic status of the case
   - Age of mother
   - Services provided to the community.

Problem Identification

Causes of neonatal death (0–4 weeks)	Causes of post-neonatal (1–12 months) death	Other causes that affects IMR
• Low birth weight (LBW) • Birth injury • Congenital anomalies • Hemolytic disease of newborn • Acute respiratory infection (ARI) • Diarrhea • Tetanus • Condition of placenta and cord	• Malnutrition • Congenital anomalies • ARI • Diarrhea • Other communicable diseases	**Biological:** • Early marriage (<18 years) • Age of mother (both increased and decreased age) • Birth spacing • Birth order • Multiple birth **Socioeconomic factors:** • Economic condition • Sociocultural condition • Maternal education • Environment and sanitation

Define the Objectives

Situation	Objective
Deaths are more in neonatal period	• Better ANC coverage regarding IFA tablets and TT2 • Better INC coverage during childbirth [Promotion of institutional deliveries and 7Cs *(clean hands+ fingernails + surface + blade + tie + birth canal + no application on cord stump)* to be followed in home deliveries/conducted by trained personnel] • Proper treatment of ARI and diarrhea
Deaths are more in post-neonatal period	• Proper treatment of ARI and diarrhea • Ensure availability of ORS in the health facility • Increase all vaccination coverage emphasizing on measles vaccination • Prevention of malnutrition

Identification of Available Resources and Whether Additional Resources are Available/Needed

Manpower

A. Based on available internal resources:
   – Supervisory functions: Supportive supervision regarding all work done by subordinates (such as BPHN, MO, etc.).

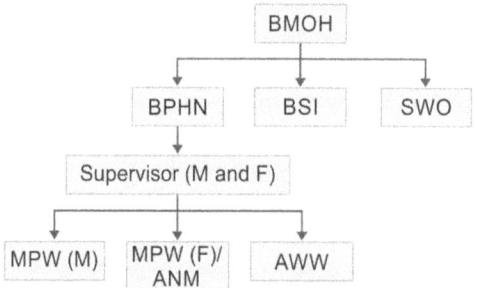

(BMOH: Block medical officer of health; BPHN: Block primary health nurse; BSI: Block sanitary inspector; SWO: Social welfare officer; MPW: Multipurpose worker; M: Male; F: Female; ANM: Auxiliary nurse midwife; AWW: Anganwadi worker)

– Administrative functions: Includes taking decision of number of workers to be appointed, their work division, etc.

B. Additional resources that can be utilized (if required):

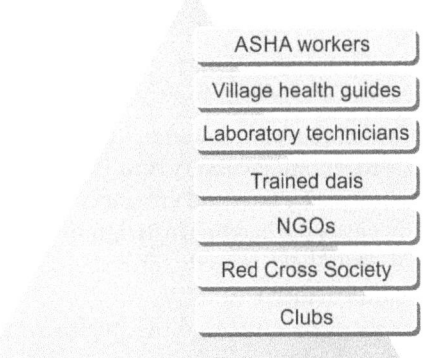

Additional manpower resources
(NGOs: Nongovernmental organizations)

Materials

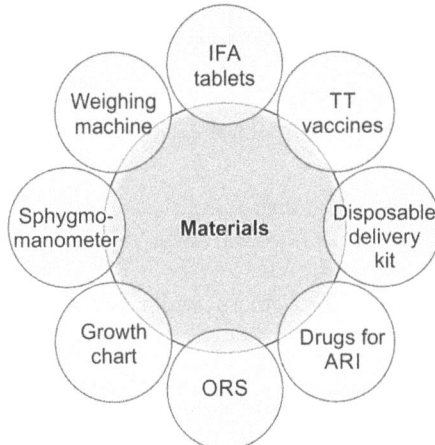

(ORS: Oral rehydration salt; ARI: Acute respiratory infections; TT: Tetanus toxoid; IFA: Iron and folic acid)

Money
An action plan is given to the CMOH for sanctioning a fund.

Writing up the Formulated Plan
❖ Detailed information about the plan
❖ Detailed information about the resources (needed and available)
❖ Interventions to be taken.

Fixing Priorities
Areas with high IMR should be prioritized at first.

Programming and Implementation
Short-term measures

Awareness programme to be arranged to:

1. Advice on early registration, at least 3 antenatal check-ups, one extra meal a day, TT vaccination, taking IFA tablets on a regular basis
2. Advice to promote institutional deliveries/delivery by trained birth attendants
3. Proper advice on colostrum feeding, exclusive breastfeeding, supplementary feeding, no prelacteal feeding
4. Advice about the benefits of immunization.

Proper training:

1. All the health workers of subcenters are called to PHC
2. The BMOH/MOs of PHC give them necessary training
3. MPHW (F) supervises deliveries by dais and ensures 7 cleans during delivery
4. MPHW (M) must identify cases of diarrhea/ARI/tetanus/diphtheria, etc. communicable diseases and notify BMOH/MOPHC immediately
5. ORS has to be given in all diarrheal cases
6. Danger signs of diseases must be known to the health workers and they must give the knowledge to the mothers.

Case management:

1. As a BMOH, I have to attend OPD/IPD/ER routinely
2. Referral cases should be dealt properly
3. Prompt treatment of ARI/diarrhea/other communicable diseases
4. Supervision on EPI (Expanded program of immunization) and IPPI (Intensified pulse polio immunization)
5. Supervision on ICDS to prevent PEM
6. Ensure supply of safe water to prevent diarrheal diseases.

Long-term Measures

Ongoing training of health workers and dais.

❖ IEC activities to promote community awareness regarding ANC/INC/diseases that are common causes of infant mortality
❖ Intersectoral coordination with NGOs/mass media/Gram Panchayats
❖ Improvement in female literacy.

Monitoring and Evaluation

❖ ANC coverage
❖ No. of deliveries attended by TBAs
❖ Proper supply of DDK/TT/ORS/antibiotics
❖ Identification and investigation of every case of infant mortality.

Report

A proper and detailed report should be prepared by the BMOH and sent to higher authorities for further actions to be taken.

Duties of BMOH Regarding High MMR

1. Maternal mortality rate (MMR) is rising in your block area. (12)

• **Define MMR**
• **As BMOH, suggest measures to improve this situation.**

Maternal mortality rate (MMR) is defined as, "Total no. of female deaths due to complications of pregnancy, childbirth or within 42 days of delivery from puerperal causes in an area during a year divided by the total no. of live births in same area and year expressed as a rate per 100,000 live births."

Situation Analysis

❖ Data collection from:
  - Hospital records
  - Subcenter record
  - House-to-house survey
  - PHCs.
❖ Analysis of data on the basis of:
  - Geographical distribution of MMR
  - Socioeconomic status of the case
  - Age of mother
  - Services provided to the community
  - Mortality and morbidity due to puerperal causes.

Problem Identification (Causes of High MMR)

Obstetric causes	Nonobstetric causes	Other causes
• Toxemias in pregnancy • Hemorrhage • Infection • Obstructed labor • Unsafe abortion	• Anemia • Associated diseases of the mother	• Inadequate healthcare services • Sociocultural factors • Lack of awareness • Lack of trained personnel and lack of Institutions

Define the Objectives

Identification of available resources and whether additional resources are available/needed

Goal: According to National Health Policy 2000 decrease in MMR below 100/1 lac mother within 2010.

Objective:

General	Specific
Elimination of determinants	• Utilization and coverage of safe motherhood intervention • Promote IEC activities • Increase training facilities for delivery practices • Increase and promote institutional deliveries

Manpower

1. Available internal resources:

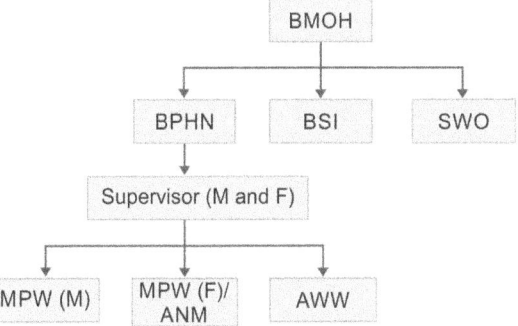

(BMOH: Block medical officer of health; BPHN: Block primary health nurse; BSI: Block sanitary inspector; SWO: Social welfare officer; MPW: Multipurpose worker; M: Male; F: Female; ANM: Auxiliary nurse midwife; AWW: Anganwadi worker)

2. Additional resources that can be utilized:

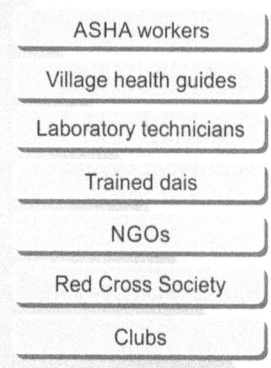

Additional manpower resources

(NGOs: Nongovernmental organizations)

Materials

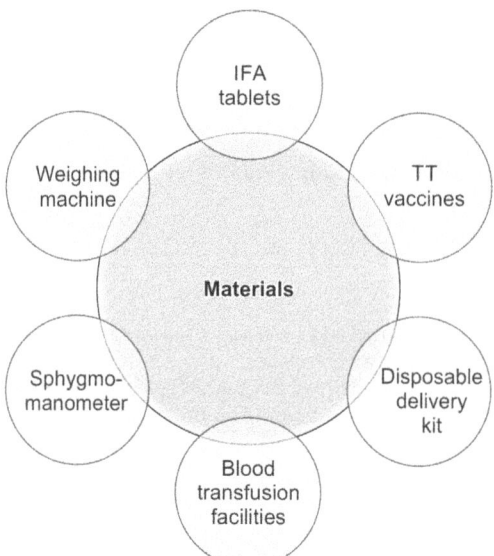

(TT: Tetanus toxoid; IFA: Iron and folic acid)

Money

An action plan is given to the CMOH for sanctioning a fund.

Writing up the Formulated Plan

a. Detailed information about the plan
b. Detailed information about the resources (needed and available)
c. Interventions to be taken.

Fixing Priorities

Areas with high IMR should be prioritized at first.

Programming and Implementation

Short-term measures

Awareness program to be arranged to promote:

A. Curative measures:
   - Attend OPDs
   - Attend emergency cases at the earliest
   - Referral to FRUs for obstructed emergencies
   - Laboratory services
   - Medical termination of pregnancies under proper supervision.
B. Preventive measures:
   a. MCH services:

Maternity services	Delivery services	Postpartum services
• Early registration • Antenatal check-up • Correction of anemia • Tetanus prophylaxis • Prevention of complications	• 5 clean delivery practices • Delivery by trained personnel • Institutional delivery of cases with bad obstetric history	• Prevention of infection and hemorrhage during puerperium • Promotion of family planning

   b. Implementation of ICDS and RCH program.

Long-term measures
1. Training of TBA, HW, AWW, MPW/HA
2. Promotion of IEC activities by:
   - Directly through meeting with mothers and community to increase awareness
   - By slide shows, pamphlets, leaflets, posters, plays and video
   - IEC activities regarding family planning practices
   - Prevention of unwanted pregnancy
   - By providing contraceptive devices
   - Social marketing of OCPs and condoms
   - IEC activities.
3. Intersectoral coordination:
   - With panchayat and community
   - With NGOs and voluntary organizations.
4. Administrative:
   - Supervision of services provided, i.e. supply of IFAs, TTs & other drugs
   - Financial power
   - Record, report, feedback maintenance.

Monitoring and Evaluation

1. ANC coverage
2. No. of deliveries attended by TBAs
3. Proper supply of DDK/TT/ORS/antibiotics
4. Identification and investigation of every case of maternal mortality
5. Approach to risk pregnancy.

Report

A proper and detailed report should be prepared by the BMOH and sent to higher authorities for further actions to be taken.

Duties of BMOH in Improving the Situation of High Proportion Low Birth Weight Babies

1. Proportion of low birth weight babies in your block is very high. As a BMOH, what actions you will take to tackle this situation? (12)

Definition of Low Birth Weight (LBW)

LBW is defined as a birth weight <2.5 kg (up to and including 2499 g), when measurement is taken preferably within the first hour of life.

Situation Analysis

Data collection and data analysis:
- ❖ Resource persons: MPHW-F/voluntary health agencies
- ❖ Source of the data:
  - – Institutional records
  - – Subcenter records
  - – House-to-house survey.
- ❖ Data have to be obtained:
  - – Geographical distribution and demographic distribution of LBW
  - – Total number of low birth weight babies
  - – Number of deaths among them
  - – Number of institutional deliveries and delivery by trained personnel
  - – Age and parity of mothers in the specified locality.

Problem Identification

a. For preterm babies (Mnemonic: MATH):
  - – **M**ultiple pregnancy
  - – **A**cute infection
  - – **T**oxemias in pregnancy
  - – **H**ard physical labor.
b. For small for date babies:

Maternal cause	Placental cause	Fetal cause
◆ Teenage pregnancy	◆ Placental abnormalities	◆ Intrauterine infection
◆ Multiple pregnancy	◆ Placental insufficiency	◆ Chromosomal abnormality
◆ Narrow birth space		◆ Multiple gestation
◆ Low socioeconomic status		
◆ Illiteracy		
◆ Severe anemia		
◆ Malaria		
◆ Toxemia		

Fixing the Goal

As per global strategy "HEALTH FOR ALL", at least 90% of newborn babies should have a birth weight of 2.5 kg or above. So, the BMOH should set a goal of around 90% of newborn babies having a birth weight of 2.5 kg.

Defining the Objectives

❖ Reduction of LBW babies
❖ Improvement of antenatal coverage
❖ Promotion of institutional deliveries.

Assessment of available resources and whether additional resources are needed or not:

Manpower

1. Available internal resources:

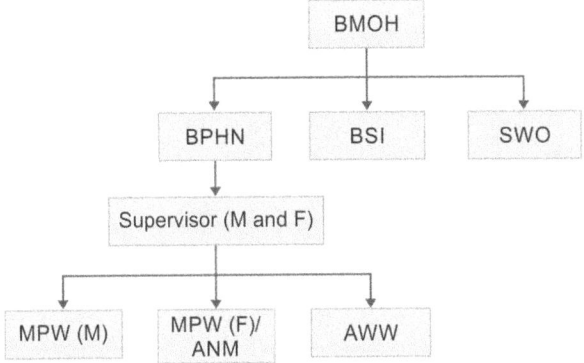

(BMOH: Block medical officer of health; BPHN: Block primary health nurse; BSI: Block sanitary inspector; SWO: Social welfare officer; MPW: Multipurpose worker; M: Male; F: Female; ANM: Auxiliary nurse midwife; AWW: Anganwadi worker)

2. Additional resources that can be utilized:

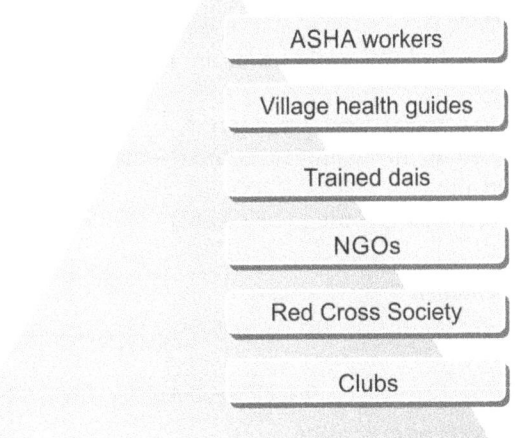

Additional manpower resources

(NGOs: Nongovernmental organizations)

Money
An action plan is given to the CMOH for sanctioning a fund.

Materials

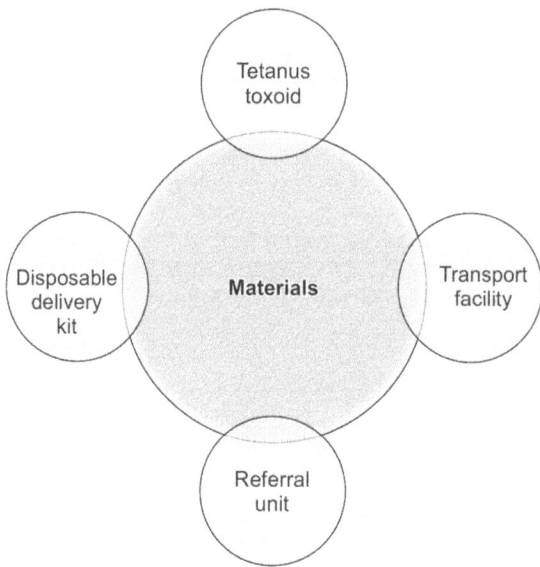

Fixing the Priorities

On the basis of initial evaluation of geographical distribution of LBW babies, the areas with greater number of LBW babies should be given priorities to implement the action plan first and to mobilize resources first to these high prevalence sites.

Writing up the Formulated Plan

The formulated plan to fight LBW problem in the block, the details of the formulated plan should be written with:
1. Detailed roadmap to achieve the defined target
2. Detailed discussion about the resources required—man, money, material, education to the manpower required, etc.
3. Details of the interventions that are to be taken.

Programming and Implementation

Short-term measures

Specific treatment	
Weight of the baby	Intervention to be taken
<2 kg	First class modern neonatal care should be given at an intensive care unit (ICU) until they reach a weight of 2 kg. The intensive care comprises of: 1. Incubatory care (monitoring of temperature, humidification and oxygen supply) 2. Maintenance of cardiorespiratory function to prevent hypothermia 3. Prevention of infection 4. Artificial feeding by nasal catheter
2–2.5 kg	Intensive care unit for 1–2 days

Kangaroo Mother Care

It is an essential element of neonatal care. It comprises primarily of four components:
1. Skin-to-skin contact of a baby on the mother's chest
2. Giving adequate nutrition to a baby through breastfeeding
3. Ambulatory care (as discussed above)
4. Support for the mother and her family in caring of the baby.

Direct Intervention Measures

The incidence of LBW can be prevented if pregnant women at risk can be identified early and treated adequately. For this purpose, *mothers health card* should be used as a powerful intervention measure by PHCs.
❖ Supplementary feeding of high-risk mothers
❖ Treatment of anemic mothers by IFA tablets
❖ Early detection and control of infections like malaria/UTI/STDs/TORCH infections, etc.
❖ Early detection and treatment of associated comorbid conditions like hypertension/diabetes/toxemia, etc.

Long-term/Indirect Intervention Measures

Establishment of first referral units (FRUs) and improvement of transport facilities. IEC activities regarding:
❖ Family planning
❖ Age of marriage
❖ Age of first pregnancy
❖ Birth spacing
❖ Avoidance of excessive smoking (by family members)
❖ Improvement of sanitation measures.

Improvement of health and nutrition condition of pregnant mothers	Category	Excess energy needed (Kcal/Day)
	Adolescent girls	+ 300
	Pregnant women	+ 350
	Lactation 0–6 months	+ 600
	Lactation 6–12 months	+ 520

Promotion of women literacy

Supervision of full functioning of ICDS

Promotion of institutional deliveries through training of manpower (ANM/ AWW/ TBA/ ASHA, etc.)

Monitoring and Evaluation

The BMOH should monitor the following to evaluate the effectiveness of the program to decrease the LBW prevalence of the area:
❖ Total number of LBW babies
❖ Number of deaths among the LBW babies
❖ Number of referred cases
❖ Percentage of institutional deliveries
❖ Percentage of antenatal coverage with 3 antenatal check-ups, 2 doses of tetanus toxoid and 100 days of IFA tablets.

Report

A proper and detailed report should be prepared by the BMOH and sent to higher authorities (CMOH) for further actions to be taken.

Duties of a BMOH in Preventing Incidence of Neonatal Tetanus

1. Few cases of neonatal tetanus (NNT) has been reported from a block of a district. As a BMOH, what measure will you take to prevent its further occurrence?   **(10)**

Situation Analysis

❖ Data collection on NNT from:
   – Birth and death records
   – ANC register
   – Maternal and child health (MCH) card
   – Subcenter record
   – House-to-house survey and enquiry of the mother whether she had taken the TT injection or not
   – Enquiry of the mother to detect what was the type of the delivery: institutional/home. If it was a home delivery, then ask who had conducted the delivery: untrained dai/ trained birth attendant (TBA)/other health service provider(s).
❖ Analysis of data on the basis of:
   – Geographical distribution of occurrence of NNT cases
   – Age of the child affected
   – Health services provided to the community.
❖ Algorithm for identification high-risk area of neonatal tetanus (based on a WHO report):

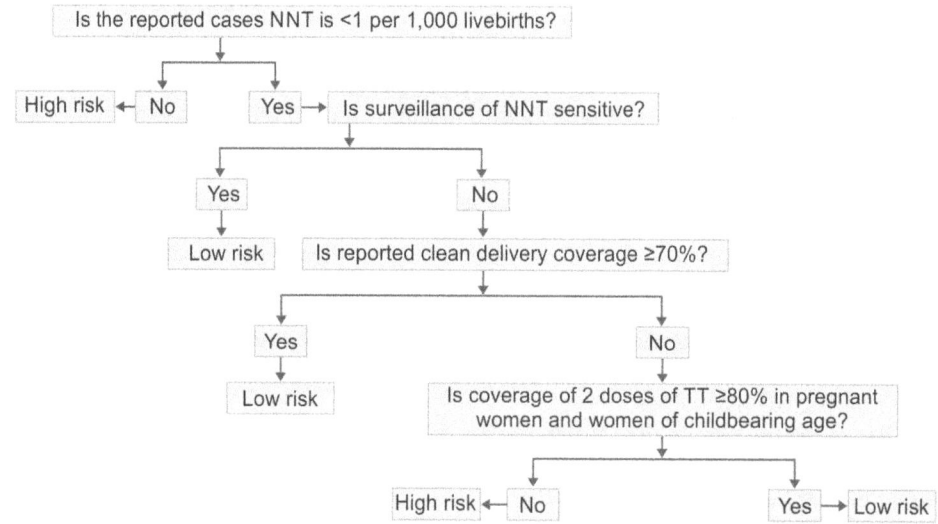

Defining the Objectives

❖ Cut down the incidence of neonatal tetanus in the community to zero
❖ Proper treatment of each present case of NNT and proper referral of all the complicated cases
❖ To achieve a TT2 coverage of >90%
❖ Dissemination of the information regarding the importance of TT immunization in pregnant mother and proper health education of the community to prevent any future incidences of NNT.

Identification of Available Resources and Whether Additional Resources are Available/Needed

Manpower

A. Available internal resources:

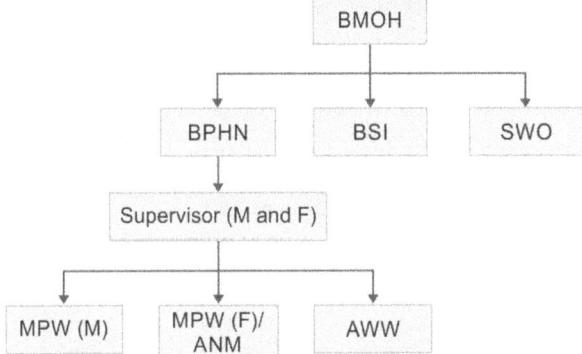

(BMOH: Block medical officer of health; BPHN: Block primary health nurse; BSI: Block sanitary inspector; SWO: Social welfare officer; MPW: Multipurpose worker; M: Male; F: Female; ANM: Auxiliary nurse midwife; AWW: Anganwadi worker)

B. Additional resources that can be utilized:

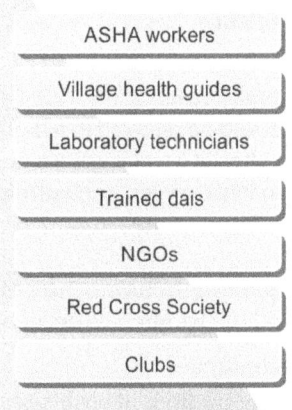

Additional manpower resources

(NGOs: Nongovernmental organizations)

Materials

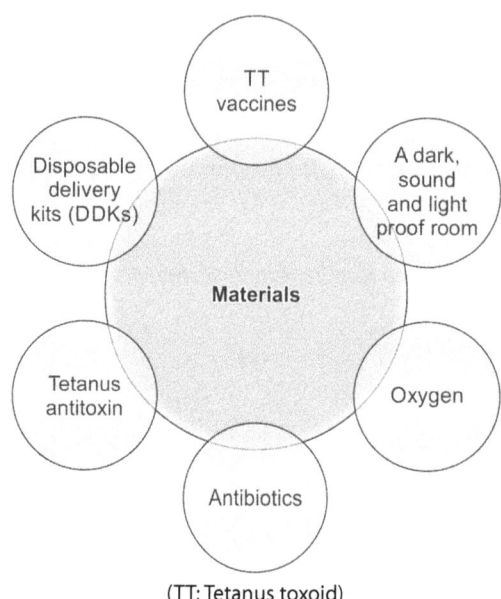

(TT: Tetanus toxoid)

Money
An action plan is given to the CMOH for sanctioning a fund.

Writing up the formulated plan
❖ Detailed information about the plan
❖ Detailed information about the resources (needed and available)
❖ Interventions to be taken.

Fixing Priorities
Areas with high prevalence of NNT should be prioritized at first.

Programming and Implementation

Short-term measures
Appropriate treatment of the case.
❖ The infected child should be referred to a higher level of health care. If prompt referral is not possible, the patient should be placed in a dark, light and sound proof room
❖ Supportive treatment with oxygen and antibiotics should be given. The antibiotic of choice is a long-acting penicillin (like *Benzathine penicillin*), given at a single IM dose of 1.2 mega units (MU)
❖ If the mother was not immunized with 2 doses of TT, then give both the mother and her baby *tetanus antitoxin (750 IU)* within 6 hours of birth.

Prevention of neonatal tetanus
Training should be given to traditional birth attendants to practice the rule of 7Cs, because this measure alone can reduce the incidence of deaths due to NNT by 90%:
1. Clean hands
2. Clean fingernails

3. Clean delivery surface
4. Clean blade for cutting the cord
5. Clean tie for the cord
6. No application on the cord stump
7. Keeping birth canal clean by avoiding harmful practices.

Administration of tetanus toxoid:

Situation	Preferable dosing schedule
Antenatal period	• 2 doses of TT to be given, 1 month apart (preferably in 4th and 5th month of period of gestation) • If not given at 5th month, 2nd dose should be given at least <3 weeks prior to delivery, so that there is enough time for good antibody titers to develop in mother and for it to be passed on to the fetus to prevent tetanus in newborn • 2 doses provide protection for subsequent pregnancies in next 5 years (only 1 booster dose is sufficient)
Pregnant woman comes at 8th month of gestation for the first time	• 2 TT doses are given irrespective of delivery time (i.e. second dose is given at the time of delivery) • This results in complete immunization of mother for subsequent 5 years but, infants remain unimmunized • In this case 750 IU heterologous serum should be administered within 6 hours of birth
Pregnant woman in labor	Give TT to a woman in labor, if she has not previously received TT

Long-term measures
❖ Sustained coverage of 2 doses of TT to pregnant mothers should be prioritized
❖ Supply of disposable delivery kits (DDKs) should be improvised
❖ Mass media should be involved to raise the awareness among the pregnant mothers and also in the community about the importance of safe delivery practices and tetanus toxoid immunization
❖ Untrained dais/traditional birth attendants should be properly trained on the aspects of safe delivery practices in an intensified scale. The provision of 7Cs should be given the utmost importance in the training.

Monitoring and Surveillance
❖ Identification and investigation of every case of neonatal deaths
❖ No. of deliveries attended by TBAs
❖ Proper supply of DDK and TT.

Report
A proper and detailed report should be prepared by the BMOH and sent to higher authorities (CMOH) for further actions to be taken.

DUTIES OF BMOH DURING FLOOD

1. **Enumerate different health hazards likely to occur during/following flood. As a BMOH, describe your preparedness plan to mitigate such hazards in future.** (4 + 8)

Health Hazards Likely to Occur During/Following Flood

A. Immediate direct effect:
   - Death due to drowning and snake bites
   - Injury
   - Accidents.
B. Damage to existing infrastructure like:
   - Water supply
   - Sanitation facilities
   - Food sources
   - Population displacement: Overcrowding
   - Damage to existing health infrastructures and interruption in routine healthcare delivery.
C. Intestinal diseases:
   - Diarrhea
   - Dysentery
   - Cholera
   - Typhoid
   - Hepatitis A and E.
D. Skin diseases.
E. Respiratory tract infections.
F. Undernutrition affecting especially:
   - Children
   - Pregnant and lactating mothers.
G. Psychological manifestations:
   - Anxiety
   - Depression
   - Post-traumatic stress disorder (PTSD).

Role of BMOH in Case of Flood

Situation Analysis

❖ Risk mapping (identify the areas affected)
❖ Vulnerability analysis (identify the population affected)
❖ Hazard mapping (identify the casualty)
❖ Opportunity mapping (Identify safe housing and drinking water supply).

Identification of Available Resources and Whether Additional Resources are Available/Needed

Manpower

A. Available internal resources:

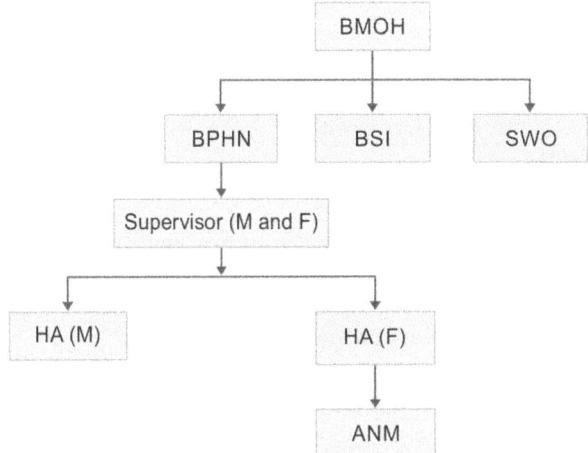

(BMOH: Block medical officer of health; BPHN: Block primary health nurse; BSI: Block sanitary inspector; SWO: Social welfare officer; HA: Health assistant; M: Male; F: Female; ANM: Auxiliary nurse midwife)

B. Additional resources that can be utilized:

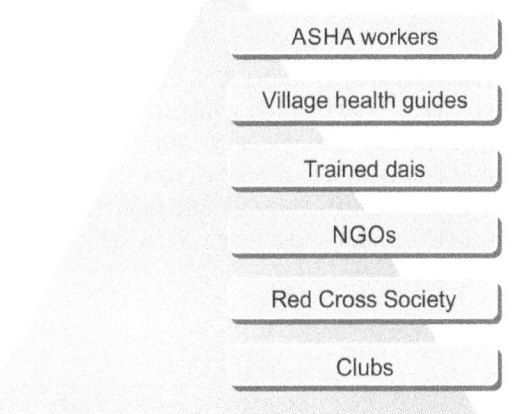

Additional manpower resources
(NGOs: Nongovernmental organizations)

Money

Funds are needed for proper rehabilitation of the victims and their families and reconstruction of the damaged infrastructures, which is usually arranged by the state and central government. An action plan is given to CMOH for sanctioning a fund.

Materials

Food, blanket, tent, tripal, clothing, shelter, sanitary engineering measures, equipment, etc.

Define the Objectives
❖ No starvation deaths
❖ No outbreaks/epidemics of water-borne/other types of diseases.

Mobilization of Resources

Writing up of Formulated Plan

The formulated plan to fight low immunization coverage in the block, the details of the formulated plan should be written with:
❖ Detailed information
❖ Discuss cost, time, manpower limit each step
❖ Intervention to be taken.

The plan should be submitted to higher officials for approval and funding.

Fixing Priorities

On the basis of:
❖ No. of people affected
❖ No. of snake bites
❖ Incidence of diarrhea, ARI, etc.

Management

1. *Inform headquarters* for rescue operations.
2. Take *rapid action on onset of crisis* including medical emergencies:
   a. Turn off electricity to reduce risk of electrocution
   b. Transfer vulnerable population to rescue camps
   c. Give provision of food, safe water, shelter and safety
   d. Ration is given by government and cooked by NGOs.

Type of ration	Calorie	Protein
Survival ration	1,200 KCal	30 g*
Maintenance ration	1,600 KCal	45 g
Regular ration**	2,000 KCal	55 g

*1/2 amount protein for <8 years
** When all are rescued, regular ration is supplied.

   The food is best cooked at the camp and served.
   e. Give first aid services to injured ones
   f. Children, old, sick, disabled should be given special attention
   g. Removal of dead bodies, shifting to the mortuary and identification
   h. Triage
   i. Tagging: With victim's name, place of origin, triage category, helps in proper diagnosis, initiation of treatment.
3. Prevention and control of outbreaks:
   a. Implement all public health measures to reduce the risk of transmission of diseases and risk of outbreaks

  b. Organize a reliable disease reporting system
  c. Investigate all reports of outbreaks and report to higher authority
  d. Arrangement of referral for emergency cases.
4. Disinfection of water sources:
  a. When tube wells/wells are submerged by floods, safe water should be distributed to families
  b. As soon as the flood water recedes, mass disinfection should be undertaken by emergency chlorination
  c. All portable water sources should be disinfected by bleaching powder within 2 km radius
  d. Potent halogen tablets has to be supplied and people should be advised how to use them.

Long-term measures
❖ Rehabilitation:
  – Reestablishment of health services.
  – *Human excreta and solid waste disposal:*
    - Advise people not to practice open air defecation
    - Use trench type of latrines
    - Employ large number of sweepers.
  – Vector control measures: Use of insecticides, investigation and control of epidemic
  – Creation of job
  – Loan for repairing buildings.
❖ Specific services to be arranged:
  – Medical care
  – Specific services for vulnerable groups, such as:
    - Growth monitoring
    - Vitamin A prophylaxis
    - Immunization.
  – Provision for first aid facilities for camps
  – Surveillance of communicable diseases specially:
    - Active surveillance
    - For presumptive treatment
    - Includes establishment of drug distribution center, fever center.

IEC Activities

Regarding safety from water contamination.

Monitoring and Evaluation

No. of deaths, casualties, victims, snake bites, electrocution should be assessed carefully to evaluate the success of the program.

Reporting

A proper and detailed report should be prepared by the BMOH and sent to higher authorities (CMOH) for further actions to be taken.

◼ DUTIES OF BMOH DURING A LOW IMMUNIZATION COVERAGE IN BLOCK

1. Percentage of fully immunized children is very low while left out and dropout rates are unacceptably high in your block. What measures you will adopt as a BMOH to improve the situation? (12)

Situation Analysis

Data Collection and Data Analysis

❖ Resource persons: MPHW-F/voluntary health agencies.
❖ Source of the data:
  – Institutional records
  – Subcenter records
  – House-to-house survey.
❖ Data have to be obtained:
  – Geographical distribution of population structure
  – Prevalence of vaccine preventable diseases
  – Community participation
  – Accessibility of existing healthcare facility.

Problem Identification

❖ Short supply of vaccines
❖ Repeated cancellation of vaccination sessions
❖ Poor acceptance
❖ Fear of adverse reaction of vaccination
❖ Too long distance
❖ Unawareness
❖ Lack of information
❖ Lack of manpower
❖ More emphasis on pulse polio immunization
❖ To identify prejudices in the community.

Fixing the Goal

Vaccination against 6 vaccine preventable diseases of children <1 year of age, i.e. TB, polio, whooping cough, diphtheria, tetanus, measles.

Defining the Objectives

❖ Immunization coverage should reach a figure of >80%
❖ Herd immunity should be achieved
❖ Make routine immunization service available in regular basis on fixed days readily or freely accessible sites.

Assessment of Available Resources and Whether Additional Resources are Needed or Not

Manpower

A. Available internal resources

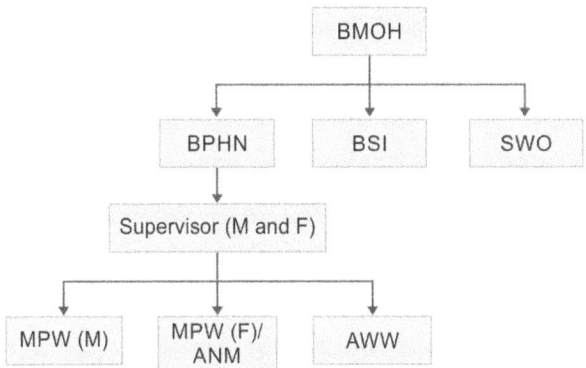

(BMOH: Block medical officer of health; BPHN: Block primary health nurse; BSI: Block sanitary inspector; SWO: Social welfare officer; MPW: Multipurpose worker; M: Male; F: Female; ANM: Auxiliary nurse midwife; AWW: Anganwadi worker)

B. Additional resources that can be utilized

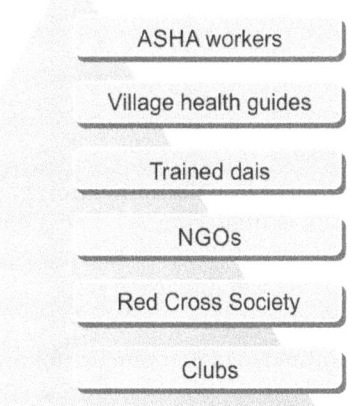

Additional manpower resources

(NGOs: Nongovernmental organizations)

Money

An action plan is given to the CMOH for sanctioning a fund.

Materials

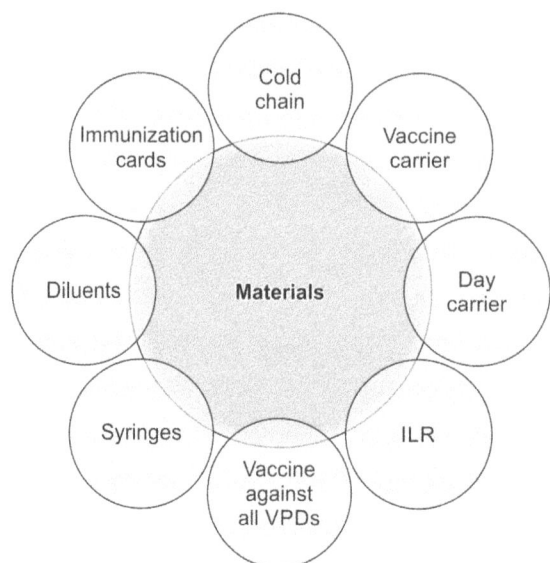

(VPDs: Vaccine preventable diseases; ILR: Ice lined refrigerator)

Fixing the Priorities

❖ Where immunization is very poor
❖ Where epidemic occurs
❖ Remote areas
❖ AFP surveillance.

Writing up the Formulated Plan

The formulated plan to fight low immunization coverage in the block, the details of the formulated plan should be written with:

❖ Detailed information
❖ Discuss cost, time, manpower limit each step
❖ Intervention to be taken.

The plan should be submitted to higher officials for approval and funding.

Programming and Implementation

❖ Administrative duty:
  – Distribution of vaccination in all centers
  – Every subcenter must take adequate vaccine
  – Sufficient no. of syringes, needles, diluents must be provided.
❖ Supervisory duty:
  – If low coverage due to long-term vacancy—special immunization are taken by sources from higher centers to meet the vacancy
  – If low coverage due to cancellation of immunization program, then reschedule them
  – Catch up immunization: Twice a month for covering up the missed cases
  – IEC activities:
    - To overcome the problem of poor acceptance by plays, posters, videos, etc.

- Meeting to be organized with the community to assure the population based on the fear of adverse reaction due to vaccination.
– If religious beliefs are one of the factors of low coverage: Religious leaders must to be involved to enlighten the people from the darkness of ignorance and false beliefs
– Support of peripheral health staffs of PHC, subcenters—in case of re-occurrence
– Training of HW, AWW and other healthcare providers
– The health workers are adequate, patronized the joining of voluntary workers
– Supervision on:
  - If ICDS is fully functional or not
  - ANC coverage
  - Mopping up
  - Ring immunization.

Monitoring and Evaluation

❖ Of adverse reaction and reporting to the higher authorities with urgent detailed investigation of cases
❖ On immunization program
❖ Check the vaccine regularly on scheduled day, check the temperature of ILR on Monday and Saturday
❖ % of children (<1 year) fully/partially immunized
❖ % of pregnant women taking TT2 vaccine
❖ % of cold chain monitoring.

Report

A proper and detailed report should be prepared by the BMOH and sent to higher authorities (CMOH) for further actions to be taken.

DUTIES OF BMOH IN SOLVING PROBLEMS OF MALNUTRITION IN BLOCK

Situation Analysis

❖ Verification of diagnosis: Done by:
  – Clinical examination:
    - Pallor
    - Edema
    - Bitot's spot
    - Angular stomatitis
    - Muscle wasting (if any).
  – Anthropometric measurement:
    - Height
    - Weight
    - Skin fold thickness
    - Mid-arm circumference
    - Weight for age
    - Height for age.
❖ Estimation of magnitude of problem: Done by counting the number of under 5 children who are suffering from/at risk of severe malnutrition.

❖ Assessment of determinants:
  – Water supply
  – Basic sanitation
  – Maintenance of proper food hygiene
  – Mode of excreta disposal
  – Housing standards.

Identification of Causal Factors

❖ Diet survey: It will provide information about:
  – Dietary intake pattern
  – Specific foods consumed
  – Estimated nutrient intake
  – EBF practiced/not
  – Weaning.
❖ Information regarding infectious disease: Like measles, diarrhea, ARI, TB, worm manifestation, etc.
❖ Information regarding cultural influences like:
  – Cultural
  – Religion
  – Customs and belief
  – Cooking procedure
  – Tradition and attitude.
❖ Assessment of socioeconomic conditions by:
  – Poverty
  – Ignorance
  – Illiteracy
  – Lack of knowledge
  – Inadequate sanitary environment
  – Improper family planning methods, family size, no birth spacing
  – Inadequate distribution of food in the family.
❖ Information regarding morbidity and mortality data of population particularly concerned about:
  – Rate of LBW babies
  – <5 mortality rate
  – Life expectancy and causes of mortality.
❖ Detailed information regarding:
  – ANC of mother
  – Place of delivery and done by whom
  – Immunization status of the children
  – Knowledge and practice of mother regarding—colostrum feeding, prelacteal feeding, EBF, feeding during illness, initiation of proper weaning in proper time, proper weaning food.
❖ Evaluation of healthcare delivery system in locality like nutritional surveillance, nutritional rehabilitation, nutritional supplementation, health education.

Assessment of Resources

Manpower

A. Available internal resources:

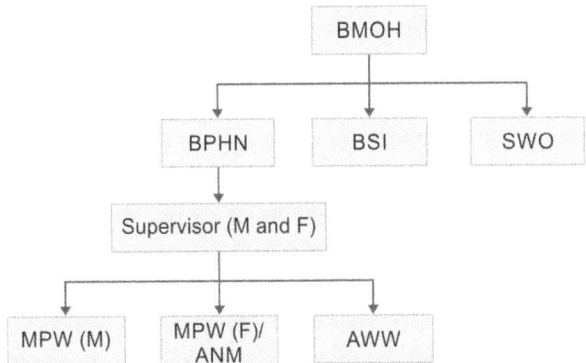

(BMOH: Block medical officer of health; BPHN: Block primary health nurse; BSI: Block sanitary inspector; SWO: Social welfare officer; MPW: Multipurpose worker; M: Male; F: Female; ANM: Auxiliary nurse midwife; AWW: Anganwadi worker)

B. Additional resources that can be utilized:

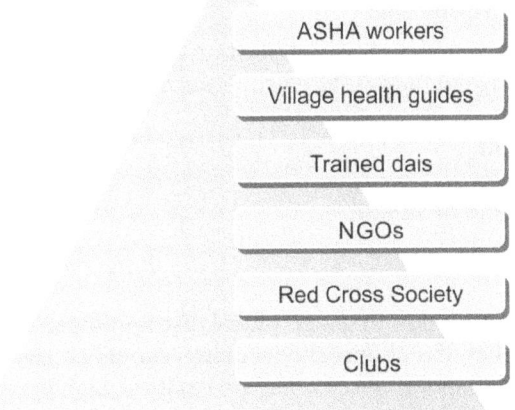

Additional manpower resources

(NGOs: Nongovernmental organizations)

Money

An action plan is given to the CMOH for sanctioning a fund.

Materials

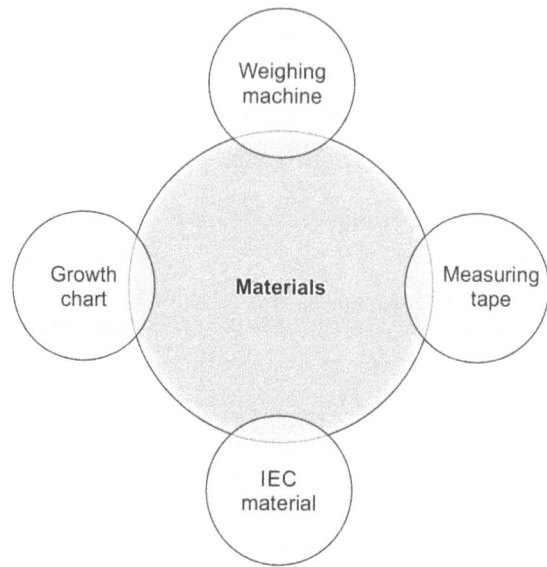

(IEC: Information, Education and Communication)

Establishment of Objective and Goal

❖ Goal: To decrease the incidence of malnutrition to a large extent
❖ Target: Proper management of children suffering from malnutrition
❖ Objectives:
  – Health promotion
  – Specific protection
  – Early diagnosis and treatment.

Fixing the Priorities

On the basis of initial evaluation of geographical distribution of malnourished children, the areas with greater number of malnourished children should be given priorities to implement the action plan first and to mobilize resources first to these high prevalence sites.

Formulation of Plan

The formulated plan to fight malnutrition problem in the block, the details of the formulated plan should be written with:
❖ Detailed roadmap to achieve the defined target
❖ Detailed discussion about the resources required—man, money, material, education to the manpower required, etc.
❖ Details of the interventions that are to be taken.

Mobilization of Resources

Programming and Implementation of Control Measures

A. Short-term measures:
  - Treatment measures for cases: According to severity of malnutrition, supplementary and therapeutic nutrition should be given:

Grade	Weight for age (%)	Treatment measures
I	71–80	Dietary modification + nutritional education to mother
II	61–70	Supplementary nutrition under ICDS scheme
III	51–60	Therapeutic nutrition under ICDS scheme
IV	<50	Hospitalization

  - Measures to control infectious diseases:
    - Proper implementation of RCH program to control diarrhea and ARI
    - Deworming
    - PHC, subcenter and other local health center should be equipped with measures to tackle diarrhea.
B. Long-term measures:
  - *Health education*: Mother should be educated about:
    - Importance of no prelacteal feeding, colostrum feeding, EBF
    - Weaning at proper time
    - Home treatment of diarrhea and respiratory illnesses
    - Proper immunization against vaccine preventable diseases (VPDs)
    - Mother should be given information about cheap locally available nutritious food.
  - *Implementation of family planning*: Regarding
    - Small family norm
    - Birth spacing
    - Cafeteria choice.
  - Proper ANC for mother
  - Water supply and proper sanitation to improve housing standards
  - Administrative supports
  - Proper supervision of:
    - Surveillance at regular interval
    - Quality of service provided should be checked and revised regularly
    - Feedback from the respondents should be considered and steps to be taken per demand.

IEC Activities

❖ Regarding warning signs and proper treatment of diarrhea and ARI
❖ Community awareness about proper nutrition
❖ Awareness about proper age of marriage, birth spacing, no. of children.

Monitoring and Evaluation

❖ No. of cases suffering from PEM
❖ No. of deaths due to malnutrition
❖ No. of LBW babies.

Reporting

By BMOH to the higher authority for proper further actions to be taken.

DUTIES OF BMOH IN PREVENTING LOW COUPLE PROTECTION RATE

1. **Define couple protection rate (CPR). What are the causes of low CPR? As a BMOH suggest some measures to increase low CPR in your block.** (4 + 8)

Couple protection rate (CPR) is defined as: *"Couples effectively protected against childbirth by one or other approved methods of family planning."*

It is an indicator of *prevalence of contraceptive practice in the community.*

❖ Causes of low couple protection rate:
   – *Unmet need for contraception*: Due to:
      - Inconvenient or unsatisfactory services
      - Lack of information
      - Fear about side effects of contraceptives
      - Opposition from husbands or relatives.
   – *Limited access to quality health services*:
      - Near about 1/3 of rural women live in a village with PHC or subcenter
      - Important subgroups such as adolescent are neglected or under served.
   – *Socioeconomic constrains*:
      - High levels of illiteracy
      - Poverty and gender biased disparities
      - Lack of male partner involvement in family planning
      - Continuous open discrimination against the girl child, adolescent girls and woman.
   – *Programmatic constrains*:
      - Limited resources
      - Lack of multisectorial approach
      - Insufficient IEC support
      - Weak health information system.
   – *Limited awareness of reversible methods*: Most of the providers have a bias towards sterilization. Only small proportion of clients are informed of reversible methods.
   – *Staff shortage and limitations*: Shortage of staff is an important cause of promoting any program intending towards lowering of CPR in the community. Poorly trained staff have little knowledge of the methods they are promoting. Women without any children are least likely to receive a home visit.

Situation Analysis

❖ Data collection: By active and passive surveillance:
   – Rapid survey involving HW, NGOs
   – Subcenter record
   – House-to-house survey.

❖ Analysis of data on the basis of:
  – Population, age, sex and structure
  – Proportion of eligible couples and adolescent girls
  – Target couple using contraceptive device
  – Socioeconomic status of the family
  – No. of eligible couples or adolescent girls
  – Services provided to the community
  – Attitude and belief of the community.

Problem Identification

Maternal cause	Health service related	Social/familial cause
• Illiteracy	• Inadequacy of training staff	• Religious belief
• Lack of awareness	• Non-motivated training staff	• Low socioeconomic condition
• Fear and side effects from contraceptive measures	• Inadequate material supply	• Opposition of husband
• Misconception		• Caste and religion
• Religious barriers		• Less involvement of community
		• Fear of infertility
		• Preference of male child

Define the Objectives, Goal and Target

Objectives	• Delaying birth • Spacing birth • Limiting birth • Providing cafeteria choice • Addressing the unmet needs of family planning
Goal	Obtaining net reproduction rate (NRR) = 1
Target	Increase couple production rate to >60%

Identification of Available Resources and Whether Additional Resources are Available/Needed

Manpower
1. Available internal resources:

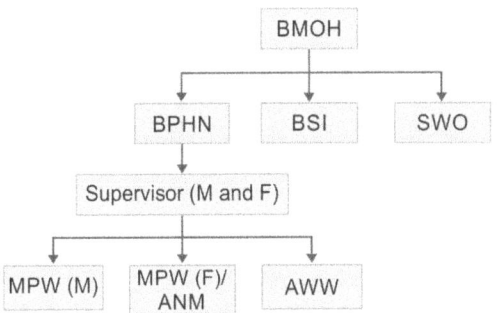

(BMOH: Block medical officer of health; BPHN: Block primary health nurse; BSI: Block sanitary inspector; SWO: Social welfare officer; MPW: Multipurpose worker; M: Male; F: Female; ANM: Auxiliary nurse midwife; AWW: Anganwadi worker)

2. Additional resources that can be utilized:

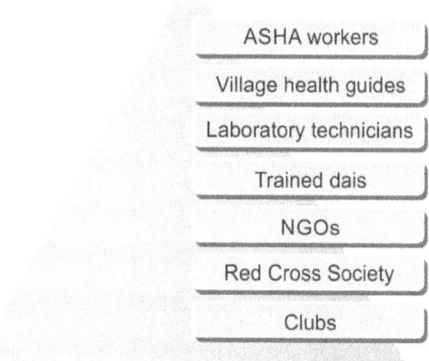

Additional manpower resources
(NGOs: Nongovernmental organizations)

Materials

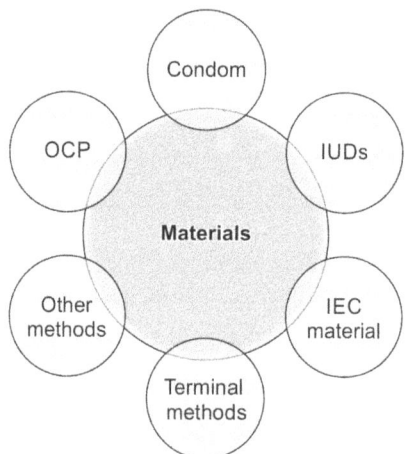

(IEC: Information, education and communication; OCP: Oral contraceptive pills; IUDs: Intrauterine devices)

Money
An action plan is given to the CMOH for sanctioning a fund.

Writing up the Formulated Plan
❖ Detailed information about the plan
❖ Detailed information about the resources (needed and available)
❖ Interventions to be taken.

Fixing Priorities
Areas with high CPR should be prioritized at first.

Programming and Implementation

Short-term measures

Family planning services and materials (like condom and OCP) should be made widely available through social marketing.

❖ Condom: It is of low cost, good quality, widely available on time and place
❖ OCP: MALA-N (given free of cost)
❖ IUD insertion
❖ DMPA
❖ Male and female sterilization: Promotion of male sterilization should be encouraged
❖ Counseling for MTP.

Long-term measures

❖ Activities: Promoting cafeteria choice
❖ IEC activities: Through posters, banners, television, playing regarding:
  – Sexuality and gender information
  – Birth spacing
  – Small family norm
  – Health education
  – Opposition from husband and other family members should be managed.
❖ Unmet need of family planning: Should be essentially met
❖ Education and counseling of eligible couples and target couples for:
  – Regular motivation to take pill or to check IUD tail
  – Male sterilization when ones family is completed
  – Fear of side effects of contraceptives should be removed.
❖ Adolescent education
❖ Quality of care to be given
❖ Training of MPHW (M/F), village health guide, trained dais
❖ Intersectoral communication
❖ Storage and supply of essential kits.

Monitoring and Evaluation

Degree of objectives and goal fulfilled.

❖ % of eligible couple using condom, IUD, OCP and sterilization procedures
❖ Practice of birth spacing of 3 years
❖ Age at 1st pregnancy.

Report

A proper and detailed report should be prepared by the BMOH and sent to higher authorities for further actions to be taken.

DUTIES OF BMOH IN PREVENTING ANEMIA IN PREGNANT WOMEN

1. What is nutritional anemia? What are the causes of nutritional anemia? Prepare an action plan to conduct an IEC campaign in your block to reduce anemia among pregnant women. (2 + 3 + 7)

According to WHO

"Nutritional anemia is a condition in which content of blood is lower than normal as a result of deficiency of one or more essential nutrients, regardless of the cause of such a deficiency."

Causes of Nutritional Anemia

A. Related to supply and demand:

Causes of nutritional anemia

Inadequate intake	Low absorption	Increased demand
• Poverty • Low socioeconomic status • Poor dietary content of iron	• Intestinal parasitism • Tropical sprue • Improper food habits	• Pregnancy • Lactation • Children <12 years • Heavy menstruation

B. Other causes:
  – Too early pregnancy
  – Too frequent pregnancy/improper spacing of birth
  – Lack of female literacy.

Role of BMOH in Controlling Anemia in Pregnancy in a Block

Situation Analysis

1. Collection of data:
  – Numbers of anemic pregnant women in the block
  – Numbers of anemic lactating mothers and children
  – Detection of high burden areas (with greater number of anemic pregnant women, lactating mothers and children)
  – Sources of iron in the foods of anemic population.
2. Analysis of data on the basis of:
  – Geographical distribution
  – Socioeconomic status of the cases
  – Services provided to the community.

Define the Objectives

A practical and achievable objective has to be defined which is to be completed with a predetermined time period.

Example
❖ Screening of at least 50% of pregnant women for anemia.
❖ Reduction of prevalence of anemia in the pregnant women of the block by 20% within 6 months.

Identification and Quantification of Available Resources and Whether Additional Resources are Needed

These resources include:
A. Manpower
B. Material
C. Money

Manpower

Existing manpower in a PHC:

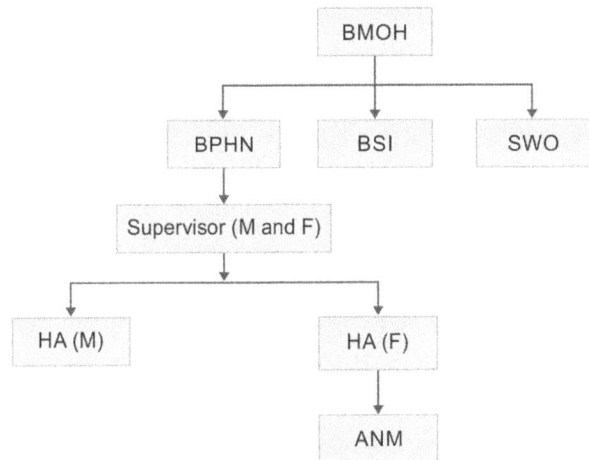

(BMOH: Block medical officer of health; BPHN: Block primary health nurse; BSI: Block sanitary inspector; SWO: Social welfare officer; HA: Health assistant; M: Male; F: Female; ANM: Auxiliary nurse midwife)

Additional manpower which may be mobilized from external sources:

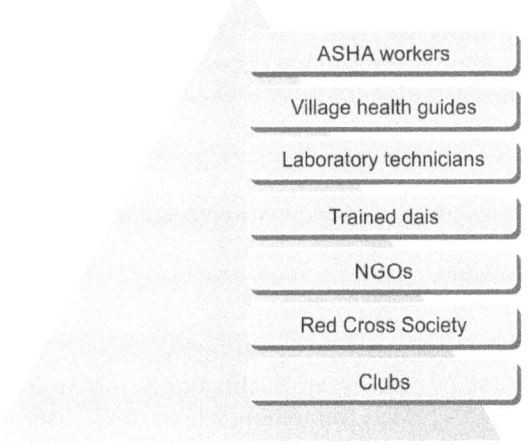

Additional manpower resources

(NGOs: Nongovernmental organizations)

Materials

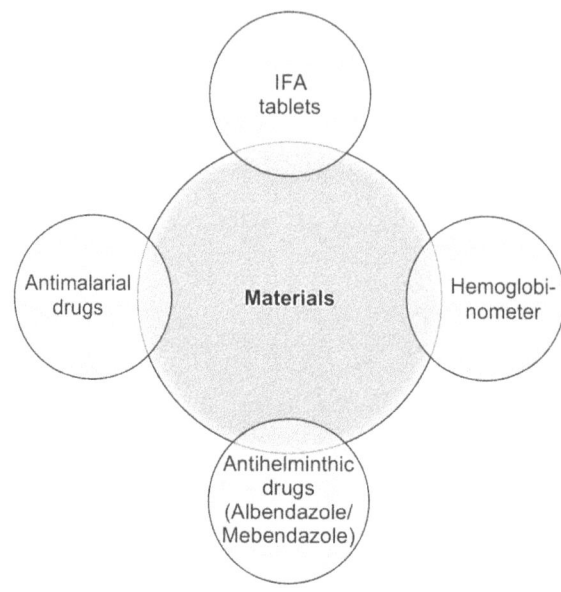

(IFA: Iron and folic acid)

Money

An action plan is given to the CMOH for sanctioning a fund.

Writing up the Formulated Plan

❖ Detailed information about the plan
❖ Detailed information about the resources (needed and available)
❖ Interventions to be taken.

Fixing Priorities

Areas with high numbers of pregnant anemic women should be prioritized at first.

Programming and Implementation

Short-term measures

Intensified National Iron Plus Initiative (I-NIPI) of the Anemia Mukt Bharat campaign is a recently launched program by Ministry of Health and Family Welfare, Government of India in April, 2018 under POSHAN (PM's Overarching scheme for holistic nourishment) abhiyaan.

Beneficiaries	Intervention/dose	Regime
Children of 6–59 months	1 mL of IFA syrup containing 20 mg of elemental iron and 100 µg of folic acid	Biweekly throughout the period 6–60 months of age and deworming for children 12 months and above
School children 5–10 years	Tablets of 45 mg elemental iron and 400 µg of folic acid	Weekly throughout the period 5–10 years of age and biannual deworming
Adolescents of 10–19 years	60 mg elemental iron and 500 µg of folic acid	Weekly throughout the period 10–19 years of age and biannual deworming

Contd..

Contd..

Beneficiaries	Intervention/dose	Regime
Pregnant and lactating women	60 mg elemental iron and 500 µg of folic acid	1 tab daily starting from 14th week of gestation, continued throughout pregnancy (minimum 180 days during pregnancy) and to be continued for 180 days postpartum: a total of 1 year
Women in reproductive age group	60 mg elemental iron and 500 µg of folic acid	Weekly throughout the reproductive period

Educate the pregnant women and all other vulnerable groups of the population about:
1. The importance of iron to prevent anemia.
2. Dietary changes:
   - Liver/meat/poultry/fish (Contain mainly heme iron)
   - Cereals/green leafy vegetables/legumes/nuts, etc. (non-heme iron)
   - Indian vegetable foods contain large amounts of inhibitors of iron absorption (phytate and oxalate mainly) so their bioavailability are poor
   - Vitamin C enhances iron absorption from these vegetable foods in the stomach by converting Fe^{3+} ion to Fe^{2+} ion. So educate people to eat fresh fruits that contain vitamin C (Amla/Guava/Cabbage/Amaranth/Cauliflower/Orange, etc.).
3. Antihelminthic drugs:
   - Ensure adequate supply of antihelminthic drugs as hookworm infestation is an important cause of anemia in rural areas
   - Educate people about general symptoms of anemia so that they can immediately come to the nearby health facility to treat them:
     - Pallor of eye/lips/tongue
     - Light yellow appearance of skin
     - Puffy face
     - Ankle edema
     - Variable symptoms of progressing anemia: Weakness/palpitation/dizziness/fainting/headache/dyspnea, etc.
4. IUD users are highly susceptible to chronic blood loss. So, they should be one important target for the campaign and should receive IFA tablets on a regular and uninterrupted basis.
5. Adequate laboratory technicians should be recruited to screen a significant proportion of the pregnant women in the locality for anemia.

IEC campaign
- All the above educational measures should be told in several IEC campaigns with the help of:
  - Banners
    - Festoons
    - Posters
    - Short play
  - Mass media should be utilized to create awareness among people. Short play can be broadcasted on local television and radio channels
  - Short ads can be published in local newspapers informing the people:
    - Danger signs of anemia
    - Danger of anemia in pregnant women and her child
    - What the health services are available in the locality to prevent and treat anemia.

Long-term measures

❖ Additional laboratory technicians should be employed step by step to continue screening for anemia in pregnant women
❖ Continuation of uninterrupted supply of IFA tablets and antihelminthic drugs
❖ Continue educating health workers about danger signs of anemia and transmit the knowledge to the local population (especially to newly pregnant women) through them
❖ Maintenance and expansion of diagnostic and screening infrastructure.

Monitoring and Surveillance

❖ IFA coverage
❖ Proportion of anemic pregnant mother in the community
❖ Search and investigation of each case of anemia in children.

Report

A proper and detailed report should be prepared by the BMOH and sent to higher authorities for further actions to be taken.

DUTIES OF BMOH IN PREVENTING INCIDENCE OF ACCIDENTS IN A BLOCK

1. **Your BPHC is situated by the side of a busy highway. Cases of road traffic accidents are common. Describe the measures you would take as BMOH to reduce the problem.** (12)

Situation Analysis

a. *Verification of situation* is done by analyzing the data from records of hospital, subcenter, PHC, etc. This includes:
   – Actual number of all accidents
   – In depth surveys to identify the *chain of events* that had led to accidents. This includes:
      - Environmental condition at the time of accident
      - Condition of the car and the driver
      - Condition of the road, etc.
b. *Estimation of the magnitude of the problem*: There are two factors affecting road traffic accidents (RTA):
   1. Human factors:
      - Age
      - Sex
      - Education
      - Medical conditions (sudden illness/heart attack/dizziness/fatigue, etc.)
      - Psychological factors
      - Lack of body protection (helmet/safety belt, etc.)
      - Alcohol and drug abuse.
   2. Environmental factors:
      - Related to road (defects in road/bad material/poor lighting, etc.)
      - Related to vehicle (high speed/poorly maintained cars/overloading, etc.)
      - Related to driver (poor experience)
      - Bad weather.

After finding out the proper causative factor(s) responsible for most of the incidents of RTA, it becomes easy to mobilize the resource accordingly to the causative factors in decreasing order.

Identification of Available Resources and Whether Additional Resources are Available/Needed

Manpower

1. Available internal resources:

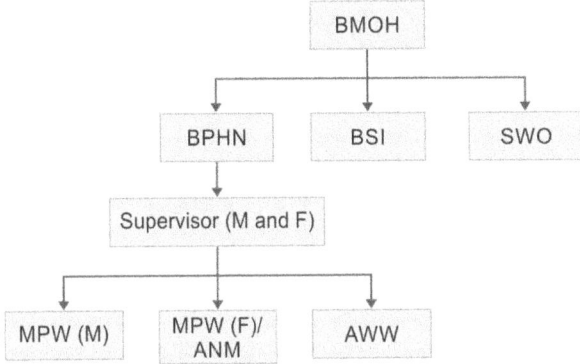

(BMOH: Block medical officer of health; BPHN: Block primary health nurse; BSI: Block sanitary inspector; SWO: Social welfare officer; MPW: Multipurpose worker; M: Male; F: Female; ANM: Auxiliary nurse midwife; AWW: Anganwadi worker)

2. Additional resources that can be utilized:

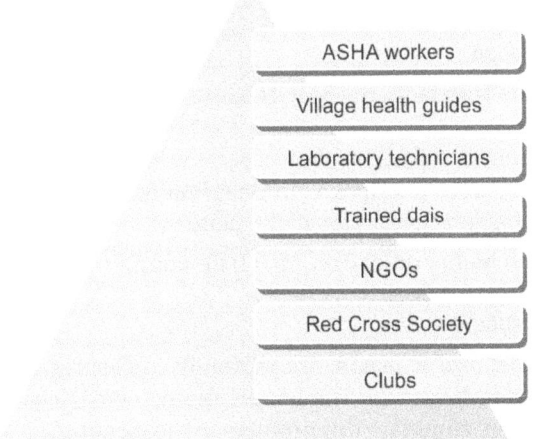

Additional manpower resources

(NGOs: Nongovernmental organizations)

Materials

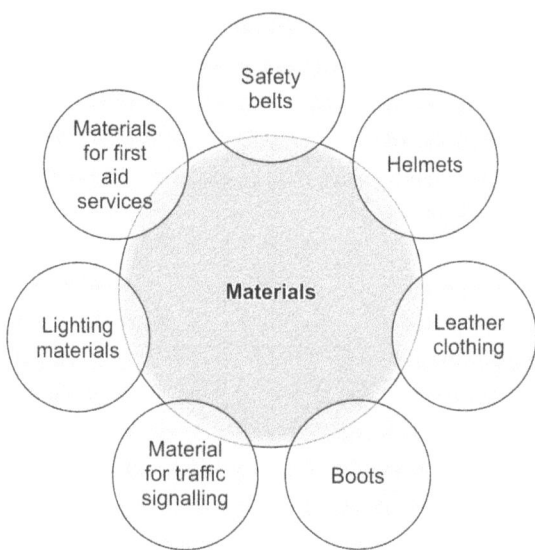

Money

An action plan is given to the CMOH for sanctioning a fund.

Establishment of Objectives and Goals

❖ The objective is set to improve the condition of the road, traffic signaling system and proper lighting of the road to decrease the incidents of road traffic accidents
❖ The goal is set to reduce the incident of RTA and to decrease mortality and morbidity associated with RTA.

Writing up the Formulated Plan

After considering all the above facts, the BMOH has to write up a precise, accurate and effective plan, which will include:
❖ Every major and minor detail of the plan
❖ Details about the resources (manpower/money/material used)
❖ Interventions to be taken at every step of the plan.

This plan is submitted to higher officials (CMOH) for approval and funding.

Programming and Implementation

As *accidents are multifactorial in origin,* the preventive measures cannot be completed with efforts from the side of a BMOH only. The BMOH should effectively establish an *intersectoral coordination* to completely eliminate this problem in the locality.

Short-term measures

Primary care:
❖ It includes initial management of trauma and emergency care, which should start at the site of accident, continued during transportation and should be completed by admission of the patient to the emergency department of a hospital
❖ To save the life of patients, there should be an Accident Services Organization/Agency with 1 fully equipped trauma care hospital at every major city.

Promotion of safety measures:
Through use of posters/banners/festoons/advertisement/short play/drama with active involvement of local newspaper and local television channels, people should be educated about proper use of effective safety measures:
❖ Use of safety belts and helmets
❖ Use of door locks and highly resistant wind screen globe
❖ Not more than 2 persons should be allowed on 2 wheelers.

Strict enforcement of laws:
❖ Driving tests
❖ Medical fitness tests
❖ Enforcement of speed limits at vulnerable points
❖ Compulsory wearing of helmets and seat belts
❖ Check of blood alcohol concentration at accident prone zones by roadside breath analysis. In case of blood alcohol concentration >0.05 g/dL, punishments should be given at the point
❖ Periodic medical check-up of drivers >55 years of age
❖ Regular inspection of vehicles.

Health education
❖ It is correctly said that, *"If accident is a disease, education is its vaccine".*
   The false belief that accidents are inevitable should be eliminated from the common people. They should be educated that every accident arises from a set of correlated etiological factors and if proper measures are taken effectively, accidents can largely be prevented
❖ Safety education must start at the level of school children
❖ The drivers should be trained properly in proper maintenance of vehicles, periodic check-up of themselves and their vehicle, safe driving, traffic rules
❖ Vehicles should not be overloaded
❖ Alcohols and other drugs like sedative-hypnotics should better be avoided before and at the time of driving.

Long-term measures
❖ Roads should be broadened
❖ Old and poorly maintained vehicles should be phased out serially
❖ Speed breakers should be placed at regular intervals in national highways
❖ Signboards showing *"Drive slow"* should be placed at vulnerable points like school crossings
❖ Proper lightening of the roads should be done for prevention of night-accidents
❖ Pedestrian lane should be separated.

Rehabilitation
The aim is to prevent/reduce/compensate disability/handicap.

Monitoring and Evaluation

The BMOH should himself supervise the monitoring process properly by taking account of:
❖ No. of accidents after implementation measures
❖ Evaluation of danger zones at periodic intervals.

Reporting

A proper and detailed report should be prepared by the BMOH and sent to higher authorities for further actions to be taken.

DUTIES OF BMOH IN REDUCING POPULARITY OF QUACKS IN A BLOCK

1. **As a BMOH you know that in certain villages, people prefer quacks rather than your service. Should you be concerned? If yes, why? What will you do about it?** (4 + 8)

It is a well-known problem in our country that some villagers prefer quack rather than the existing health services and infrastructure provided by the government. The reasons behind this situation are as follows:

❖ Some villages are at a remote distance from the PHC/subcenters which make the villagers make the quack as a quick choice in case of emergencies (*Communication gap*)
❖ The villagers get the quacks for 24 hours as they live there and share the same life of the villagers
❖ It seems to the poor villagers that treatment by quacks is quite cost-effective than the existing health services
❖ Some people prefer quacks because of the ill-behavior and ignorance they got from a previous visit to a government health facility.

The preference to quacks by villagers is of concern because:

❖ Quacks are not medically educated, so in most of the cases (especially in critical situations), their wrong treatment makes the life of patient endangered. The patient, when come to the health facility, is often in complicated states, which makes the treatment difficult
❖ Because of their illiteracy, they are not aware of the conditions where referral is of utmost importance
❖ In the eye of the villagers, the cost of treatment may be less with quacks, but ultimately it leads to more damage to the health of patient and more cost of treatment.

Duty of a BMOH to Tackle Such a Problem

A. *Problem analysis*: As a BMOH, one should first fight the inborn causes of preference to the quacks in a locality, which are:
   – Misconception
   – Illiteracy
   – Communication gap
   – Ignorance
   – Poverty.

B. *Identification of available resources and whether additional resources are available/needed:*

Manpower

Available internal resources:

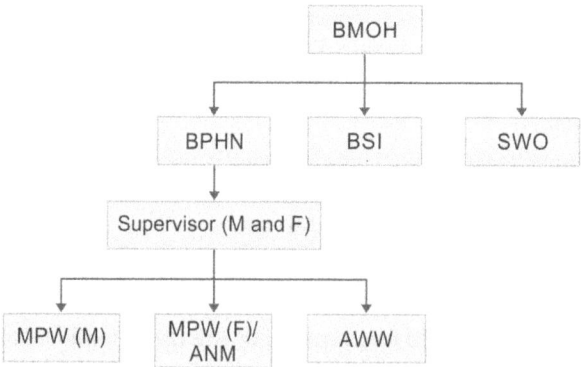

(BMOH: Block medical officer of health; BPHN: Block primary health nurse; BSI: Block sanitary inspector; SWO: Social welfare officer; MPW: Multipurpose worker; M: Male; F: Female; ANM: Auxiliary nurse midwife; AWW: Anganwadi worker)

Additional resources that can be utilized:

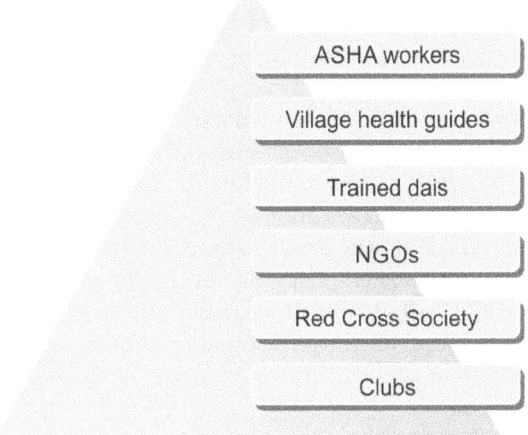

Additional manpower resources
(NGOs: Nongovernmental organizations)

Money
An action plan is given to the CMOH for sanctioning a fund.

Defining the Objectives

The main objective is to successfully promote an IEC campaign in the community to:
❖ Educate the whole "susceptible" population about dangers of treatment by quacks
❖ To educate the people about the health facilities government is providing them.

Setting a Goal

To get most of the cases of the community to the nearest health facility and to educate all the quacks in the locality for common diseases.

Writing up the Formulated Plan

The formulated plan to fight the quack problem in the block, the details of the formulated plan should be written with:
❖ Detailed roadmap to achieve the defined target
❖ Detailed discussion about the resources required—man, money, material, education to the manpower required for the IEC campaign, etc.

Programming and Implementation

Involve mass media of the locality (radio/local TV channels/local newspapers) to deliver the following messages:
❖ Quacks are not medically educated, so they do not know the actual treatment protocols and there is a good chance that whatever the treatment they deliver to the community be wrong and there are high risks to the health of the patient

❖ If the people go to the quacks for emergency conditions, which the quacks are unable to handle, there are high risks of getting permanent damages/impairments and also chances of being handicapped and death is high

❖ Quacks actually delay the proper treatment of the patient, so when the patient actually comes to the nearby healthcare provider, he may present with complications/advanced phase; which are hard to manage at that time even by a healthcare professional

❖ If it seems to the community that quacks are decreasing the cost of the treatment, then they are to be educated that actually this concept is wrong because after the damages to the patient the quack has done, when he comes to the health facility, the cost of treatment increases highly due to the additional damages done by the quack/complication of the condition

❖ Various types of communication strategies can be utilized to effectively deliver the message to the community like banners, posters, festoons, short drama, street play, advertisements, etc.

❖ Health workers of the PHC/subcenters should be educated so that they can disseminate the knowledge about the services that the government is providing to the community to ensure community participation in effective utilization of the basic health services like:
  – Immunization program
  – Antenatal, natal and postnatal check-up of pregnant mothers
  – Free transportation of pregnant mothers to the FRU in case of any complications associated with pregnancy
  – Supplementary nutrition programs
  – Janani Suraksha Yojana (JSY)/Janani Shishu Suraksha Karyakram (JSSK), etc.
  – Nutritional deficiency prevention programs
  – Family planning and family welfare programs
  – Treatment of common diseases like cough and cold/diarrhea/ARI/malaria/tuberculosis, etc.

❖ Mothers meeting/school camp, etc. should be organized to aware the mothers and children about the impact and prevention of the problem regarding quacks

❖ For some people the preference to quacks comes from the ill behavior they got in any of their visits to the nearby health facility. Those health workers should be identified and strictly warned and if they are determined not to change, they should be punished

❖ The higher authority should be informed if the main cause is a communication gap between the villagers and the health facility. There should be ideas how this gap can be eliminated (like establishing new PHC and subcenters/establishing effective transportation systems/ training of village health guides, etc.).

Monitoring

The BMOH should himself monitor the effectiveness of the IEC campaigning program. If the results are not satisfactory, he should investigate the cause of failure of the campaign and take necessary steps thereafter.

Report

A proper and detailed report should be prepared by the BMOH and sent to higher authorities (CMOH) for further actions to be taken.

Chapter
4

Short Notes

Authors' Note

In this chapter, we have given all the short notes important for university examinations. For the less commonly asked short notes, we have given a separate heading "Try Yourself" in the content, which you may read from any of the standard textbook of community medicine.

MAN AND DISEASE

Family Physician

Family physician is the specialist who provides comprehensive and continuous primary health care to all members of the family.

Roles and Main Functions of a Family Physician

A. *Patient care role*:
   - Comprehensive health care
   - Primary health care
   - Continuous care (womb to tomb)
   - Referral services
   - First aid
   - Medicolegal services.
B. *Coordinating role*: Between patient and their families, with hospital specialists to whom the patient is referred for specific care, as well as with all community agencies, welfare agencies, national health program, developmental program, etc.
C. *Community care role*: Identify problems and felt needs of the community and take necessary actions, in order to equip the community so that they can demand and utilize appropriate health and allied interventions like water supply, sanitation, nutrition, reproductive and child health services.

Social Medicine

Definition

Social medicine is the study of man as a social being in his total environment comprising physical, biological and social environment.

Its focus is on the health of the community as a whole.

Meaning of Social Medicine (According to McKeown)

Social medicine is an expression of humanitarian tradition in medicine and people read into it any interpretation consistent with their own aspirations and interests.

In broad sense	In restricted sense
• Care of patients • Prevention of disease • Administration of medical services • Any subject in the extensive field of health and welfare	• A body of knowledge embodied in epidemiology • The study of medical needs or medical care of society

❖ *Nomenclature*: The term coined by Jules Guerin.
❖ Concept first developed by Neumann and Virchow.
❖ *Social medicine deals with*:
  – Understanding how social and economic conditions impact health, disease and the practice of medicine and
  – Fostering conditions in which this understanding can lead to a healthier society.

Components

Social anatomy, physiology, pathology and therapy.

Application

❖ Development of epidemiological methods
❖ Their application to the investigations of disease.

Limitation

Social medicine was criticized because it was mostly virtually isolated from the service world and confined mostly to academic study of health services and chronic disease.

Significance

The field of social medicine is most commonly addressed today by public health efforts to understand what are known as social determinants of health.

Community Diagnosis

Definition

Community diagnosis generally refers to the identification and quantification of health problems in a community as a whole in terms of mortality and morbidity rates and ratios, and identification of their correlates for the purpose of defining those at risk or those in need of health care.

Aim: To provide preventive and promotive interventions to the community.

Method of collection of data from the community:
❖ Discussion with local community decision maker, community member, health and health-related personnel
❖ Observational visit to the community: To observe environmental situation
❖ Sample surveys and scrutiny of health service records
❖ Transect walk.

(*Transect walk* is defined as an exploratory walk undertaken by the team along with local community member to observe, discuss and understand local matters with them, e.g. sanitary measures system, water source, exposure to social life and the culture, customs of the community members).

Type of Information to be Collected
- ❖ Demographic characteristics
- ❖ Mortality and morbidity
- ❖ Socioeconomic factors
- ❖ Physical environmental factors
- ❖ Health problems felt by the community.

Tools of Data Collection
- ❖ Interview schedule
- ❖ Questionnaire
- ❖ Observational checklists.

Methods of Data Collection
- ❖ Survey
- ❖ Discussion
- ❖ Observation
- ❖ Record analysis
- ❖ Interview
- ❖ Clinical examination.

Significance
Community diagnosis helps to prioritize the health problems and implement control measures.

CONCEPT OF HEALTH AND DISEASE

Quality of Life

Definition
WHO (1997) defines Quality of Life as individuals' perception of their position in life in the context of the culture and value systems in which they live and in relation to their goals, expectations, standards and concerns.

Difference between Quality of Life and Level of Living
Quality of life comprises one individual's subjective evaluation about "well-being" and level of living comprises some objective criteria of the concept of well-being.

Measurement of "Quality of Life"
Quality of life is measured by means of some indices. The most important of those are:
- ❖ Physical quality of life index (PQLI) and
- ❖ Human development index (HDI).

Physical Quality of Life Index (PQLI)

(Mnemonic: ILL-1)

Components of PQLI	Upper limit	Lower limit
Infant mortality	100	0
Life expectancy at age 1	100	0
Literacy	100	0

So, PQLI also has an upper limit of 100 and a lower limit of 0.

India: PQLI-65

Note:

❖ PQLI is a subjective component.

❖ PQLI does not calculate economic growth of a country (PQLI does not consider income) but it measures the results of social/economic/political policies undertaken by a country.

Human Development Index (HDI)

How to calculate HDI:

Dimension	A long and healthy life	Knowledge	A decent standard of living
Indicator	Life expectancy at birth	Mean years of schooling and expected years of schooling	GNI per capita in purchasing power parity [PPP] in US $
Dimension index	Life expectancy index	Education index	GNI index

HDI = (Life expectancy index × Education index × GNI index)⅓

How to calculate dimension indices:

$$\text{Dimension index} = \frac{(\text{Actual value} - \text{Minimum value})}{(\text{Maximum value} - \text{Minimum value})}$$

The "Maximum value" refers to the highest values observed in between the years 1980–2011 in one of the countries. The lowest values are set as follows:

Dimension	Minimum values
Life expectancy	20
Mean years of schooling	0
Expected years of schooling	0
Combined education index	0
Per capita income [PPP US $]	100

Interpretation

❖ The HDI ranges from 0 to 1; 1 being the maximum and 0 the minimum

❖ HDI comparison may be done among various countries; a country with a high HDI indicates a high quality of life.

Physical Quality of Life Index (PQLI)

Write from the previous question.

Human Development Index (HDI)

Definition

HDI is defined as a composite index combining indicators representing 3 dimensions:
1. Longevity (Life expectancy at birth)
2. Knowledge (Mean years of schooling and expected years of schooling, it does not consider adult literacy rate) and
3. Income [Gross national income (GNI) per capita in purchasing power parity in US $].

How to calculate HDI:

Dimension	A long and healthy life	Knowledge	A decent standard of living
Indicator	Life expectancy at birth	Mean years of schooling and expected years of schooling	GNI per capita in purchasing power parity [PPP] in US $
Dimension index	Life expectancy index	Education index	GNI index
Calculation	HDI = [Life expectancy index × Education index × GNI index] ⅓		

How to calculate dimension indices:

$$\text{Dimension index} = \frac{(\text{Actual value} - \text{Minimum value})}{(\text{Maximum value} - \text{Minimum value})}$$

The "Maximum value" refers to the highest values observed in between the years 1980–2011 in one of the countries. The lowest values are set as follows:

Dimension	Minimum values
Life expectancy	20
Mean years of schooling	0
Expected years of schooling	0
Combined education index	0
Per capita income (PPP US $)	100

Interpretation

❖ The HDI ranges from 0 to 1; 1 being the maximum and 0 the minimum
❖ HDI comparison may be done among various countries; a country with a high HDI indicates a high quality of life.
❖ According to the value of HDI, countries may be grouped into 4 categories:

HDI value of countries	Interpretation
>0.8	Very high HDI
0.7– 0.8	High HDI
0.5– 0.7	Medium HDI
<0.5	Low HDI

❖ The ultimate goal of a country should be to achieve a HDI of 1.0
❖ India has a medium HDI value (0.645), rank 131th out of 189 countries (UNDP report, 2020).

Disability-Adjusted Life Year

Definition

The disability-adjusted life year (DALY) is a measure of overall disease burden, expressed as the number of years lost due to ill-health, disability or early death.

Development

Originally developed by Harvard University for the World Bank in 1990, the WHO subsequently adopted the method in 1996.

According to WHO: It "extends the concept of potential years of life lost due to premature death...to include equivalent years of 'healthy' life lost by virtue of being in states of poor health or disability".

In doing so, mortality and morbidity are combined into a single, common metric.

Calculation/Measurement

1 DALY = 1 year of healthy life lost

$$\text{Formula: DALY = YLL + YLD}$$

YLL = 'Years of Life Lost' measured by →

No. of deaths at each age × The expected remaining years of life (according to the global standard life expectancy)

YLD = 'Years Lived with Disability' measured by →

No. of incident cases due to injury and illness × Average duration of the disease and a weighing factor reflecting the severity of the disease on a scale from 0 (perfect health) → 1 (dead)

The value of weighing factor depends on age.

Commonly years lived as a young adult is valued more highly than years spent as a young child or older adults.

Importance

1. DALY is the best indicator of burden of disease.
2. DALY will be increased by both mortality and disability
3. If a disease is affecting younger age group we will lose more DALY.
4. DALY can be used to compare effectiveness between 2 interventions.

Example: Suppose in case of road traffic accident if use of helmets can prevent 40 DALY and if use of seatbelt can prevent 20 DALY, then use of helmets will be regarded as better intervention than seatbelts.

Note: Japanese life expectancy statistics are used as the standard for measuring premature death, as the Japanese have the longest life expectancies.

Criticism

DALYs are essentially an economic measure of human productive capacity for the affected individual, and consequently do not capture other aspects of diseases, such as emotional effects on the individual, friends and families.

For instance mentally-ill people are sometimes able to continue working normally whilst suffering great distress.

Millennium Development Goals (MDGs)

Introduction

The Millennium Development Goals (MDGs) are 8 international development goals that were established following the Millennium Summit of the United Nations in 2000, following the adoption of the United Nations Millennium Declaration.

Countries Involved

All 189 United Nations member states at the time (there are 193 currently) and at least 23 international organizations committed to help achieve the Millennium Development Goals by 2015.

Global Challenge

- ❖ Nearly half the MDGs relate to health and nutrition
- ❖ The targets cover a large share of the burden of disease and deaths among poor people
- ❖ Illness, death, malnutrition impede economic growth and contribute to income poverty.
- ❖ Baseline year for MDG: 1990
- ❖ Deadline year for MDG: 2015.

Goals

The goals follow:
1. To eradicate extreme poverty and hunger
2. To achieve universal primary education
3. To promote gender equality and empowering women
4. To reduce child mortality rates
5. To improve maternal health
6. To combat HIV/AIDS, malaria, and other diseases
7. To ensure environmental sustainability
8. To develop a global partnership for development
   - Goal 4, 5, and 6 are "directly health related".
   - Goal 2 and 3 "do not pertain to health".
   - 3 out of 8 goals, 8 out of 18 targets required to achieve them and 18 out of 48 indicators of progress are directly health related.

Reasons for Short Fall

- ❖ Availability
  - Adequacy of supply: Not satisfactory
  - Periodicity: A bottleneck
  - Quality of equipment/drugs: Need improvement.
- ❖ Accessibility
  - Remote areas: Neglected
  - Gender and socioeconomic discrimination
  - Round the clock services: Questionable
  - Accessibility of government services in urban areas.

- ❖ Utilization
  - – Lack of awareness about services
  - – Irregularity of services
  - – Quality not always maintained.
- ❖ Adequate coverage
  - – Dropouts: A common factor.
- ❖ Effective coverage
  - – Skills of workers always not up to the desired level.

Costs and Benefits

- ❖ Existing system takes into account supplies, staff and minimal on infrastructures
- ❖ Five country assessments and estimates indicate that annual public investments or MDGs will be 80 US $ per person in 2005–2006 scaling up to 124 US $ in 2015.

Epidemiological Triad

Introduction

Epidemiological triad is a model developed to explain the mode of causation of disease insufficiently explained by 'germ theory model'.

Definition

Epidemiological triad consists of an external agent; a host and an environment in which host and agent are brought together, causing the disease to occur in the host in equilibrium.

Explanation of the Model

- ❖ A state of equilibrium occurs between the agent, host and environment
- ❖ When a disease agent reaches a susceptible host in favorable environment it results in the disease state
- ❖ When a disease agent reaches a semi-resistant host and when the agent is not much virulent, then it results in carrier state
- ❖ It also explains that some persons do not suffer from the disease even though they harbor the pathogens because an equilibrium is established between host and agent in fully resistant host.

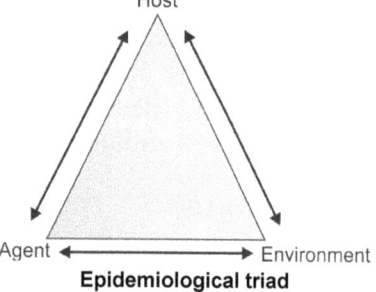

Epidemiological triad

According to this model agent, host and environmental factors are as follows:

Agent factors	
1. Biological	Microorganisms
2. Physical	Temperature, radiation, trauma and others
3. Chemical	Acids, alkalis, poisons, tobacco and others

Contd...

Contd...

Agent factors	
4. Nutrient	Protein, fat, carbohydrate deficiency or excess
5. Physiological	Hormone, enzymes, etc.
6. Mechanical	Friction, pressure, etc.
7. Social	Poverty, etc.
Host factors	
1. Demographic characteristics	Age, sex, ethnicity
2. Biological characteristics	Genetic factor, blood level of important constituent, blood enzyme, immunological factors
3. Lifestyle factor	Smoking, alcoholism, drug abuse
4. Literacy level	↑ Literacy level →↓ Disease
5. Marital status	Ca cervix more common in married woman
6. Income	Low socioeconomic status →↑ Infectious disease High socioeconomic status →↑ Noncommunicable disease
7. Occupation	Pneumoconiosis
Environmental factors	
1. Physical environment	Air, water, soil, etc.
2. Biological environment	Plant, animal, insect, etc.
3. Psychological environment	Depression, anxiety, etc.

Significance

The mission of an epidemiologist is to break at least one of the sides of the epidemiological triad, disrupting the connection between the environment, the host, and the agent; thus stopping the continuation of disease.

The Iceberg Concept of Disease

Introduction

According to this concept, disease in a community may be compared with an iceberg. The tip of the iceberg is only visible whereas rest is submerged, only people manifesting clinical signs and symptoms are thought to be diseased.

Explanation

❖ The floating tip of the iceberg represents what the physician sees in the community, i.e. *clinical cases*
❖ The vast submerged portion of the iceberg represents the hidden mass of the disease, i.e. *latent, inapparent, presymptomatic* and *undiagnosed* cases and carriers in the community.
❖ The "waterline" represents the demarcation between apparent and inapparent disease.

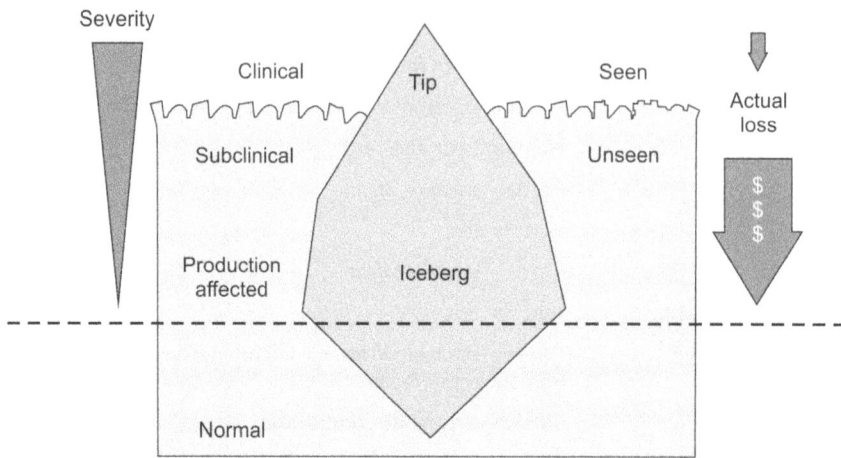

Schematic diagram showing Iceberg phenomenon of diseases

Significance of the Iceberg Phenomenon

❖ In some diseases (e.g. hypertension, diabetes, anemia, malnutrition, mental illness) the unknown morbidity (i.e. the submerged portion of the iceberg) far exceeds the known morbidity

❖ The clinician is concerned with the '*tip of the iceberg*' and the epidemiologist with the '*hidden portion of the iceberg*'

❖ *Screening is done for hidden portion of the iceberg whereas diagnosis is done for tip of the iceberg*

❖ Iceberg phenomenon is not shown by measles, tetanus, rubella, rabies (mnemonic: MTR2).

Natural History of Disease

Definition

It is the sequence of events in a disease from the earliest stage to its termination as recovery, disability or death in absence of any intervention in form of treatment or prevention.

Methods

Natural history of disease is established by cohort, cross-sectional and retrospective studies.

Components

Prepathogenesis phase:

It is a phase before the onset of disease in man. Man yet not involved but is in the "midst of disease". In this phase:

❖ Causative factors are present in the environment (Risk factors are before man)

❖ Person is susceptible to the risk of disease occurrence

❖ Due to interaction among the components of epidemiological triad host enters into the pathogenesis phase from prepathogenic phase.

Agent → Infective agent
Host → Man
Environment → Route of transmission

Pathogenesis phase:
❖ This phase begins with entry of disease agent into human host (Risk factor is into man).
❖ Sequence of events in pathogenesis phase:
   – Infection → Disease → Complication → Death

Sequence	Measured by	Definition
Infection	Infectivity	Invasion and multiplication of agent in body
Disease	Pathogenicity	Ability to produce clinical sign and symptoms
Complication and Death	Virulence	Ability to produce complication and death (given by Case Fatality Rate)

❖ Incubation period: In this phase there will be subclinical changes.
❖ After this, disease agent multiplies and induce tissue and physiologic response.
❖ Sequence of event of natural history of disease

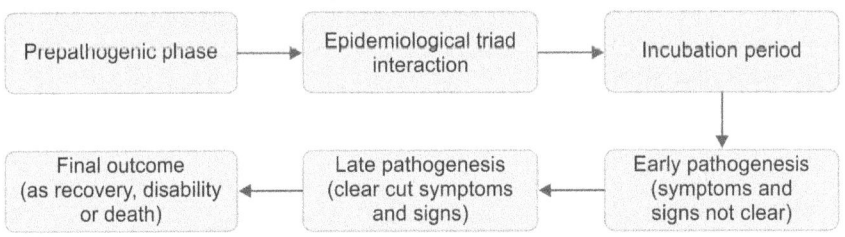

Sequence of events of natural history of disease

Sentinel Surveillance

Definition

A surveillance system in which a designated group of *reporting sources* (e.g. hospitals, agencies) agrees to provide complete, timely and regular reporting of all cases of one or more notifiable conditions to higher authority.

Aim

❖ To identify the missing cases
❖ Supplementing the notified cases.

Principle

The sentinel data is extrapolated on the entire population to estimate the disease prevalence in the total population.

Type of Prevention

It is a type of secondary prevention.

Components

Interested and competent physician (or institution) in selected areas are given responsibility to report the cases of the disease in their areas.

Advantages

❖ Reporting biases are minimized
❖ Feedback of the information to the providers is simplified
❖ Provides more valuable and detailed information than would be obtained from traditional notification system.

Example:

❖ Use of health practitioners to monitor trends of a health event in a population
❖ Sentinel surveillance is done in National AIDS Control Program (NACP) whereas STD clinics, ANC clinics are sentinel sites to monitor trends.

Healthy Lifestyles

❖ Lifestyle is often denoted by the phrase "the way people live"
❖ Considerable evidences have been accumulated which indicates that there is an association between health and lifestyles
❖ So, lifestyles are of 2 types:
   a. Those which are *harmful to health*:
      - Smoking
      - Alcoholism
      - Drug addiction
      - Poor sanitation
      - Poor personal hygiene
      - Poor nutritional habits
      - Customs and religious beliefs those are detrimental to health, etc.
   b. Those which *promote health*:
      - Adequate nutrition
      - Enough sleep
      - Sufficient physical activity, etc.
❖ Health requires the promotion of healthy lifestyle.
   – The achievement of optimum health demands adoption of healthy lifestyle.

EPIDEMIOLOGY

Case Fatality Rate

Definition

Case fatality rate is the proportion of deaths within a designated population of "cases" (people with a medical condition), over the course of the disease.

Formula

$$Case\ fatality\ rate = \frac{Total\ no.\ of\ deaths\ from\ a\ specific\ disease\ in\ a\ specific\ time\ period}{Total\ no.\ of\ cases\ of\ that\ disease\ during\ the\ same\ time\ period} \times 100$$

A CFR is conventionally expressed as % and represents a measure of risk.

Relation between Case Fatality Rate and Survival Rate

CFR is the "complement of survival rate".
CFR = 1 - survival rate.

Applicability

CFRs are most often used for diseases with discrete, limited time courses, such as outbreaks of acute infections.

Significance

❖ Represents the killing power of the disease
❖ It is closely related to virulence of organism
❖ It can be used to measure benefits of new therapy.

Limitation

❖ Time interval not specified
❖ Not useful in chronic infections
❖ Variable in same disease.

Epidemic
Nomenclature

"Epi" = "upon or above" and "Demos" = "people"

Definition

Epidemic is defined as occurrence of number of cases of a disease 'clearly in excess of normal expectancy'.

How to Confirm an Epidemic?

❖ "Normal expectancy/Endemic frequency" is derived by looking at average of number of cases of the disease in previous 3–5 years in that geographical area
❖ If normal expectancy is 0, even 1 case can be considered epidemic, e.g. yellow fever in India.
❖ Statistical expression:
  Epidemic is confirmed when:

  Epidemic frequency ≥ Endemic frequency + 2 Standard errors

❖ Reoccurrence of an eliminated or eradicated disease in a population is considered as epidemic [as Normal expectancy (NE) = 0].

Cause of Epidemic

❖ Increased virulence
❖ Changes in host susceptibility to the infectious agent
❖ Though epidemic disease is not always required to be contagious, West Nile fever, obesity epidemic, etc.

Epidemic Curve

It is the graphical representation of time distribution of epidemic cases.

Provides information about:

❖ Onset of epidemic
❖ Duration of epidemic
❖ Mode of reaching the peak of epidemic
❖ Timing of reaching the peak.

Types of Epidemic

Types	Subtypes	Features with example
Common source epidemic	Single exposure/ point source epidemic	• Sharp rise and sharp fall in number of cases • Clustering of cases in narrow interval of time • All cases develop within one incubation period Example: Food poisoning, measles, chickenpox
	Continuous/ multiple exposure epidemic	• Sharp rise in number of cases • Fall in number of cases interrupted by secondary waves Example: Prostitute in gonorrhea outbreak, contaminated well in a village
Propagated epidemic	Person-to-person Arthropod vector Animal reservoir	• Gradual rise • Gradual fall (tail off) • Transmission continues till number of susceptibles is depleted/ susceptibles are no longer exposed to infected individuals Example: TB, HIV
Slow/modern epidemic		Few noncommunicable diseases Example: Obesity

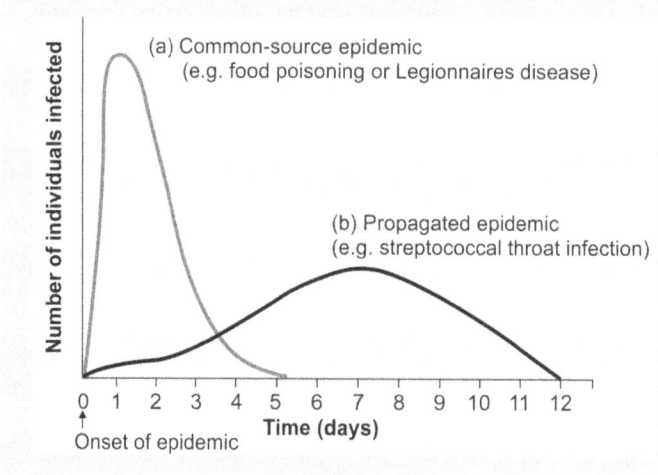

Epidemic curve

Application of Epidemic Curve

❖ To study time relationship with exposure to a suspected source
❖ To find out type of epidemic based on cyclic/seasonal pattern of particular infection.

Carriers

Definition

A carrier is defined as, "an infected person or animal that harbors specific infectious agent in the absence of discernible clinical disease and serves as a potential source of infection to others".

Elements of Carrier State

The elements of a carrier state are as follows:
- Disease agent is present in the body of the individual
- Any recognizable symptom and sign is absent
- Continuous shedding of the infectious disease agent may occur through excretions and discharges, which may act as potential source of infection for other susceptible individuals.

Example: "Typhoid Mary" was a classical example.

Types of Carrier

According to type:
- Incubatory
- Convalescent
- Healthy.

According to duration:
- Temporary
- Chronic.

According to portal of exit:
- Urinary
- Intestinal
- Respiratory, etc.

Discussion about Different Types of Carriers

Type	Description	Example
According to type		
Incubatory	They shed the infectious agent during the incubation period	Measles
Convalescent	They shed the infectious agent during the period of convalescence (recovery)	Typhoid
Healthy	They are those subclinical cases, who never experienced the disease but acting as carriers	Polio
According to duration		
Temporary	They shed the infectious agent for a short period of time	Cholera
Chronic	They shed the infectious agent for infinite period of time	Gonorrhea
According to portal of exit		
Urinary	Typhoid	
Intestinal	Helminthiasis	
Respiratory	Whooping cough/Common cold	

Importance of Carriers

Carriers are dangerous than cases from the epidemiological point of view, because:
- ❖ They escape recognition
- ❖ They continuously persist in the community as the individual leads a normal life
- ❖ They readily infect the susceptible individual over a wider area and a longer time under favorable conditions.

BCG Vaccine

Full name: BCG stands for Bacillus Calmette-Guérin.

Types

- ❖ Live attenuated vaccine
- ❖ Liquid (fresh) vaccine
- ❖ Freeze dried lyophilized vaccine (more stable than liquid vaccine).

How to keep it?

The vaccine is light sensitive, so it should be kept in amber colored vial.

WHO Recommended Strain

DANISH 1331; derived from *Mycobacterium bovis* and prepared by BCG lab, Guindy, Chennai.

Reconstituent

- ❖ Normal saline
- ❖ Water, if used as diluents, can cause irritation
- ❖ Reconstituted vaccine must be used within 3 hours
- ❖ Left over vaccine should be discarded.

Dosage

- ❖ Strength: 0.1 mg in 0.1 mL
- ❖ <4 weeks of age: 0.05 mL
- ❖ >4 weeks of age: 0.1 mL
- ❖ Because skin of newborn is thin, hence it may penetrate into deeper tissue and give rise to local abscess, resulting in enlarged axillary lymph nodes.

Indications

- ❖ Active immunization against TB
- ❖ Can be given in tuberculin negative patients.

Storage: 2°–8°C.

Administration

- ❖ Route—Intradermal (if given subcutaneously chance of abscess formation is more)
- ❖ Syringe—Tuberculin syringe (omega microstat syringe fitted with a 1 cm steel 26 gauge i.d. needle)

❖ Site—Just above the insertion of left deltoid (if proper positioning is not done adjacent lymph nodes may be affected)
❖ Alcohol should not be used to swab skin and vaccine must not be contaminated with antiseptic or detergent.

Age for Vaccinations

❖ At birth (for institutional deliveries)
❖ At 6 weeks (with other vaccines like OPV/DPT)
❖ Direct BCG: It is administered up to 1 year of age, without Mantoux test
❖ Indirect BCG: Beyond age of 1 year, it is recommended after prior Mantoux test.

Phenomena after Vaccinations

Sequel	Associated phenomena
Immediately	Small swelling persists for 6–8 hours, then disappears
2–3 weeks	Papule formation
5 weeks	4–8 mm diameter of papule
6–8 weeks	Breaks into shallow ulcer, seen to be covered with crust
6–12 weeks	Permanent tiny, round scar forms, typically 4–8 mm in diameter
8–14 weeks	Mantoux test becomes positive
Sometimes, this process of ulceration and healing recurs 2–3 times. The ultimate typical puckered scar is formed which remains for lifetime	
If ulceration occurs within 7 days of injection, one must report to the doctor, as it may be a sign of tuberculosis in the child	

Protective Efficacy

Disease/condition	Protective efficacy
Pulmonary TB	0%
Severe forms of TB	0–80%
Leprosy	20–40%

Protection Duration

Starts from 15 days and lasts for 15–20 years.

Complications

Local	Prolong severe inflammation (ulcer, abscess, keloid at the site of vaccination) maximum in 28 days
Regional	Axillary lymphadenitis
General	Disseminated BCG infection (<1 per million vaccinations)/osteomyelitis

Uses

❖ Protection from severe form of TB in children (however it does not protect child from adult form of TB)
❖ It also protects from:
  – TB meningitis
  – Miliary TB
❖ In treatment of carcinoma bladder.

Contraindications

❖ Patient suffering from generalized eczema
❖ Infective dermatosis
❖ Hypogammaglobulinemia
❖ Patients with history of deficient immunity (symptomatic HIV/leukemia/other congenital immune deficiency disorders)
❖ Patient undergone immunosuppressive treatment (corticosteroid/anticancer drugs)
❖ Pregnancy.

WHO Recommended Policy on BCG Vaccination in HIV

Asymptomatic HIV (+) infants in:
❖ High endemic areas: BCG can be given
❖ Low endemic areas: BCG need not to be given.

Hepatitis B Vaccine

Type: Recombinant vaccine.

Active substance: Hepatitis B surface antigen (HBsAg).

Available Formulation

❖ Monovalent formulation
❖ Fixed combination with other vaccines (DPT/IPV/Hepatitis A vaccine/Hib vaccine, etc.).

Route of administration: Intramuscular.

Site of Administration

❖ Adults: Deltoid region
❖ Children aged <2 years: Anterolateral aspect of thigh
❖ Gluteal region is not recommended due to poor seroconversion rates because of absorption of vaccine in gluteal fat rather than muscle.

Dosage

❖ Adults: 1.0 mL
❖ Children aged <10 years: 0.5 mL.

Vaccination Schedule

❖ Adults: 0, 1, 6 months
❖ In children, the schedule of HepB vaccination can be divided into 2 categories:
  1. Schedule including birth dose.
  2. Schedule excluding birth dose.

Category	Schedule*
Including birth dose	Birth dose + 6 weeks + 14 weeks
	Birth dose + 6 weeks + 10 weeks + 14 weeks
Excluding birth dose	6 weeks + 10 weeks + 14 weeks

* At 6, 10 and 14 weeks; the Hep B vaccine can be given as a monovalent formulation/as fixed combination with DPT.

❖ The minimum interval between 2 doses is 4 weeks.

Note:

❖ *In countries where the prevalence of chronic HBV infection is >8%, the first dose of Hep B vaccine should be given within 24 hours after birth to prevent perinatal transmission*

❖ In low birth weight (<2000 g) babies, the birth dose should not be counted and 3 additional doses should be given according to National Immunization Schedule

❖ The duration of protection is at least 15 years

❖ Interruption of the vaccination schedule does not require restarting of the schedule. If the schedule is interrupted after the 1st dose, the 2nd dose should be administered as soon as possible and the 2nd and 3rd dose should be separated by a minimum interval of 4 weeks.

Contraindication

Individuals with a history of allergic reactions to any of the components of the vaccine.

Who should be vaccinated with Hep B vaccine?

All aged <18 years who has not been previously vaccinated should be vaccinated with emphasizing over the following high risk groups:

❖ Partners and household contacts of HBsAg positive persons

❖ Injecting drug users

❖ Persons who frequently receive transfusion of blood/blood products

❖ Recipients of solid organ transplantation

❖ Healthcare workers

❖ International travelers.

Heat Sensitivity of Vaccines

Introduction

❖ Not only cold but both excessive heat or cold exposure can damage vaccines, resulting in reduced potency

❖ Once potency is lost, it cannot be restored

❖ Each time vaccines are exposed to excessive heat or cold, the potency decreases

❖ Eventually, if the vaccine cold chain is not properly maintained, all potency will be lost, and the vaccines become useless

❖ Especially when a vaccine is damaged by freezing, the potency lost can never be restored — the damage is permanent

❖ Freeze-damaged vaccines have lower immunogenicity and are more likely to cause local reactions, such as sterile abscesses.

Mechanism

After freezing, the lattice (made up of bonds between the adsorbent and the antigen) in a vaccine is broken. Separated adsorbent tends to form larger, heavier granules that gradually settle at the bottom of the vial and the potency decreases subsequently.

Note:

While exposure to both warm and cold temperatures can affect the potency of refrigerated vaccines, a single exposure to freezing temperatures will destroy some refrigerated vaccines. HepB and DPT/DT/dT vaccines are especially sensitive to freezing temperatures.

Relative Risk

Definition

In epidemiology, relative risk (RR) is the ratio of the probability of an event occurring (e.g. developing a disease) in an exposed group to the probability of the event occurring in a non-exposed group.

Derivation

Risk factor (exposure)	Disease		Total
	Present	*Absent*	
Present	a	b	a + b
Absent	c	d	c + d

$$\text{Relative risk} = \frac{\text{Incidence of disease among exposed}}{\text{Incidence of disease among non-exposed}}$$

$$= \frac{\dfrac{a}{a+b}}{\dfrac{c}{c+d}}$$

A relative risk of 2 means that the incidence of disease among exposed is 2 times higher than the incidence of disease among nonexposed.

Interpretation

In a simple comparison between an experimental group and a control group:
* A relative risk of 1 means there is no difference in risk between the two groups
* An RR of <1 means the event is less likely to occur in the exposed group than in the non-exposed group
* An RR of >1 means the event is more likely to occur in the exposed group than in the nonexposed group.

Use

Relative risk is commonly used in:
* Cohort study
* Randomized controlled trials (RCT).

Significance

* Estimation of RR is important in figuring out the etiological association between suspected risk factor and occurrence of a specific disease/event
* *RR is a direct measure of the strength of association*
* The greater the RR, the greater the strength of association.

SCREENING

Lead Time

Definition

"Lead time refers to the interval between the time when the disease can be first diagnosed by screening and when it is usually diagnosed in patients presenting with symptoms".

—WHO (2006)

Derivation

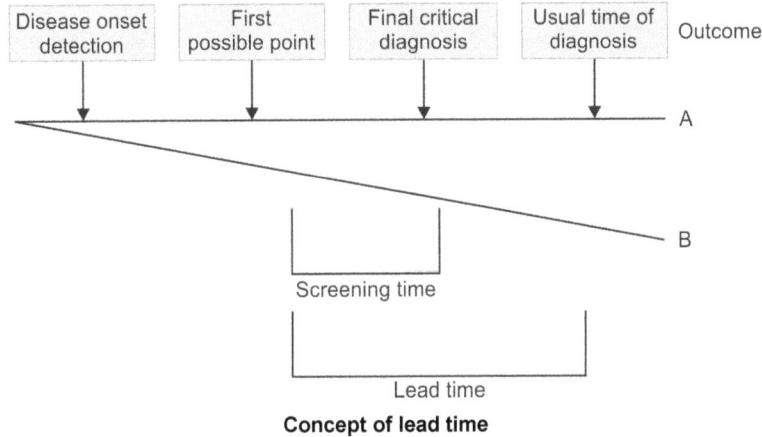

Concept of lead time

Significance

❖ For effective screening of a disease, it must have a long lead time; so that it gives the clinician a sufficient time to diagnose and treat the condition

❖ A short lead time implies a rapidly progressing disease, and treatment initiated after screening is unlikely to be more effective than that begun after the more usual diagnostic procedures. So, these diseases are not suitable for screening.

Example

Noise-induced hearing loss has a very long lead time; pancreatic cancer usually has a short one.

Multiphasic Screening

Definition

Multiphasic screening is defined as the application of two or more screening tests *applied to a large number of people* at one time than to carry out separate screening tests for single diseases.

Various types of tests have been suggested for inclusion in the screening unit. They are conducted in series.

Example:

1. Registration, chiefly for identification, is the first step, with a record of age, sex, marital status, weight and height
2. BP
3. A urine sample for albumin, sugar, sediment
4. A chest X-ray
5. A blood test–Hb, blood group and other tests based on local prevalence data
6. A test of visual acuity
7. A test for acuity of hearing
8. Pap smear for early detection of CA cervix
9. Simple muscle function tests
10. Exercise tolerance tests
11. ECG.

Advantages

❖ Per capita costing is low
❖ Many cases previously undiagnosed are uncovered.

Disadvantages

❖ Evidence from clinical trials has suggested that multiphasic screening has no added benefit accruing to the population in terms of mortality and morbidity reduction.
❖ It has increased the cost of health services without any observable benefit.

Conclusion

Comprehensive multiphasic screening programs require careful, detailed planning and coordination.

EPIDEMIOLOGY OF COMMUNICABLE DISEASES

Biological Transmission

Introduction

The chain of infection is not an independent event, but it relies on 3 important components as follows:

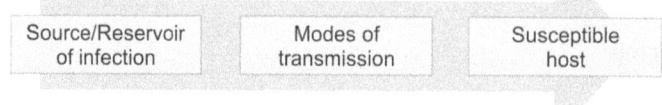

| Source/Reservoir of infection | Modes of transmission | Susceptible host |

Mode of biological transmission of disease

Definition

When the disease agent undergoes replication/development/both inside the vector, it is called "Biological transmission".

Note:

The agent needs to spend a specific time period within the vector to effectively transmit the disease to the host. This time is called as *"Extrinsic incubation period".*

Types

Biological transmission is of three types:

Types	Description	Example
Propagative transmission	Disease agent only multiplies but does not undergo developmental changes within the vector	Plague bacilli within rat flea
Cyclopropagative transmission	Disease agent multiplies and also undergoes developmental changes within the vector	Malaria parasite within mosquito
Cyclodevelopmental transmission	The disease agent does not multiply but undergoes developmental changes within the vector	Microfilaria within mosquito

Strategies of Measles Elimination Campaign

Catch-up

❖ Goal: *Rapid interrupt of transmission*
❖ *One-time-only* vaccination campaign
❖ Conducted during seasons of low transmission
❖ Conducted over short time period (One week to one month)
❖ Target age: All children *9 months to 14 years* of age.

Keep-up

❖ Goal: *>90% coverage of birth cohort*
❖ Strategies:
  – To improve routine coverage
  – Improve access to vaccination services
  – Integrate with routine health services
  – Tracking systems
  – Outreach activities
  – School-based programs
  – Reduce missed opportunities.

Follow-up

❖ Goal: *Prevent accumulation of susceptible*
❖ Measles vaccine is not 100% effective and coverage is not 100%, so long-time follow up is necessary
❖ Usually done once every 3–5 years
❖ Target age: *1–4 years* of age.

Mop-up

❖ Goal: *Intensive vaccination efforts to reach unvaccinated children*

❖ Target:
 - High-risk/low coverage areas
 - Recent measles cases
 - Poor surveillance
 - Crowding, poverty and migration.

Recent Updates in Measles Vaccination Strategy

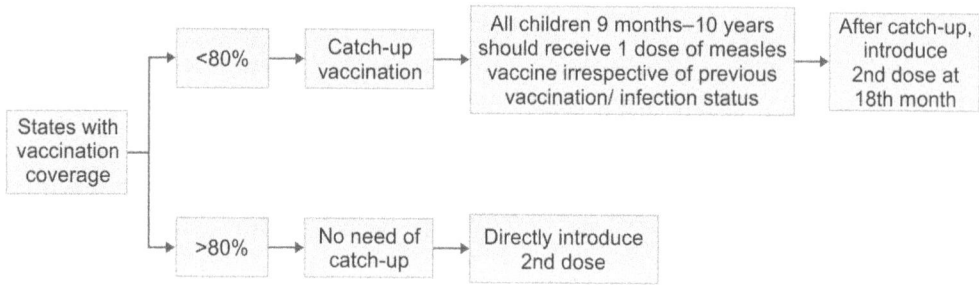

Common Homemade ORS

Description

These are used when the WHO mixture of salts is not available. These include:
❖ Table salt (1 level teaspoon) + Sugar (6 level teaspoon) + 1 liter of water
❖ Rice water
❖ Unsalted soup
❖ Yoghurt drinks
❖ Green coconut water
❖ Weak tea, etc.

Recommendations to be Read before Preparing a Homemade ORS

A. Wherever possible these should contain at least one fluid that contains salt.
B. Fluids which are sweetened with sugar should be avoided because they can cause osmotic diarrhea and hypernatremia.
 Example
 - Commercial carbonated beverages (cold drinks)
 - Commercial fruit juices
 - Sweetened tea.
C. Fluids that have stimulant purgative/diuretic effect should also be avoided like coffee.

Multidrug Therapy (MDT) for Leprosy

Before going into details of multidrug therapy of leprosy, we should first discuss the characteristics to classify leprosy into paucibacillary and multibacillary types.

Characteristics	PBL	MBL
Skin lesion	1–5	>5
Peripheral nerve involvement	0–1	>1
Skin smear	Negative at all sites	Positive at any site

MDT for leprosy in adults (National Leprosy Eradication Programme Guidelines, 2019)

Type	Drug	Dosage	Frequency	Duration
PBL	Dapsone	100 mg	Once daily	6 months
	Rifampicin	600 mg	Once monthly	
MBL	Dapsone	100 mg	Once daily	12 months
	Rifampicin	600 mg	Once monthly	
	Clofazimine	50 mg	Once daily	
	Clofazimine	300 mg	Once monthly	

MDT for leprosy in children 10–14 Years

Type	Drug	Dosage	Frequency	Duration
PBL	Dapsone	50 mg	Once daily	6 months
	Rifampicin	450 mg	Once monthly	
MBL	Dapsone	50 mg	Once daily	12 months
	Rifampicin	450 mg	Once monthly	
	Clofazimine	50 mg	Once daily	
	Clofazimine	150 mg	Once monthly	

Management of a Case of Leprosy

As per the new Leprosy treatment guidelines by WHO (2018):

Age group	Drug	Dosage and frequency	Duration	
			PBL	MBL
Adult	Rifampicin	600 mg once a month	6 months	12 months
	Clofazimine	300 mg once a month and 50 mg daily		
	Dapsone	100 mg daily		
Children (10–14 years)	Rifampicin	450 mg once a month	6 months	12 months
	Clofazimine	150 mg once a month and 50 mg daily		
	Dapsone	50 mg daily		

Rabies Vaccine

First use: Louis Pasteur.

Types of Rabies Vaccines Currently being used for Humans

❖ Vaccines for humans prepared in human diploid cells (HDC)
❖ Purified Vero cell rabies vaccine (PVRV)
❖ Purified chick embryo cell rabies vaccine (PCECV).

Indication for Rabies Vaccination

In postexposure prophylaxis against rabid animal.

Category	Postexposure prophylaxis
1	Local treatment only
2	Local treatment + Rabies vaccination
3	Local treatment+ Rabies vaccination + Rabies immunoglobulin.

Schedule for Rabies Vaccination in Postexposure Prophylaxis of Rabies

Intramuscular schedules

❖ *Single site schedule*: One dose of the vaccine should be administered on days 0, 3, 7, 14 and 28. All intramuscular injections must be given into the deltoid region or, in small children, into the anterolateral area of the thigh muscle. Vaccine should never be administered in the gluteal region.

❖ *Abbreviated multisite schedule*: In the abbreviated multisite schedule, the 2-1-1 regimen, one dose is given in the right arm and one dose in the left arm at day 0, and one dose applied in the deltoid muscle on days 7 and 21. The 2-1-1 schedule induces an early antibody response and may be particularly effective when postexposure treatment does not include administration of rabies immunoglobulin (e.g. Category 2).

Intradermal schedule

WHO recommended the following intradermal regimen and vaccines for use by the intradermal route:

❖ *2-site intradermal method*:
  – The regimen is (2-2-2-0-1-1)
  – The volume per intradermal site is: 0.1 mL.

Brain-tissue vaccines

The use of brain-tissue vaccines should be discontinued. WHO does not recommend any schedule using brain-tissue vaccines.

Active Surveillance in Malaria

Definitions

❖ *Surveillance*: *"Surveillance is the ongoing systematic collection, analysis and interpretation of outcome-specific data for use in planning, implementing and evaluating public health policies and practices".*
  Source: WHO (2006).

❖ *Active surveillance*: Public health surveillance in which the health agency solicits reports (CDC).

Objectives of Malaria Surveillance

❖ The main purpose of surveillance is to detect changes in trends or distribution in malaria and other vector-borne diseases in order to initiate investigative or control measures

❖ It provides a basis for measuring the effectiveness of antimalaria programme

❖ The ultimate objective of malaria surveillance is prevention and control of malaria in the community.

Purpose of Active Surveillance in Malaria

If all the detected cases are given radical treatment early, it will certainly lead to depletion of the human reservoir of malaria parasite in the community.

Components of Malaria Active Surveillance

There are currently 2 strategies in the active surveillance of malaria:
1. Active case detection (ACD) by fortnightly domiciliary visits.
2. Fever treatment depots (FTDs) as a supplementation of ACD.

Active case detection by fortnightly domiciliary visits

❖ Under the National Vector Borne Diseases Control Program (NVBDCP), the active case detection is carried out by *multipurpose health workers (male)* under primary health care system.
❖ Components of the activities under the active case detection during fortnightly visits are:
   - Search for a fever case or who had fever in between the visits of MPW
   - Collection of blood smears from such cases
   - Administration of appropriate antimalarial(s).

Technical viewpoint of a fortnight visit
❖ Technical justification for a fortnightly blood smear collection is based on transmission dynamics of malaria
❖ The incubation intervals of *P. vivax* and *P. falciparum* are 22 days and 35 days, respectively.

Thus, surveillance cycle of <1 incubation interval will catch most of the secondary cases before the commencement of next cycle. So, the fortnightly periodicity of domiciliary visits suits the technical requirement of malaria disease management. By fortnightly visits a large number of secondary cases can be avoided in the community where malaria transmission is seasonal but well established.

Fever treatment depots (FTDs): As a Supplementation of ACD

❖ To avoid delay in detection of cases which occur in between visits of MPW, it can be supplemented with establishment of Fever Treatment Depots in villages especially in areas which are remote/inaccessible and have low population density (e.g. in hilly terrain).
❖ The FTD holder should be given training for 1-2 days at the PHC Headquarters in:
   - The collection of blood smears
   - Administration of presumptive treatment
   - Impregnation of bed nets
   - Promotion of larvivorous fish, etc.

Recommendations about manpower involved in malaria active surveillance:
Health care system in our country provides 1 MPW (male) per 3000 population in hilly and tribal areas and 1 per 5000 population in other areas. The manpower envisaged under the plan is adequate to cater to the needs of the active case detection for malaria control *if all the positions of MPW are filled.*

Integrated Counseling and Testing Center

Introduction

Under NACP-III (National AIDS Control Programme), Voluntary Counseling and Testing Centers (VCTC) and facilities providing Prevention of Parent to Child Transmission of HIV/AIDS (PPTCT) services are remodeled as a hub or 'Integrated Counseling and Testing Center' (ICTC) to provide services to all clients under one roof.

$$ICTC = VCTC + PPTCT$$

An ICTC is a place where a person is counseled and tested for HIV, of his own free will or as advised by a medical provider.

Functions of ICTC

The main functions of an ICTC are:
- ❖ Conducting HIV diagnostic tests
- ❖ Providing basic information on the modes of HIV transmission, and promoting behavioral change to reduce vulnerability
- ❖ Link people with HIV prevention, care and treatment services.

Location of ICTC

- ❖ Ideally, each health facility should have one integrated counseling and testing center for all groups of people
- ❖ However, an ICTC is located usually in facilities that serve specific categories such as pregnant women. Accordingly, an ICTC is located in the Obstetrics and Gynecology Department of a medical college/a district hospital/in a maternity home where the majority of clients who access counseling and testing services are pregnant women. The justification for such a center is the need for providing medical care *to prevent HIV transmission from infected pregnant women to their infants*
- ❖ Similarly an ICTC is located in a TB microscopy center/in a TB sanatorium, where the majority of clients are TB patients. As *TB is the most common coinfection in people with HIV*, availability of HIV counseling and testing can help patients to diagnose their status for accessing early treatment.

Target group of ICTC

It is not the mandatory of an ICTC to counsel and test everyone in the general population. The sub-populations that are more vulnerable or practice high-risk behavior or have higher HIV prevalence levels are the target group for counseling and testing services in the country.

Conclusion

- ❖ HIV counseling and testing services are a key entry point to prevention of HIV infection and to treatment and care of people who are infected with HIV
- ❖ When availing counseling and testing services, people can access accurate information about HIV prevention and care and undergo HIV test in a supportive and confidential environment

❖ People who are found HIV negative are supported with information and counseling to reduce risks and remain HIV negative
❖ People who are found HIV positive are provided psychosocial support and linked to treatment and care.

Zoonoses

Definition

Zoonoses is defined as those diseases and infections which are naturally transmitted between vertebrate animals and man (FAO/WHO definition).

According to direction of transmission zoonoses can be categorized in 3 groups:

Type of zoonoses	Direction	Example
Anthropozoonosis	Animal → Human	Rabies, anthrax, plague
Zooanthroponosis	Human → Animal	Human TB in cattle
Amphixenosis	Human ↔ Animal	*Trypanosome cruzi, Schistosoma japonicum*

Spectrum of Zoonotic Diseases

Some common zoonoses

Disease	Causative agent	Animal reservoir	Mode of transmission
Helminthic			
Tapeworm infestation	*Dipylidium caninum*	Dogs	Ingestion of larvae transmitted in dog saliva
Fasciola infestation	*Fasciola hepatica*	Sheep, cattle	Ingestion of contaminated vegetation
Protozoan			
Malaria	*Plasmodium species*	Monkeys	Bite of *Anopheles* mosquito
Toxoplasmosis	*Toxoplasma gondii*	Cats and other animals	Ingestion of contaminated meat, inhalation of pathogen, direct contact with infected tissues
Fungal			
Ringworm	*Trichophyton species* *Microsporum species* *Epidermophyton species*	Domestic animals	Direct contact
Bacterial			
Anthrax	*Bacillus anthracis*	Domestic livestock	Direct contact with infected animals, inhalation
Bubonic plaque	*Yersinia pestis*	Rodents	Flea bites
Lyme disease	*Borrelia burgdorferi*	Deer	Tick bites
Salmonellosis	*Salmonella species*	Birds, rodents, reptiles	Ingestion of fecally contaminated water or food
Epidemic typhus	*Rickettsia prowazekii*	Rodents	Louse bites
Viral			
Rables	*Lyssavirus species*	Bats, skunks, foxes, dogs	Bite of infected animal
Hantavirus pulmonary syndrome	*Hantavirus species*	Deer, mice	Inhalation of viruses in dried feces and urine
Yellow fever	*Flavivirus sp.*	Monkeys	Bite of *Aedes* mosquito

Control of Zoonoses

❖ Control of infection in animals:
  – Immunization of animals
  – Proper diagnosis and treatment of zoonotic diseases
  – Destruction of source of infection
❖ Control of vehicles of transmission:
  – Maintenance of proper hygiene
  – Proper disposal of animal excreta and waste
❖ Early detection of zoonotic diseases in man and their treatment
❖ Periodic monitoring of health status of hazardous occupations.

Integrated Vector Management

Definition

Integrated vector management (IVM) is defined by WHO as a rational decision making process for the optimal use of resources for vector control. It entails use of a range of biological, chemical and physical interventions of proven efficacy, separately or in combination, in order to implement cost-effective control and reduce reliance on any single intervention.

Goal of IVM

The ultimate goal is to prevent the transmission of vector-borne diseases such as malaria, dengue, Japanese encephalitis, leishmaniasis, schistosomiasis and Chagas disease.

Key Elements of IVM

❖ *Policy and legislation*
❖ *Collaboration within the health sector and with other sectors*
❖ *Empowerment and involvement of local communities and other stakeholders*
❖ *Integrated approach*: This involves the integration of non-chemical and chemical vector control methods that are appropriate to the local eco-epidemiology of the disease.
❖ *Evidence-based decision making*: Strategies and interventions need to take into account local vector ecology (breeding habitats, life cycles, feeding and resting behavior), pattern of disease transmission, resources and the prevailing socioeconomic conditions
❖ *Capacity building*: In order for IVM initiatives to succeed, it is important that there is development of essential infrastructure and strengthening of technical program and project management skills at national and local levels.

Summary of Vector Control Methods

Chemical-based and non-chemical vector control methods

Control method	Brief description	Disease targets	Vectors targeted
Chemical-based vector control methods			
Adulticides			
Indoor residual spraying	Timely application of long-lasting chemical insecticides on the walls and ceilings of houses in order to kill the adult vectors that land on these surfaces	Malaria, lymphatic filariasis, visceral leishmaniasis (kala-azar), Chagas disease	Indoor biting/resting female Anopheles mosquitoes; phlebotomine sandflies; reduviid bugs

Contd...

Contd...

Control method	Brief description	Disease targets	Vectors targeted
Long-lasting insecticidal nets	Sleeping under insecticide-impregnated polyethylene, polyester or cotton net to prevent bites from disease-bearing insects	Malaria, lymphatic filariasis, visceral leishmaniasis (kala-azar)	Indoor biting/resting female *Anopheles* mosquitoes; phlebotomine sandflies
Other insecticide-impregnated materials	Use of insecticide-impregnated clothing, coverings (blankets), door and window blinds, etc. to prevent human-vector contact and bites	Malaria, dengue, lymphatic filariasis, cutaneous leishmaniasis, African trypanosomiasis (sleeping sickness), onchocerciasis	*Anopheles, Aedes, Culex* mosquitoes; phlebotomine sandflies; tsetse flies; *Simulium damnosum* black flies
Molluscicides	The use of molluscicides and insecticides to kill disease vectors in the adult stages	Schistosomiasis, lymphatic filariasis, dengue	Fresh-water snails (*Biomphilaria, Bulinus, Onchomelania*); *Anopheles, Aedes, Culex* mosquitoes
Insect traps	Insecticide-impregnated traps targeting flying vectors; may also have an attractant (color or light)	Malaria, African trypanosomiasis (sleeping sickness)	*Anopheles, Aedes, Culex* mosquitoes; tsetse flies
Chemical larvicides	The release of chemicals on water bodies and surfaces to kill larvae and pupae of insect vectors	Malaria, dengue, lymphatic filariasis, onchocerciasis	*Anopheles, Aedes, Culex* mosquitoes; *Simulium damnosum* black flies
Nonchemical vector control methods			
Environmental			
Modification	Permanent environmental changes aimed at the elimination of local vector breeding areas	Malaria, dengue, lymphatic filariasis, schistosomiasis	*Anopheles, Aedes, Culex* mosquitoes; Fresh-water snails (*Biomphilaria, Bulinus, Onchomelania*)
Manipulation	Temporary environmental changes to disrupt the reproductive cycle of a vector	Malaria, dengue, lymphatic filariasis, schistosomiasis	*Anopheles, Aedes, Culex* mosquitoes; Fresh-water snails (*Biomphilaria, Bulinus, Onchomelania*)
House modification	An improvement in the housing structure to restrict entry of disease vectors	Malaria, lymphatic filariasis, Chagas disease	Indoor biting/resting female *Anopheles*, mosquitoes; reduviid bugs
Larviciding			
Larvivorous fish	Use of natural predators (tilapia and other fish) that feed on the larvae and pupae of mosquito vectors	Lymphatic filariasis	*Anopheles, Aedes, Culex* mosquitoes
Biological larviciding	The use of bacteria against mosquito larvae or pupae (e.g. *Bacillus thuringiensis*)	Malaria, dengue, lymphatic filariasis, onchocerciasis	*Anopheles, Aedes, Culex* mosquitoes; *Simulium damnosum* black flies
Nonlarvivorous natural predators	The use of natural predators against disease vectors (e.g. molluscivorous fish, crawfish and crabs)	Schistosomiasis	Fresh-water snails (*Biomphilaria, Bulinus, Onchomelania*)
Polystyrene beads	Formation of a layer on top of the breeding water body to prevent the larvae and pupae from breathing	Malaria, dengue, lymphatic filariasis	Mosquitoes

Contd...

Control method	Brief description	Disease targets Other	Vectors targeted
Topical repellents	Use of topical insecticides to repel biting insect vectors as a personal protection measure	Malaria, dengue, lymphatic filariasis; African trypanosomiasis (sleeping sickness)	Mosquitoes, tsetse flies

EPIDEMIOLOGY OF NONCOMMUNICABLE DISEASES

Risk Factors of Diabetes

Obesity and Sedentary Lifestyle

Obesity, especially central obesity remains an important risk factor for type 2 diabetes mellitus (DM). The following indices show strong association in causation of type 2 DM:
- ❖ Waist: Hip ratio
- ❖ Body mass index (BMI)
- ❖ Weight gain
- ❖ Waist circumference.

By various epidemiological studies, the following chain of events has been worked out in the causation of DM:

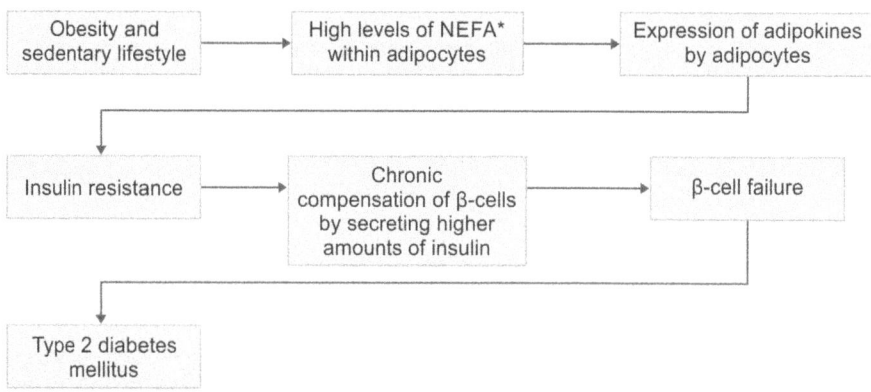

*NEFA: Non-esterified fatty acids

Obesity as an important risk factor for development of Type 2 diabetes mellitus

Dietary Habits

- ❖ A high amount of saturated fatty acid intake is associated with a higher risk of DM
- ❖ A high amount of unsaturated fatty acid and polyunsaturated fatty acid (PUFA) intake and daily dietary fiber intake at recommended levels (20 g) is associated with a reduced risk of DM
- ❖ A high amount of cyanide producing foods (cassava/beans) in the daily diet also has toxic effect on β-cells.

Malnutrition

Malnutrition at early childhood causes partial failure of β cells, pushing the individuals at higher risk of DM at a higher age.

Alcohol

Chronic alcohol intake damages the pancreatic β-cells and also predisposes the individual to obesity, subsequently increasing the risk of future DM.

Stress

Trauma, chronic disease, pregnancy, mental stress—all are thought to be risk factors of DM as they can aggravate the physiological compensation to insulin resistance and may bring out the disease.

Maternal Diabetes

Child of a diabetic mother/mother with gestational diabetes tends to develop obesity in childhood and type 2 DM in adulthood.

Modifiable Risk Factors for Hypertension

Obesity

Obesity, especially the central obesity (an increased waist: hip ratio) is the most important modifiable risk factor of hypertension. The greater the weight gain, the greater the risk of high blood pressure.

Salt (sodium) Intake

* High salt intake (7–8 g/day) increases blood pressure proportionately
* Low salt intake lowers blood pressure
* Potassium, on the other hand, antagonizes the biological effects of Na^+. Thereby, K supplements have been shown to lower BP.

Saturated Fat

A high intake of saturated fatty acids as well as a high serum cholesterol level have been shown to raise the risk of hypertension.

Dietary Fiber

Dietary fibers bind to bile salt and inhibit their reabsorption; thus more cholesterol is excreted through bile; so serum cholesterol level is decreased and subsequently, BP decreases.

Physical Activity

Physical activity decreases body weight and indirectly BP is decreased.

Stress

It is hypothesized that stress causes overactivity of sympathetic nervous system, which is responsible for a chronically higher noradrenaline level; subsequently leading to development of hypertension.

Oral Contraceptive Pill

The estrogen component of oral contraceptive pills (OCPs) is held responsible for development of hypertension in chronic OCP users.

Danger Signs of Cancer

Introduction

These are the early warning signs people should be educated about to accelerate early diagnosis and treatment because most of the cancers, when present in an early stage are preventable or curable.

Danger Signs

- ❖ An unexplained loss of weight
- ❖ A lump/hard area in the breast
- ❖ A change in a wart/mole
- ❖ A swelling/sore that is not getting better
- ❖ A persistent cough
- ❖ A persistent hoarseness of voice
- ❖ Excess blood loss at times of period/blood loss outside usual dates
- ❖ A persistent change in digestive/bowel habits.

Significance

Educating people about the early danger signs of cancer is a type of primary prevention and it should be integrated within cancer prevention programs, the aim of which is early diagnosis and treatment of cancers.

◼ HEALTH PROGRAMS IN INDIA

Adolescent Health Program

Introduction

Adolescents aged 10–19 years constitute about 21% of India's population which in absolute numbers translates to 253 million. The increasing share of adolescents and youth in India's population can translate into a demographic dividend only if policies and programs focus on the health and well-being of this large, yet very vulnerable population.

Rashtriya Kishor Swasthya Karyakram (RKSK)

Under National Health Mission (conducted by Ministry of Health and Family Welfare, Government of India)

Adolescent Health components with programs are discussed below:
- ❖ Adolescent Health component includes the:
    - Adolescent Reproductive and Sexual Health (ARSH) Programme
    - Menstrual Hygiene Scheme (MHS) and
    - Weekly Iron and Folic Acid Supplementation (WIFS) Programme components
- ❖ The newly launched RKSK subsumes these components into a comprehensive program
- ❖ RSSK is underpinned by evidence that adolescence is the most important stage of the life cycle for health interventions
- ❖ RKSK is a paradigm shift from the existing clinic-based services to promotion and prevention and reaching adolescents in their own environment, such as in schools and communities.

Achievement under each component and salient features of RKSK are as below:

Adolescent Reproductive and Sexual Health (ARSH) Programme

Introduction

ARSH focuses on reorganizing the existing public health system in order to meet health service needs of adolescents through provision of promotive, preventive and curative services at designated Adolescent Friendly Health Clinics (AFHC) across level of care.

Package of AFHC Services

Information	• IEC and IPC for nutrition, sex and reproductive health, mental health, gender-based violence, noncommunicable disease, substance misuse
Commodities	• IFA/Albendazole tablets • Sanitary napkin • Contraceptives (condoms, OCP, ECP) • Other medicines (e.g. Paracetamol, anti-spasmodic and first aid) • Pregnancy testing kits
Services	• BMI screening • Hb testing • RTI/STI management • ANC for pregnant adolescents • Counseling* • Management of menstrual problems • Management of iron deficiency anemia • Screening for diabetes and hypertension • Management of common adolescent health problems • HIV testing and counseling • Management of physical violence and sexual abuse • Linkages with de-addiction centers and referrals • Treatment by specialists • Referral services

(IEC, Information, education and communication; IPC, Interpersonal communication; ECP, Emergency contraceptive pills)

* Counseling is given on nutrition, puberty related concerns, premarital counseling, sexual problems, contraceptive, abortion, RTI/STI, substance abuse, learning problems, stress, depression, suicidal tendency, violence, sexual abuse, other mental health issues, health lifestyle, risky behavior.

Menstrual Hygiene Scheme (MHS)

Introduction

❖ The Scheme for Promotion of Menstrual Hygiene has been initiated for rural adolescent girls in the age group of 10–19 years
❖ This program aims at that girls in rural areas have adequate knowledge and information about menstrual hygiene and have access to high quality sanitary napkins along with safe disposal mechanisms.

Key activities under the scheme include:

❖ Community-based health education and outreach in the target population to promote menstrual health
❖ Ensuring regular availability of sanitary napkins to the adolescents (Central supply: 'Freedays')
❖ Sourcing and procurement of sanitary napkins
❖ Storage and distribution of sanitary napkins to the adolescent girls

❖ Training of ASHA and nodal teachers in menstrual health
❖ Safe disposal of sanitary napkins.

Weekly Iron and Folic Acid Supplementation Programme

❖ The Ministry of Health and Family Welfare has rolled out the Weekly Iron and Folic Acid Supplementation (WIFS) Programme in 2012–13 to meet the challenge of high prevalence and incidence of iron deficiency anemia amongst adolescent girls and boys
❖ WIFS programme includes:
  – Weekly supervised administration of iron and folic acid supplements (containing 100 mg elemental iron and 500 µg folic acid) to in-school adolescent girls and boys and out-of-school adolescent girls
  – Screening of target groups for moderate/severe anemia and referral to nearest centers
  – Biannual deworming (400 mg, 6 months apart)
  – Information and counseling for improving dietary intake and for taking actions for prevention of intestinal worm infestation.

Guidelines on consumption of WIFS tablets:

❖ Adolescents will be advised to take iron-folic acid tablets after meals (approximately one hour) to prevent side effects such as nausea
❖ Adolescent girls or boys who complain of side effects will be advised to take the IFA supplements after dinner and before retiring to sleep
❖ Increase intake of foods rich in vitamin C such as lemon, amla, etc. will help to absorb iron from the vegetarian Indian diet. Use of iron vessels for cooking will also be encouraged
❖ Drinking of tea or coffee within an hour of consuming main meals will be discouraged
❖ Adolescent boys and girls will be motivated to follow correct hygiene practices and the habit of using footwear to prevent worm infestation.

DEMOGRAPHY

Demographic Cycle

Introduction

Demographic cycle consists of 5 stages through which a country usually passes:

Stage no.	Name of the stage	Characterized by
1.	High stationary	High birth rate and high death rate; which cancel each other to maintain the population at a stationary level
2.	Early expanding	Birth rate unchanged and decreasing death rate, so the population is expanding
3.	Late expanding*	Decreasing birth rate and still decreasing death rate, but the birth rate is still > death rate; so that the population is still expanding
4.	Low stationary	A low birth rate and a low death rate; which maintains the population at a stationary level
5.	Declining	Birth rate is < death rate; so that the population is decreasing.

* **Note:** India is now in the stage 3 of the demographic cycle. The birth rate is decreasing due to nationwide birth control by effective family planning measures and death rate is also decreasing due to improvement in health control measures; but birth rate is still higher than death rate; so the country is in late expanding stage.

Diagrammatic Representation of Demographic Cycle in Various Stages

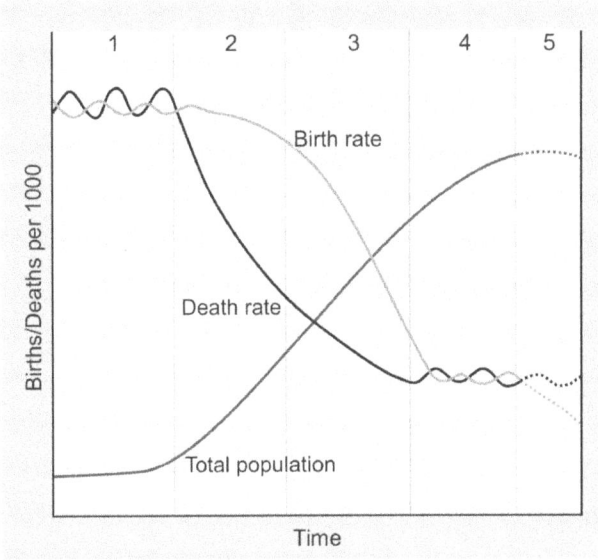

Age-Sex Pyramid/Population Pyramid

Introduction

❖ The most important demographic characteristic of a population is its age-sex structure
❖ Age-sex pyramid graphically displays this information to improve understanding and ease comparison.

Representation

❖ An age-sex pyramid typically consists of two back-to-back bar graphs, with the population plotted on the X-axis and age on the Y-axis, one showing the number of males and one showing females in a particular population in 5-year age groups
❖ Males are conventionally shown on the left and females on the right, and they may be measured by raw number/as a percentage of the total population.

Types

Age-sex pyramid is usually of three types:
1. *Expansive*: Population pyramids show larger numbers or percentages of the population in the younger age groups. These types of pyramids are usually found in populations with very large fertility rates and lower life expectancies, e.g. developing countries
2. *Constrictive*: Population pyramids display lower numbers or percentages of younger people, e.g. developed countries
3. *Stationary*: Population pyramids display somewhat equal numbers or percentages for almost all age groups, e.g., Scandinavian countries.

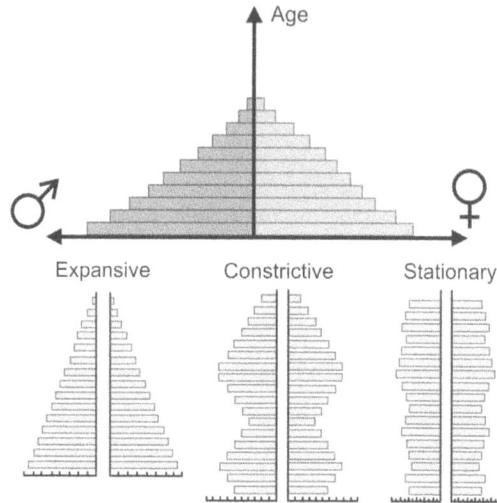

Age-sex pyramids and their types

Use of Age-Sex Pyramids

1. Population pyramids can be used to find the number of economic dependents being supported in a particular population.
   Economic dependents are measured by 'total dependency ratio'.

   Total dependence ratio

   $$= \frac{\text{Population} <15 \text{ years} + \text{Population} > 65 \text{ years}}{\text{Population between } 15 - 64 \text{ years}}$$

2. Population pyramids can also be used to observe the natural increase, birth and death rate.

Unmet Need for Family Planning

What is the "Unmet Need" for Family Planning?

Many women who are sexually active would prefer to avoid becoming pregnant although they are not using any methods of contraception (including use by their partners). These women are considered to have an "unmet need" for family planning.

Limitation of Use

Although the concept of "unmet need" may be applied to married women and sexually active unmarried women; *its measurement has been limited to married women only.*

Reasons of Unmet Need

❖ Inconvenience of unsatisfactory services
❖ Lack of information
❖ Fears about contraceptive side effects
❖ Opposition from husband/relatives.

Survey Reports

According to National Family Health Survey—3:

Age group	Unmet need is for
<20 years (27%: Highest)	Spacing of births
20–24 years	Spacing of births
25–29 years	Both for spacing and limiting of births
>30 years	Limiting of births

This survey also found out that unmet need for family planning is *higher in rural areas than in urban areas* and it also depends on education/religion/caste and wealth index.

<20 years Age Group

It should be emphasized that 15–19 years age group has the highest unmet need for contraception, not for family planning. This age group is particularly vulnerable because:

❖ Most of the pregnancies are undesired and high risk
❖ The adolescent girls often choose the risk of an undesired pregnancy and an abortion because of the fear of social exposure and shame
❖ They are uneducated about the methods of contraception and also about which ones will suite them more
❖ So this vulnerable age group should be particularly emphasized when the unmet needs have to be solved. It should be kept in mind that the suitable contraceptives for this age group are:
  – Barrier methods (especially condoms) and,
  – Hormonal contraceptives.

PREVENTIVE MEDICINE IN OBSTETRICS, PEDIATRICS AND GERIATRICS

Some definitions:
1. Infancy: Up to 1 year of age.
    a. Neonatal period: First 28 days of life.
    b. Postneonatal period: 28th day to 1 year of life.
2. Preschool age: 1–4 years of age.
3. School age: 5–14 years of age.
4. Preterm: Babies born before the end of 37 weeks gestation.
5. Term: Babies born from 37 completed weeks to less than 42 completed weeks of gestation.
6. Post-term: Babies born at 42 completed weeks of gestation or any time thereafter.
7. Low birth weight (LBW): It is defined as birth weight less than 2500 g.
8. Very low birth weight (VLBW): It is defined as a birth weight less than 1500 g.

Kangaroo Mother Care (KMC)

Introduction

KMC refers to care of preterm/low birth weight (LBW) babies by placing the infant in skin-to-skin contact with the mother/any other caregiver.

Components

1. *Kangaroo position*:
   - This consists of skin-to-skin contact between mother and infant; keeping the infant in a vertical position between the mother's breasts and under her cloths
   - Mother should keep herself in a semi-reclining position to avoid gastric reflux of the infant
   - Head of the baby should be turned to one side and slightly extended to keep the airway open
   - Hips should be flexed and abducted (frog position)
   - Arms should be flexed
   - Baby's abdomen should at the level of mother's epigastrium.

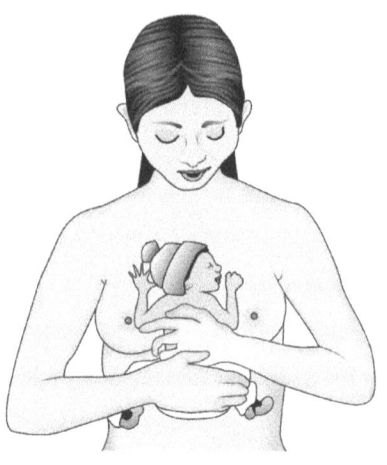

Kangaroo position

2. *Kangaroo nutrition*: Exclusive breastfeeding.
3. *Kangaroo discharge and follow-up*: Early home discharge from neonatal unit in the Kangaroo position is an important components of KMC. Mother requires adequate support and follow-up at home.

Eligibility Criteria for KMC

1. For baby:
   a. All stable LBW babies.
   b. Sick babies after hemodynamic stabilization.
2. For mother:
   a. All willing mothers in good health.
   b. Free from any serious illness.
   c. Good hygiene.
   d. Proper counseling of mother and family members.
   e. Family's support and cooperation.

Initiation of KMC

Birth weight	Initiation
<1200 g	May take days to weeks before KMC can be initiated
1200–1800 g	May take days before KMC can be initiated
>1800 g	KMC can be initiated immediately after birth

Stopping of KMC

- ❖ When the baby attains a weight of 2500 g
- ❖ When the baby completes a gestation of 37 weeks
- ❖ When the baby refuses KMC (cry/try to get out/get anxious).

Benefits of KMC

A. Physiological:
   a. Protection from cold stress and hypothermia.
   b. Stabilization of heart rate, respiratory rate, oxygenation and sleep pattern.

B. Clinical:
   a. Increased milk production in mothers.
   b. Weight gain.
   c. Thermal protection.
   d. Protection against respiratory and nosocomial infections.
   e. Emotional bonding between mother and child.
   f. Early discharge from the hospital.

First Referral Unit (FRU)

Introduction

It is a district or subdivisional hospital or community health center which has three critical determinants for being 'declared' as FRU:
   i. Availability of surgical interventions.
   ii. Newborn care.
   iii. Blood storage facility on a 24 hours basis.

To able to perform the full range of FRU function, a health facility must have following facilities:
   i. Minimum bed strength of 20–30 (10–20 in North East and underserved areas of EAG).
   ii. Fully functional OT.
   iii. Fully functional labor room.
   iv. An area embarked and equipped for newborn care in labor room and in the ward.
   v. A functional laboratory.
   vi. Blood storage facility.
   vii. 24 hours water supply and electricity supply.
   viii. Arrangements of disposal of waste.
   ix. Ambulance facility.

It provides specialist services in addition to all the services available at a PHC.

Specialist Services Available at FRU

Surgical management:
❖ Cesarean section
❖ Laparotomy and repair of ruptured uterus
❖ Surgical treatment of severe sepsis
❖ Evaluation of incomplete abortion
❖ Mid-trimester abortion
❖ Repair of cervical and vaginal tears
❖ Amniotomy with/without oxytocin
❖ Tubectomy/vasectomy.

Delivery Services

24 Hours delivery services including normal and assisted delivery.

Medical Management

❖ Severe hypertensive disorders of pregnancy, eclampsia
❖ Hemorrhagic shock

❖ Severe anemia
❖ Septicemia
❖ Use of IV oxytocin during labor.

Manual Management

❖ Manual removal of placenta
❖ Forceps delivery
❖ Vacuum extraction
❖ Partography.

Anesthesia

General, spinal.

Blood Transfusion

❖ Matching a donor and blood transfusion
❖ Performing mandatory tests.

Newborn and Pediatric Care

❖ Resuscitation
❖ Management of sick newborns and severe illnesses of young children.

Benefits of Breastfeeding

Benefits for the Infant

1. *Immunity*: Breast milk contains secretory IgA antibodies, lactoferrin (inhibits growth of intestinal bacteria) and bile salt stimulated lipase (protects from amoebic infections). It also contains macrophages, lymphocytes, lysozyme and antistreptococcal factor.
2. *Infections*: Breastfeeding benefits babies because it decreases the occurrence and/or severity of:
   – Diarrhea
   – Lower respiratory tract infections
   – Ear infections
   – Bacteremia
   – Bacterial meningitis
   – Urinary tract infections
   – Allergic diseases
   – Necrotizing enterocolitis (in premature infants).
3. *Diabetes*: Infants exclusively breastfed have less chance of developing diabetes mellitus type 1. Breastfeeding also appears to protect against diabetes mellitus type 2.
4. *Development*: Breast milk contains PUFA which are linked to early brain development. So, breastfeeding has been shown to lead to improved motor and cognitive development of the child. A breastfed baby is likely to have an IQ of 8 points higher than a nonbreastfed baby.
5. *Mental health*: Breastfeeding for more than 6 months is an independent predictor of better mental health through childhood and adolescence. The more months children are breastfed the less likely they are to suffer from depression, delinquency and other psychological problems.
6. *Childhood obesity*: Breastfeeding appears to reduce the risk of extreme obesity in children.

Benefits for the Mother

1. *Bonding*: Breastfeeding promotes emotional bonding between the mother and child.
2. *Lactational amenorrhea*: Breastfeeding delays the resumption of normal ovarian cycles by disrupting the pattern of pulsatile release of GnRH from the hypothalamus and LH from the pituitary. So, ovulation is suppressed. This lactational amenorrhea has been used as a method of natural contraception, with greater than 98% effectiveness during the first 6 months after birth if specific nursing behaviors are followed.
3. *Long-term health benefits to the mother*: Breastfeeding woman poses less risk of certain cancers (breast, ovary and endometrial CA) and postpartum hemorrhage.

Baby-friendly Hospital Initiative (BFHI)

Introduction

The original 1992 BFHI guidelines were prepared by the staff of the United Nations Children's Fund (UNICEF) and the World Health Organization (WHO) with assistance from Wellstart International in developing the Global Criteria.

Ten steps to successful breastfeeding

Every facility providing maternity services and care for newborn infants should:

1. Have a written breastfeeding policy that is routinely communicated to all health care staff
2. Train all health care staff in skills necessary to implement this policy
3. Inform all pregnant women about the benefits and management of breastfeeding
4. Help mothers initiate breastfeeding within a half-hour of birth
5. Show mothers how to breastfeed, and how to maintain lactation even if they should be separated from their infants
6. Give newborn infants no food or drink other than breast milk unless medically indicated
7. Practice rooming in—allow mothers and infants to remain together: 24 hours a day
8. Encourage breastfeeding on demand
9. Give no artificial teats or pacifiers (also called dummies or soothers) to breastfeeding infants
10. Foster the establishment of breastfeeding support groups and refer mothers to them on discharge from the hospital or clinic.

Conclusion

The baby-friendly hospitals of India are also expected to adopt and practice guidelines on other interventions critical for child survival including antenatal care, clean delivery practices, essential newborn care, immunization and ORT.

The BFHI has proved to be highly successful in encouraging proper infant feeding practices starting at birth.

Aspects of School Health Services

Health Appraisal

❖ It consists of periodic medical examination and observation of children by their teachers
❖ In 1961, the School Health Committee recommended medical examination of children at the time of entry to the school and thereafter, once in every 4 years
❖ This periodic medical checkup includes:
  – Tests for vision/hearing/speech
  – Routine examinations on blood/urine/feces

❖ The teachers have a unique potential as they look the students regularly. So, any sudden changes in appearance/any chronic change in growth can first be identified by the teachers. So, periodic teacher training program should be encouraged so that they become capable of recognizing certain danger signs/symptoms.

Remedial Measures

❖ Medical examinations should be followed by proper treatment and follow up
❖ Special clinics should be organized to examine and treat the common diseases and deformities of the school age children.

Prevention of Communicable Diseases

Vaccination against communicable diseases is the most important activity of school health services.

Nutritional Services

To decrease the drop-out rates, to provide protection against nutritional deficiency disorders and to build a proper physical and mental health of a school-age child, adequate nutrition is of utmost importance. It is given to them through the following programs:
a. Mid-day Meal Scheme (By Ministry of Human Resource Development, Government of India)
b. Applied Nutrition Program (Central and state funding with collaboration with UNICEF).

First Aid and Emergency Care

❖ Some of the common medical emergencies that may occur within the school hours are:
a. Accidents
b. Faints
c. Epileptic fits, etc.
❖ Teachers should be adequately trained to respond to these emergencies through various "*Teacher Training Programs*".

Mental Health

❖ Some of the common mental health problems in school going children are:
a. Juvenile delinquency
b. Drug addiction
c. Social maladjustment, etc.
❖ The school is the most effective place for protection from these mental disorders and for promoting proper mental health of the child, where teachers play a major role
❖ The school is also a way to achieve social equity, which is necessary for concepts of primary health care to be completely effective. No race/religion/caste/financial/intelligence prioritization should be made by the school teachers.

Dental and Eye Health Services

❖ Basic dental and ophthalmic services should be provided by every school
❖ Dental caries and periodontal diseases are most common dental diseases in school age children in India. So, dental examination should be done at least once a year for proper detection and treatment of these dental defects and diseases

❖ Refractive errors are most commonly detected during school age, so teachers should refer the child to the ophthalmologist if he/she presents with a problem in near/far vision. Any other visible abnormalities (like squint/corneal haziness) should be referred immediately.

Health Education

❖ The main objective of health education is not merely teaching the students a set of hygienic rules; but to bring a behavioral change in their knowledge, attitude and practices regarding health and hygiene
❖ Health education should cover the following things:
  – *Personal hygiene*: During the health education sessions, teacher should emphasize on the following personal hygienic measures:
    - Proper method of hand washing
    - Daily cleaning of clothes
    - Daily cleansing of teeth
    - Taking a thorough bath daily
    - Health hazards of cigarette smoking
    - Proper posture during working hours
  – *Environmental health*: The students should also be educated about the benefits of:
    - Keeping the surrounding environment clean
    - Using sanitary latrines and sanitary wells
    - Demerits of open field defecation (Fly hazards)
    - Dangers of artificial collection of water around the houses and their potential of becoming breeding places of mosquitoes
  – *Family education*: It is an important aspect of health education to provide the background for health aspects of family planning.

Education of Handicapped Children

The objective of educating a handicapped child is to assist him and his family, so that the child can live a healthy productive life as much close to a normal life as possible. This function needs intersectoral collaboration.

Maintaining School Health Records

Proper health record keeping is a duty of every educational institution, which should contain the following data:
❖ Identification particulars: Name, age, sex, date of birth, father's name, address.
❖ Past health history and findings of periodic heath examinations.

Interpretation of ICDS Growth Chart

❖ Before going into the interpretation of new ICDS growth chart, we should first discuss the salient features of it once again:
  – The new ICDS growth chart has three reference curves. They are as follows:
    - 1st curve: It depicts the median value (M); it is the top curve
    - 2nd curve: M-2SD. (SD: Standard deviation)
    - 3rd curve: M-3SD

❖ Plotted point in the ICDS growth chart for *weight-for-age* helps in assessing the nutritional status of the child
❖ Note the position of the plotted point with reference to preprinted growth curves and then interpret the position of the plotted point to identify normal growth and growth problems:
  – If plotted weight for age of a child falls much *above the 1st curve*, the child has a growth problem, probably overweight/obesity
  – If plotted weight for age of a child falls *exactly on the 1st/2nd/3rd curve*; then the child is in the less severe category of malnutrition because:
    - Plotted point on the 1st curve indicates that the child's growth is normal
    - Plotted point on the 2nd curve indicates that the child's growth is normal and he/she is not moderately underweight.
    - Plotted point on the 3rd curve indicates that the child is moderately underweight.
  – If plotted weight for age of a child falls on the *green* band, then the child's growth is *normal*; if it falls on the *yellow* band, then the child is *moderately underweight*; if it falls on the *orange* band, then child is *severely underweight*.

Position of the plotted point	Nutritional status
Plotted point is: • Exactly on/above the 1st curve • Between 1st and 2nd curve • Exactly on the 2nd curve	Child's growth is normal
Plotted point is: • Between 2nd and 3rd curve • Exactly on the 3rd curve	Child is moderately underweight
Plotted point is below the 3rd curve	Child is severely underweight

Note that:
❖ When the child is severely underweight, clinical signs of marasmus/kwashiorkor may be evident
❖ If a child has *edema of both feet*, the weight will be more due to fluid retention. So, it will mask that the baby is actually severely underweight. *The presence of edema is thus very much important and should be marked clearly close to the plotted point.* This baby will automatically be considered severely undernourished and should be referred for specialist care.

Direction of child's growth curve and its importance

Direction of curve	Pictorial depiction	Growth pattern
Upward	Good	Good: Indicates adequate weight gain for the age of the child. The child is growing well and is healthy
Flat	Dangerous	Dangerous: Indicates that the child is not gaining weight and is not growing adequately. This is called "stagnation". This should be investigated
Downward	Very dangerous	Very dangerous: Indicates loss of weight. The child requires immediate referral and health care

Juvenile Delinquency

Definitions

❖ *Juvenile*: As per 'Juvenile Justice Act, 1986', a juvenile is defined as a male below 16 years and a female below 18 years.
❖ *Delinquent*: As per 'The Children Act, 1960', delinquent is defined as 'a child who has committed an offence.'

Causes

❖ Biological causes:
  – Chromosomal abnormalities (e.g. Men with 46+ XYY genotype)
  – Physical defects
  – Hormonal imbalance, etc.
❖ Social causes:
  – Separation/deaths of parents
  – Step father/mother
  – Parental neglect/ignorance
  – Poverty
  – Alcoholism
  – Unwanted birth
  – Too many children, etc.
❖ Other causes:
  – Urbanization
  – Slum-dwelling
  – Industrialization
  – Effect of violence and crime in TV programs and movies
  – Absence of recreation, etc.

Prevention of Juvenile Delinquency

❖ Family counseling
❖ Parental education
❖ Increased availability of family planning services
❖ Proper schooling
❖ Providing recreation facilities
❖ Youth sheltering.

Battered Baby Syndrome (BBS)

Definition

Battered baby syndrome refers to injuries sustained by a child as a result of physical abuse, usually inflicted by an adult caregiver.

Description

❖ Internal injuries
❖ Cuts
❖ Burns
❖ Bruises
❖ Broken/fractured bones
❖ Sexual abuse, etc.

Incidence

The incidence of BBS is higher in families with lower socioeconomic status where caregivers suffer greater stress and social difficulties.

Symptoms

Symptoms of a battered baby may include:
* ❖ A delayed visit to the emergency room with an injured child
* ❖ An implausible explanation of the cause of a child's injury
* ❖ Bruises that match the shape of a hand, fist, belt, cigarette burns, scald marks, black eyes, etc.
* ❖ Unconsciousness
* ❖ A bulging fontanel in infants.

Diagnosis

* ❖ Physical examination will detect bruises, burns, swelling, retinal hemorrhages, etc.
* ❖ X-rays and other imaging techniques may confirm fractures or other internal injuries
* ❖ *The presence of injuries at different stages of healing (i.e. having occurred at different times) is nearly always indicative of Battered Baby Syndrome.*

Treatment

Reporting child abuse to authorities is mandatory for doctors as a way to prevent continued abuse. Both physical and psychological therapy are often recommended as treatment for the abused child.

Health Problems of Geriatric Population

The health problems in geriatric population may be divided into several subgroups as follows:
1. Problems due to aging process
2. Problems associated with long-term illness
3. Psychological problems.

Groups	Health problems
Problems due to aging process	• Senile cataract • Glaucoma • Nerve deafness • Osteoporosis • Emphysema • Diminution/failure of special senses
Problems associated with long-term illness	• Atherosclerosis • Cancer • Diabetes • Diseases of the respiratory tract (chronic bronchitis/asthma/emphysema) • Diseases of bones and joints (gout/rheumatoid arthritis/osteoarthritis/spondylitis of spine/ myositis/fibrositis/neuritis) • Disorders of genitourinary system (benign hypertrophy of prostate/dysuria/nocturia/urgency of micturition) • Accidents
Psychological problems	• Impaired memory • Irritability (due to reduced sexual activity) • Depression (due to social maladjustment) • Suicide

PNDT Act

Full Name

Prenatal Diagnostic Techniques (Regulation and Prevention of Misuse) (PNDT) Act, 1994.

Introduction

This act was enacted to stop female feticides and arrest the declining sex ratio in India. The act banned prenatal sex determination.

Main Provisions in the Act

❖ The Act provides for the *prohibition of sex selection, before or after conception*
❖ It regulates the use of prenatal diagnostic techniques, like *ultrasound and amniocentesis* by allowing them their use only to detect:
  – Genetic abnormalities
  – Metabolic disorders
  – Chromosomal abnormalities
  – Certain congenital malformations
  – Hemoglobinopathies
  – Sex-linked disorders.
❖ No laboratory or center or clinic will conduct any test including *ultrasonography (USG) for the purpose of determining the sex* of the fetus
❖ No person, including the one who is conducting the procedure as per the law, will *communicate the sex of the fetus* to the pregnant woman or her relatives *by words, signs or any other method*
❖ Any person who puts an advertisement for prenatal and preconception sex determination facilities in the form of a notice, circular, label, wrapper or any document, or advertises through interior or other media in electronic or print form or engages in any visible representation made by means of hoarding, wall painting, signal, light, sound, smoke or gas, can be imprisoned for *up to three years and fined ₹ 10,000.*

Amendment

Prenatal Diagnostic Techniques (Regulation and Prevention of Misuse) (PNDT) Act, 1994, was amended in 2003 to The Preconception and Prenatal Diagnostic Techniques (Prohibition of Sex Selection) Act (PCPNDT Act).

Aim

To improve the regulation of the technology used in sex selection.

▓ NUTRITION AND HEALTH

Dietary Goal

Introduction

All countries should develop a national nutrition and food policy setting out a 'dietary goal' for achievement.

Definition of healthy diet in adult (As per WHO recommendation 2015)

❖ Fruits, vegetables, legumes (e.g. lentils, beans), nuts and whole grains (e.g. unprocessed maize, millet, oats, wheat, brown rice)

❖ At least 400 g (5 portions) of fruits and vegetables a day. Potatoes, sweet potatoes, cassava and other starchy roots are not classified as fruits or vegetables
❖ Less than 10% of total energy intake from free sugars which is equivalent to 50 g (or around 12 level teaspoons) for a person of healthy body weight consuming approximately 2000 calories per day, but ideally less than 5% of total energy intake for additional health benefits
❖ Less than 30% of total energy intake from fats:
  – Unsaturated fats are preferable to saturated fats. Industrial trans fats are not part of a healthy diet
❖ Less than 5 g of salt (equivalent to approximately 1 teaspoon) per day and use iodized salt.

Definition of healthy diet for infants and young children (As per WHO recommendation 2015)
In the first 2 years of a child's life, optimal nutrition fosters healthy growth and improves cognitive development. It also reduces the risk of becoming overweight or obese and developing NCDs later in life.

Advice on a healthy diet for infants and children is similar to that for adults, but the following elements are also important.
❖ Infants should be breastfed exclusively during the first 6 months of life
❖ Infants should be breastfed continuously until 2 years of age and beyond
❖ From 6 months of age, breast milk should be complemented with a variety of adequate, safe and nutrient dense complementary foods. Salt and sugars should not be added to complementary foods.

Spectrum of Iodine Deficiency Disorders

Disease	Level of severity/presentations
Goiter (WHO classification)	Grade 0: Goiter is not palpable or visible even when neck is extended
	Grade 1a: When the goiter is palpable
	Grade 1b: When the goiter is visible
	Grade 2: Goiter is visible when neck is in normal position
	Grade 3: Large goiter visible from distance
Hypothyroidism	Variable clinical signs may be present in different stages of the disease
Endemic cretinism	Hypothyroid cretinism
	Neurological cretinism
Neurological effects	Subnormal intelligence
	Delayed motor milestones
	Mental deficit
	Hearing defects
	Speech defects
	Muscle weakness in legs/arms/trunk
	Spastic diplegia
	Spastic quadriplegia

Contd...

Contd...

Disease	Level of severity/presentations
Intrauterine death	Spontaneous abortion
	Miscarriage
Squint	Unilateral
	Bilateral

Pasteurization of Milk

Definition

Pasteurization is a process that kills harmful bacteria by heating milk to a specific temperature for a set period of time (FDA).

Discovery

The method of sterilization was first developed by Louis Pasteur in 1864.

Bacteria Killed by Pasteurization

Pasteurization kills harmful organisms responsible for many diseases like:
❖ Listeriosis
❖ Typhoid fever
❖ Tuberculosis
❖ Diphtheria and
❖ Brucellosis.

Methods of Pasteurization

1. *"Holder" method*: Milk is heated in a large jacketed container by steam or hot water circulating in the interspace at 60°–65.5°C, for at least 30 minutes. The milk is then cooled to 10°C or less. The batch holder vessel is then to be emptied, and there is a break in the operation of at least 1 hour before the next batch is ready for filling into the distribution bottles or cartons.
2. *"Flash" method*: Milk is heated as rapidly as possible to 75°–80°C or even above, and then cooled rapidly.
3. *"High-temperature, short-time (HTST)" continuous method*: Milk is rapidly brought to a temperature of 71°–72°C and held at that temperature for not less than 15 seconds, and is then rapidly cooled to 10°C or below.
4. *"Ultra-high temperature (UHT)" continuous method*: Milk is rapidly heated, usually in two stages (the second stage being under pressure), to 135°–150°C for a few seconds only, and is then either cooled rapidly and bottled as aseptically as possible, or bottled hot (at 75°–80°C).

Integrated Child Development Scheme

Introduction

Integrated child development scheme (ICDS) is the country's most comprehensive and multidimensional program. It is a centrally sponsored scheme of the Ministry of Women and Child Development.

Objectives

1. Lay foundation for the proper psychological, physical and social development of the child.
2. Improve nutritional and health status of children below six years.
3. Reduce incidence of mortality, morbidity, malnutrition and school dropouts.
4. Achieve effective coordination of policy and implementation amongst various departments.
5. Enhance the capabilities of the mother to look after the normal health and nutritional needs of child through proper nutrition and health education.

Focal Point to Deliver all the Services Under ICDS

Anganwadi Center (1 for 1000 population).

Beneficiaries and Services Provided

Beneficiaries	Services provided
Children <3 years	• Supplementary nutrition • Growth monitoring • Immunization • Health check-up • Referral services
Children 3–6 years	• Nonformal preschool education • Supplementary nutrition • Growth monitoring • Immunization • Health check-up • Referral services
Expectant and nursing mothers	• Health check-up • Tetanus toxoid immunization to pregnant women • Supplementary nutrition • Nutrition and health education
Other women of 15–45 years	• Nutrition and health education
Adolescent girls of 11–18 years	• IFA supplementation and deworming intervention • Nonformal education • Home-based skill training and vocational training • Supplementary nutrition

What are the Integrated Packages of Services under ICDS Scheme?

Packages	Services
Nutrition	• Supplementary nutrition • Growth monitoring • Nutrition and health education
Health	• Health check-up • Immunization

Contd...

Contd...

Packages	Services
	• Identification and treatment of common childhood illnesses • Referral services
Supportive services and convergence	• Safe drinking water • Environmental sanitation • Women's empowerment programs • Adult literacy
Early childhood care and preschool education	• Early care and stimulation of children under 3 years • Preschool education to children in the 3–6 years age group

Special Note: Supplementary Nutrition

Age	Nutrition provided
Normal children (6 months–6 years)	500 kcal and 12–15 g protein
Severely malnourished children (6 months–6 years)	800 kcal and 20–25 g protein
Pregnant and lactating mothers	600 kcal and 18–20 g protein

National Program for Prevention of Nutritional Blindness

Objective

The specific objective of the program is to reduce the disease prevalence due to vitamin A deficiency.

Activities

❖ A massive dose of vitamin A is given every 6 months to children between 6 months–5 years
❖ The recommended schedule for the mega-dose administration is:
  – *6–11 months*: 1 dose of vitamin A of 100,000 IU
  – *1–5 years*: A total of 8 doses of vitamin A of 200,000 IU every 6 months
❖ The long-term strategy emphasizes the improvement of dietary intake of vitamin A through regular consumption of vitamin A rich foods:
  – Green leafy vegetables
  – Yellow fruits
  – Dairy products and promotion of breastfeeding.

Intensified National Iron Plus Initiative (i-NIPI)

Estimation of the level of Hb in pregnant women should be done at the initial antenatal visits and again at 28 weeks.

Hemoglobin level	Designation
>11 g/dL	Normal
7–11 g/dL	Moderately anemic
<7 g/dL	Severely anemic

Intensified National Iron Plus Initiative (I-NIPI) of the Anemia Mukt Bharat campaign is a recently launched program by Ministry of Health and Family Welfare, Government of India in April, 2018 under POSHAN (PM's Overarching scheme for holistic nourishment) abhiyaan.

The beneficiaries are:
  i. Children of 6–59 months
  ii. School children of 5–10 years
  iii. Adolescents of 10–19 years
  iv. Pregnant and lactating women
  v. Women in reproductive age group.

Beneficiaries	Intervention/Dose	Regime
Children of 6–59 months	1 mL of IFA syrup containing 20 mg of elemental iron and 100 μg of folic acid	Biweekly throughout the period 6–60 months of age and deworming for children 12 months and above
School children 5–10 years	Tablets of 45 mg elemental iron and 400 μg of folic acid	Weekly throughout the period 5–10 years of age and biannual deworming
Adolescents of 10–19 years	60 mg elemental iron and 500 μg of folic acid	Weekly throughout the period 10–19 years of age and biannual deworming
Pregnant and lactating women	60 mg elemental iron and 500 μg of folic acid	1 tab daily starting from 14th week of gestation, continued throughout pregnancy (minimum 180 days during pregnancy) and to be continued for 180 days postpartum: a total of 1 year
Women in reproductive age group	60 mg elemental iron and 500 μg of folic acid	Weekly throughout the reproductive period

National Iodine Deficiency Disorders Control Programme

Introduction

India commenced the National Goiter Control Programme in 1962, which was intensified into a greater national program called National IDD Control Programme.

Objectives

The important objectives and components of National Iodine Deficiency Disorders Control Programme (NIDDCP) are as follows:
  ❖ Surveys to assess the magnitude of the iodine deficiency disorders
  ❖ Supply of iodated salt in place of common salt
  ❖ Resurvey after every 5 years to assess the extent of iodine deficiency disorders and the impact of iodized salt
  ❖ Laboratory monitoring of iodated salt and urinary iodine excretion
  ❖ Health education and publicity.

Components

a. Use of iodized salt in place of common salt
b. Monitoring and surveillance
c. Manpower training
d. Mass communication.

Use of iodized salt in place of common salt

❖ The daily requirement of iodine for adults is 150 µg
❖ According to this assumption, the Prevention of Food Adulteration Act in India has fixed the iodization level to at least 30 ppm at the production point and at least 15 ppm at the consumer level
❖ Iodization of common salt is the most effective way towards mass prophylaxis in an IDD prevalent zone
❖ Another effective way to control IDDs in the country is the use of intramuscular injection of iodized oil. Beside the advantage that it can be applied on a large scale basis, the cost is higher than that of iodized salt.

Monitoring and Surveillance

The following indicators are most commonly used to monitor the efficacy of the control program:
❖ Prevalence of neonatal hypothyroidism: It is the most sensitive indicator
❖ Measurement of urinary iodine excretion
❖ Prevalence of goiter and cretinism in a community
❖ Measurement of iodine levels in food, water and salt.

Manpower training and mass communication

They are also important components of National IDD Control Program, which include proper training of healthcare providers and peripheral health workers and at the same time, creating public awareness by collaboration with mass media to achieve effective IDD control at the fullest extent.

Mid-day Meal Scheme

Objectives

The objectives of the mid-day meal scheme are:
❖ Improving the nutritional status of children in classes I–VIII in Government, Local Body and Government-aided schools, and EGS and AIE centers
❖ Encouraging poor children, belonging to disadvantaged sections, to attend school more regularly and help them concentrate on classroom activities
❖ Providing nutritional support to children of primary stage in drought-affected areas during summer vacation.

Nutritional Content: Calorific and Nutrition Value and Food Norm Per Child Per Day

To achieve the above objectives a cooked mid-day meal with the following nutritional content is provided to all eligible children.

Items	Primary (Class I-V)	Upper primary (Class VI-XII)
Calorie	450	700
Protein	12 g	20 g
Rice/wheat	90 g (previously 100 g)	125 g (previously 150 g)
Dal	20 g	30 g
Vegetables	50 g	75 g
Oil and fat	5 g	7.5 g
Micronutrients and deworming medicine	In convergence with school health program of NRHM	

New Guidelines for Mid-day Meal Scheme

❖ Addition of additional items like milk, milk products, eggs, banana
❖ Use of double fortified salt with iodine and iron
❖ Increase in oil/fat intake
❖ The oil should be mix of three combinations:
   a. Palmolein/coconut oil/ghee
   b. Sunflower or mustard/soyabean or linseed.

Rationale of Mid-Day Meal Scheme

❖ *Promoting school participation*: Mid-day meals have great effects on school participation, not just in terms of getting more children enrolled in the registers but also in terms of regular attendance on a daily basis.
❖ *Preventing classroom hunger*: Many children reach school on an empty stomach. Even children who have a meal before they leave for school get hungry by the afternoon and are not able to concentrate—especially children from families who cannot give them a lunch box or are staying a long distance away from the school. Mid-day meal can help to overcome this problem by *preventing "classroom hunger".*
❖ *Facilitating the healthy growth of children*: Mid-day meal can also act as a regular source of "supplementary nutrition" for children and facilitate their healthy growth.
❖ *Intrinsic educational value*: A well-organized mid-day meal can be used as an opportunity to impart various good habits to children (such as washing one's hands before and after eating), and to educate them about the importance of clean water, good hygiene and other related matters.
❖ *Fostering social equality*: Mid-day meal can help to break the barriers of caste and class among school.
❖ *Enhancing gender equity*: The gender gap in school participation tends to narrow, as the Mid-Day Meal Scheme helps erode the barriers that prevent girls from going to school. Mid-Day Meal Scheme also provides a useful source of employment for women, and helps liberate working women from the burden of cooking at home during the day. In these and other ways, women and girl children have a special stake in Mid-Day Meal Scheme
❖ *Psychological benefits*: Physiological deprivation leads to low self-esteem, consequent insecurity, anxiety and stress. The Mid-Day Meal Scheme can help address this and facilitate cognitive, emotional and social development.

MEDICINE AND SOCIAL SCIENCES

Acculturation

Meaning: "Culture contact".

Definition

Diffusion of culture between individuals of different types of culture in both direction.

Factors Influencing Acculturation

Mnemonic: PEPTIC-M
❖ **P**restige of different culture and its people
❖ **E**ducation

❖ **P**ropagation of religion
❖ **T**rade and commerce
❖ **I**ndustrialization
❖ **C**onquest
❖ **M**igration.

Examples

❖ Indus valley civilization, Greek civilization, Egyptian civilization have spread to other parts of the world
❖ After renaissance the center of the world culture shifted to Great Britain, France and other European countries which spread to other countries through colonization
❖ Introduction of scientific medicine/habits through culture contact, e.g. orthodox Brahmins of India eat meat today.

Barriers of Acculturation

❖ Resistance to culture changes
❖ Mores and taboos
❖ Sense of superiority
❖ General cultural inertia
❖ Adaptability of the recipients of the new culture
❖ Physical isolation.

Effects of Acculturation

Good effect	Bad effect
• Positive changes in food habit	• Smoking, alcohol consumption
• Introduction of new ideas, concept ethics, etc.	• Drug abuse
• Increased literacy	• Sedentary lifestyle

Significance

Important for cultural growth of the community. But "culture borrowing" (borrowing ideas of different culture) is better for cultural growth of the community.

Problem Family

Introduction

Problem families are those which lag behind the rest of the community. In these families, the standards of living is usually far below the accepted minimum standards. These families are recognized as "problems in social pathology".

Underlying Factors

❖ Poverty
❖ Backwardness
❖ Chronic illness of a family member
❖ Mental and emotional instability
❖ Marital disharmony
❖ Relationship problems
❖ Character defects.

Dangers of Problem Family

Children who are reared in these families are prone to:
- ❖ Crime
- ❖ Violence
- ❖ Prostitution
- ❖ Gambling
- ❖ Drug abuse
- ❖ Vagrancy.

How to Solve this Problem in the Society?

- ❖ Usually problem families are found among lower social classes
- ❖ This problem can only be solved by active involvement of all parts of the society, where the health personnel can take an active role
- ❖ Health visitor, health inspector, midwife, social worker, medical officer—all have to work together to eliminate this problem.

Social Security

Definition

Social security is the security that society furnishes through the appropriate organizations against certain risk to which its members are exposed.

Risks Covered

Mnemonic: SOMA DI
- ❖ **S**ickness
- ❖ **O**ld age
- ❖ **MA**ternity
- ❖ **D**eath
- ❖ **I**nvalidity.

Components

- ❖ Social insurance
- ❖ Social assistance.

Topic	Social security	Social assistance
Contribution	Not only by the employees but also employers and organizations	No contribution system
Benefits	In terms of cash, not by sympathy but by a matter of right	Cash/a kind by sympathy/charity
Inferiority complex	Do not develop	May develop
Active involvement	Members are actively involved in economic planning for future	Not actively involved
Contribution	Suitable to the workers, who can contribute	Suitable to the workers who cannot contribute
Dependency	May not arise permanently	May become permanently dependent on the scheme

Contd...

Contd...

Topic	Social security	Social assistance
Legislation	Many	Hardly any legislation
Beneficiary	Industrial worker, employees of state and Central Government	Unemployed, widows, orphans, handicapped, old age people
Example	*For industrial worker*: • Workmen's compensation work • Central Maternity Benefits Act • ESI scheme *For civil servants*: • The family pension scheme *For general public*: • Public provident Fund Scheme, LIC of India	Unemployment allowance, Sanjay Gandhi Niradhar Yojana

Significance

Social security is nothing but a basis of social welfare and is essential because those who are not secured in this way, may cause social harm in fulfilling their own needs.

ENVIRONMENT AND HEALTH

Indicators of Air Pollution

Some of the most commonly used indicators of air pollution are:
❖ Sulfur dioxide
❖ Smoke
❖ Grit and dust.
❖ Air pollution index.

Sulfur Dioxide

It is a major air pollutant globally. Its concentration in air is measured in all environmental surveys.

Smoke

Its concentration is measured in microgram/cubic meter of air.

Grit and Dust

Their concentrations are monitored on a monthly basis.

Air Pollution Index

It is an arbitrary index taking account for one or more pollutants as a measure of severity of air pollution.

How the Values are Calculated?

The indicator values are measured for one population only, it is the average value measured over a specified time.

Example:

Pollutant (Unit: $\mu g\ m^{-3}$)	Indicators
Carbon monoxide	Annual maximum 8 hours running average
Lead	Annual average
Nitrogen dioxide	Annual maximum 24 hours average Annual average
Ozone	Annual maximum 1 hour average Annual maximum 8 hours running average
Particulate matter	Annual maximum 24 hours average Annual average
Sulfur dioxide	Annual maximum 24 hours average Annual average

Some commonly used air pollution indicators and their excess values

(According to the recommended revision of the WHO Air Quality Guidelines for Europe)

Indicators	Excess value
NO_2	No. of days where 1 hour average >200 $\mu g/m^3$
SO_2	No. of days where daily average >125 $\mu g/m^3$
TSP*	No. of days where daily average >120 $\mu g/m^3$
PM 10#	No. of days where daily average >70 $\mu g/m^3$
Black smoke	No. of days where daily average >125 $\mu g/m^3$ (Recommended only in areas where coal smoke from domestic fires is the dominant component of the particulate)
CO	• No. of days where 1 hour average >30 $\mu g/m^3$ • No. of days where 8 hour average >10 $\mu g/m^3$
Lead	Annual average >0.5 $\mu g/m^3$
BaP^	It has been estimated that 9 out of 100,000 people exposed to 1 ng BaP per m^3 over lifetime would be at risk of developing cancer The unit risk of BaP for developing lung cancer is 8.7 x 10–5 ng/m^3 BaP

* Total suspended particulates. #: Particulate matter of 10 μm diameter. ^: Benzo(a)pyrene.

Chlorination of water

Introduction

Chlorination of water is one of the most essential part for disinfection of water due to its fast action, broad spectrum antimicrobial action, residual effect, nontoxic nature and many other favorable properties.

Action of Chlorine in the Process of Disinfection

❖ $H_2O + Cl_2 \rightarrow$ Hypochlorous acid (HOCl) + Hydrochloric acid (HCl)
❖ $HOCl = [H] + [OCl]$

Phases of Chlorination

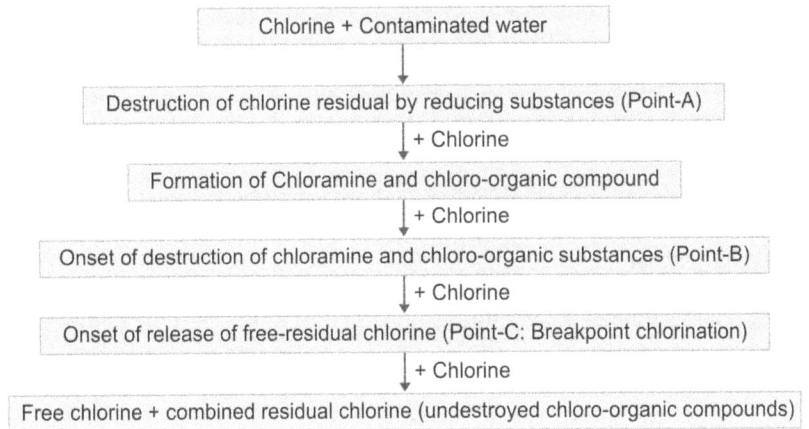

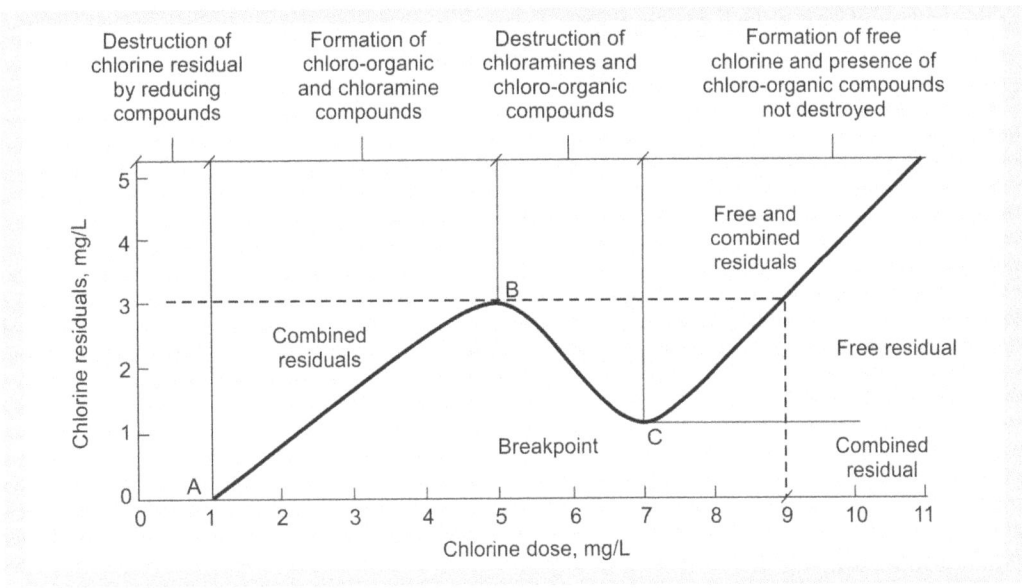

Graphical representation of Chlorine dose vs. Chlorine residuals in various phases of chlorination

Achievements of Breakpoint Chlorination Indicates

❖ Destruction of all organic compounds along with organisms
❖ Oxidation of harmful ammoniacal substances.

Breakpoint chlorination achieves same results as superchlorination (when large dose of chlorine applied for heavily polluted water; here residual chlorine is usually >1 ppm).

Recommended contact time of free residual chlorine in water: 1 hour

Recommended free residual chlorine levels:

Type of water	Recommended levels (in mg/liter*)	Recommended contact time
Drinking water	0.5	1 hour
Water bodies (post-disaster)	>0.7	1 hour
Swimming pool	>1	1 hour

* 1 mg/lit = 1 ppm

Correct dose of chlorine to be applied: chlorine demand + FRC 0.5 mg/L

Tests for Chlorination of Water

Tests	Ortho-toluidine (OT) test	Ortho-toluidine Arsenite (OTA) test
Measures level of:	• Free chlorine • Free chlorine + combined chlorine	• Free chlorine separately • Combine chlorine separately

OTA Test is Better than OT Test because:

❖ It detects combined and free chlorine separately
❖ Not affected by interfering substance.

Soakage Pit

Introduction

Soakage pit is very cheap, simple and sanitary method of disposing sullage water especially in rural set up.

Use

Soakage pits are used to soak septic tank effluent into the surrounding soil otherwise haphazard collection of water may lead to problems of fly, mosquito breeding, sight and smell nuisance and contaminated drinking water.

Principle

Soakage pits do not provide any direct treatment and are based on the principle that effluent gets treated as it passes through the surrounding soil before entering the ground water table or other water body.

Criteria

In building and using soakage pits following shall be noted:
❖ At least 18 m away from a well or other drinking water source
❖ At least 5 m from the nearest building
❖ At least 10–20 m from any other soakage pit
❖ At least 1.5 m shall be kept between the bottom of the tank to the seasonal ground water table
❖ Adequate contact area with the surrounding soil to absorb the effluent into the soil. In clayey soil, larger pits will be needed.

Alternatives

If a soakage pit cannot be constructed due to above reasons, there are following measures in place of a soakage pit:
- ❖ Anaerobic biofilters
- ❖ Soakage trench
- ❖ Soakage bed.

Model of Soakage Pit

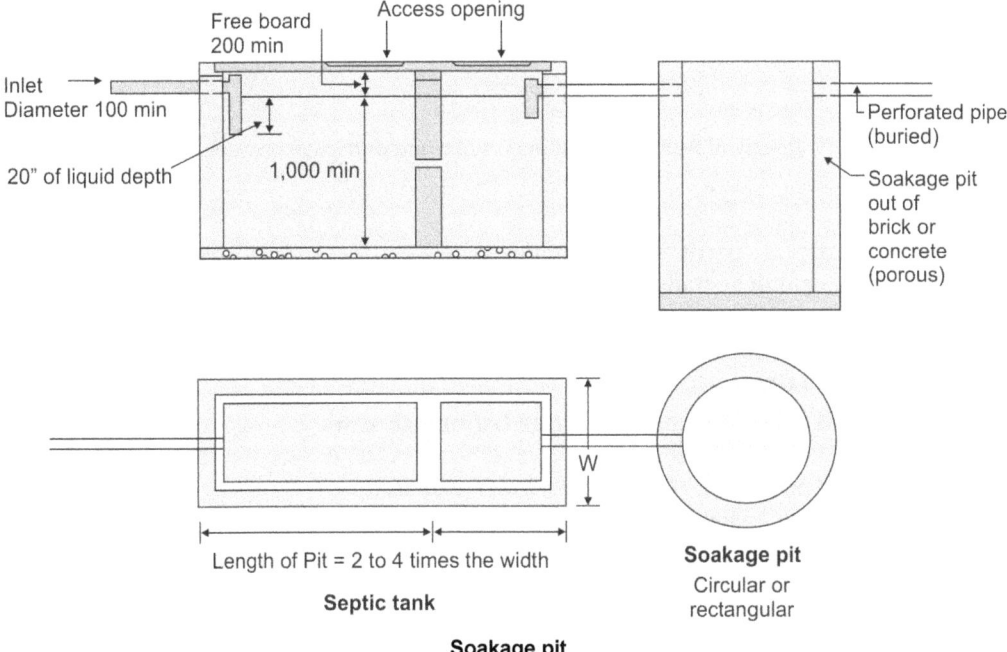

Septic tank

Length of Pit = 2 to 4 times the width

Soakage pit
Circular or rectangular

Soakage pit

Advantages
- ❖ Cheap, simple and sanitary method for sullage disposal
- ❖ Easy to build.

Sanitary Latrine

Introduction

From the feces, disease agent can be transmitted to the host through 5 channels (also known as 5 Fs):
1. Food
2. Flies
3. Fingers
4. Fluid
5. Field/fomite.

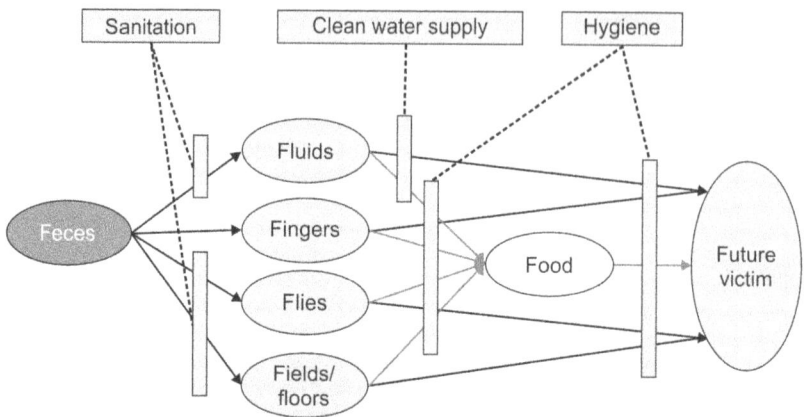

Routes of fecal disease transmission and protective barriers

Sanitation barrier is a barrier which is imposed between feces and all these channels so that the disease agent cannot be transmitted to the host through these channels. *Sanitation barrier can be effectively provided in the form of sanitary latrine.*

Criteria for a Sanitary Latrine

❖ Excreta should not contaminate the ground or surface water
❖ Excreta should not pollute the soil
❖ Excreta should not be accessible to flies, rodents or animals
❖ Excreta should not create bad odor or ugly appearance.

Some Common Types of Sanitary Latrine

❖ Bore hole latrine
❖ Dug well latrine
❖ Water seal latrine.

Short Description of Commonly used Sanitary Latrines

Bore hole latrine

It consists of a circular hole of about 16 inches in diameter dug into the ground to a depth of 20 feet. A concrete squatting place with a central opening and foot plate is placed over the hole. A suitable enclosure is put up for privacy. This type of latrine is useful for a family of 5–6 people for about 1 year.

Dug well latrine

It is an improvement over bore hole latrine. It consists of a circular pit of 30 inch diameter and 10–12 feet deep. This pit is lined with pottery rings. A concrete squatting plate is placed on the

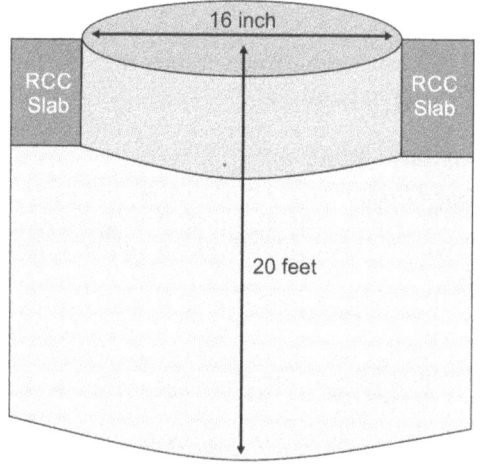

Bore hole latrine

top of the pit. The latrine is enclosed within a suitable structure for privacy. This type of latrine may serve for 5 years.

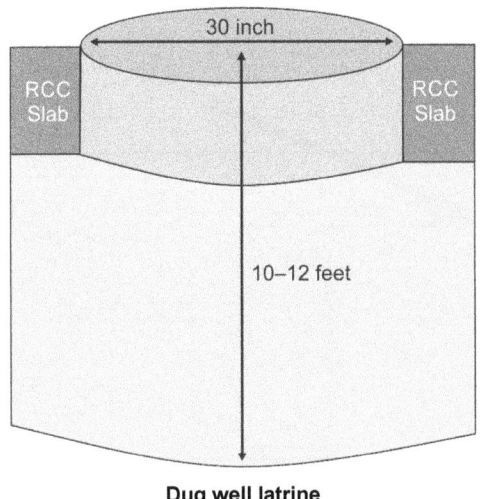

Dug well latrine

Water seal latrine

It is an improved form of sanitary latrine.

Advantages of water seal latrine

❖ It prevents access to flies
❖ It prevents the escape of foul odor and gases
❖ It requires minimum use of water.

Two types are available

A. PRAI type (evolved by Planning Research and Action Institute of Lucknow)
B. RCA type (designed by Research-Cum-Action Projects in environmental sanitation of Health Ministry).

Of these two, RCA type is most popular.

RCA latrine

Parts with Description

Parts	Description
Squatting plate with pan	The size of squatting plate is 3 ft x 3 ft. It contains raised foot rests and a pan which receives feces, urine and wash water
Trap	It is a bent pipe of about 3 inches in diameter and it is connected to the pan. *The trap contains water and acts as a water seal.* Water seal is the distance between the level of water in the trap and the lowest point in the concave surface of the trap. The water seal is usually 20–30 mm (1") in depth. The water seal prevents access to flies and also suppresses bad odor
Connecting pipe	The trap is connected to the dug well pipe by means of a connecting pipe. It is 3 inches in diameter and 3 feet in length with a bend at the end
Dug well pit	It is 30 inches in diameter and 10–12 feet deep. When one pit is full another one may be dug
Super structure	It provides both privacy and shelter

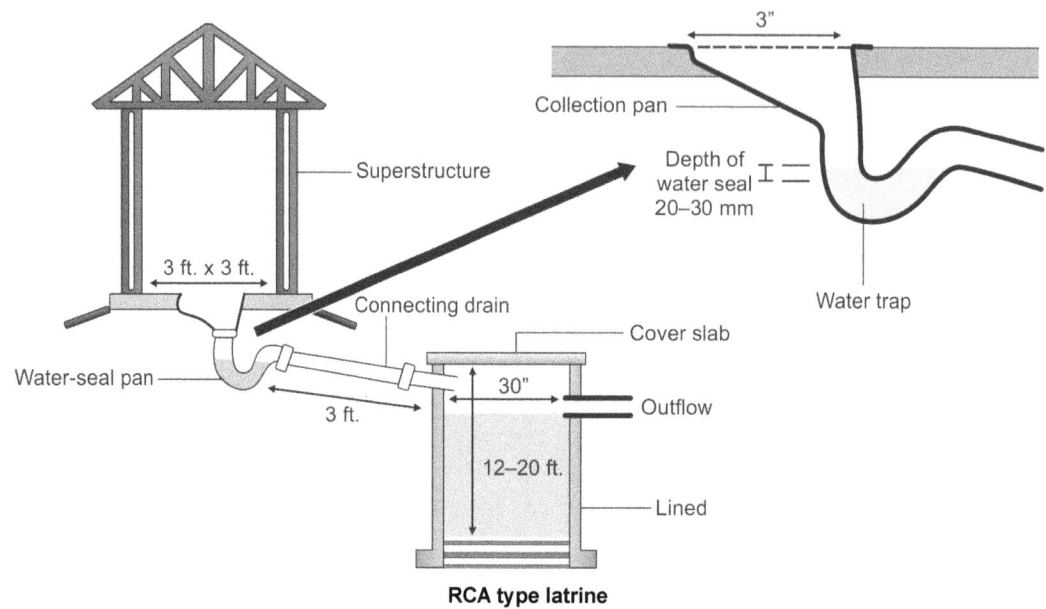

3 ft. x 3 ft.

Superstructure

Collection pan

Depth of water seal 20–30 mm

Connecting drain

Water-seal pan

3 ft.

Cover slab

30"

Outflow

12–20 ft.

Lined

Water trap

3"

RCA type latrine

Sanitary Well

Introduction

A sanitary well is one that is properly located, well-constructed, and well protected from possible locations of contamination so as to ensure supply of safe water.

Criteria

The criteria for a sanitary well are: [MNEMONIC of points: "**(PLC)2-HDQ**"]

❖ *Parapet wall:*
   – A sanitary well should have a parapet wall up to a height of at least 70–75 cm.
❖ *Platform:*
   – A cement concrete platform should be constructed around the well with a radius of at least 1 m in all directions
   – The margin of the platform should have a drain for collecting the spilled water.
❖ *Location:*
   – A sanitary well should be located at least 15 m (50 ft) away from possible sources of contamination
   – It should be located at higher level than nearby sources of contamination
   – It should not be located too far away from the people's houses—it is suggested that no user should have to carry water for more than 100 m.
❖ *Lining:*
   – The inside of the well should be lined with bricks up to a depth of at least 6 m
   – This is to ensure that the water enters the well from the bottom, not from the sides
   – Also the lining should be continued till about 60–90 cm above the ground level.
❖ *Cover:*
   – A proper cement concrete cover is essential for maintaining the quality of the water of the well
   – It increases the bacterial quality of the well water considerably.

❖ *Consumer responsibility:*
  – The people who use the well should observe certain precautions to ensure the quality of the water
  – They should not dump waste materials around the well
  – Washing of clothes and animals in the vicinity of the well should be prohibited.
❖ *Hand pump*
  – A hand pump should be installed to draw water from the well
  – It should be of good quality so as to endure the rough handling by the people
  – It should be regularly serviced and there should be provision to repair it quickly if any fault were to arise.
❖ *Drain:*
  – The spilled water should be channelled away from the well using a proper drain system
  – It should be connected to the public drain system or to a drainage pit located outside the cone of filtration of the well.
❖ *Quality:*
  – The physical, chemical and biological parameters of the well water should conform to acceptable standards.

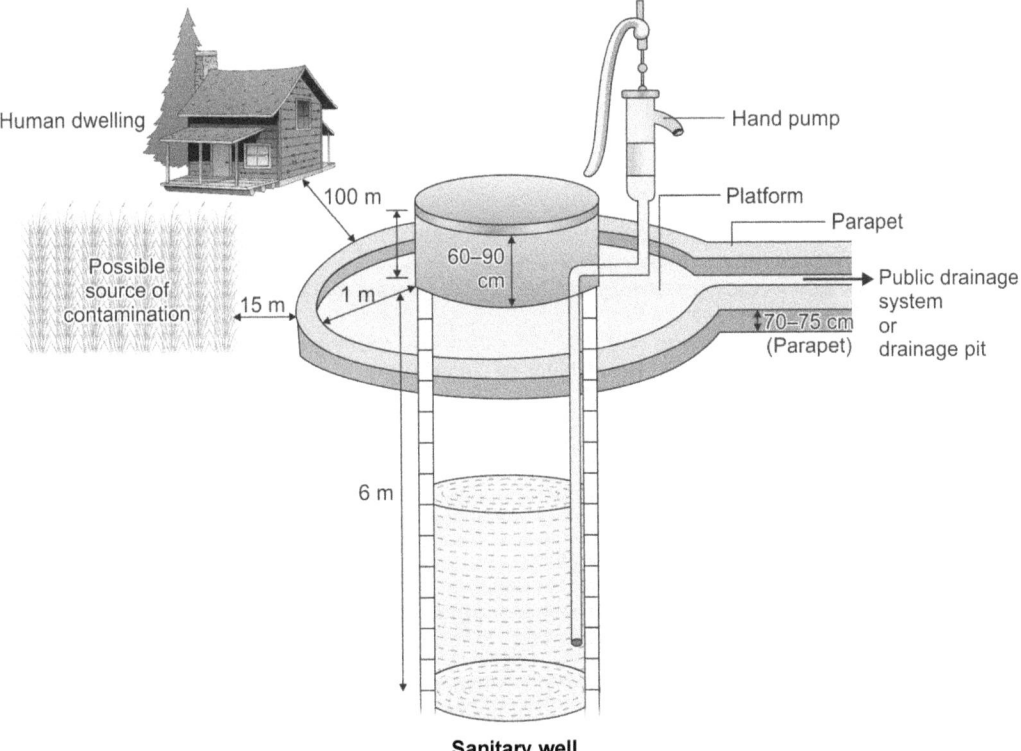

Sanitary well

Sanitation Barrier

Definition

Transmission of all prevailing endemic diseases can be prevented and controlled by preventing the contamination of physical environment such as food, soil and water by construction of a

barrier called as sanitation barrier, which is nothing but construction and use of sanitary latrines, which prevents access of pathogens from feces through 6Fs such as:
1. **Fluid** (water and milk)
2. **Food**
3. **Fruits** and vegetables
4. **Fomites** (utensils)
5. **Flies** (vectors) and
6. **Fingers**, to mouth of susceptible person.

A fecalborne disease roughly follows the transmission cycle shown below:

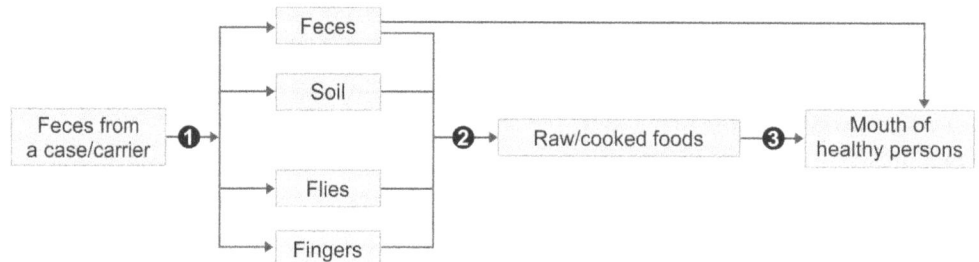

Routes of transmission of disease from feces to healthy person

To block the transmission chain shown above, we can apply sanitation barrier by taking the following measures:

Route	How can it be achieved?
Route 1	• All families should have a clean and functional latrine • The latrine should be regularly washed • If there is no latrine, family members should defecate at a distance of at least 10 meters from water supply source • Hand washing with soap after defecation/after cleaning a child who has defecated/after disposing off a child's stool should be promoted • There should be an effective excreta disposal system
Route 2	Hand should be washed thoroughly with soap: • Before preparing food • Before eating • Before feeding a child
Route 3	• Cooked hot food should be eaten • Proper food handling techniques should be used • Cooking utensils should be cleaned and dried after use • Reduction measures should be taken to reduce the number of houseflies

It should be emphasized that all these preventive sanitation measures will produce only temporary results if they are not combined with *health education*. So health education with the help of community members should be utilized and people of a community should be taught about importance of all these preventive measures in a long term.

Hazards of Noise Pollution

Introduction

"Noise" is defined as "wrong sound, at the wrong place and at the wrong time".

Sources of Noise in Daily Life

- ❖ Automobiles
- ❖ Industries
- ❖ Factories
- ❖ Aircrafts
- ❖ Railway junctions
- ❖ Bus terminuses
- ❖ Loudspeakers, etc.

Tolerable Level

A daily exposure of 85 dB is the limit people can tolerate without substantial damage to their hearing.

Permitted Daily Exposure

According to the Factory Act, 1948; the permitted level of daily exposure is as follows (Remember: A rise of 5 dB noise level will reduce the permitted daily noise exposure time to ½ times):

Noise level (dB)	Permitted daily exposure (in hours)
90	8
95	4
100	2
105	1
110	0.5
115	0.25

Effects of Noise Pollution

Effects of noise pollution are of two types:
1. Auditory effects
2. Nonauditory effects.

Type of effect	Includes	Exposure level	Deleterious effects
Auditory	Auditory fatigue	90 dB and 4000 Hz	Whistling and buzzing in the ears
	Temporary hearing loss	4000–6000 Hz	Hearing is impaired immediately after exposure but recovers after some time
	Permanent hearing loss	~100 dB	Damage to the inner ear
		~160 dB	Rupture of tympanic membrane
Nonauditory	Interference with speech		For good speech intelligibility, the speech sound level must exceed speech interference level by 12 dB. Road traffic sounds often interfere with speech
	Annoyance		Workmen exposed to higher intensity of noise are often irritated and impatient
	Efficiency		In high level of sound, mental concentration is lost and work efficiency is decreased

Contd...

Contd...

Type of effect	Includes	Exposure level	Deleterious effects
	Physiological changes	• Rise in blood pressure • Rise in intracranial pressure • Increase in heart rate • Increase in sweating • Interference with sleep • Decreased color perception and decreased night vision • Nausea and fatigue	
	Economic loss	The potential cost of noise-induced hearing loss in the industry is great	

Sanitary Land Fill

Introduction

It is the most satisfactory method of refuse disposal where suitable land is available.

Methods

There are three methods used in this operation:

Name of methods	Description
Trench method	• A long trench is dug out (Depth: 2–3 m and Width: 4–12 m) • The refuse is compacted and covered with excavated earth
Ramp method	• It is best suited to sloping land • Solid waste is spread and compacted on a slope and covered
Area method	• The refuse is compacted and packed in successive layers (2–2.5 m depth) • Each layer is sealed with mud (depth of at least 30 cm)

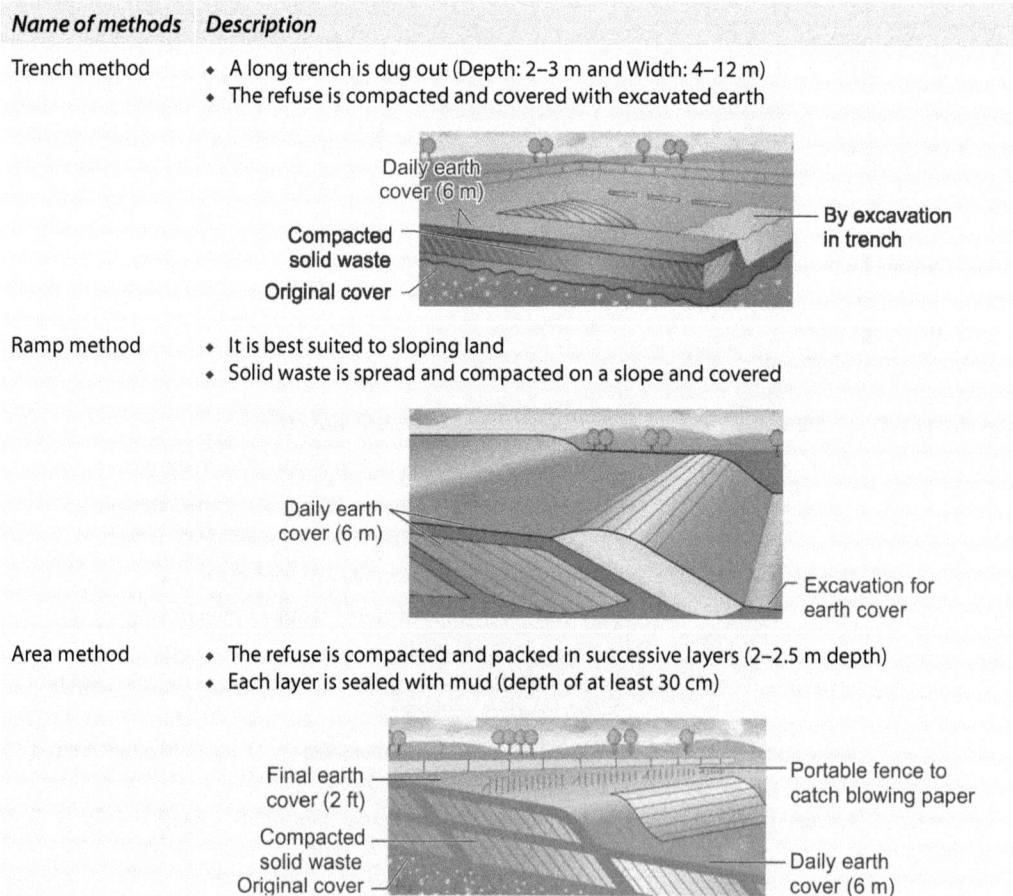

Daily earth cover (6 m)
Compacted solid waste
Original cover
By excavation in trench

Daily earth cover (6 m)
Excavation for earth cover

Final earth cover (2 ft)
Compacted solid waste
Original cover
Portable fence to catch blowing paper
Daily earth cover (6 m)

Changes in the Buried Refuse

- ❖ Temperature rises to >60°C within 7 days and kills all the pathogens
- ❖ Then it cools down for the next 2–3 weeks
- ❖ Within 4–6 months, the buried refuse is completely decomposed and it is converted into a nonoffensive mass.

Overcrowding

Definition

Overcrowding refers to the situation, in which more people are living within a single dwelling than there is space for, so that:
- ❖ Movement is restricted
- ❖ Privacy secluded
- ❖ Hygiene impossible
- ❖ Rest and sleep difficult.

Accepted Standards with Respect to Overcrowding

1. *Person per room*: Accepted standards

Room	Person
1	2
2	3
3	5
4	7
5	10
>5	Add 2 per room

2. *Floor space*: Accepted standards

Floor space (sq ft)	Persons
≥110	2
90–100	1.5*
70–90	1
50–70	0.5*
<50	0

* Children aged <12 months are not counted. Children aged 1–10 years are counted as 0.5.

3. *Sex separation*: Overcrowding is considered to be present if *2 persons aged >9 years, who are not husband and wife and of opposite sexes are obliged to sleep in the same room.*

Problems Associated with Overcrowding

Type of diseases	Name of diseases
Respiratory infections	• Tuberculosis • Influenza • Diphtheria
Psychological illness	• Irritability • Frustration • Lack of sleep • Anxiety • Violence • Mental disorders

Water-borne Diseases

Classification of Water-borne Diseases

Category		Contents
Due to presence of an infective agent	Viral	Hepatitis A, hepatitis E, poliomyelitis, rotavirus diarrhea
	Bacterial	Typhoid and paratyphoid fever, bacillary dysentery, cholera, *E. coli* diarrhea
	Protozoal	Amoebiasis, giardiasis
	Helminthic	Roundworm, threadworm, hydatid disease
	Leptospiral	Weil's disease
Due to presence of an aquatic host	Snail	Schistosomiasis
	Cyclops	Guineaworm, fish tape worm

Among the above diseases, diarrhea is the most common water-borne disease, responsible for ~8% of under 5 mortality in India.

Common Modes of Transmission in Water-borne Diseases

Fecal oral route: This is the major route of transmission of most of the water-borne diseases. It may occur in two ways:
1. Directly (Person-to-person contact)
2. Indirectly ("5 F" mechanisms: Flies/Fingers/Fomites/Food/Fluid).

Some of the Important Signs of Water-borne Diseases

In case of acute diarrheal diseases:
1. Lethargy/unconsciousness.
2. Restlessness/irritability.
3. Not able to drink/drinks eagerly.
4. Sunken eyes.
5. Skin pinch going back slowly/very slowly.

In case of dysentery: Blood in the stool.

Prevention and Control of Water-borne Diseases

1. *Immunization*: Some vaccines are recommended for high-risk populations:

Disease/Infectious agent	Name of the vaccine
Polio*	OPV/IPV
Rotavirus	Rotavac
Cholera	Dukoral/Shanchol and mORCVAX
Typhoid	ViPS/ Ty21a
Hepatitis A	Formaldehyde inactivated vaccine

* For all populations.

2. *Sanitation barrier*: The following measures should be taken to block the fecal-oral transmission:
   – All families should have a clean and functional latrine
   – The latrine should be regularly washed
   – If there is no latrine, family members should defecate at a distance of at least 10 meters from water supply source

- Hand washing with soap after defecation/after cleaning a child who has defecated/after disposing off a child's stool should be promoted

There should be an effective excreta disposal system.

- Hand should be washed thoroughly with soap:
    - Before preparing food
    - Before eating
    - Before feeding a child
- Cooked hot food should be eaten
- Proper food handling techniques should be used
- Cooking utensils should be cleaned and dried after use
- Reduction measures should be taken to reduce the number of houseflies.

3. *Health education*: It should be emphasized that all these preventive sanitation measures will produce only temporary results if they are not combined with *health education*. So health education with the help of community members should be taken and people of a community should be taught about importance of all these preventive measures in a long term.

4. *Appropriate clinical management and specific treatment*: Whether possible, the recommended therapeutic measures should be taken to reduce mortality rates. Some of the recommended drugs are:

Water-borne disease	Specific treatment
Acute diarrhea due to all etiologies	Oral rehydration therapy (ORT) in mild dehydration and intravenous rehydration in severe dehydration
Cholera	Ciprofloxacin/Tetracycline/TMP-SMX, etc.
Bacillary dysentery	Ciprofloxacin
Typhoid fever	Ciprofloxacin/Ofloxacin/Ceftriaxone/Cefixime, etc.
Amoebiasis	Metronidazole/Diloxanide furoate
Hookworm infection	Albendazole/Mebendazole

Vital Layer

Definition

In a slow sand filter, the *surface of the sand bed* gets covered with slimy gelatinous growth (biofilm) throughout the purification process (like mechanical straining, sedimentation, adsorption, oxidation), called as vital layer/zoological layer/biological layer/"Schmutzdecke" layer.

The formation of the vital layer is known as "ripening" of the slow sand filter.

Contents

❖ Thread-like algae
❖ Numerous life forms (such as plankton, diatom, aquatic insect larvae and bacteria).

Time duration for formation: 10–20 days.

Thickness: 2–3 mm.

Mode of Action

❖ The *Schmutzdecke* is the layer that provides the effective purification in potable water treatment

❖ The underlying sand provides the support medium for this biological treatment layer
❖ As water passes through the *Schmutzdecke*, particles of foreign matter are trapped in the *mucilaginous matrix* and *dissolved organic* material is adsorbed and metabolized by the bacteria, fungi and protozoa.
❖ In this way this layer:
  – Removes organic matter
  – Holds back bacteria
  – Oxidizes ammoniacal nitrogen into less harmful nitrites
  – Helps in obtaining a bacteria-free water.
❖ Thus, the water produced from a well-managed slow sand filter can be of exceptionally good quality with 90–99% bacterial reduction.

Effects on Performance

Slow sand filters slowly lose their performance as the *Schmutzdecke* grows and thereby reduces the rate of flow through the filter.

Methods for Cleaning the Vital Layer for Maintaining the Flow

❖ *Scraping*:
  – The top 1–2 cm of fine sand is scraped off to expose a new layer of clean sand
  – Water is then poured back into the filter and re-circulated for a few hours to allow a new *Schmutzdecke* to develop.
❖ *Wet harrowing*:
  – Involves lowering the water level to just above the *Schmutzdecke*
  – Stirring the sand and thereby suspending any solids held in that layer and then running the water to waste
  – The filter is then filled to full depth and brought back into service. Wet harrowing can allow the filter to be brought back into service more quickly.

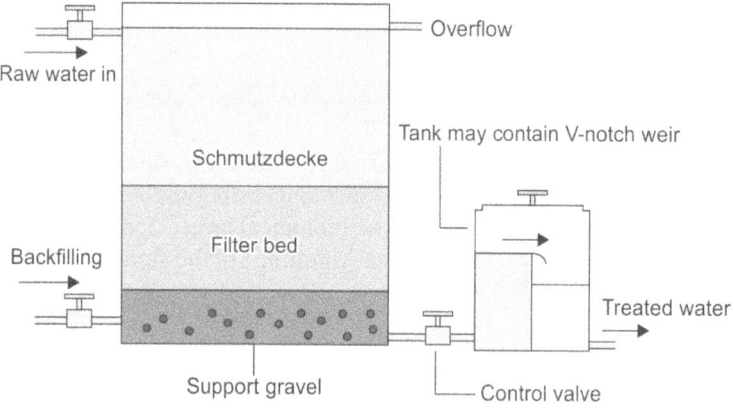

Mechanism of slow sand filter

Oxidation Pond

Definition

Oxidation pond is large and shallow pond designed to treat waste-water through the interaction of sunlight, bacteria and algae.

Other Names

❖ Waste stabilization pond
❖ Redox pond sewage lagoon.

Principle

❖ Working principle based on interaction between sunlight, bacteria and algae
❖ *Bacteria*: Oxidize the organic matter to Carbon dioxide + ammonia + water + phosphate + oxidized organic substance (by consecutive oxidative assimilation and endogenous respiration) which is utilized by algae.

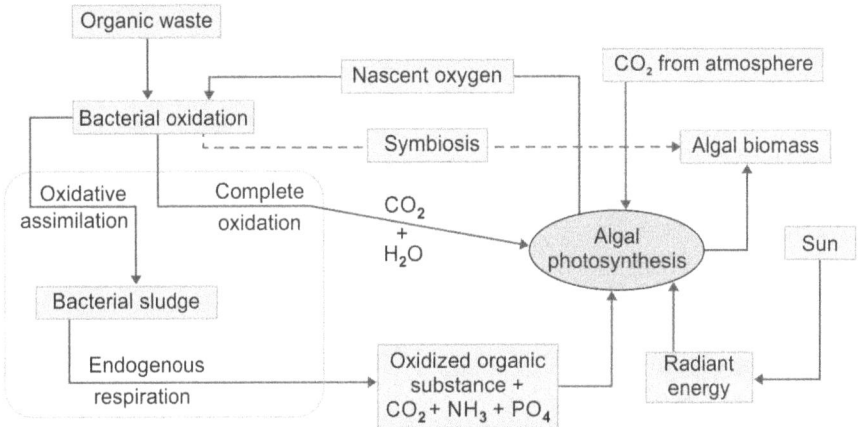

Chemical reactions in biological pond

❖ *Algae:*
  – Use oxidized products for their nutrition by photosynthesis and
  – Release nascent oxygen which is utilized by bacteria for oxidation process.
❖ *Sunlight*: Helps in photosynthesis.

Structure

❖ Open, shallow; depth: 1–1.5 m with an inlet
❖ Length, breadth: varies according to community needs
❖ Surrounding should be free from vegetation and weeds to avoid mosquito menace
❖ Actually oxidation pond ideally consists of 3 sequential ponds for different purposes.

Topic	Anaerobic pond	Facultative pond	Maturation pond
Depth (meter)	2–5	1–2	1–2
Waste received	Raw strong waste	From anaerobic pond	From facultative pond
Type of digestion of waste	Anaerobic	Upper layer: Aerobic Deeper layer: Anaerobic	Aerobic

Ultimate Disposal

Overall retention time for effluent in oxidation pond: at least 20 days. Thereafter, effluent obtained from an oxidation pond:

❖ It can be used for irrigation
❖ It may be discharged into river or sea after appropriate treatment.

Advantages of an Oxidation Pond

❖ Cheap and efficient method
❖ If maintained properly foul smelling discharge do not occur
❖ Can be used for fish farming
❖ A type of flowering plant "Water hyacinth" grow in the oxidation pond, can be used for production of good quality manure (rich in N, K, P).

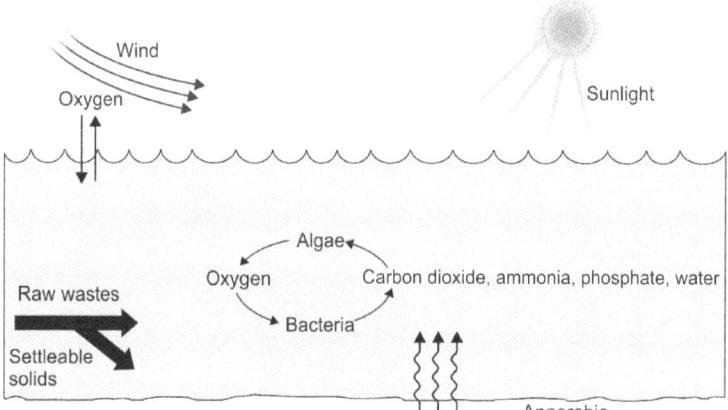

Mechanism of oxidation pond

Disinfection of Well

Needs for Well Disinfection

Wells are the most important sources of water supply in rural areas. The need for well disinfection arises in certain conditions:

❖ When coliform bacteria are present in the water
❖ After flooding of the well
❖ In the time of cholera/gastroenteritis epidemic
❖ When water taste/odor changes (from iron/sulfur reducing bacteria)
❖ As part of annual maintenance
❖ During start-up of seasonal wells.

Steps of Well Disinfection

1. *Calculate the volume of the well*:
   - Measure the depth of water column (h in meter)
   - Measure the diameter of well (d in meter)
   - Calculate the volume (V in liter)

$$V = \frac{\pi d^2 h}{4} \times 1000$$

[1 liter = 1000 cubic meter]

2. *Calculate the amount of bleaching powder required for disinfection*:
   - The chlorine demand of well water and amount of bleaching powder needed for disinfection may be measured with use of a "Horrock's apparatus".
   - If not available, the following rough estimations may be used:

$$\text{Amount of bleaching powder (in gram)} = \frac{V}{1000} \times 2.5$$

(Roughly, 2.5 g bleaching powder is needed for 1000 liter water disinfection.)

3. *Dissolve bleaching powder in water*:
   - The required amount of bleaching powder is kept in a bucket and a thin paste is prepared. A bucket should not contain >100 g powder.
   - Water is added to the paste till 3/4th of the bucket is filled
   - The contents are stirred vigorously and allowed to sediment for 5–10 minutes
   - The supernatant (chlorine solution) is transferred to another bucket and the precipitate (lime) is discarded.

4. *Delivery of chlorine solution into well*: The bucket containing chlorine solution is delivered below the water level of the well and moved vigorously in both horizontal and vertical directions so that the mixing takes place properly.

5. *Contact period*: Drawing water from the well is restricted for a period of 1 hour.

HOSPITAL WASTE MANAGEMENT

Health Hazards of Healthcare Waste

Characteristics of a Healthcare Waste (1 or more)

❖ It contains infectious agents
❖ It is genotoxic
❖ It contains toxic/hazardous chemicals/pharmaceuticals
❖ It is radioactive
❖ It contains sharps, e.g. hypodermic needles.

Persons at Risk

❖ Doctors/nurses/healthcare auxiliaries/hospital maintenance personnel
❖ Patients in healthcare establishments or receiving home care
❖ Visitors to healthcare establishments
❖ Workers in support services allied to healthcare establishments, such as laundries, waste handling, and transportation
❖ Workers in waste disposal facilities (such as landfills or incinerators) including scavengers.

Routes of Entry to Human Body

❖ Inhalation of dust/aerosol
❖ Ingestion through food/water
❖ Absorption through skin/eye/mucous membrane
❖ Through contaminated sharps (risk for medical personnel)
❖ Indirectly through contamination of water sources by sewerage system.

Hazards

1. *Infections*:

Type of infection	Examples of causative organisms	Transmission vehicles
Gastroenteric infections	Enterobacteria, e.g. *Salmonella, Shigella* species, *Vibrio cholerae*, helminths	Feces and/or vomit
Respiratory infections	*Mycobacterium tuberculosis*, measles virus, *Streptococcus pneumoniae*	Inhaled secretions, saliva
Ocular infection	Herpesvirus	Eye secretions
Genital infections	*Neisseria gonorrhoeae*; herpesvirus	Genital secretions
Skin infections	*Streptococcus* species	Pus
Anthrax	*Bacillus anthracis*	Skin secretions
Meningitis	*Neisseria meningitidis*	Cerebrospinal fluid
Acquired immunodeficiency syndrome (AIDS)	Human immunodeficiency virus (HIV)	Blood, sexual secretions
Hemorrhagic fevers	Junin, Lassa, Ebola, and Marburg viruses	All bloody products and secretions
Septicemina	*Staphylococcus* species	Blood
Bacteremia	Coagulase-negative *Staphylococcus* species; *Staphylococcus aureus; Enterobacter, Enterococcus, Klebsiella*, and *Streptococcus* species	Blood, Central lines
Candidemia	*Candida albicans*	Blood
Viral hepatitis A	Hepatitis A virus	Feces
Viral hepatitis B and C	Hepatitis B and C viruses	Blood and body fluids

2. *Hazards from chemical/pharmaceutical waste*:
   – Burns
   – Intoxication
   – Injury.
3. *Hazards from genotoxic waste*: Many cytotoxic drugs are extremely irritants and have harmful local effects after direct contact with skin or eyes. They may also cause dizziness, nausea, headache or dermatitis.
4. *Hazards from radioactive waste*: The type of disease caused by radioactive waste is determined by the type and extent of exposure. It can range from headache, dizziness, and vomiting to much more serious problems. Because radioactive waste, like certain pharmaceutical waste, is genotoxic; it may also affect genetic material. Handling of highly active sources, e.g. certain sealed sources from diagnostic instruments, may cause much more severe injuries (such as *destruction of tissue*, necessitating amputation of body parts) and should therefore be undertaken with the utmost care.

Importance of Biomedical Waste Tracking

Introduction

❖ Medical care is vital for our life and health, but the waste generated from medical activities represents a real problem of living nature and human world

❖ Improper management of waste generated in healthcare facilities causes a direct health impact on the community, the healthcare workers and on the environment

❖ Every day, relatively large amount of potentially infectious and hazardous waste are generated in the healthcare hospitals and facilities around the world

❖ Indiscriminate disposal of biomedical waste/hospital waste and exposure to such waste possess serious threat to environment and to human health that requires specific treatment and management prior to its final disposal.

Types of Biomedical Waste

Type of hazard	Route of exposure	Threat to human life
Infectious waste	Puncture/abrasion/ cut of the skin/mucous membranes, inhalation, ingestion, burns, etc.	HIV/Hepatitis B and C
Chemical and pharmaceutical waste		Intoxication
Genotoxic waste		Headache, dizziness, vomiting and cancer risk on chronic exposure
Radioactive waste		

Treatment/Disposal of Different Biomedical Waste

See Chapter 21.

DISASTER MANAGEMENT

Triage

Definition

Triage is the process of sorting injured people into groups based on the severity of their conditions, so that the most serious cases can be treated first.

Why "Triage" is Used?

The principle of "First come, First treated" cannot be followed in case of medical emergencies where the quantity and severity of injuries overwhelm the operative capacity of the available health facility. In these cases, triage is the only system which provides maximum benefit to greatest number of people needing medical attention.

Triage System

There are four color codes used in the triage system to rapidly assess the severity of injury and need for intervention:

Color code	Priority	Category	Inference
Red	Highest	Immediate	High priority treatment or transfer
Yellow	High	Delayed	Medium priority
Green	Low	Minimal	Ambulatory patients
Black	Least	Dead	Dead or moribund patients

Types of Triage

Triage is mainly of three types:

Type	Description
Simple triage	It is a triage system used in a scene of massive casualty, in order to sort the injured ones into those needing immediate medical attention and transport and those needing little medical attention
Rapid triage	It is a simplified triage system that can be performed by lightly trained personnel in times of emergencies
Reverse triage	There are some situations where less wounded persons are given priority than seriously wounded persons, e.g. In battlefield, where less wounded soldiers have to return within a short period

Phases of Triage

There are usually three phases in a modern triage system:
1. *Pre-hospital phase*: Immediate prehospital care, rapid classification and transportation if indicated.
2. *Early emergency phase*: Treatment/care by the first clinician attending the patient.
3. *Relief phase*: Triage after arrival of external assistance to the disaster site.

Disaster Preparedness

Definition

It is a programme of long-term developmental activities whose goals are to strengthen the overall capacity and capability of a country to manage efficiency of all types of disasters.

Phases in Disaster Cycle

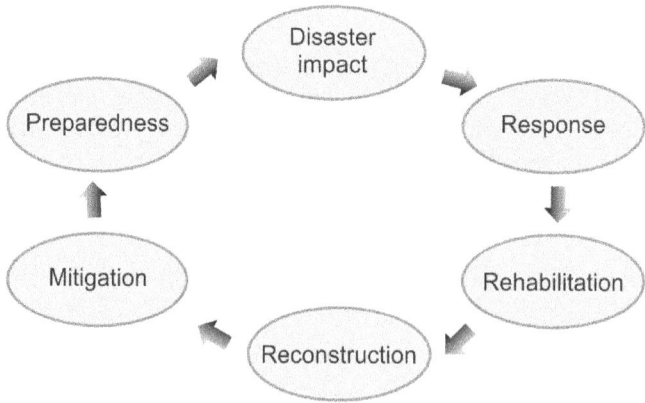

Phases in disaster cycle

Objective

To ensure that appropriate systems, procedures and resources are in place to provide effective assistance to disaster victims thus facilitating relief measures and rehabilitative services.

Basis of WHO Strategy for Disaster Preparedness

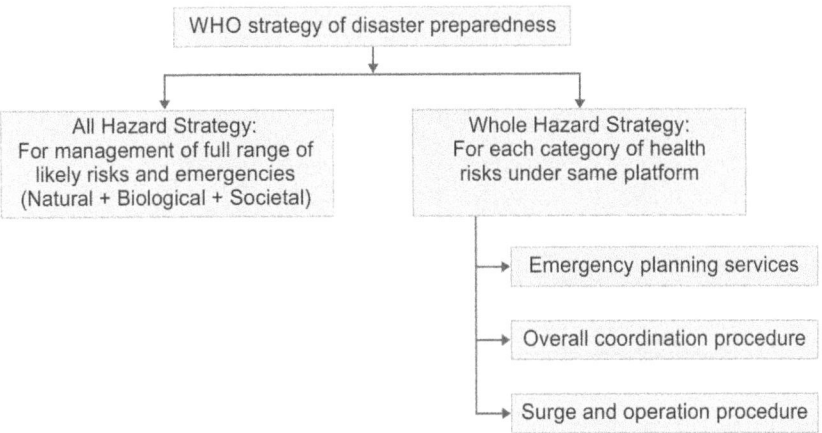

WHO strategy for disaster preparedness

Cornerstone of Organization

❖ Community members
❖ Organizations
❖ Resources
❖ Administration.

Importance of Community Members in Disaster Preparedness

❖ Those who respond to an emergency come from within the community
❖ Resources are most easily pooled at the community level.

Components

Disaster preparedness is a multisectorial organization and carries out following tasks:

❖ Evaluates the risk of country/particular region from past experiences
❖ Adopts standards and regulations
❖ Organizes communication, information and warning system
❖ Ensures coordination and response mechanism
❖ Develop public education program
❖ Coordinates information with new media
❖ Gives proper training of health worker, social worker and NGO workers
❖ Keeps stocks of the foods, drugs and other essential commodities.

Implementation Strategy

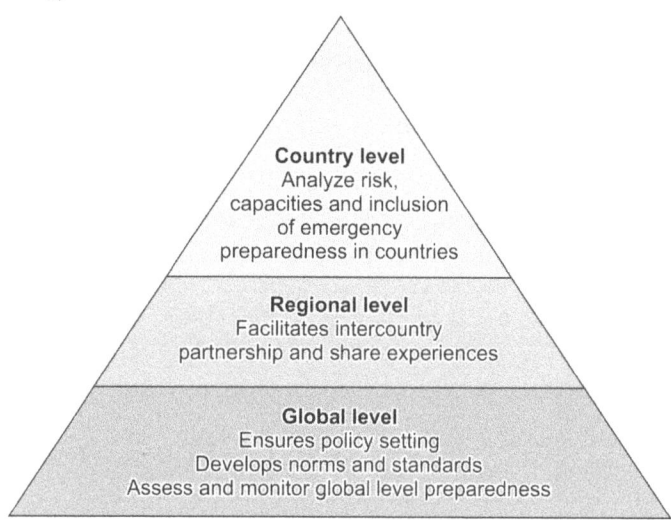

Implementation strategy of disaster preparedness at various levels

Health Hazards Likely to Occur during and Following Flood

Introduction

A flood can devastate homes, commercial buildings, agricultural and pastoral lands, public goods, and other physical properties. However, during the flood and its aftermath, there are also threats to one's health and safety.

Health Hazards of Flood

1. *Death due to damage of infrastructure*: Massive amounts of erosion can be accomplished by flood waters. Such erosion can undermine bridge structures, levees, and buildings causing their collapse.
2. *Drowning*: The most overlooked health risk is drowning while attempting to drive or walking through raising water.
3. *Electrocution and gas hazards*: Drowned power lines and other electrical sources are an obvious threat. Leaking gas lines are another threat.
4. *Cold water hazards—Cold shock (from immersion)*: Flood waters are hazardous because of the normally cold temperatures. There is a shock reaction that incapacitates many people as soon as they are immersed in cold water. There is a gasp reflex followed by hyperventilation, muscle spasm and drowning.
5. *Physical injuries*: Flood debris—such as broken bottles, woods, nails, sharp metals, stones and walls—may also cause fresh wounds and injuries.
6. *Food poisoning*: Flood waters contain disease causing bacteria, dirt, oil, human and animal wastes, and farm and industrial chemicals. Their contact with food items including food crops in agricultural lands can make that food unsafe to eat and hazardous to human health.
7. *Water-borne diseases*: Flooding impairs clean water sources with pollutants and devastates sanitary toilets. In this manner, unclean drinking and washing water and sanitation, coupled with lack of adequate sewage treatment, can lead to disease outbreaks, e.g. life-threatening cholera, diarrhea, typhoid, dysentery and some forms of hepatitis, etc.

8. *Vector-borne diseases*: Prolonged rainfall and floods provide new breeding grounds—wet areas and stagnant pools—for mosquitoes and can lead to an increase in the number of mosquito-borne diseases such as malaria, dengue, chikungunya, etc. Leptospirosis, or Weil's disease often accompanies floods.

9. *Molds and mildews*: Excessive exposure to molds and mildews can cause flood victims—especially those with allergies and asthma—to contract upper respiratory diseases and to trigger cold-like symptoms, e.g. sore throat, watery eyes, wheezing and dizziness.

10. *Wildlife*: Following floods, animals are forced out of their natural habitats and into unusual places. Snakes can easily get into damaged structures through cracks and pipes. Cases of snake bites are thus very common during flood.

11. *CO poisoning*: In the event of power outages following floods, the flood victims tend to use alternative sources of fuels or electricity for heating, cooling, or cooking inside enclosed or partly enclosed houses, garages or buildings without an adequate level of air ventilation. CO builds up from these sources and poisons the people and animals buildings inside.

12. *Chemical hazards during re-entering and cleaning flooded homes*: Containers of hazardous chemicals including pesticides, insecticides, fertilizers, car batteries, propane tanks, and other industrial chemicals may be hidden or buried under flood debris.

13. *Mental stress and fatigue*: Having experienced a devastating flood, seen loved ones lost or injured, and homes damaged or destroyed, flooding poses a long-term psychological impact on the flood victims. In addition, the cost and labor required to repair flood-damaged homes places severe financial and psychological burdens on the people affected, in particular the unprepared and uninsured. Post-flood recovery—especially when it becomes prolonged — can commonly cause mental disorders, anxiety, anger, depression, lethargy, hyperactivity, sleeplessness, and in an extreme case, suicides amongst the flood victims. Behavioral changes may also occur in children such as an increase in bed-wetting and aggression.

Vaccination in Disaster

Introduction

Natural and complex disasters dramatically increase the mortality and morbidity due to communicable diseases. The major causes of communicable diseases in disasters are categorized into four sections:
1. Infections due to contaminated food and water
2. Respiratory infections
3. Vector and insect-borne diseases
4. Infections due to wounds and injuries.

Vaccination in Disaster (As per WHO Literature Review)

The vaccination policy to be adopted should be decided at senior level only.

Consistently Recommended for Introduction Immediately

1. Measles
2. Polio
3. Tetanus (only for people with open wounds).

Recommended Only After the Outset of an Outbreak

1. Hepatitis A
2. Meningococcal meningitis
3. Yellow fever.

Influenza and typhoid vaccines are generally not recommended at all during emergencies, regardless of the phase.

Routine immunizations through national expanded programme for immunization (EPI) services should be reinstated as soon as conditions stabilize.

OCCUPATIONAL HEALTH

The Factories Act, 1948

Introduction

It is an act to consolidate and amend the law regulating labor in factories.

Definition of "Factory" According to The Factories Act

Factory is an establishment employing:
A. 10 or more workers where power is used
B. 20 or more workers where power is not used.

Recommendations Made in the Factories Act

Health, safety and welfare of the workers:
❖ A minimum of 500 cu. ft. space per worker
❖ 1 safety officer per 1000 workers
❖ 1 welfare officer per 500 workers
❖ 1 canteen in case of >250 workers
❖ 1 crèche in case of >30 women workers.

Employment of young persons:
❖ Employment is prohibited for age <14 years
❖ Old adolescents (15–18 years) to be declared "fit" by "certifying surgeons" and they will work only between 6 am to 7 pm
❖ Employment of women and children prohibited in certain dangerous occupations.

Hours of work:
❖ For adults
  – Maximum 9 hours per day
  – Maximum 48 hours per week
  – Maximum 60 hours per week including overtime.
❖ For adolescents:
  – Maximum 4.5 hours per day.

Leave with wages:

For adults	For children
1 day leave for every 20 days work	1 day leave for every 15 days work
Maximum of 30 days leave per year	Maximum of 40 days leave per year

Occupational diseases:
It is obligatory to give information regarding:
❖ Specific events which cause death/serious bodily injury
❖ Some notifiable occupational diseases contracted by employee.

Note:

The Government of India has incorporated a new chapter to the Factories Act related to hazardous processes. A site appraisal committee is to be constituted for examination of service conditions in the factory, including hazardous processes.

Ergonomics

Derivation of the Word

"Ergon" = Work
"Nomos" = Law
Ergonomics = "Fitting the job to the worker".

Objective of Ergonomics

To achieve the best mutual adjustment of man and his work, for the improvement of human efficiency and well-being.

1. Why ergonomics is important?

Industries increasingly require higher production rates and advances in technology to remain competitive and stay in business. As a result, jobs today can involve:
- ❖ Frequent lifting, carrying, and pushing or pulling loads without help from other workers or devices
- ❖ Increasing specialization that requires the worker to perform only one function or movement for a long period of time
- ❖ Working more than 8 hours a day
- ❖ Working at a quicker pace of work
- ❖ Having tighter grips when using tools.

These factors—especially if coupled with poor machine design/tool/workplace design/use of improper tools can create physical stress on workers' bodies, which can lead to injury.

So adapting tasks, work stations, tools, and equipment to fit the worker can help reduce physical stress on a worker's body and eliminate many potentially serious, disabling work-related musculoskeletal disorders (MSDs).

2. What types of work are most likely to pose ergonomic hazards?

Musculoskeletal disorders (MSDs) affect workers in almost every occupation and industry in the nation and workplaces of all sizes. The disorders occur most frequently in jobs that involve:
- ❖ Manual handling
- ❖ Manufacturing and production
- ❖ Heavy lifting
- ❖ Twisting movements
- ❖ Long hours of working in awkward positions.

3. How ergonomics can be achieved in a workplace? How ergonomic hazards can be prevented?

By taking some simple measures, we can achieve ergonomics/prevent ergonomic hazards in a workplace:
- ❖ Preplacement examination (Taking a thorough history and physical examination)
- ❖ Periodic health check-up of workers

❖ Essential healthcare services like first aid
❖ Periodic examination of working conditions
❖ Health education: Especially the importance of personal protective measures (masks/gloves/personal hygiene/hand washing, etc.)
❖ Upgradation of general environment of the workplace (like adequate ventilation and lighting/removal of excessive dust/food safety, etc.).

GENETICS AND HEALTH

Genetic Counseling

Definition

Genetic counseling *is the process, by which patients or relatives, at risk of an inherited disorder, are advised of the consequences and nature of the disorder, the probability of developing or transmitting it, and the options open to them in management and family planning.*

Types

It is of two types:
1. Prospective genetic counseling
2. Retrospective genetic counseling.

Category	Prospective genetic counseling	Retrospective genetic counseling
Indication	Heterozygotic individuals to assess the probability of having a child with genetic disorders	Usually the couples reporting voluntarily after having a child with congenital anomalies/mental retardation/inborn errors of metabolism
Timing	◆ Before the couple produce their first child ◆ Before the individual develops symptom	After birth of an affected child or other affected family member
Mode of intervention	◆ If a person is identified as heterozygotic for a genetic condition, he/she should be advised against marrying another heterozygotic individual as there is increased risk of the trait expressing itself in the phenotype ◆ Education about MTP in married couple with unfavorable prenatal diagnosis	◆ Contraception ◆ Sterilization ◆ Termination of pregnancy (depending upon attitudes and cultural environment of the couples involved)

Significance of Genetic Counseling

A. *Genetic counseling can assist women or couples who are*:
   – Concerned about first or second trimester screening results
   – Known to be at risk for carrying genetic disorders such as:
     - Thalassemia
     - Sickle cell disease
     - Hemophilia
     - G6PD deficiency
     - Cystic fibrosis
     - Muscular dystrophy
   – Pregnant and will be 35 years or older at the time of delivery
   – Increased paternal age (40 years and older).

B. *Genetic counseling can help with the implications of:*
  - Previous miscarriages or pregnancy losses
  - Either parent's diagnosis or family history of birth defect, genetic disorder or mental retardation
  - Previously having a child with a birth defect, genetic disorder or mental retardation
  - A laboratory test such as a maternal serum screening test indicating an increased risk for a genetic disorder
  - A woman's exposure to certain medications or drugs, significant radiation, and/or particular infections during her pregnancy.

In this way, genetic counseling play a very important step for prevention of transmission of some genetic diseases to the offspring.

HEALTH INFORMATION AND BASIC BIOMEDICAL STATISTICS

Sources of Health Information

Introduction

Health information is an integral part of the national health system. A health information system is defined as:

  "A mechanism for *collection, processing, analysis* and *transmission** of information required for *organizing* and *operating* health services and also for *research* and *training#*".

[Mnemonic: CPAT* and ORT#]

Sources of Health Information

1. Census
2. Registration of vital events
3. Sample registration system (SRS)
4. Notification of diseases
5. Hospital records
6. Disease registers
7. Record linkage
8. Epidemiological surveillance
9. Environmental health data
10. Health manpower statistics
11. Population surveys
12. Routine statistics related to health.

Short description

Source	Short description

Census	• Census is a massive undertaking to contact every member of a population in a given time and collect a variety of information
	• It is taken at an interval of 10 years (Started in 1881)
	• Functions of census:
	  1. It provides demographic information (such as total count of population and age and sex distribution)
	  2. It provides information about social and economic characteristics of the people
	  3. All these data provides a reference frame for future planning, action and research
	  4. With the help of census, we can calculate the much needed health, demographic and socioeconomic indicators

Contd...

Contd...

Source	Short description
Registration of vital events	The Central Births and Deaths Registration Act, 1969 provides for compulsory registration of births and deaths all over the country within 21 days
Sample registration system (SRS)	• SRS is a dual record system; consisting of continuous enumeration of births and deaths by: 1. An enumerator and 2. An independent survey taken every 6 months by an investigator-supervisor • SRS provides reliable data on birth rates, death rates and mortality rates (infant, under 5, adult and age specific)
Notification of diseases	• Usually diseases which are public health menace are included in the list of notifiable diseases. • According to IHR (International health regulation), three diseases are notifiable to WHO: 1. Cholera 2. Plague 3. Yellow fever • Some diseases are subject to international surveillance: 1. Polio 2. Malaria 3. Influenza 4. Rabies 5. Salmonellosis 6. Louse borne typhus 7. Relapsing fever • There is active participation of village health guides and multipurpose workers (male and Female) in notification system
Hospital records	A study of hospital data provides information on the following aspects: • Geographic source of patients • Age and sex distribution of diseases • Duration of hospital stay • Distribution of diagnosis • Association between different diseases • Period between disease and hospital admission • Cost of hospital care From the above information, we can calculate certain indices which are helpful for future planning of hospital services: • Bed occupancy rate • Duration of stay • Cost effectiveness of treatment
Disease registers	• Morbidity registers are maintained for only certain diseases (mainly noncommunicable diseases) like: 1. Stroke 2. Myocardial infarction 3. Cancer 4. Blindness 5. Congenital defects 6. Congenital rubella 7. Tuberculosis 8. Leprosy • Morbidity registers provide valuable information about: 1. Duration of illness 2. Case fatality 3. Survival 4. Quality of follow up

Contd...

Contd...

Source	Short description
Record linkage	• The term "Record linkage" describes the process of bringing together the records of an individual, when the records originate from different times/places. • The events commonly recorded are: 　1. Birth 　2. Death 　3. Hospital admission 　4. Discharge 　5. Marriage, etc. • Record linkage is particularly suitable for *studying associations between diseases*
Epidemiological surveillance	As a part of different disease control programs (like malaria, TB, filariasis, etc.); surveillance programs are set up for reporting of new cases/efficacy of preventive measures (immunizations)
Environmental health data	Health statistics are now approaching to provide data on: • Pollution: Air/water/noise • Harmful food additives • Industrial pollutants • Inadequate waste disposal, etc.
Health manpower statistics	These records are maintained by State Councils and Directorate of Medical Education and includes data on name/age/sex/speciality/place of work of physicians/pharmacists/dentists/veterinarians, etc.
Population surveys	These surveys may be of following types: 1. Surveys for evaluating health status of a population (community diagnosis) 2. Surveys for investigation of factors that affect health and disease (like environment/occupation, etc.) 3. Surveys for administration of health services (use of services/unmet needs/cost of services)
Routine statistics related to health	These include: 1. Population density and population movement 2. Consumption of tobacco/ dietary fat, etc. 3. Per capita income 4. Employment and unemployment data 5. Sickness absenteeism 6. Disability rates

Sampling

(May come as long question, so it is given in detail)

Definition

A sample is "a smaller (but hopefully representative) collection of units from a population used to determine truths about that population". (Field, 2005)

Basically, sampling is concerned with the selection of a subset of individuals from within a statistical population to estimate characteristics of the whole population.

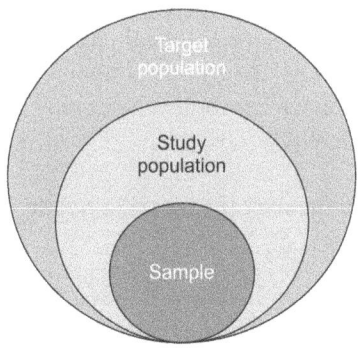

Sampling

Process

The sampling process comprises several stages:
* ❖ Defining the population of concern
* ❖ Specifying a sampling frame (sampling frame is the list from which the potential respondents are drawn, e.g. register's office)
* ❖ Specifying a sampling method for selecting items or events from the frame
* ❖ Determining the sample size
* ❖ Implementing the sampling plan
* ❖ Sampling and data collecting
* ❖ Reviewing the sampling process.

Importance of Sampling

* ❖ It is impossible to study the whole population
* ❖ Sampling provides less cost, less field time at limited resources (time, money) and workload
* ❖ Sampling also gives results with known accuracy that can be calculated mathematically.

Types of Sampling Techniques

* ❖ *Probability (Random) samples*:
  - Simple random sampling
  - Systematic random sample
  - Stratified random sample
  - Multistage sample
  - Multiphase sample
  - Cluster sample
* ❖ *Nonprobability samples*:
  - Convenience sample
  - Purposive sample
  - Quota.

Special Note

The consequence is that an unknown portion of the population is excluded (e.g. those who did not volunteer). One of the most common types of nonprobability sample is called a *convenience* sample—not because such samples are necessarily easy to recruit, but because the researcher uses whatever individuals are available rather than selecting from the entire population.

Because some members of the population have no chance of being sampled, the extent to which a convenience sample—regardless of its size—actually represents the entire population cannot be known.

Probability (Random) Sampling

Definition

* ❖ A probability sampling scheme is one in which every unit in the population has a chance (>0) of being selected in the sample, and this probability can be accurately determined
* ❖ When every element in the population *does* have the same probability of selection, this is known as an 'equal probability of selection' (EPS) design
* ❖ Such designs are also referred to as 'self-weighting' because all sampled units are given the same weight.

Simple random sampling:

❖ Applicable when population is *small, homogeneous and readily* available

❖ Each element of the frame thus has *an equal probability of selection*

❖ It provides for *greatest number of possible samples.* This is done by assigning a number to each unit in the sampling frame

❖ A table of random number or lottery system is used to determine which units are to be selected. Estimates are easy to calculate.

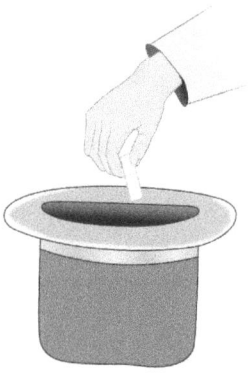

Simple random sampling is always an EPS design, but not all EPS designs are simple random sampling.

Simple random sampling

Example: Suppose N college students want to get a ticket for a movie show, but there are only $X (<N)$ number of tickets for them, so they decide to have a fair way to see who gets to go. Then, everybody is given a number in the range from 1 to N, and random numbers are generated, either electronically by lottery system or from a table of random numbers. The first X numbers would identify the lucky ticket winners.

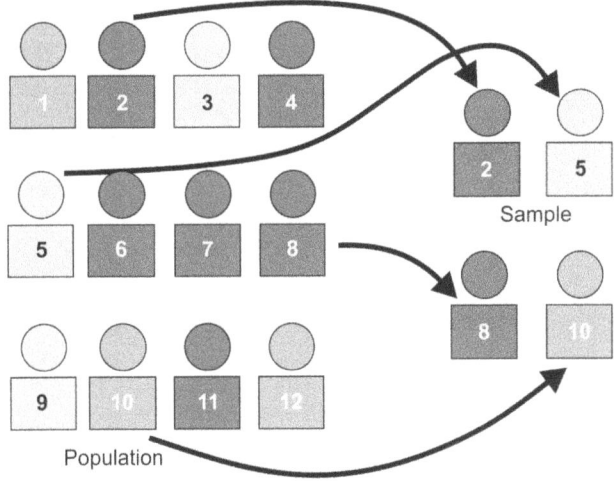

Example of simple random sampling

❖ *Advantages:*
  – Easy but scientific method
  – More cost effective
  – More representative when sample size increases.
❖ *Disadvantages:*
  – When the sample size is small, it will not be a true representative of the whole population
  – It needs complete list of the study population, which is often difficult to obtain.

Systematic random sample

❖ Preferred when the population is large, scattered and *not* homogenous

❖ Systematic sampling relies on arranging the target population according to some ordering scheme and then selecting elements at regular intervals through that ordered list

❖ Systematic sampling involves a random start and then proceeds with the selection of every element from then onwards. In this case:

$$k = \frac{\text{Population size (N)}}{\text{Sample size (n)}}$$

❖ It is important that the starting point is not automatically the first in the list, but is instead randomly chosen from within the first to the element in the list

❖ Systematic sampling is an EPS method, because all elements have the same probability of selection.

Example: Suppose we want to sample 4 students from a group of 12 students in a batch; so the sampling interval would be 12/4 = 3 (so we have to choose 'every 3rd ' sample, also referred to as 'sampling with a skip of 3').

So every 3rd student is chosen after a random starting point between 1 and 3. If the random starting point is 2, then the students selected are 2, 5, 8 and 11.

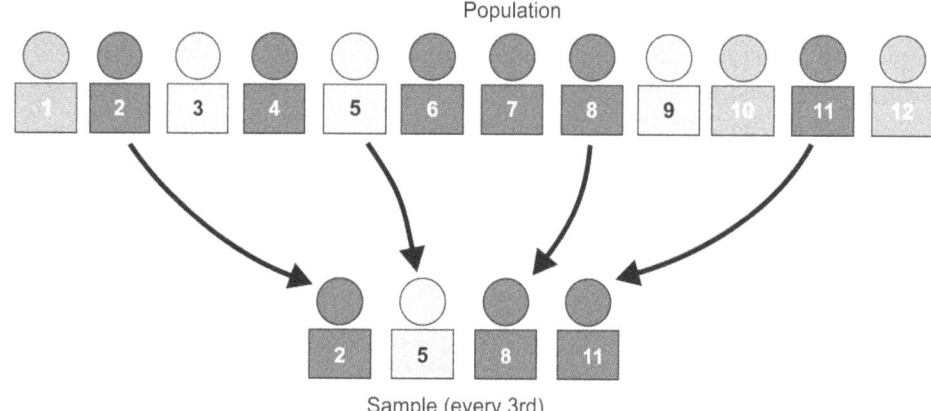

Example of systematic random sampling

❖ *Advantages*:
  – Sample easy to select
  – Suitable sampling frame can be identified easily
  – Sample evenly spread over entire reference population.

❖ *Disadvantages*:
  – Sample may be biased if hidden periodicity in population coincides with that of selection
  – Difficult to assess precision of estimate from one survey.

Stratified random sample

❖ Stratification is the process of dividing members of the population into homogeneous subgroups before sampling

❖ The strata should be mutually exclusive: every element in the population must be assigned to only one stratum

❖ The strata should also be collectively exhaustive: no population element can be excluded

❖ Then simple random sampling or systematic sampling is applied within each stratum

❖ It can produce a weighted mean that has less variability than the arithmetic mean of a simple random sample of the population

❖ Every unit in a stratum has same chance of being selected

- ❖ Types:
  - – *Proportional size*: Here the size of each stratum is proportionate to its representation within the general population

    Example: If the population X consists of m in the male stratum and f in the female stratum (where $m + f = X$), then the relative size of the two samples ($x1 = m/X$ males, $x2 = f/X$ females) should reflect this proportion.
  - – *Disproportional size*: Here the sizes of different groups may vary and not represent the percentage of the any particular group within the larger population.

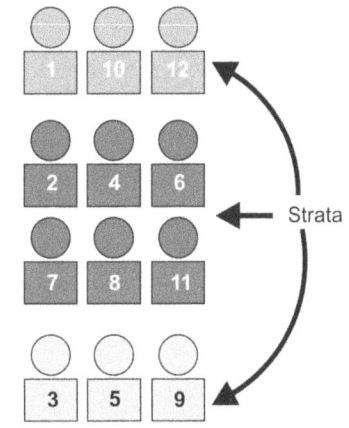

Separation of samples in different strata

Example:
- ❖ Suppose we have to sample 4 students from 12 students which are from 3 different classes.
- ❖ So at first we have to divide the 12 members according to their respective classes.
- ❖ Suppose students 1, 10, 12 are from 1st year
- ❖ Students 2, 4, 6, 7, 8, 11 are from 2nd year
- ❖ Students 3, 5, 9 are from 3rd year.

Now simple random sampling or systematic random sampling is done from every stratum (every year) to obtain 4 samples 2, 10, 8, 5.

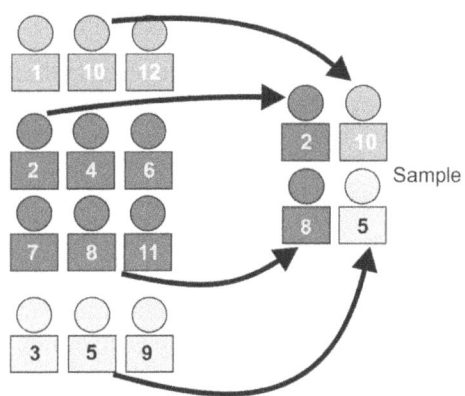

Example of stratified random sampling

- ❖ *Advantages*:
  - – More representative of the sample by reducing sampling error
  - – Important in case of skewed distribution of the population.
- ❖ *Disadvantages*:
  - – Sometimes, it is difficult to divide population in homogenous strata
  - – Not useful when the population cannot be exhaustively partitioned into disjoint subgroups (where different strata overlaps).

Multistage sample
This method consists of sampling procedure carried out in several stages, using random sampling technique.

In this method, the random selection is made of primary, intermediate, final units from a given population.

The area of investigation is scientifically restricted to a small number of ultimate units, which are representative of whole.

Example: For hookworm survey in a district, 10% of talukas are selected → followed by 10% of village in these talukas → all the people in 10th house of these village are subjected to stool examination.

Multiphase sample
The study is carried out in several phases.

Here, part of information is collected from the whole sample and part of information from subsample.

Example:

For a cross-sectional study of nutrition:

1. Phase-1 → All the families in the original sample are covered for KAP (knowledge attitude and practice).
2. Phase-2 → Subsample of families are taken for dietary intake.
3. Phase-3 → Subsample of members of 'phase-2' are subjected for anthropometric examination.
4. Phase-4 → Subsample of members of 'phase-3' are taken for biochemical examination.

Cluster sample

Cluster sampling is an example of 'two-stage sampling'.

❖ First stage a sample of areas is chosen
❖ Second stage a sample of respondents *within* those areas is selected
❖ Population divided into clusters of homogeneous units, usually based on geographical contiguity
❖ Sampling units are groups rather than individuals
❖ A sample of such clusters is then selected
❖ All units from the selected clusters are studied.

Nonprobability Sampling

Definition

Nonprobability sampling is any sampling method where some elements of population have *no* chance of selection (also called 'out of coverage'/'undercovered'), or where the probability of selection cannot be accurately determined.

Example: We visit every household in a given street, and interview the first person to answer the door. In any household with more than one occupant, this is a nonprobability sample, because some people are more likely to answer the door (e.g. an unemployed person who spends most of his time at home is more likely to answer than an employed housemate who might be at work when the interviewer calls) and it is not practical to calculate these probabilities.

Standard Normal Curve

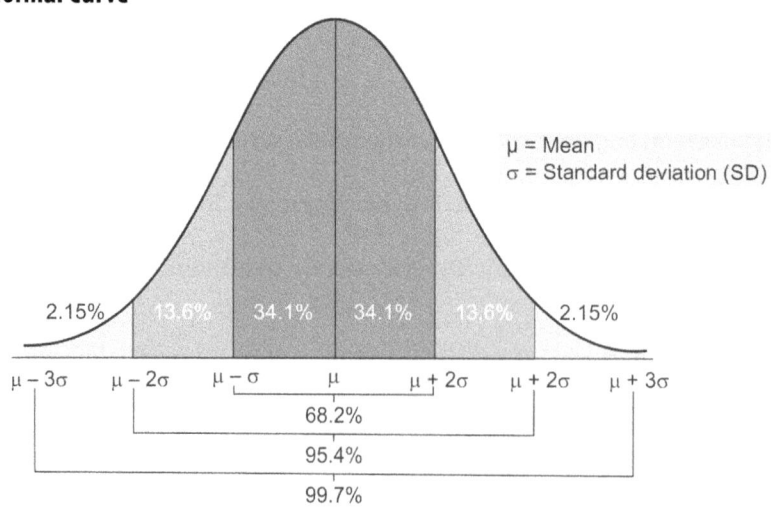

Standard normal curve

Introduction

The standard normal curve is a smooth, bell-shaped, perfectly symmetrical curve; based on an infinite number of observations.

Features

❖ The total area under the curve is 1
❖ Mean is 0 and standard deviation is 1
❖ The mean, median and mode all coincide
❖ The distance of a value (θ) from the mean (μ) in units of standard deviation (σ) is called "standard normal deviate", which is usually denoted by Z.

$$Z = \frac{\theta - \mu}{\sigma}$$

❖ A random variable (θ) is said to have been standardized when its mean is 0 and standard deviation is 1.

Interpretation and Derivation of the Concept of "P"

❖ At first the area under curve in addition of each standard deviation with mean should be discussed:

Values	Area under curve
(θ + 6) to (θ – 6) [(m – 1SD) to (m + 1SD)]	68.2%
(θ + 26) to (θ – 26) [(m – 2SD) to (m + 2SD)]	95.4%
(θ + 36) to (θ – 36) [(m – 3SD) to (m + 3SD)]	99.7%

❖ Suppose we are considering the 95% confidence limits [(m-2SD) to (m+2SD)].
When we say this, we mean 95% of the area under curve, i.e. 95% of the values in the distribution will be included between the limits (m-2SD) and (m+2SD).
Therefore, 5% of the values will be excluded between these limits.
So, the probability of a random reading falling outside the 95% confidence limits is 5 in 100, i.e. 1 in 20.
So, P = 1/20 = 0.05.

COMMUNICATION FOR HEALTH EDUCATION

Channels of Communication

Before going into detail of channels of communication, the basic concept of human communication process should be discussed. Human communication consists of 4 main components, which are interrelated as follows:

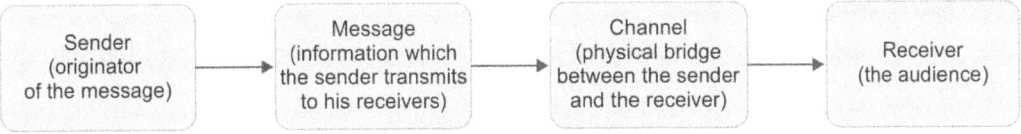

Channels of communication

Types of Channels of Communication

There are usually three channels of communication/media systems:
1. Interpersonal/face-to-face communication
2. Mass communication
3. Traditional/folk media.

Interpersonal/face-to-face communication

❖ It is the most common channel of communication
❖ As it is personal, it is more effective than any other channels of communication
❖ It is particularly important in making choice in a decision making situation.

Mass communication

❖ In mass communication, the channel is one/more mass media (TV/Radio/Printed media, etc.)
❖ Mass media have the advantage of reaching a large audience in a short period of time
❖ But it has the disadvantage that the feedback system is not well organized, so it is difficult to understand whether the message is rejected/accepted by the audience.

Traditional/folk media

❖ Every community has its own traditional/folk media which are close to the culture and customs of the rural population. These media can be utilized to deliver health messages to the community
❖ Examples of these traditional media include folk dances/singing/drama/group gathering/caste or regional meetings/festivals, etc.

Functioning of the Channels of Communication

❖ The message delivered by the mass media/traditional media is diffused into the community
❖ Then the message is picked up by the interpersonal networks
❖ Then it is subject to debate and discussion by interpersonal communications
❖ On the basis of opinion of majority, a consensus is gradually built up in the community. This opinion tells the whole community whether they will accept or reject the delivered message.

Conclusion

❖ Every channel of communication has its own advantages and disadvantages
❖ So proper selection and application of appropriate channel will result in successful communication and dissemination of a message in a community
❖ One channel seldom achieves complete effectiveness, so combination of two or more channels may be needed to successfully deliver a message to the community.

Barriers of Communication

Here also the basic concept of human communication process should be discussed.

Definition of Communication Barriers

They are defined as "difficulties involved in the process of communication which distort the message from being properly perceived by the receiver."

Various types of barriers and their examples

Types of barriers	Example
Physical	<ul><li>Defects in media</li><li>Noise in environment</li><li>Distance</li><li>Information overload</li></ul>
Physiological	Individual's personal discomfort caused by: <ul><li>Ill health</li><li>Poor eyesight</li><li>Difficulty in hearing</li></ul>
Psychological	<ul><li>Emotional disturbance</li><li>Level of intelligence</li><li>Poor communication skill</li><li>Resistance to change</li></ul>
Cultural	<ul><li>Economic and social background of the audience</li><li>Customs, beliefs and attitudes</li><li>Illiteracy</li><li>Language variations</li></ul>

Strategies to Overcome the Barriers

❖ Using multiple channels of communication
❖ Taking the receiver more seriously
❖ Thinking more clearly about the message
❖ Being prepared for probable questions coming from the audience
❖ Delivering the message skillfully.

Group Discussion

Introduction

Group discussion is a very effective method of health communication.

Definition of Group

A group is defined as, "an aggregation of people interacting in a face-to-face situation".

Conditions Required for an Effective Group Discussion

❖ The group should comprise of 6–12 members
❖ The participants should sit in a circle so that each member becomes visible and audible to others
❖ There should be a "group leader" who:
 – Initiates the subject,
 – Guides the discussion to continue in a proper manner,
 – Encourages everyone to participate,
 – Sums up and represent the discussion at the end
❖ The agreement/decision reached at the end should be based on ideas/opinions of all the members.

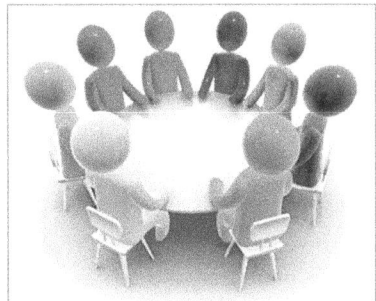

Model of group discussion

❖ A "recorder" should be present in every group discussion who will prepare a complete report on the issues discussed and agreement/decision reached.

Do's in a Group Discussion

❖ Make original points and support them by substantial reasoning
❖ Be an active and dynamic participant by listening to other participants
❖ Talk with confidence
❖ Consider the feelings of others
❖ Accept criticism.

Don'ts in a Group Discussion

❖ Don't use irrelevant material/points
❖ Don't interrupt another participant before his argument is over
❖ Don't change your opinions
❖ Don't make fun of any participants (even if his arguments are funny)
❖ Don't engage yourself in sub-group conversation.

Panel Discussion

Definition

A panel discussion is defined as, "a discussion designed to provide opportunity for a group, to hear several people having knowledge about a specific issue/topic and discuss personal views."

How to Proceed to a Panel Discussion?

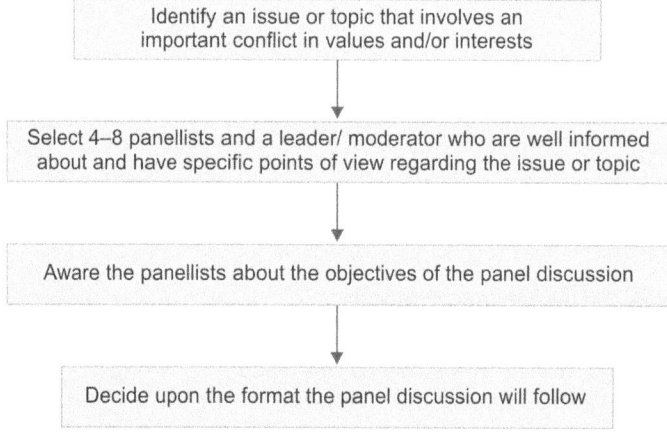

Procedure of panel discussion

Various Formats of a Panel Discussion

❖ The leader introduces a topic and the pane lists present their views and opinions about it
❖ The panelists discuss the topic actively with each other by asking questions/reacting to the views and opinions of others
❖ The leader may call for a "forum period" after panelists explore the topic completely, during which the audience may take part in the discussion and ask questions about various aspects of the topic.

Note

When a topic is explored completely by the panelists, the leader/instructor closes the discussion and provides a summary.

Conclusion

Panel discussion can be an effective method in education if it is properly planned.

HEALTH PLANNING AND MANAGEMENT

Planning Cycle

Definition of Planning

Planning is defined as, "the process of setting goals, developing strategies and outlining tasks and schedules to accomplish the goals".

Definition of Healthcare Planning

Healthcare planning is an orderly process of:
* Defining community health problems,
* Identifying unmet needs,
* Surveying resources to meet those needs,
* Establishing priority goals that are realistic and feasible and,
* Projecting administrative actions to accomplish the purpose of the proposed programs.

Steps of Health Planning

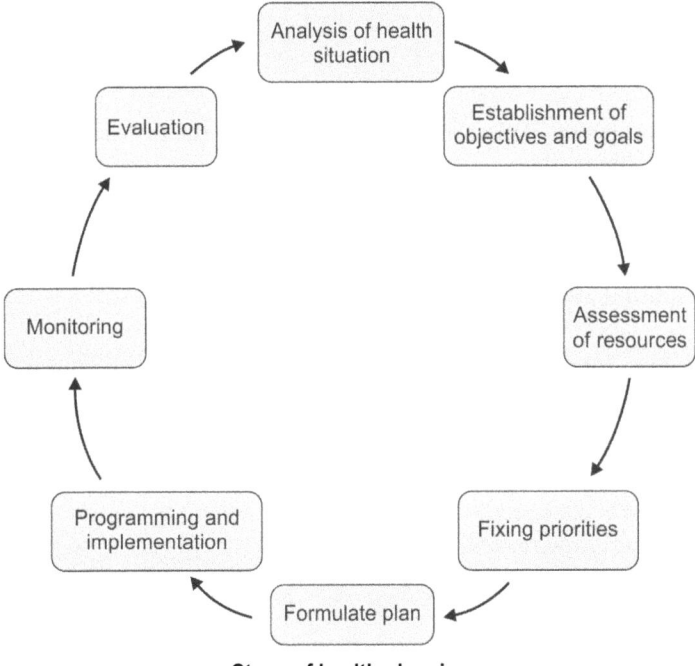

Steps of health planning

Analysis of Health Situation

It is the first step of health planning consisting of data collection regarding the following characteristics of a population:
1. Age and sex structure of the population
2. Statistics of morbidity and mortality
3. Epidemiology and geographical distribution of the prevalent diseases
4. Medical care facilities
5. Manpower
6. Attitudes and beliefs of the population towards the diseases.

Establishment of Objectives and Goals

The objectives and goals are currently set by modern methods like "cost-effective analysis" and should have the following features:
1. The goal should be realistic
2. It should be specific
3. Acceptable to the population
4. Easily measurable.

Assessment of Resources

The following resources should be assessed:
1. Manpower
2. Money
3. Materials
4. Skills and knowledge
5. Technical needs.

Fixing Priorities

It is the most important step of planning cycle. While fixing the priorities, the following points should be discussed in detail:
1. Financial requirement and constraints
2. Mortality and morbidity data regarding the problem in question
3. Saving the lives of younger people
4. Community interest and pressure.

Writing up the Formulated Plan

The formulated plan should be written in brief and comprehensive manner mentioning the following points:
1. Steps to achieve the defined target
2. Resources needed at each step
3. Time allotment to complete each step
4. A complete guidance to execution.

Programming and Implementation

This step consists of the following:
1. Assign and fix responsibilities

2. Define roles and tasks
3. Selection, training, motivation and supervision of manpower involved
4. Organization and communication
5. Efficiency of health institutions.

Monitoring

It refers to the continuous process of observing, recording and reporting on the activities of the organization or project.

Evaluation

It assesses the degree to which objectives and targets are fulfilled and the quality of results obtained.

Bhore Committee, 1943

Chairman: Sir Joseph Bhore

Aim:
❖ To survey the then existing position regarding the health condition and health organizations
❖ To make future recommendations.

Submission of report: 1946

Principles

❖ No individual should be denied to secure adequate medical care because of inability to pay.
❖ Facilities for proper diagnosis and treatment
❖ Health program must lay special emphasis on preventive work
❖ As much medical relief and preventive health care should be provided to the vast rural population
❖ Health services should be located close to the people to ensure maximum benefit to the community
❖ Doctor should be a social physician protecting the people
❖ Medical services should be free to all, without distinction.

Observation

The committee observed that....

"If the nation's health is to be built, the health program should be developed on a foundation of preventive health work and that such activities should proceed side-by-side with those concerned with the treatment of patients".
❖ Mortality rates were very high. IMR = 162/1000 LB, MMR = 20/1000 LB
❖ Life expectancy at birth was about 27 years
❖ Incidence of communicable diseases was very high
❖ Many of the health problems were preventable
❖ Committee stated that health and development are interdependent
❖ Improvement in sector other than health will also lead to improvement in health like water supply, sanitation improvement, nutrition, elimination of unemployment.

Recommendations

❖ Integration of preventive and curative services at all administrative levels

❖ Minimum required ratio 567 hospital beds, 62 doctors and 151 nurses per 100,000 population
❖ The committee visualized the development of PHC in 2 stages.

Short-term measure (to be implemented within 5–10 years)

❖ Each PHC: Supported by 3 subcenter and a secondary health center
❖ Population norm—40,000
    – 2 MOs
    – 4 PHN
    – 1 nurse
    – 2 midwives
    – 4 trained dais
    – 2 sanitary inspectors
    – 2 health assistants
    – 1 pharmacist and
    – 15 other class IV employees.

Long-term program (3 million plan)

Consist of health care system in 3 tiers:
❖ *Primary unit*
    – Population norm: 10,000–20,000 population
    – Highly dense province: 20,000/PU
    – Highly dispersed province: 10,000/PU
        - 75 hospital beds
        - 6 MOs
        - 6 PHN
        - 2 sanitary inspectors
        - 2 health assistants and
        - 6 midwives.
❖ *Secondary unit*
    – 60 primary units under a secondary unit (650 bedded)
    – First level referral hospital.
❖ *Tertiary unit (District hospital)*
    – District hospitals with 2,500 beds to serve the needs of about 3 million
    – Deals with nutrition, health education, professional/UG/PG education, population problem
    – 2 grades in nursing profession
    – Village health committee, medical research
    – Special attention to diseases like malaria, TB, small pox, leprosy, plague, cholera, venereal disease, filariasis, mental illness
    – Special programs for health of mothers and children, environmental hygiene and occupational health for industrial workers
    – Major changes in medical educations which include 3 months training in preventive and social medicine.

Significance and Importance of Bhore Committee Report

❖ Important landmark in public health in India
❖ Initiated the concept of integrated development and comprehensive health care
❖ Idea of primary healthcare
❖ The three tier pattern of healthcare services.

HEALTH CARE OF THE COMMUNITY

Primary Health Care

Definition

"Primary health care is essential health care made universally accessible to individuals and acceptable to them, through their full participation and at a cost the community and country can afford".

Elements of Primary Health Care

❖ Education concerning prevailing health problems and the methods of preventing and controlling them
❖ Promotion of food supply and proper nutrition
❖ An adequate supply of safe water and basic sanitation
❖ Maternal and child health care, including family planning
❖ Immunization against major infectious diseases
❖ Prevention and control of locally endemic diseases
❖ Appropriate treatment of common diseases and injuries
❖ Provision of essential drugs.

Principles of Primary Health Care (PHC)

❖ *Equitable distribution*: This is the first and foremost key to PHC. Healthcare services must be shared by all the people of the community irrespective of their race, religion, cast or economic status. This concept clearly indicates the need to shift the accessibility of healthcare from the urban areas to the rural areas where the most needy and vulnerable groups of the population live.
❖ *Community participation*: Universal coverage of health services cannot be achieved without the involvement of local community. The term "community participation" includes meaningful involvement of the community in planning, implementing and maintaining their health services. Through the involvement of the community, maximum utilization of local resources, such as manpower, money and materials can be achieved to fulfil the goals of PHC.
❖ *Intersectoral coordination*: Improvement of the health status of a population needs not only the participation of health sector, but also the involvement of other sectors like agriculture, education and housing.
❖ *Appropriate technology*: It is defined as, "technology that is scientifically sound, adaptable to local needs and acceptable to those who apply it and for those whom it is used and that can be maintained by the people themselves".
Example: ORS.

Elements of Primary Health Care

❖ Education concerning prevailing health problems and the methods of preventing and controlling them
❖ Promotion of food supply and proper nutrition
❖ An adequate supply of safe water and basic sanitation
❖ Maternal and child health care, including family planning
❖ Immunization against major infectious diseases
❖ Prevention and control of locally endemic diseases
❖ Appropriate treatment of common diseases and injuries
❖ Provision of essential drugs.

Voluntary Health Agencies

Definition

A voluntary health agency is defined as, "a nonprofit, nongovernmental agency, governed by lay or professional individuals, organized on a national, state or local level whose main purpose is health related and supported by voluntary public contributions".

Services Rendered by Voluntary Health Agencies

❖ Supplementing and guiding the work of governmental agencies.
❖ Health education and research, e.g. the voluntary health agencies pioneered the family planning program of India at the very beginning, the government accepted it as a national policy after realizing the importance of family planning.
❖ Demonstration of experimental projects, e.g. demonstration of bore hole latrines by Rockfeller Foundation to solve the problem of Hookworm infestation in India.

Voluntary Health Agencies of India

Name	Activities
Indian Red Cross Society	• Relief work at times of disaster • Supply of milk powder, medicines, vitamins, etc. • Care of the sick and wounded of the armed forces • Maternal and child welfare services • Guiding the family planning services • Blood bank and first aid services
Hind Kusht Nivaran Sangh	• Financial assistance to leprosy homes and clinics • Health education and research • Training of medical workers
Indian Council for Child Welfare	• Child protection • Child survival • Developmental rights • Disaster management
Tuberculosis Association of India	• Providing quality diagnostic and treatment services • Supplementing the Directly Observed Treatment Short Course (DOTS) services of Revised National Tuberculosis Control Program (RNTCP) by Government of India • Health education aimed at increasing public awareness about TB, involvement of community leaders, seeking cooperation of patients and their families
Bharat Sevak Samaj	• Improvement of sanitation in villages • Help people to achieve health by their own actions and efforts
Central Social Welfare Board	• Social education • Creation and training of self-help groups • Literacy classes • Maternity aid for women • Play centers for children
Family Planning Association of India	Training of doctors and social workers about: • Gynecological services • Infertility services • Services for male sexual and urinary disorders

Contd...

Contd...

Name	Activities
	• Contraceptive services • MTP services • HIV-related services • Maternal and child care services • Reproductive cancer-related services
All India Women's Conference	Most of the branches are running: • MCH clinics • Medical centers • Adult education centers • Family planning clinics
The All India Blind Relief Society	It organizes eye relief camps and other measures for the relief of the blind
Professional Bodies, e.g. Indian Medical Association	• Conducting annual conferences • Publication of journals • Arrangement of scientific exhibitions • Setting up standards of professional education • Organizing relief camps at times of natural calamities

AYUSH

❖ It is an indigenous system of medicine constitutes:
  - A = Ayurveda
  - Y = Yoga
  - U = Unani system of medicine
  - S = Siddha system of medicine and
  - H = Homeopathy.

These together termed as AYUSH

❖ Government of India is studying to avail the services of these medicines for effective and total health coverage
❖ Integration of AYUSH: By National Health Mission
❖ AYUSH village: One village per block
❖ Advantages:
  - Most of the AYUSH practitioners are local residents
  - They mingle with people socially and culturally.

Intersectoral Coordination

Defining Intersectoral Coordination

❖ In the health literature, the term intersectoral coordination/collaboration refers to the *"collective actions involving more than one specialized agency, performing different roles for a common purpose"*
❖ Declaration of Alma Ata (1978), Article VII said that: *"Primary health care involves, in addition to health sector, all related sectors and aspects of national and community development, in particular agriculture, food, industry, education, housing, public works, communications and other sectors; and demands the coordinated efforts of all those sectors"*
❖ Declaration of Alma Ata (1978), Article VIII said that: *"All governments should formulate national policies, strategies and plans of action to launch and sustain primary health care as part of a comprehensive national health system and in coordination with other sectors".*

❖ More recently (1997), the WHO promoted the concept of intersectoral action for health as, *"a recognized relationship between part or parts of the health sector with parts of another sector which has been formed to take action on an issue to achieve health outcomes in a way that is effective, efficient or sustainable than could be achieved by the health sector alone".*

The Place of Intersectoral Coordination in Primary Health Care

The WHO defined health as "a state of complete physical, mental and social well-being and not merely an absence of disease or infirmity." But the fact is that these broad concepts of well-being cannot be achieved by the health sector alone. Some examples are as follows:

❖ Literacy improvement and school health programs are mainly a task of education sector
❖ Developing an appropriate technology is mainly a task of technology and industrial sector
❖ Poverty reduction is mainly a task of economic planning sector
❖ Storage of huge information on utilization of Govt. health services is mainly a task of information technology (IT) sector.

So, Primary health care fundamentally calls for multisectoral inputs.

MDG and Intersectoral Coordination

❖ The Millennium Development Goals (MDGs) include some goals related to health sector like reduction of maternal, infant and under 5 mortality; combat HIV/AIDS, malaria and other communicable diseases as well as some goals like achieving universal primary education and eradication of extreme hunger and poverty which are not directly related to health sector
❖ All these goals are highly dependent on intersectoral coordination, without which all these goals will be failed
❖ As for an example, an effective electricity system is required for efficient maintenance of cold chains. Otherwise it may lead to loss of potency of vaccines and subsequently to an increased neonatal and infant mortality
❖ So, to achieve the goals of MDG in time, intersectoral coordination is a must.

Recommendations

Intersectoral coordination has been neglected in most parts of the health sector, but fortunately this trend is presently declining. Strong political will, as well as reduction of fatigue in seeking help from other sectors should be prioritized. Formation of suitable legislative acts can be an effective way to ensure intersectoral coordination in health sectors.

Central Government Health Scheme (CGHS)

Objectives

Providing comprehensive medical care facilities to Central Government employees, pensioners and their dependents residing in CGHS covered cities (17 cities).

Beneficiaries

❖ All Central Government Servants paid from Civil Estimates (other than those employed in Railway Services and those employed under Delhi Administration except members of Delhi Police Force)
❖ Pensioners drawing pension from Civil Estimates and their family members (Pensioner residing in non-CGHS areas also may obtain CGHS Card from nearest CGHS covered city)

❖ Honorable Members of Parliament
❖ Honorable Judges of Supreme Court of India
❖ Ex-Members of Parliament
❖ Employees and Pensioners of Autonomous Bodies covered under CGHS (Delhi)
❖ Ex-Governors and Ex-Vice Presidents
❖ Former Prime Ministers
❖ Former Judges of Honorable Supreme Court of India and Honorable High Courts
❖ Freedom Fighters.

Medical Facilities Provision

It provides service through following categories of systems:
❖ Allopathic
❖ Homeopathic
❖ Indian System of Medicines, e.g.
 – Ayurveda
 – Unani
 – Yoga
 – Sidha system.

Components of the Scheme

❖ Dispensary services including domiciliary care.
❖ FW and MCH services
❖ Specialists consultation facilities both at dispensary, polyclinic and hospital level including X-ray, ECG and laboratory examinations
❖ Hospitalization
❖ Organization for the purchase, storage, distribution and supply of medicines and other requirements
❖ Health education to beneficiaries.

ASHA Scheme

Introduction

❖ Under the ASHA (Accredited social health activist) scheme, there is an ASHA worker for a population of 1000
❖ The guidelines for selection of ASHA worker are:
 – ASHA must be a resident of the village, preferably a woman
 – She should have a formal education of at least 8th standard
 – She should be preferably in the age group of 25–45 years
 – She should have communication skills and leadership qualities.

Roles and Responsibilities of an ASHA Worker

Roles	Description
Awareness and information to the community/women of the community about	• Importance of nutrition/basic sanitation/personal hygiene as determinants of health • Need for utilization of health and family welfare services • Importance of breastfeeding/immunization/complementary feeding/family planning/prevention of STDs

Contd...

Contd...

Roles	Description
Referral services	ASHA will arrange escort/accompany pregnant women/child requiring referral to the nearest PHC/CHC/FRU
Primary health care for minor illnesses	• Diarrhea • Fever • First aid services
Depot holder and provider of:	• DOTS • ORS • IFA tablets • Chloroquine • Disposable delivery kits • Oral pills • Condoms
Facilitation of utilization of government health services	• Antenatal check-up • Postnatal check-up • Immunization • Supplementary nutrition
Development of a comprehensive village health plan	ASHA will develop it working with: • Village health guides • Anganwadi workers • Sanitation committee of Gram Panchayat
Notification services	ASHA will notify nearby PHC/Subcenter about: • Birth • Death • Disease outbreaks in the community • Any unusual health problem in the community

INTERNATIONAL HEALTH ORGANIZATIONS

Indian Red Cross Society (IRCS)

Introduction

Indian Red Cross Society is a leading member of the largest independent humanitarian organization in the world, the International Red Cross and Red Crescent Movement.

Mission

The mission of IRCS is to inspire, encourage and initiate all forms of humanitarian activities so that human suffering can be minimized and even prevented and thus contribute to create more congenial climate for international peace.

Establishment

The IRCS was established in 1920 under the Indian Red Cross Society Act and incorporated under the Parliament Act XV of 1920.

Branches

The IRCS has 35 state/union territories branches with their more than 700 district branches and subdistrict branches.

Highest Members

The Honorable President of India is the president of IRCS and the honourable Union Health Minister is the chairman of the IRCS.

Seven Fundamental Principles

1. Humanity
2. Impartiality
3. Neutrality
4. Independence
5. Voluntary service
6. Unity
7. Universality.

Programs and Activities

IRCS's programs are grouped in 4 main core areas:
1. Promoting humanitarian principles and values
2. Disaster response
3. Disaster preparedness
4. Health and Care in the community.

Other major activities include:
- Hospital service
- Blood bank
- HIV/AIDS program
- Home for disabled servicemen
- Vocational training centers
- Maternal, child and family welfare services
- Nursing
- Junior Red Cross activities: Junior Red Cross is one of the most active sections in the society. It gives opportunity to millions of boys and girls of India to be associated with village uplift/first aid/antiepidemic work/building up an international fraternity of youth
- Prevention of communicable diseases
- Relief operations in case of accidents and disasters.

CARE INDIA

Full name: Cooperative for Assistance and Relief Everywhere.

Founding: North America, 1945.

Organization Type

It is one of the world's largest independent, nonprofit, nonsectarian international relief and development organization.

Function

CARE provides emergency aid and long-term developmental assistance.

Role in India

From mid 1980s, CARE India focused its food support in the ICDS program and in development of program in the areas of health and income supplementation.

It is now helping in the following projects:
❖ Integrated Nutrition and Health Project
❖ Better Health and Nutrition Project
❖ Anemia Control Project
❖ Improving Women's Health Project
❖ Improved Health Care for Adolescent Girls' Project
❖ Child Survival Project
❖ Improving Women's Reproductive Health and Family Spacing Project.

UNICEF

History

❖ UNICEF (United Nations International Children's Emergency Fund) was established in 1946 by the United Nations General Assembly to deal with rehabilitation of children in 2nd World War ravaged countries
❖ In 1953, when the war and the need for emergency functioning were over, it was renamed as "United Nations Children's Fund" by the General Assembly.

Functioning

❖ UNICEF is governed by a 36 member Executive Board
❖ The headquarters of UNICEF is at United Nations, New York
❖ The regional office of South Central Asia Region is located at New Delhi, India
❖ UNICEF works in close collaboration with various international health agencies like WHO, The United Nations Development Program (UNDP), Food and Agricultural Organization of the United States (FAO) and The United Nations Educational, Scientific and Cultural Organization (UNESCO).

Approach of Functioning: Country Health Programming

UNICEF is currently paying greater attention to the "whole child" approach, i.e. not only to the improvement of health and nutrition of children; but also to the long-term intellectual development of them and development of the country they live in. The aim of this "Country Health Programming" is to meet the demand of children as an integral part of a country's developmental effort.

Services Provided by UNICEF

Child health
❖ UNICEF is supporting India's BCG vaccination campaign from its inception.
❖ UNICEF has helped creating the following plants:
  - A penicillin plant
  - A DDT plant
  - A plant for manufacturing Iodized salt
  - A plant for manufacturing Triple Vaccine (DPT).
❖ Currently, UNICEF is focusing on the primary health care given to the mother and child such as:
  - Immunization

- Infant and young child care
- Family planning
- Safe water and basic sanitation.

❖ These services are delivered through part time volunteers/primary health workers who are selected from the local community in which the services are to be delivered.

Child nutrition

❖ UNICEF supplied equipment for modern dairy firms to many states of India
❖ UNICEF is also working to decrease the prevalence of nutritional deficiency diseases:
  - By providing large doses of vitamin A to prevent xerophthalmia
  - Enrichment of salt with iodine to prevent endemic goiter
  - Provision of IFA tablets to prevent nutritional anemia, etc.

GOBI-FFF campaign

Currently, UNICEF is promoting a campaign for *"Child health revolution"* incorporating 3-F named as GOBI-FFF campaign. GOBI-FFF stands for:

G	Growth charts for monitoring growth of a child
O	Oral rehydration to treat mild and moderate dehydration
B	Breastfeeding for adequate growth of child and protection from childhood infections
I	Immunization against vaccine preventable diseases (Tuberculosis, Diphtheria, Pertussis, Tetanus, Polio, Measles)
F	Family education
F	Family spacing
F	Family supplementation

Formal and nonformal education

UNICEF is supplying many necessary things to the educational institutions in collaboration with UNESCO:

❖ Library books
❖ Laboratory equipments
❖ Workshop tools
❖ Audiovisual aids, etc.

Family and child welfare

UNICEF is working to improve the *care of children* by means of:

❖ Parent education
❖ Daycare centers
❖ Promoting child welfare and youth agencies.

Urban basic services (UBS)

UNICEF is participating in UBS since 1976 to upgrade the basic services for children and women in selected cities and towns in order to improve the quality of development of children from low-income urban families. Those basic services include improvement of:

❖ Health
❖ Nutrition
❖ Water supply
❖ Sanitation
❖ Education.

Authors' Note

These questions may come as a part of long essay type questions, short notes and may be asked in viva exam. These 'Explain Why' questions will also help the students understanding the basics and minute details of this subject with a clear concept.

CONCEPT OF HEALTH AND DISEASE

1. Definition of Health by WHO is idealistic than realistic.

2. According to the WHO definition of health, we are occasionally healthy.

According to WHO

"Health is a state of complete physical, mental and social well-being and not merely an absence of disease or infirmity and ability to lead a socially and economically productive life."

In reality "a state of complete physical, mental and social well-being" cannot be achieved, because these are almost absolute concept.

According to Dubos:

"...man will never be so perfectly adopted to his environment that his life will not involve struggles, failures, and sufferings".

On the other hand, some argue that health cannot be defined as "a state" but must be seen as a *process of continuous adjustment to the changing demands of life. So health is "dynamic".* Hence, definition of Health by WHO is idealistic than realistic.

3. Health of an individual is not static.

The spectral concept of health emphasizes that the health of an individual is not static, but is a dynamic phenomenon.

It is a continuous process, subject to frequent subtle variations, what is considered maximum today may be minimum tomorrow.

The "spectrum" may vary from optimum positive health to ultimate death like this order: Positive health → better health → freedom from sickness → unrecognized sickness → mild sickness → severe sickness → death.

It implies that health is a state not to be attained once and for all, but never be renewed. There are such degrees (also known as "level of health") as there are degrees or severity of illness; so it can never be static.

4. Lifestyle and customs are important in prevention of disease.

Lifestyle means *"the way people live"* reflecting a whole range of social values, attitudes and activities.

Healthy lifestyle can prevent several diseases, whereas, harmful lifestyle can lead to different diseases.

❖ Healthy lifestyle:
  – Adequate nutrition
  – Enough sleep
  – Sufficient physical activity, etc.
❖ Harmful lifestyle:
  – Personal habits like smoking, alcoholism (increase risk of coronary artery disease, COPD, chronic liver disease, etc.)
  – Lack of sanitation
  – Poor nutrition (predisposes to several infective diseases including tuberculosis)
  – Poor personal hygiene
  – Lack of physical activity (leads to obesity—increased risk of cardiovascular diseases)
  – Drug addiction.
  In this way lifestyle and customs are important in prevention of disease.

5. Rehabilitation is not only a medical issue.

Rehabilitation is defined as, "combined or coordinated use of physical, social, vocational and psychological measures of training and retraining the individual to the highest possible level of functional ability".

It is not just a medical issue but a social issue, so that the individual becomes useful to himself, to the family, and to the community at large.

In rehabilitation it is essential to identify the remaining capacities in such an individual and adopt measures to make him fit, independent, productive, useful and an active member in the family as well as in the community.

It cannot be possible only by medical care but following different positive aspects are very much essential:

Type of rehabilitation	Meant for restoration of
Physical	Function
Vocational	Earning capacity
Social	Relationship in the society
Psychological	Personal dignity and confidence

6. Community medicine is best taught in the community.

Community medicine is a branch of medicine that is concerned with promoting, maintaining and when necessary restoring health of the community (Mnemonic: PMR).

❖ Objectives of community medicine:
  – To identify the health need and the problem in the community, i.e. community diagnosis
  – To plan, implement and evaluate health measures effectively to meet those need.
❖ Practice of the community medicine requires:
  – A defined community
  – Understanding the community health problems

- Management oriented approach to solve the problem
- Comprehensive and integrated health service.

❖ Community diagnosis is made by:
  - Interviewing the community people
  - Transect walk
  - Going through the health records
  - Sample survey.

To do all these, we have to go in the community not only to learn the methods of community diagnosis but also to understand the community problems and implement different measures for solution of the problems.

7. Submerged part of the iceberg disease has immense importance to an epidemiologist.

According to this concept, disease in a community may be compared with an iceberg.

Tip of the iceberg is only visible, whereas rest is submerged, only people manifesting clinical sign and symptoms are thought to be diseased.

Explanation

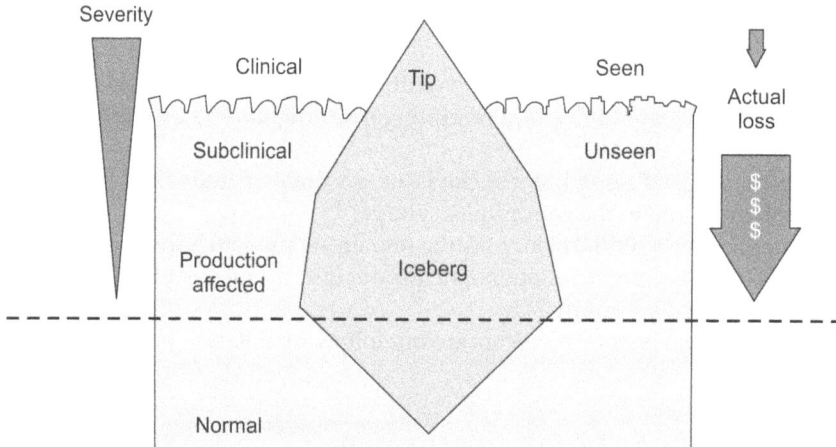

The floating tip of the iceberg represents what the physician sees in the community, i.e. clinical cases.

The vast submerged portion of the iceberg represents the hidden mass of the disease in the community, i.e.

❖ Latent cases
❖ Inapparent cases
❖ Presymptomatic cases
❖ Undiagnosed cases and
❖ Carriers.

The "waterline" represents the demarcation between apparent and inapparent disease.

Significance of the Iceberg Phenomenon

❖ In some diseases (e.g. hypertension, diabetes, anemia, malnutrition, mental illness), the unknown morbidity (i.e. the submerged portion of the iceberg) far exceeds the known morbidity.

❖ The clinician is concerned with the 'tip of the iceberg' and the epidemiologist is concerned with the 'hidden portion of the iceberg'.

❖ Screening is done for hidden portion of the iceberg, whereas diagnosis is done for the tip of the iceberg.

❖ Iceberg phenomenon is not shown in: Rabies, tetanus, measles and rubella.

8. Sentinel surveillance of disease is better than periodic mass screening. Explain.

At the very beginning, there should be a clear idea of what these 2 terms mean.

Sentinel Surveillance

It is a reporting system for identifying the missed cases and supplementing the notified cases for the purpose of identifying all the cases of a particular disease.

Example

❖ Use of health practitioners to monitor trends of a health event in a population.

❖ Sentinel surveillance is done in National AIDS Control Program wherein STD clinics, ANC clinics are sentinel sites to monitor trends.

Periodic Mass Screening

It means the screening of a whole population/subgroup at a regular interval irrespective of the individual risk of contracting that disease.

Example

❖ Cancer screening.

❖ Pap smear or liquid-based cytology to detect potentially precancerous lesions and prevent cervical cancer.

❖ Mammography to detect breast cancer.

Sentinel Surveillance has the following Advantages Over Periodic Mass Screening

❖ Reporting biases are minimized.

❖ Feedback of the information to the providers is simplified.

❖ Provides more valuable and detailed information than that could be obtained from periodic mass screening.

❖ Less costly.

❖ There is little jurisdiction of use of periodic mass screening in many instances.

PRINCIPLES OF EPIDEMIOLOGY AND EPIDEMIOLOGICAL METHODS

1. Epidemiologically carriers are more dangerous than cases.

A case is defined as, "a person in the population or study group identified as having the particular disease, health disorder or condition under investigation".

A carrier is defined as, "an infected person or animal that harbors specific infectious agent *in the absence of discernible clinical disease* and serves as a potential source of infection to others".

The elements of a carrier state are as follows:

❖ Disease agent is present in the body of the individual.

❖ Any recognizable symptoms and signs are absent.

❖ Continuous shedding of the infectious disease agent may occur through excretions and discharges, which may act as potential source of infection for other susceptible individuals, e.g. "Typhoid Mary" was a classical example.

Though from clinical point of view, carriers are less dangerous than cases, but from the epidemiological point of view, carriers are more dangerous because:
❖ They escape recognition.
❖ They continuously persist in the community as the individual leads a normal life.
❖ They readily infect the susceptible individual over a wider area and for a longer time under favorable conditions.

2. Carrier state of a disease is not amenable to control. Explain.

❖ The elements of a carrier state are:
  – Presence of the disease agent in the body.
  – Absence of recognizable signs and symptoms.
  – Shedding of the disease agent in discharges/excretions; acting as a source of infection to others.
❖ This carrier state is not amenable to control because:
  – They escape recognition.
  – They live a normal life among the community.
  – They readily infect susceptible individuals over a wide area.
  – They remain a source of infection to others for a long period of time.

Note: The most important type of carriers in this aspect is chronic carriers who excrete the infectious agent for an infinite period.

Chronic carrier state exists in the following diseases:
❖ Typhoid fever
❖ Hepatitis B
❖ Malaria
❖ Gonorrhea
❖ Dysentery, etc.

3. Different types of epidemiological studies are indicated to measure frequency, distribution and determinants of health.

Epidemiology is the study of distribution and determinants of health-related states or events for specified populations and application of the study to control of health problems.

Epidemiological studies to measure frequency, distribution and determinants of health:

		Epidemiological studies
1. Frequency of disease (measured in terms of rate, ratio, normal range, incidence rate, prevalence rate)	Incidence rate	Longitudinal study
	Prevalence rate	Cross-sectional study
	Formulation of hypothesis/rate determination	Case control and cohort study
2. Distribution of disease		Descriptive study (in respect to time, place, person)
3. Determinants of disease		Analytical study

4. Randomization is the heart of clinical trial; Justify.

Introduction

Clinical trials are research studies that explore whether a medical strategy, treatment or device (or any other intervention) is safe and effective for humans.

Criteria of a Good Clinical Trial

A good clinical trial minimizes variability of the evaluation and provides an unbiased evaluation of the intervention.

Randomization in Clinical Trials

Randomization ensures that each patient will have an equal chance of receiving any of the treatments under study.

Example

In concurrent parallel randomization in clinical trials:
- ❖ Aim: To know effectiveness or efficacy of a new antihypertensive drug
- ❖ Procedure:

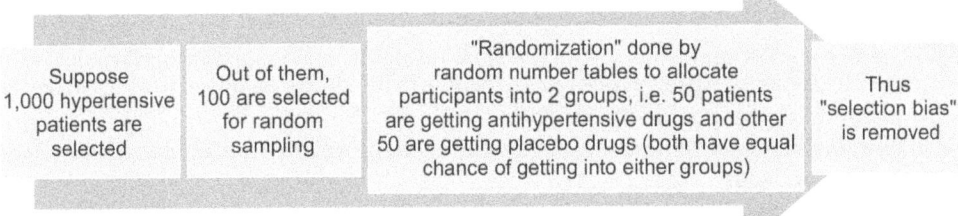

- ❖ In case of cross over RCT, ethical issues can be cut-off as all the patients get cross over in one point of time.
  - – If we take the above mentioned example, those in phase-1 survey who will receive treatment in phase-2 will get placebo and vice versa.

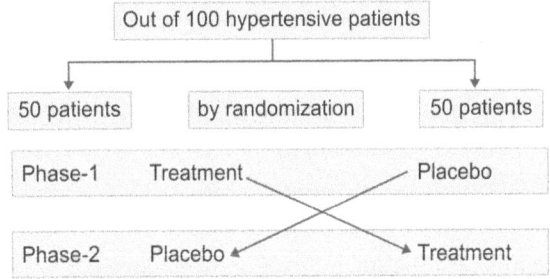

Role of Randomization in Clinical Trials

The advantages of proper randomization in RCTs include:
- ❖ It eliminates bias in treatment assignment, specifically selection bias and confounding.
- ❖ It facilitates blinding of the identity of treatments from investigators, participants, and assessors.

❖ It permits the use of probability theory to express the likelihood that any difference in outcome between treatment groups merely indicates chance.

In general, a randomized trial is an essential tool for testing the efficacy of the treatment.

Goals of an Ideal Randomization
❖ Maximize statistical power.
❖ Minimize selection bias.
❖ Minimize allocation bias (confounding).

5. Prevalence of a specific health problem depends on the incidence and duration of the problem.

Prevalence refers specifically to all current cases (old and new) existing at a given point of time (point prevalence) or over a period of time (period prevalence).

Whereas, incidence refers to number of NEW cases occurring in a defined population during a specific period of time.

So, for a stable population:

$$P = I \times D$$
Prevalence = Incidence × Mean duration of disease

This equation shows that longer the duration of a disease the greater its prevalence.

Example
❖ Tuberculosis has high prevalence rate in relative to incidence because new cases may come throughout the year but old cases persist.
❖ On the other hand, for acute disease (short duration) prevalence rate is relatively low because of recovery or death.

This way, prevalence of a specific health problem depends on the incidence and duration of the problem.

6. Surveillance is an integral part of any effective disease control.

❖ Surveillance is defined as, *"the continuous scrutiny of the factors that determine the occurrence and distribution of disease and other conditions of ill-health".*
❖ The main role of disease surveillance is to: *Predict, observe, and minimize the harm caused by outbreak, epidemic, and pandemic situations, as well as increase knowledge about which factors contribute to such circumstances. A key part of modern disease surveillance is the* practice of disease case reporting.
❖ So for control of a specific disease, the knowledge of pattern of distribution of a disease and its contributing factors in the community should be known and this can only be known by effective disease surveillance.

7. Diseases with short incubation period are easy to control.

Incubation period is defined as the time interval between invasion by an infectious agent and appearance of first symptom of the disease in question.

If the IP is short → sign/symptom appears more quickly → early and easy detection and treatment of the disease → less chance to spread in the community.

In case of a disease with short IP ranging from a few hours to few days, it is relatively simple to trace the source of infection and "follow the trail" of the spread of infection as in cases of food poisoning, bacillary dysentery and typhoid fever, etc. (But in case of rabies short IP makes the disease more fatal).

8. Unsafe injection can harm recipient, provider and community.

Unsafe may not only cause cuts and punctures but also infect these wounds if they are contaminated with pathogens.

Most common infections are: Hep B, Hep C and HIV

	Effects of unsafe injections
To the recipient	Iatrogenic infection
	Delay treatment
	Comorbidity
To the provider	Unnecessary burden to the health care facility
To the community	Hinders overall development of the community

9. Case-control study is superior to cross-sectional study for establishment of association.

❖ A cross-sectional study measures exposure and disease at one point of time. It can be described as a snapshot of the study population (*Example*: A patient survey).

❖ This study design provides weak evidence of causal association between exposure and outcome because the exposure may not have preceded the disease.

❖ On the other hand, a case-control study identifies individuals who develop the disease (cases) and individuals without the disease (controls), and then determines the previous exposure of both cases and controls.

❖ The case group is composed only of individuals known to have the outcome; the control group is drawn from a comparable population who have not experienced the outcome. Then we compare the odds of exposure between cases and controls.

❖ A case-control study is stronger than a cross-sectional study in establishing individual-level causality because we are certain that exposure preceded the disease outcome. This association is reported as an odds ratio.

10. The term source and reservoir of infection are not always synonymous.

Transmission of communicable disease starts with source or reservoir of infective agent.

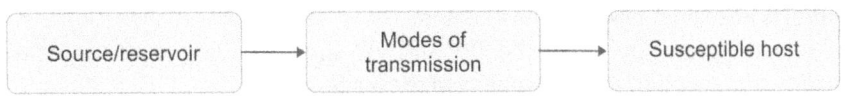

Chain of transmission of infection

A "source" of infection is defined as, "the person, animal, object or substance from which an infectious agent passes or is disseminated to the host".

A "reservoir" is defined as, "any person, animal, arthropod, plant, soil or substance (or combination of these) in which infectious agent lives and multiplies on which it depends primarily on survival, and where it reproduces itself in such a manner that it can be transmitted to a susceptible host."

Reservoir is nothing but the natural habitat in which the organism metabolizes and replicates, but the term source refers to the immediate source of infection which may be or may not be the part of infection.

So, the term "source" and reservoir of infection are not always synonymous.

For example:

Example	Reservoir	Source
Hookworm infestation	Man	Soil contaminated with infective larvae
Tetanus	Soil	Soil
Typhoid	Case/carrier	Feces and urine of patient/contaminated food, milk or water

SCREENING FOR DISEASE

1. Predictive values are more important than sensitivity and specificity in the view of a clinician.

The positive predictive value (PPV) is formulated as:

$$PPV = \frac{\text{Number of true positives}}{\text{Number of true positives + number of false positives}}$$
$$= \frac{\text{Number of true positives}}{\text{Number of test positives}}$$

It is more important than sensitivity and specificity in the view of a clinician because:

❖ When evaluating a clinical test, the terms sensitivity (ability to identify true positives) and specificity (ability to identify true negatives) are used because they are independent of the population of interest subjected to the test.

❖ The terms positive predictive value and negative predictive value (NPV) are used when considering the value of a test to a clinician because **they are dependent on the prevalence** of the disease in the population of interest.

❖ The PPV of a test is a proportion that is useful to clinicians since it answers the question: 'How likely is it that this patient has the disease given that the test result is positive?'

❖ The NPV of a test is also important to the clinician because it answers the question: 'How likely is it that this patient does not have the disease given that the test result is negative?'

So, the predictive value of a test is of more importance in the view of a clinician than sensitivity and specificity.

2. Positive predictive value depends on prevalence.

This question is answered best with an example.

Unlike sensitivity and specificity, the PPV and NPV are dependent on the population being tested and are influenced by the prevalence of the disease.

$$PPV = \frac{TP}{TP + FP}$$

(TP: True positive, FP: False positive)

Consider the following example:

❖ Screening for SLE in a general population using the antinuclear antibody (ANA) has a low PPV because of the high number of false positives it yields.

❖ However, if a patient has signs of SLE (e.g. malar flush and joint pain) and these signs are used as diagnostic criteria (or test), then PPV of the test increases because the population from which the patient is drawn is different (from general population with a low prevalence of SLE to a clinically suspicious population with a much higher prevalence).

So, PPV is dependent on prevalence in population.

3. Lead time is the advantage gained by screening.

❖ The intention of screening is to diagnose a disease earlier than it would be without screening. Without screening the disease may be discovered later, when symptoms appear.

❖ As we diagnosed the disease earlier with screening, the survival time since diagnosis is longer with screening.

❖ As described above, lead time is this advantage gained in due to the screening test where the disease is identified in the incipient stage so as to treat it appropriately in the early stage of natural history of that disease.

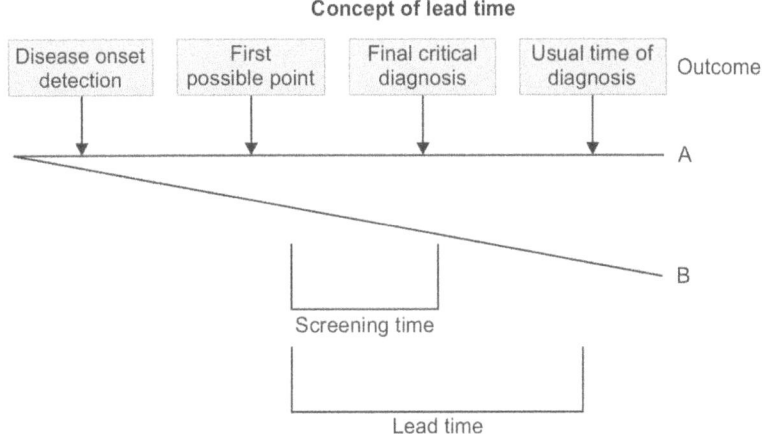

4. Screening is not exactly case finding.

Please see the Chapter 6: Page no. 336.

5. Sensitivity may be increased only at the expense of specificity and vice versa.

OR

6. Sensitivity and specificity are inversely proportional.

Sensitivity and specificity are inversely proportional meaning that as the sensitivity increases, the specificity decreases and vice versa.

What do we mean by this? Let us say that an intraocular pressure (IOP) of ≥25 mm Hg is test positive and <25 mm Hg is test negative.

❖ Very few normal subjects would have IOP more than 25 mm Hg, and hence the specificity would be very high

❖ But as a significant number of glaucoma subjects would have an IOP <25 mm Hg (normal-tension glaucomas), the sensitivity of IOP >25 mm Hg in the detection of glaucoma would be low.

Another example:

Suppose we take the IOP cut-off for test positive to be 35 mm Hg. Almost no normal subject would have this high an IOP, and the specificity would be very high (>99%); and a highly specific test if positive (for *example*, an IOP >35 mm Hg), rules in the disease.

Remember this as **SpPIN**: a highly **S**pecific test if **P**ositive, rules **IN** disease.

7. Disease should possess certain criteria before it is considered suitable for screening.

Following criteria of a disease should be fulfilled before it is considered suitable for screening: (Mnemonic: Public recognizes natural history by diagnosis and treatment and agrees on early detection for cost benefit)

❖ Serious and constitutes a *public health problem*

❖ *Recognizable latent period* (early asymptomatic phase) or high prevalence of preclinical stage

❖ *Natural history* well-understood (to identify the stage at which the disease ceases to be irreversible)

❖ *Effective facilities for diagnosis* available

❖ *Effective treatment* available

❖ Agreed on policy for confirmation of diagnosis available (e.g. lower ranges of BP, borderline DM)

❖ Evidence that early detection and treatment reduces mortality and morbidity

❖ Expected *benefits of early detection* should exceed *costs and risks.*

8. An important attribute of an ideal screening test is its repeatability or reliability.

Repeatability (or reliability) means a screening test must give consistent results when repeated more than once on the same individual under same conditions.

Determinant of repeatability:

1. *Observer variation:*
   - Intraobserver variation:
     - Single observer takes multiple measurements in the same subject, at the same time and each time obtained results are different, e.g. BP measurement
     - Correction: By taking average of several measurements.
   - Interobserver variation:
     - Different observers take multiple measurements in the same subject, but obtained results are different, e.g. blood smear examination for malaria parasite detection.
     - Correction:
       * By standardization of procedures for obtaining measurements and classifications
       * Intensive training of all the observers.
2. *Subject (biological) variation:*
   Due to variability associated with many physiological variables.
   - Causes:
     - Changes in the parameter observed
     - Individual variation of patients in their perception and expression
     - Regression to the mean.
   - Correction: By repetition of observation over time.
3. *Technical errors:*
   - Correction:
     - By using reliable instruments, reagents and best probable test techniques
     - By repetition of observation over time.

9. **When screening for a disease, a prior decision on cut-off point has to be made.**

OR

10. **In case of a screening test for a lethal disease, a greater degree of sensitivity is desired.**

Sensitivity is a statistical index of *"diagnostic accuracy"*.
It is the ability of a test to identify correctly all those who have disease (i.e. true positive).

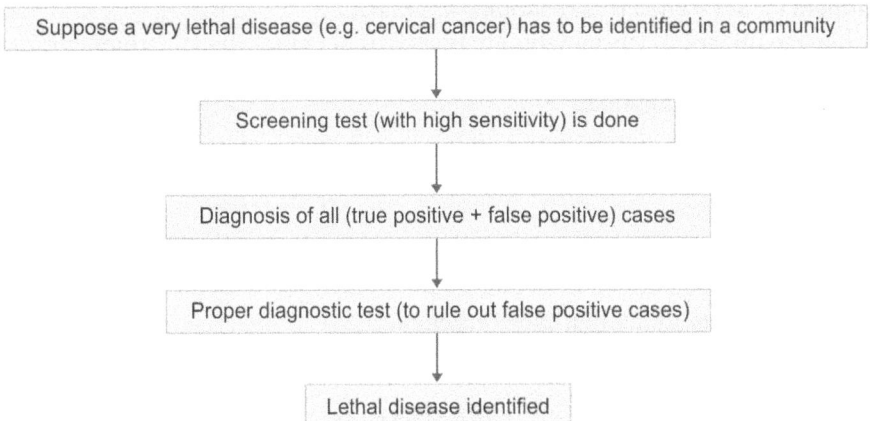

So, a proportion of false positive results are tolerable but not false negatives in case of identification of lethal diseases.

That is why greater degree of sensitivity is required for a lethal disease even at the expense of specificity is desired.

11. **In case of a screening test for a prevalent disease for which treatment does not markedly alter the outcome, a greater degree of specificity is desired.**

❖ *Specificity means the ability of a test to identify correctly those who do not have the disease (i.e. "true negatives").*
❖ In prevalent diseases (like diabetes) for which the treatment does not markedly alter the outcome, specificity must be high. Here, early cases may be missed, but false positives should be limited.
❖ Otherwise, the health system will be overburdened with diagnostic demands on the positives, both true and false.

That is why high specificity is necessary when false positives errors must be avoided.

(An important index in making this decision is the predictive value of a positive test which measures the percentage of positive results that are true positive).

EPIDEMIOLOGY OF COMMUNICABLE DISEASE

1. **Syndromic management of STD is most appropriate approach in India.**

Early diagnosis and treatment is one of the most important steps to prevent and control a disease and transmission.

Previously, in STD Control Program, the diagnosis was based on microscopic and laboratory finding. But this type of laboratory diagnostic approaches had the following *limitations:*

❖ Expensive
❖ Time-consuming—leads to delay in treatment
❖ Require sophisticated equipment and trained manpower
❖ Clients of STD are lost as they may not come again
❖ Most of the patients go to the private practitioners who have limited facility for diagnosis.

For these limitations of this approach a new approach was developed for early diagnosis and treatment for STDs known as *syndromic approach.*

According to this approach, patients are treated as per prescribed treatment protocol.

Advantages of Syndromic Approach

❖ Diagnosis and treatment is done on visit.
❖ It can be implemented in large scale even at PHC levels as it is:
  – Simple
  – Rapid
  – Inexpensive
  – Requires minimum training and equipment
  – Patients are treated for possible mix infection by addressing all important causes of the presenting symptoms
  – Gives a unique opportunity for preventing AIDS
  – Prevent development of complications.
❖ For all patients of STD syndromic approach is based on (5C's) which are as follows:
  – Counseling and education
  – Condom promotion
  – Compliance of treatment
  – Contact tracing and treatment of the patient
  – Follow-up, to come again after 7 days
  – Encourage voluntary counseling and testing centers (VCTC).

So for India, which is a developing country having limited resources, manpower, literacy, economic condition and community participation with huge population syndromic approach is the most appropriate to cope up with STD.

3. Vitamin A supplementation is necessary after measles infection. Explain.

❖ All cases of severe measles and all cases of measles in areas with high case fatality rates should be treated with vitamin A because a large portion of these children develop acute deficiency of vitamin A which may lead to keratomalacia and blindness.
❖ The dosage of vitamin A is as follows:

No. of dose	Timing of administration	Dosage
1st	Immediately on diagnosis	<6 months: 50,000 IU
2nd	Given on the next day	6–11 months: 100,000 IU
3rd	If the child has clinical sign of vitamin A deficiency (xerosis/Bitot's spots, etc.) give 4–6 weeks later	>12 months: 200,000 IU

4. HIV is a behavioral disease. Explain.

HIV is transmitted through certain body fluids. Behaviors that increase a person's contact with the body fluids of another person increases the chance of HIV transmission. These behaviors include:

❖ Unsafe sexual behavior
❖ Unsafe drug use behavior
❖ Combining sex and drug/alcohol
❖ Not taking antiretroviral drugs properly.

Unsafe Sexual Behavior

❖ Unprotected sexual intercourse with a HIV positive partner is the most common route of transmission of HIV.
❖ Any factor that causes trauma/scratch in the mucous membrane of genital organs can increase the chance of infection like:
  – Anal intercourse
  – A previous or ongoing episode of STD (syphilis/chancroid/herpes, etc.)
  – Women who are very young (cervix is not fully developed).

Unsafe Drug use Behavior

❖ Sharing of needles and syringes by injecting drug abusers increases the chances of HIV transmission markedly.
❖ As the risk of HIV transmission increases proportionately with "dose of the infection", the chance is considerably lower in case of only a needle prick injury; but it gets higher where needle sharing becomes a habit.

Combining Sex and Drug/Alcohol

❖ When people use drugs/alcohol, their decision-making abilities and awareness to the surroundings become considerably lower; making them less likely to practice safer sex.
❖ In addition, these substances can increase sexual desire; making them more vulnerable to injury to the genital organs leading to HIV transmission.

Not Taking Antiretroviral Drugs Properly

❖ Antiretroviral therapy (ART) decreases the virus load in the body fluids; making the person less likely to infect other people.
❖ When they do not take antiretroviral drugs properly, they have more virus load and they become more likely to infect others.
So, HIV is correctly called as a "behavioral disease".

5. PEP should be given within 72 hours of exposure to HIV.

❖ The WHO considers 72 hours post-exposure as the upper limit of opportunity to initiate PEP and a delay of that scale is believed to compromise PEP efficacy.

❖ The 72 hour limit recommendation is based on animal studies; no human data are available.
❖ It takes a few days for HIV to become established in the body following exposure. PEP drugs given at this time may help the body's immune system to stop the virus from replicating (multiplying) in the infected cells of the body.
❖ The cells originally infected would then die naturally within a short period of time without producing more copies of the HIV virus. When there is a risk of HIV transmission, post-exposure prophylaxis should be initiated as soon as possible, within hours and no later than 72 hours following the potential exposure.

According to WHO:
❖ When there is a risk of HIV transmission, post-exposure prophylaxis should be initiated as soon as possible within hours and no later than 72 hours following the potential exposure.
❖ According to the results of animal studies, initiating PEP within 12, 24 or 36 hours of exposure is more effective than initiating it 48 or 72 hours following exposure. Such studies have also established that PEP is not effective when given more than 72 hours following exposure and these are the basis of the recommendations that individuals presenting more than 72 hours after potential exposure would not be eligible for it.

6. Role of pretest counseling of HIV/AIDS is useful. Explain.

Counseling before an HIV testing is important because it provides critical information about HIV itself and about the testing process. It should also help clients feel more relaxed during the test procedure.

The purpose of pretest counseling is to provide the client with information on the technical aspects of testing and the possible personal/medical/social/psychological/legal/ethical impacts of being diagnosed as HIV positive/HIV negative.

The counselor should follow the guidelines stated below in pretest counseling:
❖ Reasons for testing
❖ Assessment of risk
❖ Beliefs and knowledge about HIV infection and safer sex:
  – Client should be given information about how HIV is transmitted and how one can protect himself from infection. So questions about recent/previous sexual intercourse(s)/intravenous drug use/history of any needle prick injury should be carefully asked.
❖ Information regarding the test:
  – Information about the HIV test: What it tests for, what it might not tell and how long it will take to give the results?
❖ A clear and easily understandable explanation of what the test results mean.
❖ The possible impacts of an HIV test result (positive/negative).
❖ Anticipate with a positive result.
❖ Confidentiality of test results.
❖ Informed consent.
❖ Information about giving the result and ongoing support.
❖ Relieve the stress of the client in the waiting period.

7. OPV at birth is considered as "zero" dose.

The first dose of oral polio is considered as "zero" dose because the "zero" refers to the first moment in "time" when the vaccine is given (the next dose might be called "the 1 month" or "3-month" dose). If a child had never had the oral polio vaccine before, then at the time of his/ her zero dose, a tested serum sample of his/her blood should show NO antibodies against the polio virus while future sample would give him a positive protective titer.

8. Explain the criteria for certification of polio eradication.

❖ Zero cases for consecutive 3 years
❖ Reliable and effective surveillance
❖ Absence of wild polio virus from the environment
❖ All serological tests done for AFP should show positive results are not compatible
❖ After eradication nonpolio AFP rate should be ≤1 per 1 lakh population for consecutive 3 years.

9. Routine immunization alone cannot eradicate polio.

Because:
❖ Routine immunization (5 doses of bivalent OPV) cannot percolate through every corners of the country due to remoteness.
❖ Pulse polio is carried out to give repeated doses to build up immunity against infective stains of polio virus.
❖ This program is carried out for all children <5 years of age.
❖ Done between November to February (as between July to September there is high rate of transmission)
❖ Objectives of pulse polio immunization:
  – Not a single child should miss the immunization, leaving no chance of polio occurrence
  – Cases of acute flaccid paralysis (AFP) to be reported in time and stool specimens of them to be collected within 14 days. Outbreak response immunization (ORI) to be conducted as early as possible
  – Maintaining a high level of surveillance
  – Performance of good mop-up operations where polio has disappeared.
❖ Mopping up program is done for those children who are not attending the regular session.
❖ Intensified pulse polio immunization (IPPI) is undertaken to supplement cancelled sessions and nonimmunization due to inconvenience of time regular sessions.

10. Line listing of AFP cases are essential steps for polio eradication.

Line listing is relevant because:
❖ To check duplication of cases.
❖ To check the year of onset of illness for screening the children for residual paralysis who develop polio prior to the year of reporting.
❖ Identification of high-risk pockets.
❖ Documentation of high-risk age groups.
❖ Line listing helps to take appropriate follow-up action in all areas of all AFP reported cases at 60 days to check for paralysis.

❖ Provide useful epidemiological data for program purposes as, for example, urgency for early completion of OPV immunization in high-risk age groups and areas.
❖ Helps in documentation of all AFP cases due to polio and nonpolio etiology which is essential for taking containment measures for outbreak control.

11. Surveillance is carried out for all cases of AFP not just for poliomyelitis.

❖ Acute flaccid paralysis is defined as any case of new onset hypotonic weakness in a child aged less than 15 years.
❖ Beside polio (which is the major contributor to AFP cases in India), this includes possible illness due to:
  – Guillain-Barré syndrome
  – Transverse myelitis
  – Traumatic neuritis
  – Viral infections caused by other enteroviruses
  – Toxins and tumors.
  The early stages of polio may be difficult to differentiate from other forms of AFP. Therefore, to ensure that no case of polio goes undetected; surveillance targets a symptom (AFP) rather than a specific disease (e.g. polio).

12. Congenital anomalies due to TORCH are preventable.

Several vertically transmitted infections are included in the TORCH complex which stands for:
TO—**To**xoplasmosis/*Toxoplasma gondii*
R—**R**ubella
C—**C**ytomegalovirus
H—**HE**rpes simplex virus 2 or neonatal herpes simplex
(Sometimes **O** refers to Other infections)

The "other agents" under **O** include:
❖ Coxsackie virus
❖ Chickenpox (caused by varicella zoster virus)
❖ Parvovirus B19
❖ Chlamydia
❖ HIV
❖ Syphilis.

("**TORCHES**" refers to: **TO**xoplasmosis, **R**ubella, **C**ytomegalovirus, **HE**rpes simplex, **S**yphilis)

Clinical Features

❖ Symptoms
  – Fever
  – Poor feeding
  – Petechial rash
  – Small for gestational age
  – Blueberry muffin spots (in CMV).
❖ Signs
  – Features of VSD

- Hepatosplenomegaly
- Hearing impairment
- Eye problems (cataract, glaucoma, retinopathy, optic atrophy)
- Mental retardation
- Autism
- IUGR
- Cerebral palsy.

Prevention

❖ Primary prevention:
- Rubella and varicella zoster can be prevented by vaccinating the mother prior to pregnancy
- Vaccination strategy should be undertaken **for high-risk areas**.
- For rubella vaccination priority should be given to the women of childbearing age group (15–34 or 39 years) and then to interrupt transmission of rubella by vaccinating all children aged 1–14 years, and subsequently all children at 1 year age.
- Health education of mother regarding proper hygiene and nutrition to avoid infections.
❖ Secondary prevention:
- Some of the vertically transmitted infections, such as toxoplasmosis and syphilis, can be effectively treated with antibiotics (if the mother is diagnosed early in her pregnancy). But many of the viral vertically transmitted infections have no effective treatment.
- If the mother has active herpes simplex (suggested by a Pap test), delivery by cesarean section can prevent the newborn from contact, and consequent infection with this virus.

13. India is yellow fever receptive country.

OR

14. India needs an international certification against yellow fever.

India is yellow fever receptive country. Yellow fever receptive area means where yellow fever does not exist but *favorable conditions may permit its development in future.*

India is yellow fever receptive country because: (Mnemonic: VVCC)

❖ *Vaccination status:* The population is unvaccinated and susceptible to yellow fever.
❖ *Vector:* The vector *Aedes aegypti* is found in abundance.
❖ *Climatic condition*: Suitable for its transmission.
❖ *Other host: Common monkey* is found to be susceptible.

Thus entry of yellow fever virus in India would lead to a massive epidemic. But India is protected probably due to:

❖ Cross immunity with other widely prevalent flavivirus
❖ Repeated mosquito bites of *Aedes aegypti* may stimulate antibody production against the mosquito which may somehow prevent attack of yellow fever.

15. From time to time influenza epidemic or pandemic is expected.

Because:
- ❖ *Frequent antigenic variation* leads to incapability of treatment resulting in outbreak of infection
- ❖ *Large no. of subclinical infection* is present
- ❖ *Incubation period* is very short (18–72 hours)
- ❖ *Cross immunity* is absent
- ❖ *Immunity* is short-lasting.

16. Clinical diagnosis is sufficient for treatment of leprosy.

A case of leprosy is diagnosed by eliciting cardinal signs of leprosy through systematic clinical (and wherever required bacteriological) examination. At least one of the following signs must be present to diagnose leprosy:

1. Hypopigmented or reddish skin lesion(s) with definite sensory deficit
2. Involvement of the peripheral nerves, as demonstrated by definite thickening with loss of sensation and weakness/paralysis of the corresponding muscles of the hands, feet or eyes
3. Demonstration of *Mycobacterium leprae in the lesions.*

   The first two cardinal signs can be identified by clinical examination alone, while the third can be identified by examination of the slit skin smear.

   Leprosy is classified as paucibacillary or multibacillary, based on the number of skin lesions, presence of nerve involvement and identification of bacilli on slit-skin smear.

Characteristics	PBL	MBL
Skin lesion	1–5	>5
Peripheral nerve involvement	0–1	>1
Skin smear	Negative at all sites	Positive at any site

17. Leprosy is not amenable to eradication.

Because:
- ❖ Incubation period:
  - – Long and variable
  - – For lepramatous cases 3–5 years (average) for tuberculoid type IP is shorter
  - – Symptoms may appear even after 20 years.
- ❖ Modes of transmission:
  - – Disputed modes of transmission. Probably by:
    - - Droplet infections (most evidences for it)
    - - Contact transmission
    - - By insect vectors, tattooing, etc.
- ❖ Subclinical cases: Present
- ❖ Detection of cases in community: Usually failed as early symptoms and signs remain undiagnosed for a long period (due to long IP)
- ❖ Spectrum of disease manifestation: Complicated

- ❖ Immunity: In lepramatous leprosy CMI completely breaks down
- ❖ Bacterial resistance and persistence in human
- ❖ Vaccine: Absent
- ❖ Social stigma: Cultural and social taboos, economic problems are related to leprosy
- ❖ Extra-human reservoir: Recently discovered.

18. Smallpox eradication was possible.

- ❖ No known animal reservoir
- ❖ No long-term carrier of virus
- ❖ Lifelong immunity after recovery from the disease
- ❖ Detection of case is simple due to presence of characteristic rashes on visible parts of the body
- ❖ Persons with subclinical cases does not transmit the disease
- ❖ Vaccine is:
  - – Highly effective
  - – Easily administered
  - – Heat stable
  - – Provides long-term immunity.
- ❖ International cooperation and good political will.

19. Tetanus cannot be eradicated from the world.

Because:
- ❖ Extra-human reservoir:
  - – The natural habitat of the organism is soil and dust
  - – The bacilli are found in the intestine of many herbivorous animals (e.g. cattle, horse, goat and sheep) and excreted through their feces
  - – Spores survive for years in nature.
- ❖ Lifelong immunity does not arise as a result of previous infection. As a general rule a patient who have recovered from tetanus must be actively immunized because the amount of toxin responsible for the disease in man do not stimulate protective immunity.
- ❖ Vaccine:
  - – No effective lifelong vaccine is available
  - – Herd immunity does not protect the individual.

20. Measles may be eradicated in future.

Because:
- ❖ Only source of infection is a case of measles.
- ❖ Carriers are not known to occur.
- ❖ Measles immunization has its favor in the light of the following facts:
  - – Only 1 dose is needed.
  - – Vaccine is heat stable.
  - – Vaccine efficacy: 95%.

❖ It requires:
  – Achieving an immunization coverage of at least 96% of children under 1 year of age.
  – That the cumulation in the immunity gap be prevented.
❖ Only 1 serotype of measles virus is known
❖ Measles virus cannot survive outside the human body for longer time.

21. Man is dead end host for Japanese encephalitis. Or, Incidence of Japanese encephalitis is very small compared to the population exposed to mosquito bite.

Japanese encephalitis (JE)is a zoonotic disease. Natural hosts of JE virus include water birds of Ardeidae family (mainly pond herons).

Pigs serve as an **amplifier host**, since they allow many fold virus multiplication without suffering from the disease and maintain prolonged viremia.

Due to the long period of viremia, mosquitoes get opportunity to pick up infection from pigs easily.

Probable basic cycles of transmission:
❖ Pig → Mosquito → Pig
❖ Ardeid bird → Mosquito → Ardeid bird

But man is an accidental host, i.e. dead end due to:
❖ Low and short lived viremia
❖ No cyclo-propagative and cyclo-developmental stage is recorded in human.

So, mosquitoes do not get infection from JE patient.

22. Explosive outbreaks are rare in filariasis.

Because:
❖ Restricted multiplication:
  – The parasite does not multiply in the insect vector
  – The infective larvae do not multiply in the human host.
❖ Long life cycle: Relatively long, 15 years or more.
❖ Lack of source:
  – In human the source of infection is a person with circulating microfilariae in peripheral blood. But in filarial disease (in late obstructive stage) microfilariae are not found in the blood.
  – Microfilariae of infected person come in peripheral blood between 10–2 pm. So, mosquito bites apart from this time period cannot harbor microfilariae in their body hence cannot infect other human.
❖ The minimum level of microfilariae will permit the infection of the mosquitoes is unknown (it was reported that a man with 1 microfilaria/40 cu mm of blood was infective to only 2.6% of the mosquitoes feed on them).
❖ When mosquitoes feed on carriers with huge concentration of microfilariae (as many as 180+ microfilariae/20 cu mm of blood), they die. Because a huge number of microfilariae began to reach maturity at a time.
❖ Filarial disease appears only in small % of infected individual (commonly >10 years of age).

23. DOTS is not only supervised swallowing.

❖ During continuation phase patient is issued medicine for 1 week in a multiblister pack of which the 1st dose (administered by swallowing) is supervised by health worker or trained person and consumption of rest of the medicine of the continuation phase is checked by return of empty multiblister combi pack when patient comes to collect medicine for the next week.

❖ DOTS ensures that the patient adheres to treatment. The responsibility of treating the patient and ensuring that the patient does not miss even a single dose falls on the health provider.

❖ Directly Observed Treatment, Short-course (DOTS) does not just mean supervised swallowing but the building of a human bond with the patient. It means that the *right drugs* in the *right doses* are taken at the *right interval* for the *right duration*.

24. DOTS is the only strategy which has been documented to be effective worldwide.

DOTS is a community based tuberculosis (TB) treatment care strategy which combines the benefits of supervised treatment and benefits of community based care and support.

According to WHO:

"The most cost-effective way to stop the spread of TB in communities with a high incidence is by curing it. The best curative method for TB is known as DOTS."

It ensures high cure rates through its basic three components:
1. Appropriate medical treatment
2. Supervision and motivation by health worker or nonhealth worker.
3. Monitoring of disease status by health services.

Thus, it has been universally accepted and effective strategy ensuring its success on the following five components:
1. Government commitment (including political will at all levels, and establishment of a centralized and prioritized system of TB monitoring, recording and training).
2. Case detection by sputum smear microscopy.
3. Standardized treatment regimen of six to eight months directly observed by a healthcare worker or community health worker for at least first 2 months.
4. A regular, uninterrupted drug supply.
5. A standardized recording and reporting system that allows assessment of treatment results.

25. Diagnosis of TB is more difficult in HIV patients.

Making diagnosis of TB in HIV-infected individuals can be challenging.

Clinical Diagnosis

❖ Clinical presentation of pulmonary TB can vary widely in both immunocompetent and immunocompromised hosts.

❖ In general, the presentation in HIV-infected patients is similar to that seen in HIV-uninfected patients, although the signs and symptoms (such as fever, weight loss, and malaise) may be attributed to HIV itself and the possibility of TB overlooked.

❖ Symptoms usually are present for weeks to months, and *an acute onset of fever and cough are more suggestive of a nonmycobacterial pulmonary process.*

Laboratory Diagnosis

❖ HIV patients have higher rates of sputum smear-negative disease.

❖ Smear-negative, culture-positive TB is more common and occurs more frequently with advanced immunosuppression.

❖ Rates of smear-negative disease vary widely but have been reported as high as 66%.

❖ In general, the rate of smear positivity correlates with radiographical extent of the disease.

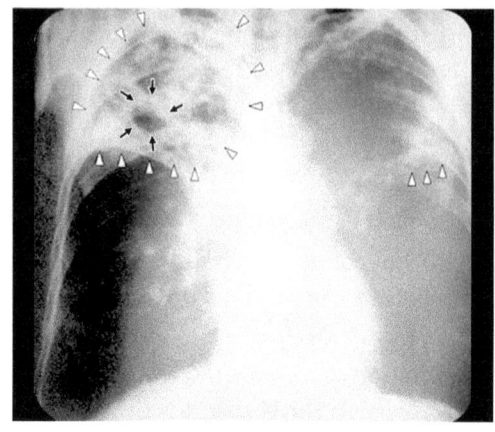

For example, patients with cavitary lesions caused by active TB will more commonly have positive smear results, whereas a negative smear in a patient with minimal disease on chest radiograph would not be unusual, and would not rule out active TB.

However, in HIV-infected patients, positive smear results may be seen with relatively little radiographic evidence.

Diagnosis of TB in HIV infection also becomes more difficult by the higher rates of extrapulmonary disease and necessitates the need to distinguish TB from other infectious and neoplastic complications of HIV.

26. Multidrug-resistant TB is posing to be a serious health problem.

Multidrug-resistant TB (MDR-TB) is defined as resistance to two of the most important and effective "first-line" drugs, *rifampicin* and *isoniazid* which are the preferred option for treatment.

About 3.3% of all TB disease cases are MDR-TB. 50% of MDR-TB cases are estimated to occur in China and India and 27 countries account for 86% of cases.

Problems associated with MDR-TB

1. Difficulty in treatment:
   - All cases of MDR-TB must be treated with second-line drugs which are less effective, but more expensive and having more serious side effects than first-line drugs.
   - However, the cost of drugs for treating the average MDR-TB patient is 50–200 times more than normal TB.
   - It takes 3 times more time to cure, i.e. 18–24 months.
2. Difficulty in diagnosis:
   - Diagnosis of drug resistance is difficult, especially in low resource countries
   - Diagnosis may take anywhere from 6 to 16 weeks and
   - Requires sophisticated laboratory equipment.
3. Mortality rate: Much higher than drug-susceptible TB patients.

27. Chemotherapy is not the only mean for prevention and control of TB in India.

Tuberculosis is a communicable disease so mere chemotherapy cannot prevent and control TB in India. It has several components:

For protection of the susceptible:

❖ General measures:
  – Health promotion:
    - Improvement in general health of the individual to improve resisting power
    - Improvement in living conditions with good lighting and ventilation, personal hygiene, good food, adequate nutrition.
  – Health education:
    - Health education of community about the mode of transmission of the disease, its hazards and availability of drugs to cure it completely
    - Educate the mothers about importance of BCG vaccination
    - Motivate TB patient and defaulters to take treatment regularly and continuously.
❖ Specific measures:
  – Vaccination: By BCG vaccination at birth (but can be done up to 6 weeks).

28. A partially blocked flea is more dangerous than a completely blocked flea or, a partially blocked flea is an efficient transmitter of plague.

Transmission of plague occurs as follows:

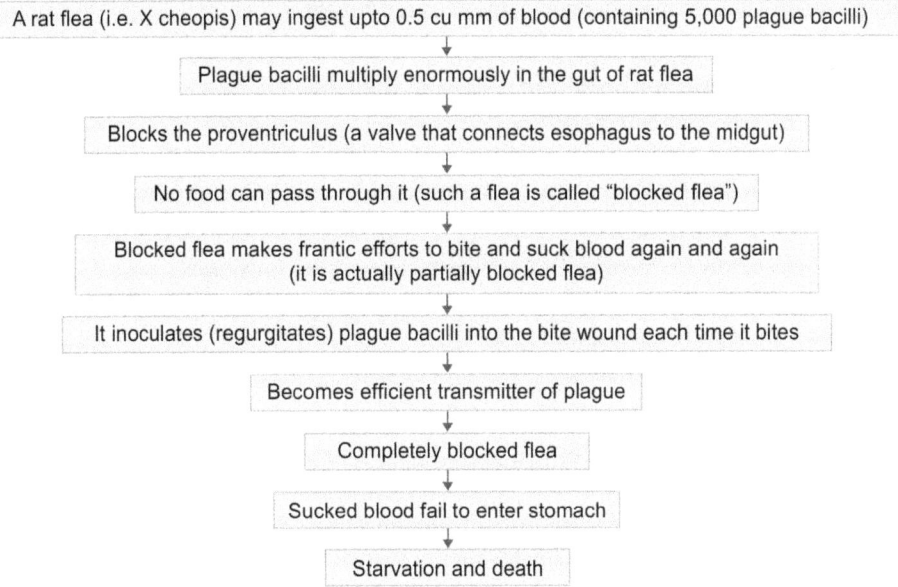

As the partially blocked flea lives longer (up to a year; and certain species survive as long as 4 years) it infects huge number of individuals. So, a partially blocked flea is more dangerous than a completely blocked flea.

29. ORS is the best treatment for diarrhea.

Because:

❖ Composition of ORS (WHO) is very effective and scientific in controlling dehydration state (it has been experienced that as many as 90–95% of cholera and diarrhea can be treated by ORS alone)

❖ Cost-effective
❖ Easy to administer, do not need medical personnel
❖ Can be undertaken at home for management of diarrhea by the mother
❖ It also ensures proper utilization of appropriate technology (a component of primary health care).

Criteria for "appropriate technology"	Reason
Scientifically sound	◆ ORS can be safely and scientifically used in treating acute diarrhea due to all etiology in all age group, in all country ◆ 90–95% of all cases of diarrhea can be completely treated by ORS
Acceptable to those who apply it	◆ Easy to prepare ◆ Easy to administer ◆ Can be prepared at home ◆ No boiling/sterilization needed
Acceptable to those on whom it is applied	◆ Orally administrated ◆ Self-administrated ◆ Less expensive ◆ Minimum side effects

30. Low osmolarity ORS for management of diarrhea is valuable.

❖ In 2003, clinical trials and comparisons with rice water led to a reduction in the recommended osmolarity of ORS by joint activity of WHO and UNICEF
❖ The guidelines were updated in 2006
❖ The recommended osmolarity of ORS was reduced from 311 mmol/L to 245 mmol/L
❖ But the concentration of glucose and sodium chloride were reduced, while that of potassium and citrate remained the same.

Basic advantages of low osmolarity ORS in diarrhea over previous one:
❖ It decreases vomiting
❖ It decreases stool volume by about 25%
❖ It decreases the need for IV therapy by about 30%.

31. Zinc therapy is beneficial in management of diarrhea.

When a zinc supplement is given during an episode of acute diarrhea it shows following beneficial effects:
  i. It reduces the duration and severity of diarrheal episodes
  ii. When given for 10–14 days it lowers the incidence and risk of diarrhea in the following 2–3 months.
❖ Dosing schedule:
  – WHO and UNICEF recommendation of zinc supplement:
    - <6 months—10 mg daily } for 10–14 days
    - >6 months—20 mg daily
❖ Zinc acts by following ways in diarrhea:
  – Thorough physiological effect of zinc on intestinal ion transport has not yet been established
  – Probably zinc inhibits cAMP-induced, Cl-dependent fluid secretion by inhibiting specifically basolateral potassium (K^+) channels

- *Improves the absorption of water and electrolytes*
- Improves regeneration of the intestinal epithelium
- Increases the levels of brush border enzymes, and enhances the immune response, allowing for a better clearance of the pathogens
- Zinc inhibits toxin-induced cholera
- It also plays a critical role in metalloenzymes, polyribosomes, and cell membrane and cellular function giving credence to the belief that it plays a central role in cellular growth and in the function of the immune system.

32. Carriers have an important role in transmission of typhoid fever.

❖ Mode of transmission of typhoid fever: Usually by fecal-oral route/urine oral route.
❖ Direct transmission: Through soiled hands contaminated with feces or urine of cases/carriers
❖ Indirect transmission: Ingestion of contaminated water, milk and/or food, or through flies.

The chronic typhoid carrier state can occur following symptomatic or subclinical infections of *Salmonella typhi.*

Chronic carriers of typhoid are, by definition, asymptomatic. So, they do not go to the doctors, but spreads the disease to the community.

Since humans are the only known reservoir for *S. typhi.* So among untreated cases, 10% will shed bacteria for 3 months after initial onset of symptoms and 2–5% will become chronic carriers (the chronic carrier state occurs most commonly among middle-aged women).
So, carriers play an important role in transmission of typhoid fever.

33. Indoor residual spray is not very effective to control dengue and chikungunya.

Aedes mosquitoes act as vector both for dengue and chikungunya. It breeds in artificial collection of water in and around human dwellings such as in discarded bins, broken bottles, flower pots, coconut shells, etc.

So indoor residual spray is not very effective as it involves spreading only on the walls and other surfaces of house where mosquitoes are presumed to be sit.

Hence,
❖ Cleaning up of surrounding environment
❖ Disposal of water holding containers, such as empty pots, broken bottles, coconut shells, tyres and similar other artificial collection of water shows effective result to control dengue and chikungunya.

34. Integrated vector control measures should be adopted wherever possible.

Integrated vector management (IVM) is the appropriate coordinated biological, environmental and chemical interventions of proven efficacy, separately or in combination as appropriate to the area through the optimal use of resources.

Advantages of using different methods at a time in IVM are:
❖ Cost effectiveness
❖ Synergistic actions
❖ Less chance of development of resistance
❖ Highly effective for full population coverage.

35. Knowledge about breeding habits of mosquito is necessary for undertaking control measures.

Type of mosquito	Breeding habit	Transmission of disease	Control measures
Anopheles	Clean water	Malaria	• Filling and drainage operation • Planned water management • Paris green (as anophiline larvae are surface feeder) • Mineral oil to kill larvae and pupa
Culex	Dirty, polluted water	Bancroftian filariasis, Japanese encephalitis, West Nile fever	• Filling and drainage operation • Planned water management • Mineral oil to kill larvae and pupa
Aedes	Artificial collection of water	Dengue, DHF, chikungunya, yellow fever, Rift Valley fever	• Artificial containers turn upside down to drain away the water • Oiling is useless • Paris green is unnecessary
Mansonia	Water bodies containing aquatic plants	Brugian filariasis	• Physical removal of aquatic plants or use of herbicides • Oiling useless • Paris green can be used

So, main focus should be on the source reduction based on their specific breeding habit according to local epidemic of mosquito-borne diseases.

36. Slide positivity rate is a better malariometric index than annual parasite incidence (API).

Slide positivity rate (SPR) is a much better malaria metric index than API.

Because
Annual parasite incidence (API) in malaria is defined as:

$$API = \frac{Confirmed\ cases\ during\ 1\ year}{Population\ under\ surveillance} \times 1000$$

SPR in malaria is defined as:

$$SPR = \frac{Slides\ positive\ for\ malaria\ parasite}{Total\ slides\ taken\ for\ examination} \times 100$$

❖ In both the definitions, numerators are almost same in meaning; so denominators are important in differentiating between these two indices.
❖ In the definition of API, the denominator "population under surveillance" is important in this question because it is very difficult to cover the whole susceptible population to detect the API.
❖ On the other hand, SPR detection is much more accurate because the denominator "total slides taken for examination" is suitable for measuring the index without any difficulty.
❖ So, SPR is taken as an operational indicator in active and passive case detection; whereas API is a basis of environmental surveillance (space/area spraying) in malaria.

37. What are the setbacks of malaria control in India?

Most important setbacks of malaria control in India are:
❖ Excessive breeding of mosquitoes due to favorable tropical climate.
❖ Lack of clearance of water clogged places that helps in breeding due to lack of:
  – Political cooperation
  – Public awareness
  – Health education.
❖ Lack of social hygiene and awareness.

38. Aedes aegypti index should be kept zero at all ports.

Aedes aegypti index is defined as:
  "The ratio expressed as percentage between the no. of houses in a limited well-defined area on the premises of which actual breeding of Aedes aegypti are found, and total no. of houses examined in that area".

$$\text{Aedes aegypti index} = \frac{\text{No. of houses in which actual breeding of } Aedes\ aegypti \text{ are found in a limited well-defined area}}{\text{Total no. of houses examined in that area}} \times 100$$

This index is kept zero at all ports.

According to WHO, International Health Regulations (IHR) all international airports and seaports are kept free from all types of mosquitoes for a distance of 400 meters around the perimeters of the ports. Because:
  1. *Aedes aegypti* do not fly over a long distance (usually <100 mts)
  2. It breeds in artificial collection of water around human dwellings, and
  3. India is a yellow fever receptive country.

So, keeping *Aedes aegypti* index zero at all ports we can prevent international transmission of different diseases in which *Aedes aegypti* acts as vector like yellow fever, dengue, chikungunya fever, Rift Valley fever, etc.

39. Local treatment of wound in case of post-exposure prophylaxis of rabies is the first requisite.

Immediate and adequate local treatment of all bite wounds and scratches is the first requisite and of utmost importance. Because:
❖ Rabies virus replicates in muscle or connective tissue cells at or near the site of inoculation (site of bite or scratches), then attaches to the nerve endings and enters peripheral nerves.
❖ Immediate local treatment helps to remove and inactivate as much virus as possible from the site of inoculation before it can be absorbed on the nerve endings.
❖ Animal experiments have shown that local treatment of wound can reduce the chances of developing rabies by up to 80%.

Local treatment includes:
❖ Cleansing:
  – Immediate flushing and washing of wounds, scratches and adjoining areas with plenty of water (preferably under running tap) for at least 15 minutes is very useful.

- – If soap unavailable simple flushing with water should be done
  - – In case of punctured wound irrigation by catheter should be done.
- ❖ Chemical treatment:
  - – For inactivation of residual viruses
  - – Done by alcohol (400–700 mL/L) or tincture or 0.01% aqueous solution of iodine or povidone iodine.
- ❖ Suturing:
  - – Should not be sutured as it may help to spread the virus into deeper tissue
  - – If needed done after 1–2 days, undercover of antirabies immunoglobulin with minimum sutures.
- ❖ Antibiotics and antitetanus measures:
  - – Should be done when indicated.

40. Intradermal regimes of antirabies vaccine are superior to intramuscular regimes.

Because:
- ❖ Efficacy and immunogenicity: It has been found that both type of vaccine regimes against rabies [i.e. intradermal (ID) and intramuscular] have equal efficacy and they are equally immunogenic
- ❖ Intradermal regimes involve less no. of vials and sites. As per 5-dose IM regime or 5 vials of vaccine are required, whereas intradermal 2-dose regime only involves <2 vials
- ❖ Patient compliance (like abscess, swelling, etc.) with ID regime is less than that of IM regime.

41. A biting animal should be watched for at least 10 days.

A biting animal should be observed for at least 10 days because:
- ❖ It is found that the rabies virus may be present in saliva 3–4 days before onset of symptoms and animal usually dies within 5–6 days of developing the disease (4 + 6 = 10 days).
- ❖ If the animal remains healthy after this period there is no risk of rabies and thus no need for vaccination which if already started may be discontinued (though this, of course, does not take account of the rare possibility of the carrier state in dogs).

42. AIDS is no longer limited to the high-risk of population.

AIDS is caused by HIV which is an emerging disease and known as our modern pandemic affecting both developed and developing countries.

Population Groups for AIDS/HIV

Risk	At risk persons
High-risk group	• Commercial sex worker • Homosexual men • IV drug user
Bridge population	• Clients of sex worker • STD patient • Partners of IV drug user • Migrant population
General population	• Common people

❖ AIDS epidemic has shifted from one population to next population when the prevalence of AIDS in high-risk group reaches >5%.
❖ The lag time of shifting one group to next is 2–3 years
❖ The trend indicates that HIV infection spreads in 2 ways:
  1. From urban to rural population
  2. From individual practicing high-risk population to general population.

The spreading of infection from high-risk group to others is due to *increasing bridge population* as:
❖ Social factors like prostitution, broken home, emotional immaturity, easy money, sexual disharmony, industrialization are responsible for increased prevalence in bridge population
❖ AIDS is recognized as an emerging disease since 1983. So, this long-lasting epidemic was enough for shifting of HIV infection from high-risk group to general population
❖ Limited use, accessibility and availability of antiretroviral drugs
❖ Fear of social stigma.

43. STD control is linked to HIV/AIDS control.

Because:
❖ *Behavior:* Leading to transmission of STD and AIDS are same.
❖ *Relation in transmission:* Transmission in HIV is increased 7–8 times in presence of STD.
❖ *Early diagnosis and treatment* of STD is now recognized as one of the major strategies to control spread of HIV.
❖ *Condom promotion:* Plays an important role in primary prevention of both STD and HIV.
❖ *Health education and individual counseling* are more or less same for both the cases.

44. Why mosquito is not carrier of AIDS?

For the transmission of HIV from an infected individual to a normal one through mosquito the virus need to be alive inside the mosquito. But HIV virus neither can survive nor can reproduce inside a mosquito. So, the virus cannot invade the salivary gland of the mosquito. That is why mosquito is not the carrier of AIDS.

45. In an STD patient the risk of transmission of HIV is 8–10 times higher.

❖ The first thing to focus is the conditions which allows an easy invasion by HIV, they are:
  – Epithelial breaches and
  – Virus load.
❖ In an episode of STD, there are two types of changes to the genital area:
  – There are areas of mucosal epithelial damages and breaches caused by infection which permits an easy entry by the HIV, and
  – Due to decreased local immunity caused by the residing STD infection, the area which first serves the attack of HIV cannot provide an effective resistance to the organism.
❖ Together these two factors act in such a way that relatively lower amount of virus load increases the chance of infection.

EPIDEMIOLOGY OF CHRONIC NONCOMMUNICABLE DISEASE AND CONDITION

1. Mass strategy is better than individual approach for prevention of noncommunicable disease.

❖ Mass strategy/population strategy is based on the principle that a small change in the risk factor levels in total population can achieve the biggest reduction in mortality and this strategy should be based on mass approach not on individual approach.

❖ Thus, the aim should be to shift the whole risk factor distribution on the direction of biologically normality which requires the mobilization and involvement of the whole community to alter lifestyle practises associated with different noncommunicable diseases in addition to medical measures.

2. Hypertension is an iceberg disease.

At first describe the iceberg phenomenon of disease as given in Chapter.

Hypertension in the community can be demonstrated by "Rule of halves" which is the direct representation of "iceberg phenomenon of a disease".

❖ Rule of halves: Demonstrated in 1970.

States that: Only about 1/2 of the hypertensive subjects in the general population of most developed countries are aware of this condition → Only about 1/2 of those aware of the problem are being treated → Only about 1/2 of those treated may be considered adequately treated.

That is how it represents the iceberg phenomena of the disease.

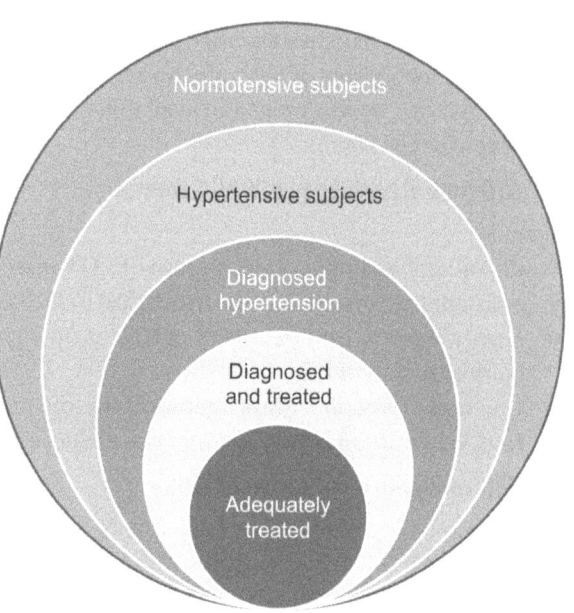

3. Diabetes mellitus is a public health issue.

Diabetes is now one of the most common noncommunicable disease globally. It is the fourth or fifth leading cause of death in most high-income countries and there is substantial evidence that it is epidemic in many low- and middle-income countries.

Some Salient Features of Diabetes Epidemiology Representing as Public Health Issue

❖ Globally, as of 2010, an estimated 285 million people had diabetes with type 2 making up about 90% of the cases.

❖ In 2011, it resulted in 1.4 million deaths worldwide making it the 8th leading cause of death.

❖ This is an increase from 1 million deaths in 2000.

❖ Its rate has increased, and by 2030, this number is estimated to almost double.

❖ Diabetes mellitus occurs throughout the world, but is more common (especially type 2) in more developed countries.

❖ The greatest increase in rates is, however, expected to occur in Asia and Africa, where most people with diabetes will probably be found by 2030.

❖ The increase in rates in developing countries follows the trend of urbanization and lifestyle changes, perhaps most importantly a "Western-style" diet.

❖ This has suggested an environmental (i.e. dietary) effect, but there is little understanding of the mechanism(s) at present, though there is much speculation, some of it most compellingly presented.

4. Application of different levels of prevention of DM.

Different levels of prevention of DM:

Levels of prevention		Modes
Primary prevention	Population strategy	Improvements of nutritional habits like: • Avoiding sweets, fatty foods, alcohol • Regular intake of proteins, dietary fiber rich in foods
	High-risk strategy	Preventive cares like: • Correction in obesity • Avoiding overnutrition and alcohol • Changing lifestyle • Regular exercise
Secondary prevention	Early diagnosis	High-risk screening in people with: • Age >40 years • Obesity • Family history of diabetes • Sedentary worker with lack of exercise • History of babies weighing >4.5 kgs • Typical clinical features
	Treatment	• Diet • Antidiabetogenic drugs
Tertiary prevention	Disability limitation and rehabilitation	• By providing supportive medical and social cares

5. Cancer can be prevented by primary prevention.

Strategy for prevention of cancer by primary prevention:

Health Education

Can be given by:
- Individual approach
- Mass approach
- Group approach.

❖ Aim: To prevent people from adopting harmful lifestyle and making them aware of early signs of cancer so that they can seek timely help.

❖ Education to be given about:
- Harmful effects of smoking, alcohol consumption through means of mass media, street plays, lectures, etc.
- The available treatment facilities for cancer

   – Warning signs of cancer
   – Time of seeking medical advice.

Specific Prevention

❖ Control of tobacco consumption
❖ Immunization against Hep B
❖ Food hygiene—preventing use of food colors and additives
❖ Control of air pollution
❖ Preplacement examination for preventing occupational cancers.

6. Accident is a noncommunicable disease.

Accident is defined as "an unexpected, unplanned occurrence which may involve injury"/"unpremeditated event resulting in recognizable damage".
As accidents have:
❖ Their own natural history and
❖ Follow the same epidemiological pattern as any other disease, e.g. agent, host and environment interacting together, so it is considered as a noncommunicable disease.

7. BMI is a measure of obesity.

❖ Body mass index (BMI) is a simple and widely used tool for estimating body fat mass. BMI is an accurate reflection of body fat percentage in the majority of the adult population.

   (Though it, however, is less accurate in people such as bodybuilders and pregnant women.)

WHO standards for Asian population according to BMI:

Value	Interpretation
<18.5	Underweight
18.5–23	Normal weight
23–27.5	Overweight
≥27.5	Obese

HEALTH PROGRAMS IN INDIA

1. ASHA links healthcare delivery with community. Explain.

Role of ASHA linking healthcare delivery with community:

Roles	Description
Awareness and information to the community/women of the community about	• Importance of nutrition/basic sanitation/personal hygiene as determinants of health • Need for utilization of health and family welfare services • Importance of breastfeeding/immunization/complementary feeding/family planning/prevention of STDs

Contd...

Contd...

Roles	Description
Referral services	ASHA will arrange escort/accompany pregnant women/child requiring referral to the nearest PHC/CHC/FRU
Primary health care for minor illnesses	<ul><li>Diarrhea</li><li>Fever</li><li>First aid services</li></ul>
Depot holder and provider of	<ul><li>DOTS</li><li>ORS</li><li>IFA tablets</li><li>Chloroquine</li><li>Disposable delivery kits</li><li>Oral pills</li><li>Condoms</li></ul>
Utilization of government health services	<ul><li>Antenatal checkup</li><li>Postnatal checkup</li><li>Immunization</li><li>Supplementary nutrition</li></ul>
Development of a comprehensive village health plan	ASHA will develop it working with:<ul><li>Village health guides</li><li>Anganwadi workers</li><li>Sanitation committee of gram panchayat</li></ul>
Notification services	ASHA will notify nearby PHC/subcenter about:<ul><li>Birth</li><li>Death</li><li>Disease outbreaks in the community</li><li>Any unusual health problem in the community</li></ul>

DEMOGRAPHY AND FAMILY PLANNING

1. India is in the late expansion phase (3rd phase) of demographic cycle.

Demography focus on three observable phenomenon, i.e.

1. Change in population size
2. Composition of population
3. Distribution of population.

So considering three vital features, India in the demographic cycle stands in late expansion phase. Because:

❖ The birth rate of India tends to fall
❖ The death rate declines further
❖ The population continues to grow because birth exceeds death
❖ The age and sex composition of India reveals a typical of underdeveloped country with broad base and tapering top.
For more details, please see Chapter 4, "Short Notes".

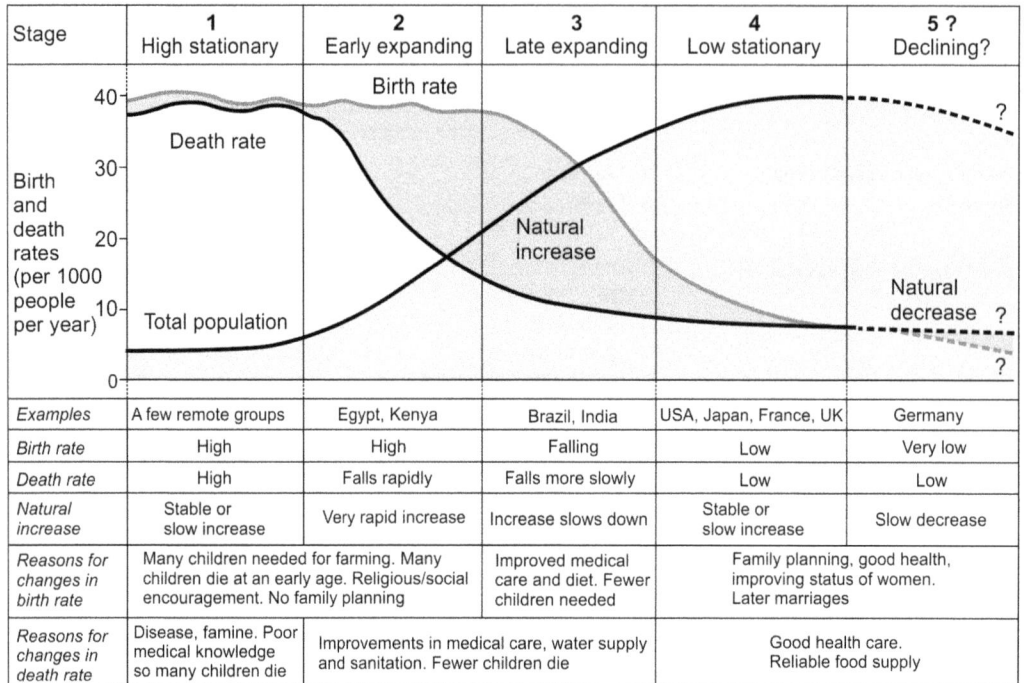

Stage	1 High stationary	2 Early expanding	3 Late expanding	4 Low stationary	5 ? Declining?
Examples	A few remote groups	Egypt, Kenya	Brazil, India	USA, Japan, France, UK	Germany
Birth rate	High	High	Falling	Low	Very low
Death rate	High	Falls rapidly	Falls more slowly	Low	Low
Natural increase	Stable or slow increase	Very rapid increase	Increase slows down	Stable or slow increase	Slow decrease
Reasons for changes in birth rate	Many children needed for farming. Many children die at an early age. Religious/social encouragement. No family planning		Improved medical care and diet. Fewer children needed	Family planning, good health, improving status of women. Later marriages	
Reasons for changes in death rate	Disease, famine. Poor medical knowledge so many children die	Improvements in medical care, water supply and sanitation. Fewer children die		Good health care. Reliable food supply	

PREVENTIVE MEDICINE IN OBSTETRICS, PEDIATRICS AND GERIATRICS

1. Institutional delivery can reduce maternal mortality to a great extent. Explain.

❖ According to WHO, **maternal death** is defined as:
"The death of a woman while pregnant/within 42 days of termination of pregnancy, irrespective of the duration and site of pregnancy from any cause related to/aggravated by the pregnancy/its management **but not from accidental/incidental causes.**"

Major causes of maternal deaths in India are as follows:

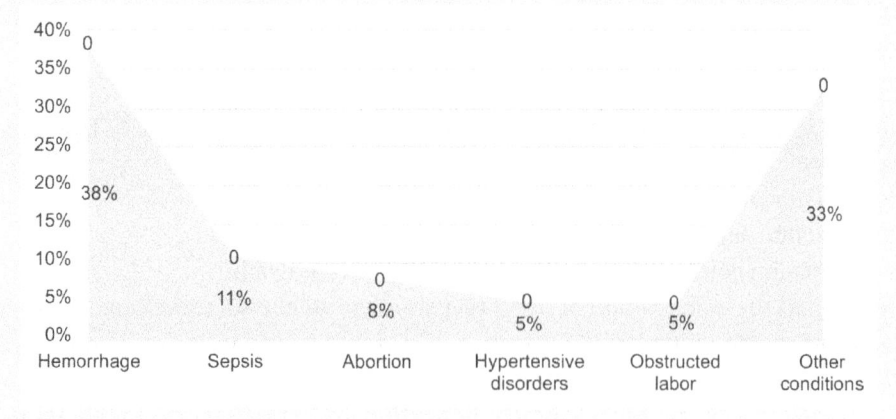

Major causes of maternal deaths in India

The disadvantages of home deliveries are:
1. The mother has less medical and nursing supervision than in the hospital.
2. Septicemia may result from unskilled/septic manipulations.
3. Tetanus neonatorum may result from the use of unsterilized instruments.
4. If the mother presents with any complications/danger signs of pregnancy, then home delivery is never recommended and she should be immediately referred to the nearby health institution.
5. The mother may take less rest.
6. She may resume her domestic daily duties too soon.
7. Her diet may be neglected.

So, the institutional deliveries reduce maternal mortality to a great extent by providing asepsis and assistance in complicated pregnancies.

2. FRUs will reduce maternal mortality rate. Explain.

The major causes of maternal mortality rate (MMR) in India are:
❖ Hemorrhage
❖ Sepsis
❖ Abortion
❖ Hypertension
❖ Obstructed labor.

We can see from the above list that the major causes of maternal mortality in India are from complications of pregnancy.

It occurs because despite best possible antenatal care, some women develop complications without any warning signs and require emergency care.

For this reason, establishment of first referral units (FRUs) for emergency obstetric care should be prioritized under the safe motherhood component of RCH program.

Remember: Specialist Services Available at FRU

Surgical Management
❖ Cesarean section
❖ Laparotomy and repair of ruptured uterus
❖ Surgical treatment of severe sepsis
❖ Evaluation of incomplete abortion
❖ Mid-trimester abortion
❖ Repair of cervical and vaginal tears
❖ Amniotomy with/without oxytocin
❖ Tubectomy/vasectomy.

Delivery Services
24 hours delivery services including normal and assisted delivery.

Medical Management
❖ Severe hypertensive disorders of pregnancy, eclampsia

❖ Hemorrhagic shock
❖ Severe anemia
❖ Septicemia
❖ Use of IV oxytocin during labor.

Manual Management

❖ Manual removal of placenta
❖ Forceps delivery
❖ Vacuum extraction
❖ Partography.

Anesthesia

General/spinal.

Blood Transfusion

❖ Establishment of blood transfusion services in FRUs
❖ Performing mandatory tests
❖ Newborn and pediatric care
❖ Resuscitation
❖ Management of sick newborns and severe illnesses of young children.

Referral Services

So, FRUs definitely have an impact on reduction of MMR by:
❖ Provision of clean delivery practice/aseptic intranatal care
❖ Prevention and/or treatment of complications of pregnancy
❖ Treatment of coexisting medical conditions (like hypertension/diabetes, etc.)
❖ Prevention of anemia and hemorrhage
❖ Provision of safe abortion services.

3. Under-five mortality rate is the best indicator for social development.

The under-five mortality rate (U5MR) is used as the principal indicator of social development.

The U5MR has several advantages which are as follows:

❖ It *measures an end result of the development process rather than an 'input'* such as school enrollment level/per capita calorie availability/number of doctors per 1,000 population—all of which are means to an end.
❖ The *U5MR is known to be the result of a wide variety of inputs*:
   – The nutritional health and the health knowledge of mothers
   – The level of immunization and ORT use
   – The availability of maternal and child health services
   – Income and food availability in the family
   – The availability of clean water and safe sanitation
   – The overall safety of the child's environment.

❖ The U5MR is less susceptible than, say, per capita GNP to the fallacy of the average. This is because the natural scale does not allow the children of the rich to be one thousand times as likely to survive, even if the manmade scale does permit them to have one thousand times as much income.

In other words, it is much more difficult for a wealthy minority to affect a nation's U5MR, and it therefore presents a more accurate picture of the health status of the majority of children (and of society as a whole).

For these reasons, the U5MR is chosen by UNICEF as its single most important indicator of the state of a nation's children.

NUTRITION AND HEALTH

1. Parboiled rice is nutritionally superior to milled rice. Explain.

It should be mentioned that the rice grain consists of three parts:

Layer	Nutritive element
Rice germ	Vitamin (mostly B-complex vitamins) and proteins
Outer pericarp and aleurone grain layer	Most of the essential nutrients
Inner endosperm	Starch
White rice	Carbohydrates

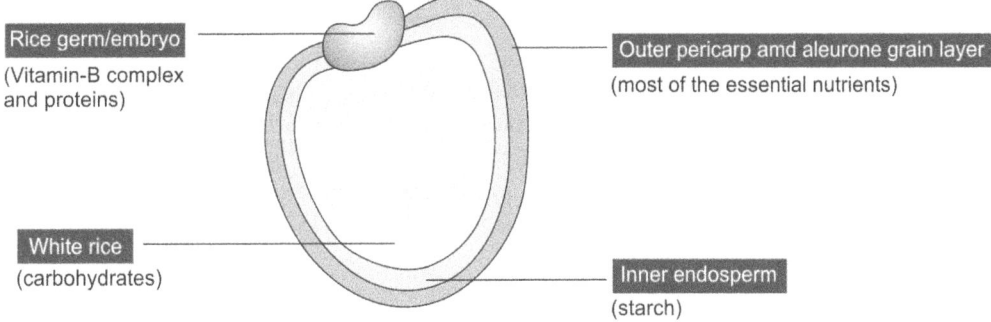

Effect of Milling on Rice

❖ The milling process deprives the rice grain of its valuable nutritive elements like:
   – Thiamine
   – Riboflavin
   – Protein.
❖ So, the resulting white/polished rice is poor in nutritive value and people consuming it for a long time become prone to *beriberi*.

Advantage of Parboiling over Milling of Rice

Parboiling is partial cooking of rice in steam. It has the following advantages:
❖ **During the steaming process**, *a greater part of vitamins and minerals present in the outer pericarp and aleurone grain layer of rice grain are driven into the inner endosperm.*

- ❖ **During the drying process,** *the germ gets attached firmly to the grain*
- ❖ In addition, heat used in drying *hardens the rice grain, so the grain becomes resistant to insect invasion and suitable for storage*
- ❖ *The starch gets gelatinized which also improves the keeping quality of rice.*

2. Growth chart may play multiple roles. Explain.

Roles of Growth Chart

- ❖ **Growth monitoring.**
- ❖ **As a diagnostic tool:** Malnutrition can be detected long before signs and symptoms of it become apparent.
- ❖ **Planning and policy making:** Growth chart provides an objective basis for planning and policy making in relation to child health care at local/state/central levels.
- ❖ **Educating mothers:** The mother can be easily educated in the care of her own child and she is encouraged for participating more actively in growth monitoring.
- ❖ **Tool for action:** Growth chart guides the health worker to take appropriate intervention (like nutritional interventions and referrals) at the right time.
- ❖ **Tool for evaluation:** Growth chart provides an effective tool for evaluating the effect of the intervention measures.
- ❖ **Tool for teaching:** The growth chart can be used to teach importance of adequate feeding/ effects of diarrhea and ARI on child health, etc.

3. Interpretation of ICDS growth chart.

- ❖ Before going into the interpretation of new ICDS growth chart, we should first discuss the salient features of it once again:
  - – The new ICDS growth chart has three reference curves. They are as follows:
    - - 1st curve: It depicts the median value (M); it is the top curve.
    - - 2nd curve: M-2SD. Standard deviation (SD)
    - - 3rd curve: M-3SD.
- ❖ Plotted point in the ICDS growth chart for weight-for-age helps in assessing the nutritional status of the child.
- ❖ **Note** the position of the plotted point with reference to pre-printed growth curves and then interpret the position of the plotted point to identify normal growth and growth problems:
  - – If plotted *weight-for-age* of a child falls much *above the 1st curve*, the child has a growth problem, probably overweight/obesity.
  - – If plotted weight-for-age of a child falls *exactly on the 1st/2nd/3rd curve;* then the child is in the less severe category of malnutrition because:
    - - Plotted point on the 1st curve indicates that the child's growth is normal.
    - - Plotted point on the 2nd curve indicates that the child's growth is normal and he/she is not moderately underweight.
    - - Plotted point on the 3rd curve indicates that the child is moderately underweight.
  - – If plotted weight-for-age of a child falls on the **green** band, then the child's growth is **normal**; if it falls on the **yellow** band, then the child is **moderately underweight**; if it falls on the **orange** band, then child is **severely underweight**.

Position of the plotted point	Nutritional status
Plotted point is: • Exactly on/above the 1st curve • Between 1st and 2nd curve • Exactly on the 2nd curve	Child's growth is normal
Plotted point is: • Between 2nd and 3rd curve • Exactly on the 3rd curve	Child is moderately underweight
Plotted point is below the 3rd curve	Child is severely underweight

Note that:

❖ When the child is severely underweight, clinical signs of marasmus/kwashiorkor may be evident.

❖ If a child has edema of both feet, the weight will be more due to fluid retention. So, it will mask that the baby is actually severely underweight. The presence of edema is thus very much important and should be marked clearly close to the plotted point. This baby will automatically be considered severely undernourished and should be referred for specialist care.

Direction of child's growth curve and its importance

Direction of curve	Pictorial depiction	Growth pattern
Upward	Good	**Good:** Indicates adequate weight gain for the age of the child. The child is growing well and is healthy
Flat	Dangerous	**Dangerous:** Indicates that the child is not gaining weight and is not growing adequately. This is called "**stagnation**". This should be investigated
Downward	Very dangerous	**Very dangerous:** Indicates loss of weight. The child requires immediate referral and health care

4. Revised ICDS growth chart currently in operation differ from the earlier one. Explain.

Points	Old ICDS growth chart	New ICDS growth chart
Standard	Developed based on National Center for Health Statistics (NCHS) standard	Based on WHO 2006 child growth standard
Based on:	It is based on a cross-sectional study on American children	It is based on a Multicentre Growth Reference study (MGRS) organized over 6 countries (Brazil, Ghana, India, Norway, Oman, USA)
No. of reference curves	There are four reference curves present in the chart	There are three reference curves present in the chart

Contd...

Contd...

Points	Old ICDS growth chart	New ICDS growth chart
Position of the reference curves	Topmost: 80% of median 2nd curve: 70% of median 3rd curve: 60% of median 4th curve: 50% of median	Topmost: Median 2nd curve: M-2SD 3rd curve: M-3SD Standard deviation (SD)
Categorization of nutritional basis (by measurement of weight)	≥80%: Normal 70–80%: Mild (**grade 1**) 60–70%: Moderate (**grade 2**) 50–60%: Severe (**grade 3**) <50%: Severe (**grade 4**)	Above 2nd curve: **Normal** Below 2nd curve to 3rd curve: **Moderately underweight** Below 3rd curve: **Severely underweight**
Sex	It was valid for both sexes	Separate for boys and girls (Pink for girls and blue for boys)
Plotting	Plotting was done at the middle of the boxes	Plotting is done on the line for each completed months
Differences in interpretation	*Stunting will be greater throughout the childhood in the new growth chart.* *Underweight will be greater during the first 6 months of delivery in the new growth chart.* *Wasting will be higher during infancy in the new growth chart*	

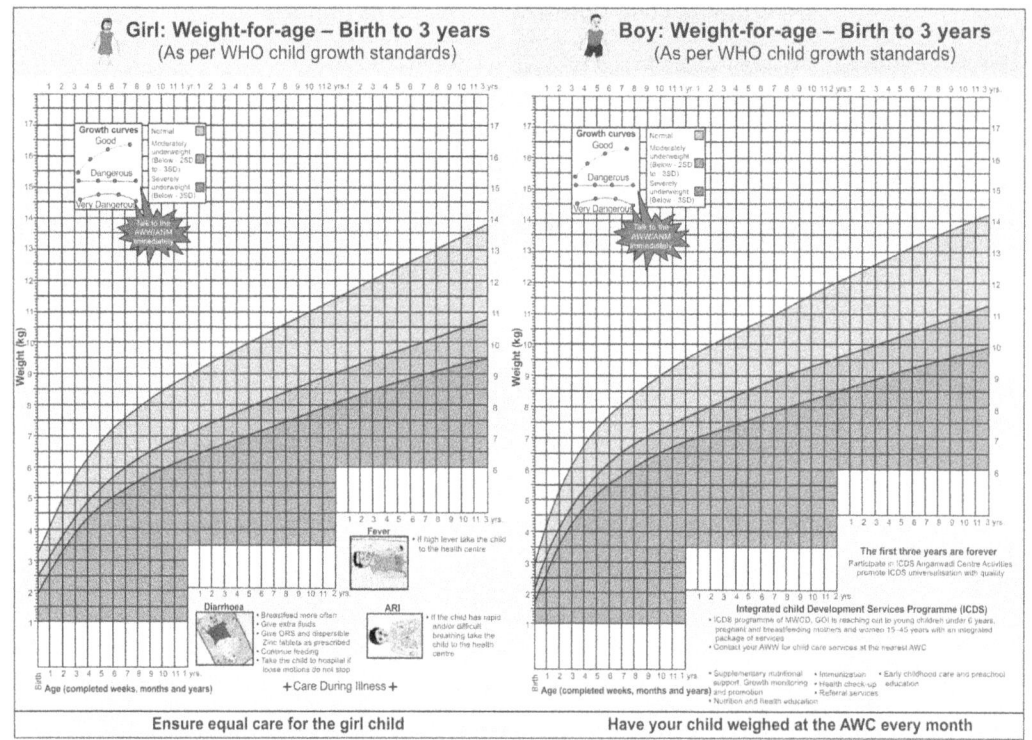

5. Public health significance of iodine deficiency disorder (IDD) is much larger than that of goiter only.

Spectrum of iodine deficiency disorders (IDD) is as follows according to WHO:

Disease	Level of severity/presentations
Goiter	• Grade 0: Goiter is not palpable or visible even when neck is extended • Grade 1a: When the goiter is palpable • Grade 1b: When the goiter is visible • Grade 2: Goiter is visible when neck is in normal position • Grade 3: Large goiter visible from distance
Hypothyroidism	• Variable clinical signs may be present in different stages of the disease
Endemic cretinism	• Hypothyroid cretinism • Neurological cretinism
Neurological effects	• Subnormal intelligence • Delayed motor milestones • Mental deficiency • Hearing defects • Speech defects • Muscle weakness in legs/arms/trunk • Spastic diplegia • Spastic quadriplegia
Intrauterine death	• Spontaneous abortion • Miscarriage
Squint	• Unilateral • Bilateral

According to IDD problem pyramid goiter and cretinism together possess a small portion at the top of it.

It contains at about 1–10% of all IDD spectrum.

Remaining 90% remain hidden but they can show several neurological, developmental, etc. damages in the community people just as seen in the "iceberg phenomena" of the disease. Most of the times they remain undiagnosed and untreated making a huge burden of disease over the community.

So, public health significance of iodine deficiency disorder is much larger than that of goiter only.

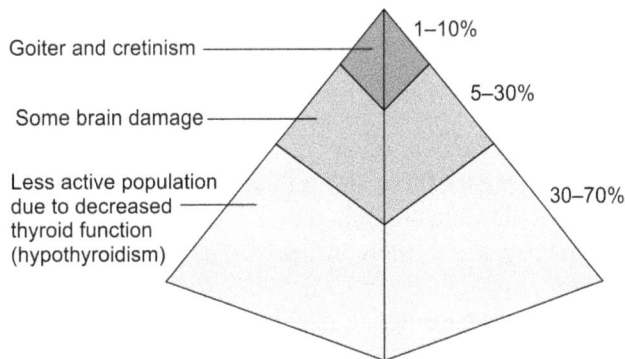

• It is worldwide major public health problem. Globally 1.5 billion people are at the risk of iodine deficiency disorders
• The pyramid shows the visible effects of ioding deficiency disorders. Goiter and cretinism account only for 1–10% of these
• Whereas 90% of the effects remain hidden

Goiter and cretinism — 1–10%

Some brain damage — 5–30%

Less active population due to decreased thyroid function (hypothyroidism) — 30–70%

IDD problem pyramid

6. Only iodized salt should be available for consumption universally.

According to WHO, nearly 30% of world population are living in iodine deficiency conditions.

According to this assumption, the Prevention of Food Adulteration Act (PFA) in India has fixed the iodization level to at least 30 ppm at the production point and at least 15 ppm at the consumer level.

Importance of Availability of Only Iodized Salt for Consumption

❖ Iodization of common salt is the most effective way towards mass prophylaxis in an IDD prevalent zone.
❖ Consumption of iodized salt has many benefits which are as follows:
  – Improved thyroid function: Thus help to regulate the metabolism and growth and development of the body.
  – Improved brain function such as memory, concentration and the ability to learn. An iodine deficiency can lower the IQ by as much as 15 points.
  – Healthy pregnancies: Iodized salt in moderation can help to prevent miscarriages and stillbirths. It can also help to avoid cretinism.
  – Fights depression.
  – Controls weight: By regulating the metabolism.
  – Prevents irritable bowel syndrome (IBS).
  – Improved appearance: By curing dry and flaky skin, and improve the growth of the hair and nail.
  – Fights cancer.
❖ If only iodized salt is available universally then people will be compelled to take iodine through taking salts. So, there will be decreased in incidence of IDD.

7. Fluorine is a double edged sword.

Because:
Both deficiency and excess of fluorine leads to different health hazards.

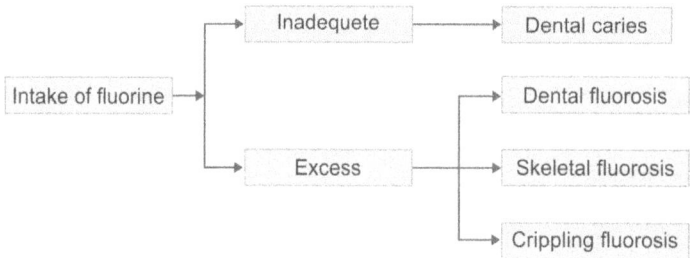

❖ Inadequate intake of fluorine:
  – Leads to "dental fluorosis" as fluorine is an important component of cement formation of teeth (fluorohydroxyapatite)
  – Characterized initially by opaque white patches, staining, mottling and pitting of teeth.
❖ Excess intake of fluorine:

Type of fluorosis	Level of fluorine in water	Characteristics
Dental fluorosis	>1.5 ppm	• Due to excess fluorine intake in 1st 7 years of life (time of tooth calcification) • "Mottling" (best seen in incisor of upper jaw)

Contd...

Contd...

Type of fluorosis	Level of fluorine in water	Characteristics
Skeletal fluorosis	3–6 ppm	• Leads to an increase in bone density, calcification of ligaments • Rheumatic or arthritic pain in joints and muscles along with stiffness and rigidity of the joints • Bending of the vertebral column
Crippling fluorosis	>10 ppm	• Severe form of skeletal fluorosis • During skeletal fluorosis, both cortical and cancellous bones undergo structural and biochemical changes, and • In advanced stages of the disease, the changes are irreversible leading to crippling fluorosis

So, recommended level of fluorides in drinking water in India (0.5–0.8 ppm) must be strictly followed.

8. Vitamin A supplementation is necessary after measles infection.

❖ Several studies have shown that, measles virus (MV) can be transmitted from infected immune cells to epithelial cells via an epithelial cell receptor located on the basolateral surface of the latter. Mutant MV that lacks the ability to use epithelial cell receptors fails to infect epithelial cells. The unidentified receptor may be a molecule related to tight junctions.

❖ Progeny MV particles bud exclusively from the apical surface of the epithelium and are thus actively released into the airway.

As a result measles virus shows a huge damage of the epithelial cells by their invasion and transmission process into the body tissue.

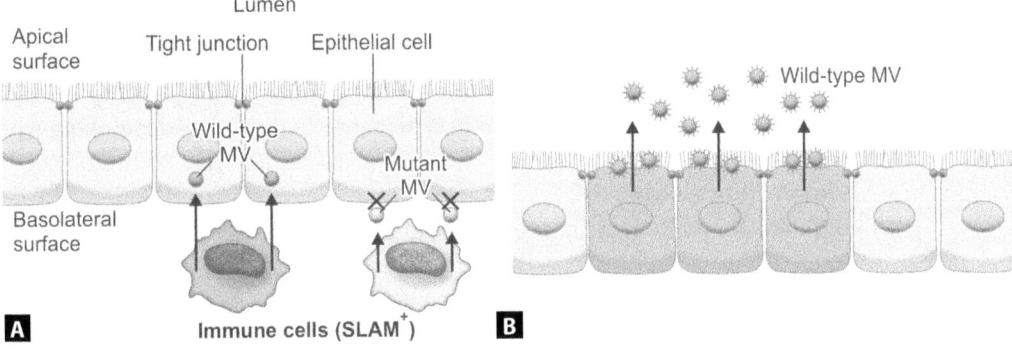

Here vitamin A acts as a necessary substrate in fighting measles, because:

❖ It helps in preserving epithelial cell integrity

❖ Enhances epithelization

❖ Prevent vomiting initiated after measles vaccination

❖ Vitamin A is fat soluble vitamin, helps to improve fat absorption

❖ Vitamin A indirectly helps to protein absorption from gut

❖ Helps to prevent protein-energy malnutrition (PEM), and grass root level implementation of it decreases occurrence of xerophthalmia

❖ Vitamin A if initiated too early in infant, there may cause impairment with the function of maternal antibodies. Thus, it plays a very vital role in immune modulation.

So, vitamin A is administered in measles.
(Reference: The Journal of Clinical Investigation: http://www.ncbi.nlm.nih.gov/pmc/articles/PMC2430502/figure/F3/)

9. Dietary fibers are essential components of a balanced diet.

Benefits of consuming dietary fibers are as follows:
❖ It reduces constipation:
  – As it absorbs water which increases the bulk of the stool and helps to reduce the tendency of constipation by encouraging bowel movements
  – They are resistant to digestion in the gastrointestinal (GI) tract
  – In large intestine, the bacterial action causes emulsification of these fibers thus making the stool soft and passage easier
  – By reducing the intestinal transit time of the food, it drastically reduces the possibilities of putrefaction and formation of gases and toxic substances.
❖ Fibers also inhibit fecal mutagens synthesis by changing colonic pH and bacterial metabolism.
❖ Helps maintain bowel health:
  – Lowers the risk of developing hemorrhoids and diverticular disease of colon.
❖ Lowers blood cholesterol levels:
  – Soluble fiber found in beans, oats, flax seed and oat bran may help lower total blood cholesterol levels by lowering low-density lipoprotein, cholesterol levels
  – Probably, it happens as dietary fiber binds to bile salts and prevents resorption thus reduces circulating cholesterol level.
❖ Helps control blood sugar levels:
  – In people with diabetes, fiber: Particularly soluble fiber (gum and pectin)—can lower the absorption of sugar and help to improve blood sugar levels.
  – A healthy diet that includes insoluble fiber may also reduce the risk of developing type 2 diabetes.
❖ Aids in achieving healthy weight:
  – High-fiber foods generally require more chewing time which gives the body time to register when it is no longer hungry, thus making people less likely to overeat. Also, a high-fiber diet tends to make a meal feel larger and linger longer, so people stay full for a greater amount of time. High-fiber diets also tend to be less "energy dense" which means they have fewer calories for the same volume of food.
❖ Another benefit attributed to dietary fiber is *prevention of colorectal cancer*. However, the evidence that fiber reduces colorectal cancer is mixed.

Daily requirement of dietary fiber for adult:

	Age < 50 years	Age >50 years
Men	38 g	30 g
Women	25 g	21 g

So, dietary fibers are essential components of balanced diet.

10. Milk and egg protein are considered as biologically complete.

A biologically complete protein (or whole protein) is a source of protein that contains an adequate proportion of all nine essential amino acids necessary for the dietary needs of humans or other animals. Some incomplete protein sources may contain all essential amino acids, but a complete protein contains them in correct proportions for supporting biological functions in the human body.

Nearly milk and egg protein contains all nine essential amino acids (phenylalanine, valine, threonine, tryptophan, methionine, leucine, isoleucine, lysine and histidine) in adequate amount and proportion meeting biological functions of the human body adequately. So, these are considered as biologically complete protein.

11. Mixing cereals with pulses improves the quality of diet.

Cereals have poor nutritive value as they are deficient in the very essential amino acid, lysine. The proteins of maize are still poorer as they are deficient in both lysine and tryptophan. But cereals contains methionine and cysteine in adequate amount.

On the other hand, pulses contain 20–25% of proteins which is 2 times than wheat and 3 times than that of rice. It has been seen that pulses are poorer in methionine and to lesser extent in cysteine, but very rich in lysine.

So, if cereals are taken with pulses, it will definitely improve the quality of food and also act as a complete protein.

12. Mid-day meal is a substitute for family diet.

Now the mid-day meal scheme (MDMS) is the largest school lunch program in the nation. It has been reported that MDMS has catered to the nutritional needs of school children in both rural and urban areas.

It has been seen that:

	MDMS provides	Overall body requirement
Energy	350–386 Kcal	450 Kcal
Protein	10.9–11.9 g	12 g

The comparison of average daily nutrient intake of school children with RDA showed that intake of all the nutrients was inadequate.

The mid-day meal was found to be a substitute rather than a supplement for the home meal, as:

❖ The percent contribution of energy, protein and fat by the MDM to actual nutrient intake of children was 28.2, 51.7 and 27.5, respectively.

❖ The percent contribution of other nutrients was β-carotene (22.7), thiamine (28.3), riboflavin (25.3), niacin (28.7), folacin (23.6), vitamin C (15.2), iron (25.7) and calcium (27.7).

So MDMS is considered as substitution of family diet, not supplementary.

ENVIRONMENT AND HEALTH

1. Sanitation barrier aims at breaking the transmission cycle of fecal-borne diseases. Explain.

A fecal-borne disease roughly follows the transmission cycle which is shown below:

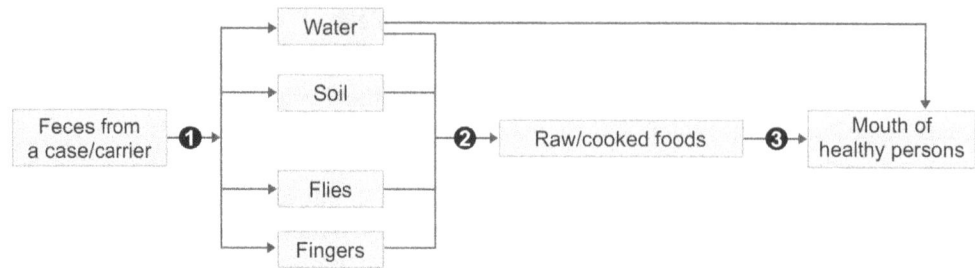

To block the transmission chain shown above, we can apply sanitation barrier by taking the following measures:

Route	How can it be achieved?
Route 1	• All families should have a clean and functional latrine • The latrine should be regularly washed • If there is no latrine, family members should defecate at a distance of at least 10 meters from water supply source • Hand washing with soap after defecation/after cleaning a child who has defecated/after disposing off a child's stool should be promoted • There should be an effective excreta disposal system
Route 2	Hand should be washed thoroughly with soap: • Before preparing food • Before eating • Before feeding a child
Route 3	• Cooked hot food should be eaten • Proper food handling techniques should be used • Cooking utensils should be cleaned and dried after use • Reduction measures should be taken to reduce the number of houseflies

It should be emphasized that all these preventive sanitation measures will produce only temporary results if they are not combined with *health education*. So, health education with the help of community members should be taken and people of a community should be taught about importance of all these preventive measures in a long-term.

2. Chlorine is the best disinfectant for purification of water on large scale.

Because:
❖ Broad spectrum: Chlorine has wide antimicrobial spectrum (it is a potent bactericidal, fungicidal, sporicidal, tuberculocidal and virucidal agent) within the contact time
❖ Fast acting: Produce a rapid kill
❖ Residual effect of free residual chlorine prevents recontamination (minimum recommended concentration of free residual chlorine for drinking water is 0.5 mg/L for 1 hour)
❖ Nontoxic: On safe and accurate application
❖ Unaffected by environmental factors or organic matters (like blood, sputum, and feces)
❖ Odorless: Not disgraceful in appropriate concentration
❖ Easily available
❖ Easily soluble

❖ Easy to use
❖ Amenable to detect: By practical, rapid, simple and analytical techniques even in small concentration
❖ Ecofriendly.

3. The mere addition of chlorine is not chlorination.

OR

4. Break point chlorination must be achieved for disinfection of water. Explain.

Break point chlorination is the point at which chlorine demand is met and the free residual chlorine starts appearing.

In other words, it is the point when ALL combined chlorine has been completely destroyed. The corresponding dosage is called as break point dosage.

Method for Achievement of Break Point Chlorination

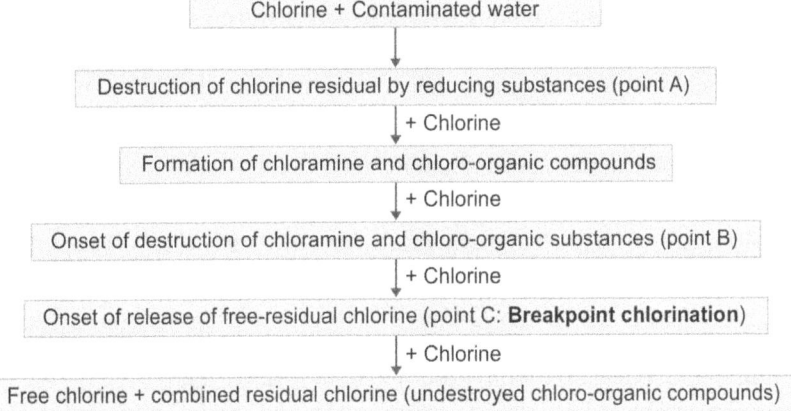

Chlorine + Contaminated water

↓

Destruction of chlorine residual by reducing substances (point A)

↓ + Chlorine

Formation of chloramine and chloro-organic compounds

↓ + Chlorine

Onset of destruction of chloramine and chloro-organic substances (point B)

↓ + Chlorine

Onset of release of free-residual chlorine (point C: **Breakpoint chlorination**)

↓ + Chlorine

Free chlorine + combined residual chlorine (undestroyed chloro-organic compounds)

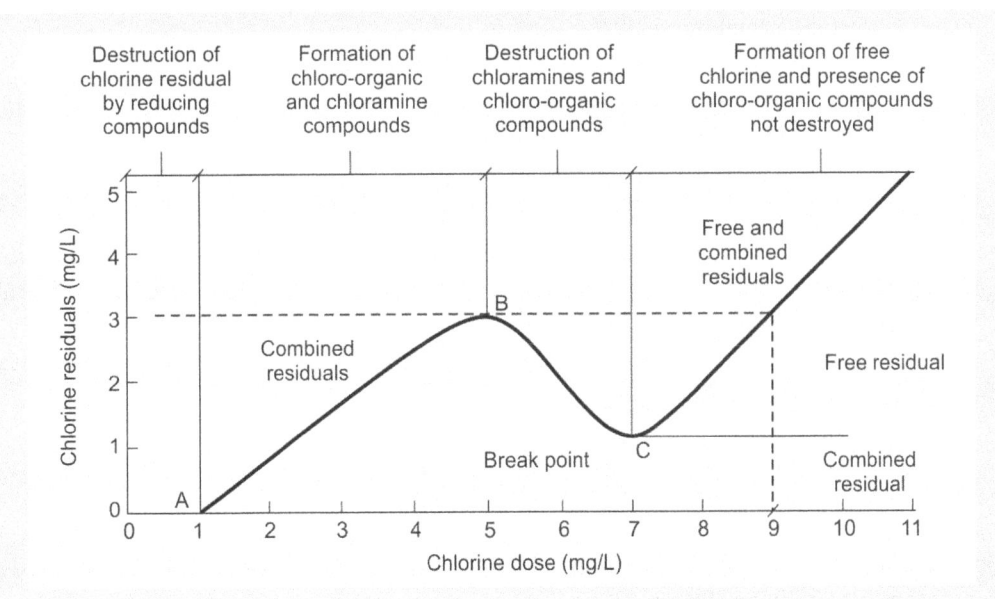

Achievements of Break Point Chlorination Indicates

❖ Destruction of all organic compounds along with organisms
❖ Oxidation of harmful ammoniacal substances
❖ Break point chlorination achieves same results as super chlorination (when large dose of chlorine applied for heavily polluted water; here residual chlorine is usually >1 ppm). So, break point chlorination should be achieved for disinfection of water.

5. Boiling is an important method of purification of water on small scale.

❖ Bringing water to its boiling point (at 100°C/212°F), is the oldest and most effective way of killing any ova, bacteria and viruses present in contaminated water.
❖ It eliminates most microbes causing intestine related diseases (for human health, complete sterilization of water is not required, since the heat resistant microbes does not affect intestine).
❖ Water should be boiled till it comes to a rolling boil (large bubbles continuously coming to the surface of the water) which should be maintained for 1 minute. It is an excellent method of purification of water provided boiling is done in a neat and clean vessel and after boiling it is stored in a clean covered container. Preferably water should be boiled in the same container in which it is to be stored. Only that much amount of water should be boiled which can be used within a few hours.

6. Coliform organisms are chosen as an indicator of fecal contamination.

Indicator organisms are used to measure such things as potential fecal contamination of environmental samples. The presence of coliform bacteria, such as *E. coli*, in surface water is a common indicator of fecal contamination.
Because:

❖ *Abundance in human intestine:* The coliform are constantly present in the human intestine in huge number (average excretion—200–400 billion/head/day).
❖ As the coliform organism are foreign to natural water body so finding them in environmental water indicates fecal contamination.
❖ *Easy detection and culture:* Sensitivity—1 bacteria in 100 mL water.
❖ *Survival:* Longer as compared to other bacteria.
❖ *Resistance to natural purification of water:* Greater than other bacteria.

7. OTA test is better than OT test to detect chlorination.

Because:

❖ Orthotolidine (OT) test measures both free and combined chlorine in water, when the reagent is added to water, it turns yellow, the intensity of color varying according to the concentration of chlorine.
❖ Whereas Orthotolidine arsenite test (OTA) measures free and combined chlorine separately.

8. Vital layer is the heart of slow sand filter.

Please see Chapter 4: Page no. 219.

9. Housing is important for a man's health and well-being.

Housing does not just include 'physical structure' but is expanded in terms of "all places in which a group of people reside and pursue their life goals; the size of settlement may vary from a single family to millions of people."

Thus healthful housing is important in:

- ❖ Providing physical protection and shelter
- ❖ Space for adequate cooking, eating, drinking and excretory function
- ❖ Preventing spread of communicable diseases
- ❖ Providing protection from noise and pollution
- ❖ Is free from unsafe toxic harmful chemicals and physical arrangements
- ❖ Encourages personality and community development.

10. Off-site sanitation is better than on-site sanitation in urban areas.

- ❖ Introduction:
  - – For practical purposes, sanitation can be divided into on-site and off-site technologies.
  - – On-site systems, store/treat excreta at the point of generation, e.g. latrines.
  - – In off-site systems, excreta is transported to another location for treatment, disposal or use, e.g. sewerage.
- ❖ Explanation:
  - – The main selection criteria for on-site or off-site sanitation are *population density and water volume.*
  - – High population density and high water volume (in urban areas) require off-site systems.
  - – Low population density and low water volume (in rural areas) require on-site sanitation.
- ❖ Factors that are in support for construction of off-site sanitation in urban areas:
  - – Very less space is required
  - – Good adapted for urban cities
  - – High removal of organic waste
  - – Good control of waste disposal.
- ❖ Factors that are not in support for construction of off-site sanitation in rural areas:
  - – High cost
  - – Highly skilled personnel
  - – Imported materials
  - – High water demand
  - – High energy demand.

HOSPITAL WASTE MANAGEMENT

1. Color coding of biomedical waste is important for its management.

According to Biomedical Waste (Management and Handling) Rules, 1998 of India, "Any waste which is generated during the diagnosis, treatment or immunization of human beings or animals or in research activities pertaining thereto or in the production or testing of biologicals."

Importance of this Color Coding for BMW in Hospital

See Chapter 21 Biomedical Waste Management.

It helps in:

- ❖ Segregation of clinical waste at the point of generation which is very critical to the safe management of healthcare wastes
- ❖ Aiding the management costs of these wastes

❖ Ensures proper storage, transportation and ultimately correct disposal of waste in a cost-effective manner.

2. Improper handling of biomedical waste can pose several health hazards.

Exposure to hazardous healthcare waste can result in several health hazards according to their nature.

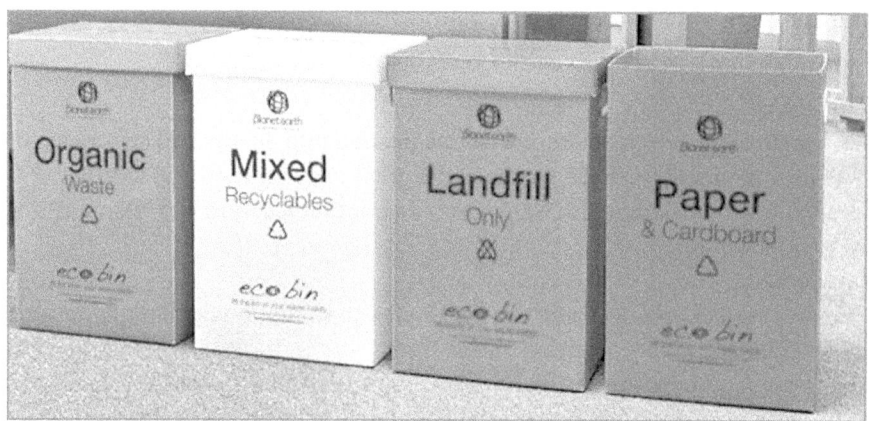

❖ High-risk groups:
  – Medical personnel (doctor, nurse, healthcare auxiliaries, etc.)
  – Patients and visitors to healthcare establishments
  – Supportive health workers in laundries, waste handling and transportation
  – Staffs in disposal facility.

Heath hazards are as follows:
Hazards from:
❖ Infectious waste and sharps:
  – Enters through puncture/abrasion/skin cut/mucous membrane or by ingestion/inhalation
  – HIV, Hep B are main infections of concern.
❖ Chemical and pharmaceutical waste:
  – Mainly disinfectants
  – Can cause burn, corrosion of skin.
❖ Genotoxic waste:
  – Effect depends on toxicity of the substance and period of exposure
  – Route of exposure: Inhalation of dust/aerosol, absorption through skin, ingestion of food, accidental contamination with cytotoxic drugs, chemicals.
❖ Radioactive substances:
  – Effect depends on type and extent of exposure
  – Can cause headache, vomiting, etc.
  – Even cause genetic mutation.
❖ Public sensitivity:
  – Huge sensitivity towards visual impact of healthcare wastes mainly anatomical wastes.

DISASTER MANAGEMENT

1. Triage is of maximum benefit in disaster management

Triage is the process of sorting injured people into group based on the severity of their conditions, so that the most serious cases can be treated first.

Why "Triage" is used?

The principle of "First come, First treated" cannot be followed in case of medical emergencies where the quantity and severity of injuries overwhelm the operative capacity of the available health facility. In these cases, triage is the only system which provides maximum benefit to greatest number of people needing medical attention.

Triage System

There are four color codes used in the triage system to rapidly assess the severity of injury and need for intervention:

Color code	Priority	Category	Inference
Red	Highest	Immediate	High priority treatment or transfer
Yellow	High	Delayed	Medium priority
Green	Low	Minimal	Ambulatory patients
Black	Least	Dead	Dead or moribund patients

Types of Triage

Triage is mainly of three types:

Type	Description
Simple triage	It is a triage system used in a scene of massive casualty, in order to sort the injured ones into those needing immediate medical attention and transport and those needing little medical attention
Rapid triage	It is a simplified triage system that can be performed by lightly trained personnel in times of emergencies
Reverse triage	There are some situations where less wounded persons are given priority than seriously wounded persons. For example: In battlefield, where less wounded soldiers have to return within a short period

Phases of Triage

There are usually three phases in a modern triage system:
1. Prehospital phase: Immediate prehospital care, rapid classification and transportation if indicated.
2. Early emergency phase: Treatment/care by the first clinician attending the patient.
3. Relief phase: Triage after arrival of external assistance to the disaster site.

Importance of Record-keeping and Post-event Analysis

❖ The chaotic environment at the casualty site can easily lead to losing track of casualties, which can be prevented by a pre-planned record-keeping system.

❖ Written documentation of casualty management is an essential tool for maintaining continuity of care during a mass casualty event.

❖ The quality and accuracy of triage decisions and the impact of these decisions on casualty outcome are the key elements of any post-event analysis.

❖ These results should be used to further train triage officers and add to the body of knowledge of triage decision-making in future disasters.

OCCUPATIONAL HEALTH

1. Periodical examination is effective in prevention of occupational diseases. Explain.

❖ Most of the occupational diseases develop slowly over a long period of time, leading to their nonrecognition in early stages.

❖ For this reason, periodic medical checkup is necessary for workers especially when the work is associated with handling of toxic/harmful substances.

❖ The frequency of periodic medical checkup depends on the toxicity of the substance and duration of exposure. For *example*:

Substance	Frequency of checkup
Ordinary workers	Yearly
Occupational exposure to lead/toxic dyes/radium	Monthly
Irritant chemical like dichromates	Daily

❖ Particular care should be given to workers returning from medical leave to assess any disability, if present, caused by the exposure.

2. Industrialization is a serious health hazard.

Industrialization means the transformation of peasant society into a community dependent upon the industries. But it can give rise to several health hazards, enumerated as follows:

❖ Environmental pollution:
  – Housing:
    - Increased no. of slums and insanitary dwelling
    - Migration of people from country side
  – Water pollution:
    - Due to discharge of industrial wastes without treatment
  – Air pollution:
    - Due to discharge of toxic fumes, gases, smoke and dusts into air
  – Noise pollution
  – Thermal pollution
  – Sewage disposal:
    - Lack of facilities for proper disposal of industrial wastes leads to contamination of water, soil and an increased burden for existing sanitation system

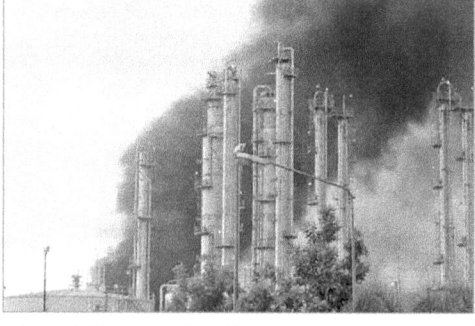

❖ Transmission of communicable diseases: Like TB, venereal diseases, and food and water-borne diseases.

❖ Deterioration of food sanitation: May lead to food-borne disease like typhoid, hepatitis

❖ Alteration of mental health
❖ Accidents: In factories and surrounding locality, due to congestion of traffic
❖ Social problems: Alcoholism, drug addiction, prostitution, etc.
❖ Morbidity and mortality rate: Increased.

3. **Preplacement examination of workers is an example of ergonomics.**

OR

4. **Preplacement examination is the foundation of efficient occupational health service.**

Ergonomics simply means "fitting the job to the worker".

Purpose of it is "*to achieve the best mutual adjustment of man and his work, for improvement of human efficiency*" *by placing* "*the right man for the right job*", so that the worker can perform his duties efficiently without hampering his health.

Preplacement examination:
❖ Is done at the time of employment
❖ A thorough physical examination along with biological and radiological examination (e.g. electrocardiography (ECG), vision test, urine, stool, blood) are carried out
❖ A fresh recruit may be totally rejected or given a job suitable of his mental and physical ability
❖ Serves as benchmark for future comparisons.

Arrangement should be made in such a way that the shortcoming or disability of the worker does not affect productivity. That is why, preplacement examination is done for appointing appropriate man for appropriate job.

Hazards	Undesirable conditions/contraindication to placement
Lead	Anemia, hypertension, nephritis, peptic ulcer
Dyes	Asthma, skin, bladder and kidney diseases, precancerous lesions
Silica	Healed or active TB of lungs, chronic lung disease
Solvents	Liver and kidney diseases, dermatitis, alcoholism
Radium and X-rays	Ill-health, blood disorder

5. **In view of prevention and compensation pneumoconiosis is an important occupational disease.**

Inhalation of dust within the size range of 0.5–3 micron can cause health hazards like a lung disease after a variable period of exposure. This is known as pneumoconiosis.

❖ Prevention of pneumoconiosis:
  – *Dust control measures:*
    - Substitution
    - Complete enclosure of apparatus
    - Isolation
    - Hydroblasting
    - Good housekeeping
    - Unique exhaust ventilation.
  – *Personal protection:*
    - Personal protective equipment like:
      * Masks
      * Respirators with mechanical filters
      * Equipment with oxygen or air supply (if necessary).

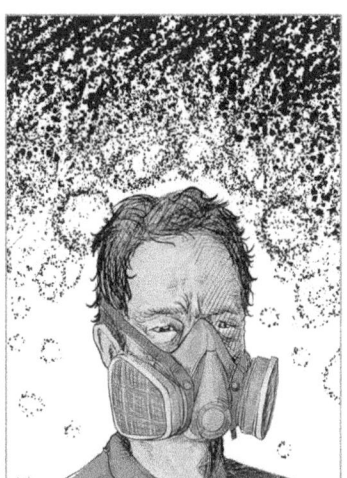

Fu Yexing/for China Daily

- Medical control:
  - Preplacement examination
  - Periodic examination
  - Medical and healthcare services.
- Specific protection:
  - For bagassosis: Bagasse control by keeping moisture content >20% and spraying the bagasse with 2% propionic acid
  - For asbestosis: Using safer types of asbestos like (chrysolite and amosite) and substitution of other insulants: Glass fiber, mineral wool, Ca silicate, etc.
❖ Compensation of pneumoconiosis:
  Pneumoconiosis is liable for compensation as per:
  - Workmen's Compensation (amendment) Act of 1959 for anthracosis
  - Amendment of Factories Act of 1976 for asbestosis.

6. Sickness absenteeism does not reflect true morbidity pattern.

Sickness absenteeism is the number of days in a year that is spent without attending job/work per individual worker.

The unit of sickness absenteeism is number of absent days in work/head/year.
❖ Causes of sickness absenteeism:
  - *Medical cause:* Constitutes about 10% of total lost days due to ill health (mainly due to respiratory and alimentary cause).
  - *Nonmedical cause:*
    - Economic cause: Paid leave of workers
    - Social cause: Cultural, social and family festivals of workers like weddings, festivals, etc.
    - Nonoccupational cause: Alcoholism, drug abuse, nutritional disorder, etc.
  Whereas "morbidity" is ONLY related to ill health conditions, so while measuring morbidity it should only focus on the medical cause of sickness absenteeism, not other nonmedical causes.

  So, sickness absenteeism does not reflect true morbidity pattern as it has multiple non-medical causes.

7. Human factors are much more important than environmental factors in causation of industrial accidents.

Human factors are responsible for 85% of all accidents.
❖ Physical factor: The physical power of the worker may not be enough for work.
❖ Physiological factors:
  - Sex: Female, less accidents
  - Age: Young, more accidents
  - Time: Less accidents at the beginning of work
  - Experience: Less in experienced
  - Working hours: More accidents in longer hours of work.
❖ Psychological factors: Careless.

GENETICS AND HEALTH

1. Genetic counseling is an important step for prevention of some genetic diseases.

Genetic counseling is the process by which patients or relatives at risk of an *inherited disorder* are advised of the consequences and nature of the disorder, the probability of developing or transmitting it, and the options open to them in management and *family planning*.

❖ It is of two types:
  1. Prospective genetic counseling
  2. Retrospective genetic counseling

Category	Prospective genetic counseling	Retrospective genetic counseling
Indication	Heterozygotic individuals to assess the probability of having a child with genetic disorders	Usually the couples reporting voluntarily after having a child with congenital anomalies/mental retardation/inborn errors of metabolism
Timing	• Before the couple produce their first child • Before the individual develops symptom	After birth of an affected child or other affected family member
Mode of intervention	• If a person is identified as heterozygotic for a genetic condition, he/she should be advised *against marrying another heterozygotic individual* as there is increased risk of the trait expressing itself in the phenotype • *Education about MTP* in married couple with unfavorable prenatal diagnosis	• Contraception • Sterilization • Termination of pregnancy (depending upon attitudes and cultural environment of the couples involved)

Significance of Genetic Counseling

❖ *Genetic counseling can assist women or couples who are:*
  – Concerned about first or second trimester screening results
  – Known to be at risk for carrying genetic disorders such as:
    - Thalassemia
    - Sickle cell disease
    - Hemophilia
    - G6PD deficiency
    - Cystic fibrosis
    - Muscular dystrophy.
  – Pregnant and will be 35 years or older at the time of delivery
  – Increased paternal age (40 years and older).
❖ Genetic counseling can help with the implications of:
  – Previous miscarriages or pregnancy losses
  – Either parent's diagnosis or family history of birth defect, genetic disorder or mental retardation
  – Previously having a child with a birth defect, genetic disorder or mental retardation
  – A laboratory test such as a maternal serum screening test indicating an increased risk for a genetic disorder

- A woman's exposure to certain medications or drugs, significant radiation, and/or particular infections during her pregnancy.

In this way, genetic counseling play a very important step for prevention of transmission of some genetic diseases to the offspring.

MENTAL HEALTH

1. Rehabilitation is cornerstone for treatment of drug addiction.

Drug rehabilitation (often drug rehab or just rehab) is a term for the processes of medical or psychotherapeutic treatment, for dependency on psychoactive substances such as alcohol, prescription drugs, and street drugs such as cocaine, heroin or amphetamines.

Aim of Rehabilitation

The general intent is to enable the patient to cease substance abuse in order to avoid the psychological, legal, financial, social and physical consequences that can be caused especially by extreme abuse.

Modes of Treatment

Treatment includes medication for depression or other disorders, counseling by experts and sharing of experience with other addicts. Some rehab centers include meditation and spiritual wisdom in the treatment process.

Medical Treatment

Medication used in opiates addiction → Methadone and buprenorphine
For behavioral therapies → Stimulants, benzodiazepines and other drugs.

Behavioral Therapy Include

❖ Cognitive-behavioral therapy (CBT): It helps patients to recognize, avoid and cope with situations in which they are most likely to relapse.
❖ Multidimensional family therapy: It is designed to support recovery of the patient by improving family functioning.
  - Motivational interviewing: It is designed to increase patient motivation to change behavior and enter treatment.
  - Motivational incentives: It uses positive reinforcement to encourage abstinence from the addictive substance.

HEALTH INFORMATION AND BASIC BIOMEDICAL STATISTICS

1.   Birth registration cannot be done at any time.

According to the Central Births and Deaths Registration Act, 1969 the time limit for registering event of births is 14 days. In case of default a fine up to ₹ 50/- can be imposed.

2. Median is more important than mean for calculating statistical average.

Median is obtained by arranging data in ascending or descending order of magnitude and then the value of the middle observation is located.

Whereas, mean is obtained by dividing the arithmetic summation of individual observations by number of observations.

So, mean value may be unduly influenced by "abnormal" values in the distribution.

For example, if we consider runs of 7 batsmen in a cricket match as follows: 102, 3, 5, 5, 10, 4 and 11.

$$\text{Mean} = \frac{102 + 3 + 5 + 5 + 10 + 4 + 11}{7} = 20$$

Median = 5

Increasing order	3	4	5	5	10	11	102

In this example, runs scored by the first batsman (102) has seriously affected the mean, whereas median remain unaffected.

So, in this example median is nearer to the truth, and therefore, median is more important than mean for calculating statistical average.

3. Diagrammatic form of data presentation is more appropriate for mass media.

Because:
Diagrammatic representation:
❖ Has a powerful impact on the imagination of common people
❖ Is better retained in the memory
❖ Provides less chance of misunderstanding of the fact due to its simplicity.
    However, simplicity can be obtained only at the expense of details and accuracy
    – So, diagrammatic form of data presentation is more appropriate for mass media, especially in the newspaper and magazines.

4. Standard deviation is better than range or mean deviation in measuring dispersion.

Advantages of SD over others in measuring the dispersion are as follows:
❖ The standard deviation is a measure that summarizes the amount by which every value within a dataset varies from the mean.
❖ Effectively it indicates how tightly the values in the dataset are bunched around the mean value.
❖ It is the most robust and widely used measure of dispersion since, unlike the range, it takes into account every variable in the dataset.
❖ When the values in a dataset are pretty tightly bunched together the standard deviation is small.
❖ When the values are spread apart the standard deviation will be relatively large.
❖ Standard deviation is the baseline for defining the concept of standardized score/Z score.

5. Hospital records are not ideal source of information.

Because:
❖ Hospital records are not the true representation of the general population as cases does not come according to prevalence but according to *severity of symptoms*
❖ Attendance to the hospital depends on the awareness of the patient and various *hurdles in approaching the hospital*, e.g. transport irregularities in remote areas

❖ *Etiological hypothesis needs* confirmation from community studies.
❖ *Subclinical cases* are not reported
❖ Not true representation due to *lack of catchment area,* hence not sensitive and specific
❖ Admission to hospital are *not according to the community involvement.*

COMMUNICATION FOR HEALTH EDUCATION

1. Two-way communication is better approach than one-way communication.

Two-way communication is a form of transmission in which both parties involved transmit information.

Whereas, in one-way communication, transmission of a message does not call for or require a response.

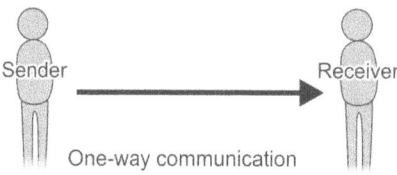

One-way communication

Two-way communication is better approach than one-way communication because:
❖ It permits individuals to learn by freely exchanging their knowledge, ideas and opinions
❖ Provides wider interaction among members than is possible with other methods
❖ Provides opportunity to rectify some confusions by exchanging ideas.

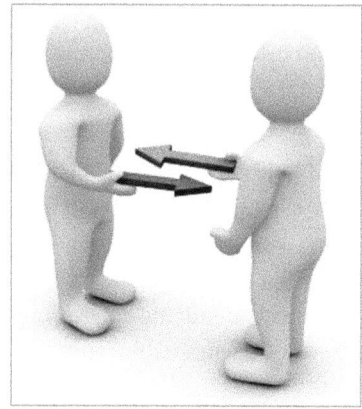

Two-way communication

2. Group discussion provides a wider interaction among members than other methods.

OR

3. Group discussion is considered as very effective way for health education.

In this method, there is discussion on a particular topic, its benefits, and adverse effects among a group that is an aggregate of people interacting in face-to-face situation.

Thus, it naturally provides a wide interaction among members. People learn by freely exchanging their opinion, knowledge and idea.

In other type of discussions like panel discussion, play, symposium, conference/mass communication, there is a less chance of participation of all the members in front whom the subjects are discussed and these methods also provide less interaction among the participants important for exchanging their views.

So, group discussion is much better approach because:

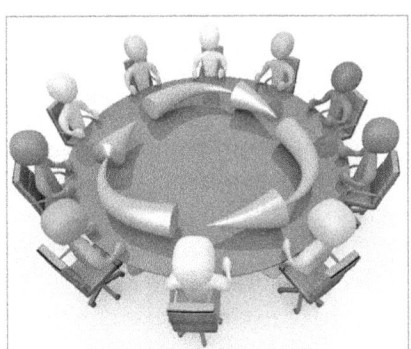

❖ Persons learn by exchanging their knowledge, idea
❖ All members take part in forming opinion so acceptance is good
❖ Pressure of group leader keeps the discussion on the specific topic
❖ Conclusion is not based on the opinion of a single person.
❖ A well-conducted group discussion can change life-style and behavior.

4. As a measure of behavioral change group discussion is better approach than lecture.

Because:

Lecture has several disadvantages like:

❖ Minimum audience involvement
❖ Passive learning
❖ Does not stimulate thinking power of the audience for solving problems
❖ Comprehension of lecture varies according to audience.

As a result of authoritative nature of lecture, it is not suitable for general population.

But, a group discussion based on the ideas of all people is very effective in reaching decisions, which is more acceptable. Because of:

❖ Active participation of the audience
❖ Effective exchange of views and experiences in group discussion
❖ Encouragement of participants to express their views freely to group leader provides a sum of the topic discussion which helps to acquire the knowledge discussed more comprehensively.

5. Interpersonal communication is considered as one of the best methods of communication.

Because:

❖ It provides ample opportunity to discuss, argue and persuade the individual to change his behavior
❖ It provides opportunities to ask questions in terms of specific interactions.

6. Health education is not health propaganda.

OR

7. Health propaganda is short-lasting.

Health education is not health propaganda, because it is more than mere information.
To educate means to cause or facilitate learning.

Meaning of Health Education

According to Alma-Ata declaration (1978)

"A process aimed at encouraging people to want to be healthy, to know how to stay healthy, to do what they can individually and collectively to maintain health, and to seek help when needed."

According to John M Last

"The process by which individuals and groups of people learn to behave in a manner conducive to the promotion, maintenance or restoration of health."

Whereas, propaganda means to spread particular systemized doctrine. Propaganda generally means that:

❖ Knowledge is instilled in the mind of the people discouraging independent thinking.
❖ It can only develop a reflexive behavior, aiming at impulsive actions.
❖ Appeals to emotions rather than reasoning.
❖ Develops a standard pattern of attitude acceptable to moulds not individual personality or self-expression.

Thus, it is clear that above criteria of propaganda do not make it suitable for internalization by a subject. Thus, rendering it short lasting.

8. Panel discussion and group discussion are not the same.

Topic	Panel discussion	Group discussion
Definition	It is a setting where 4–8 qualified people talk about the topic, sit and discuss a given problem or the topic in front of a large group/audience	A group is an aggregation of people interacting in face-to-face situation
Procedure	• A chairman/moderator opens the meeting, welcomes the group and introduces panel speakers • He introduces the topic briefly • Then panel speakers expresses their view in front of the audience	• A group leader initiates the subject, helps the discussion in proper manner involving all the members equally, by preventing side-conversations, encouraging everyone to participate
Advantages	• Audience can be involved actively • Provides views from different speakers which helps to achieve a solution more easily	• Every individual/members can take part exchanging their views • Provides wider interaction among members
Disadvantages	• Success depends on efficiency of chairman as he/she determines the flow of conversation	• Shy people may not take part in the discussions • Some may dominate the discussion
Significance	Very effective	• Properly planned and guided • Helps in changing behaviors

HEALTH PLANNING AND MANAGEMENT

1. Prioritization is an important step in health planning. Justify.

❖ A health planning cycle involves the following steps:

❖ Once the problems, resources and objectives have been determined, the next important step in planning is establishment of priorities in order of importance/magnitude.

❖ In fixing priorities, attention is paid to:
  – Financial constraints
  – Mortality and morbidity data
  – Diseases which can be prevented at low cost
  – Saving the people with younger age
  – Political and community interests and pressures.

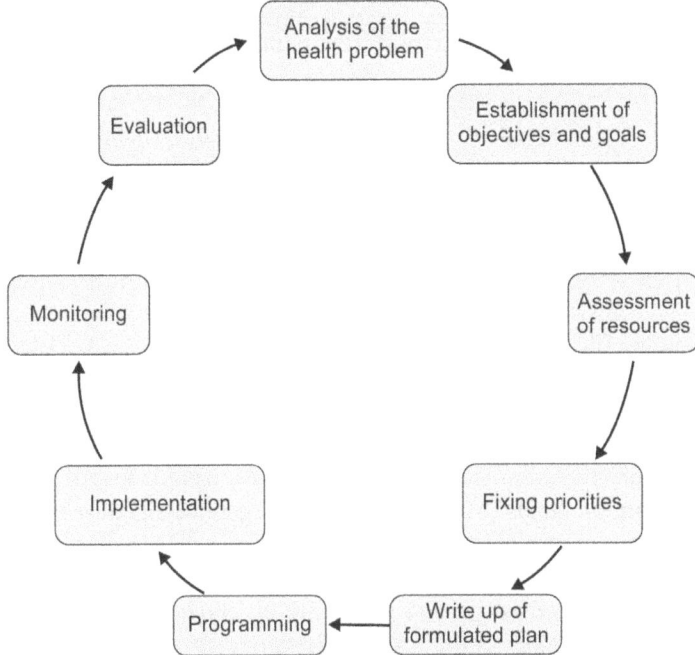

❖ Once priorities have been established, alternate plans for achieving them are formulated and assessed to determine whether they are practicable and feasible.
❖ An alternate plan with greatest effectiveness is chosen.

2. Management consists of four basic activities. Explain.

❖ Management can be defined as, "the purposeful and effective use of resources for fulfilling a predetermined objective".
❖ The resources include manpower, materials and financial support.
❖ Management consists of four basic activities:
  1. *Planning:* To determine what is to be done.
  2. *Organizing:* To set-up the framework and make it possible for groups to do the work.
  3. *Communicating:* To motivate people to do the work.
  4. *Monitoring:* To check that the work is progressing satisfactorily.
❖ The current emphasis of WHO is to improve the efficiency of healthcare delivery systems through appropriate application of modern management methods and techniques.

HEALTH CARE OF THE COMMUNITY

1. Medical care and health care are not synonymous.

Health care concerns for human being.

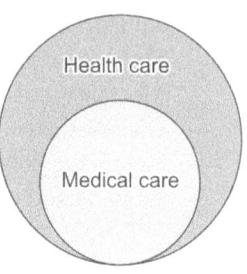

It is defined as multitude of services rendered to individuals or family or community by the agents of health services to promote, maintain, monitor and restore health.

Medical care is a subset of healthcare system which ranges from domiciliary care to hospital care.

Topic	Health care	Medical care
Aims at	Promoting, maintaining, monitoring and restoring health	Only restoring health and recovery from the disease
Services provided	Preventive, educative, curative and rehabilitative	Only curative
Service provider	Healthcare staff, organization, administration, epidemiologist	Physician only

2. "Primary health care is basically the responsibility of the state."

Constitution of India states that health is a state responsibility.

India is a signatory to Alma-Ata Declaration (1978), Health for All (HFA) by 2000 and Millennium Development Goals (MDG). But all the targeted objectives in these can only be achieved by concept of primary health care.

Primary health care (PHC) is defined at the Alma-Ata Conference as *"Primary health care is essential care made universally accessible to individuals and acceptable to them, through their full participation and at a cost the community and country can afford."*

PHC is based on its four principles:
1. Equitable distribution
2. Community participation
3. Intersectoral coordination
4. Appropriate technology.

All the four principles of PHC have to be followed by the states to achieve the targets of HFA and MDG. So, basically primary health care is a state responsibility.

3. Subcenter is considered as pivot of healthcare delivery system in rural area. Explain.

❖ Subcenter is the peripheral outpost of the existing healthcare delivery system as it provides health care to the community at the grass root level.

❖ There is 1 subcenter for every 5,000 rural population and for 3,000 population in hilly/tribal/backward areas.

❖ Subcenter delivers the following important basic health services to the community:
   – Immunization
   – Antenatal, intranatal and postnatal care
   – Prevention against malnutrition and common childhood diseases
   – Prevention of nutritional deficiency diseases
   – Treatment of common diseases like diarrhea, ARI, cough and cold, uncomplicated fever, worm infestation, etc.

- Family planning and contraception services
- National health programs

So, subcenter is considered as pivot of healthcare delivery system in rural areas.

4. Coordination with Panchayati Raj institution is essential for delivery of primary health care in India.

The Panchayati Raj is a three tier structure of rural local self-government of India linking village healthcare delivery system to district health care.

There are accepted agencies for public welfare. All development programs are channelled through three bodies. Three levels are as follows:

Panchayati Raj institution	Level	Importance in healthcare delivery system
Panchayat	Village	Covers entire field of civic administration including sanitation, public health and social and economic development of the village
Panchayat samiti/ janapada panchayat	Block	Execution of the community development program in the block
Zila parishad/zila panchayat	District	Supervisory and coordinating body. In Gujarat, family planning and district MCH officers are under control of Zilla parishad

5. Networking with voluntary health agencies plays an important role in healthcare delivery. Explain.

- ❖ Voluntary health agencies have played a major role in delivering and upgrading health care to the community.
- ❖ Some of the well-known voluntary agencies working in India are:
  - WHO
  - UNICEF
  - USAID
  - World Bank
  - Indian Red Cross.
- ❖ Other voluntary health agencies include:
  - Indian Medical Association
  - Ford Foundation
  - Lions Clubs
  - Rotary Clubs
  - Citizens Forum
  - Christian Missionaries
  - Private Hospitals.
- ❖ Some of the important works by these voluntary agencies are:
  - **UNICEF** has supported India's BCG vaccination programs from its inception and had also developed two plants for manufacture of triple vaccine and iodized salt.
  - Currently, UNICEF is focusing attention on providing primary health care to mothers and children.
  - **World Bank** gives loans for projects that will lead to economic growths (electricity/roads/railways/agriculture/water supply/education/family planning, etc.).
  - **Danida** is providing assistance for National Blindness Control Program.
  - **Rockefeller Foundation** helped establishing the "All India Institute of Hygiene and Public Health" at Kolkata. At present, the foundation is directing its support in improvement of agriculture, family planning and rural training centers.

– **Junior Red Cross** is one of the most active sections in the society. It gives opportunity to millions of boys and girls of India to be associated with village uplift/first aid/anti-epidemic work/building up an international fraternity of youth.

6. ORS is an example of appropriate technology.

Appropriate technology has been defined as technology that is scientifically sound, adaptable to local needs and acceptable to those who apply it and for those on whom it is applied.

This can be maintained by the people themselves in keeping with the principle of self-reliance with the resources, community and country can easily afford.

In single word, appropriate technology is the name of that process in which there is maximum output obtained by giving minimum input.

Now ORS is an appropriate technology because:

Criteria for appropriate technology	Reason
Scientifically sound	• ORS can be safely and scientifically used in treating acute diarrhea due to all etiology in all age group and in all countries • About 90–95% of all cases of diarrhea can be completely treated by ORS
Acceptable to those who apply it	• Easy to prepare • Easy to administer • Can be prepared at home • Needed no boiling/sterilization
Acceptable to those on whom it is applied	• Orally administrated • Self-administrated • Less expensive • Minimum side effects

The technology can be maintained with the resources that is affordable by community or country.

Due to above reasons ORS is said to be an example of appropriate technology.

7. DDK is an example of appropriate technology.

Appropriate technology is defined as a technology that is scientifically sound, adaptable to local needs and acceptable to those who apply it and for those on whom it is applied.

This can be maintained by the people themselves in keeping with the principle of self-reliance with the resources, community and country that can easily afford.

Appropriate for	Reason
User	• Easy to use • No complicated calculation and adjustment needed • Minimum skill/education of user needed
Beneficiary	• Important for 5 cleans (clean surface, hand, cord tie, cord stump, blade) • Intranatal care • Neonatal tetanus elimination
Manufacturers	• Low cost of production • Easily distributable • Maximum benefit with minimum cost

DDK is scientifically approved, easily accessible and acceptable, hence undoubtedly it is an appropriate technology.

8. Disposable delivery kit is helpful in prevention of neonatal tetanus.

To reduce incidence of neonatal tetanus the aim must be prevention of wound contamination due to birth in a neonate with tetanus spore.

Contamination must be prevented by sterilized equipments and environment.

To achieve this sterilized condition the birth process must maintain 5 C's (rather 7 C's). These are:

❖ 5 C's:
  – Delivery surface: Plastic sheet
  – Hands: Soap and clean water of birth attendant
  – Cord cut: A new razor blade
  – Cord tie: A clean piece of thread
  – Cord stump: Nothing applied to cord.
❖ 7 C's: 5 C's + Clean:
  – Water
  – Towel for hand washing.
❖ As DDK is:
  – Easy to apply
  – Inexpensive
  – Can be provided in spite of minimum resources
  – Scientifically sound

So, disposable delivery kit (DDK) is an appropriate technology, thus it is so much significant in reducing the incidence of tetanus.

9. Anganwadi worker and trained birth attendant are examples of community participation.

Community participation means involvement of individual, families, and communities in promotion of their own health and welfare as an essential ingredient of PHC.

Basis of Community Participation

❖ Achieving universal coverage of PHC is not possible without the involvement of local community
❖ It provides maximum reliance on the local resources such as manpower, money and materials
❖ It promotes social awareness and self-reliance of the community
❖ It increases community acceptance of the PHC programs and reduces distance between provider and consumer
❖ It also provides PHC the way that is acceptable to the society by overcoming the cultural and communication barrier.

Health care provider	Selection criteria
AWW	• Local resident • Studied up to class 10
TBA	• Female • Local permanent resident • Acceptable to all sector of the community

They are selected locally, trained locally, and provide service locally (to the area they belong) free of cost. They get honorarium. Above all, they provide care to the community by overcoming the cultural and other barriers.

So, they are the examples of community participation.

Chapter

6

Differences

Authors' Note

There are some terms in community medicine which apparently seems similar, but carries a huge difference. To aware the students of these basics, this chapter has been included in this book. These questions do not come as direct questions in most university examinations but may come as part of long essay type questions or as 'Explain why/justify' type questions (e.g. 'A' and 'B' are not same/synonymous) or may be asked in viva voce. So, this chapter is necessary for concept building purpose of students.

COMMUNITY DIAGNOSIS VS. CLINICAL DIAGNOSIS

Topic	Clinical diagnosis	Community diagnosis
Made by	Physician	Epidemiologist
Concerned with	Individual	Defined population
Deals with	Only sick people	Sick + healthy people
Duty	Doctor examines the patient and decides the treatment	Epidemiologist conducts surveys and decides the plan of action
Basis	It is arrived based on signs and symptoms	It is arrived based on natural history of disease
Aim	Treatment	Prevention and promotion of health
Investigations	Laboratory investigations	Epidemiological investigations
Involves	Follow-up of the case	Evaluation of the program
Field of interest	Doctor is interested in technological advances	Epidemiologist is interested in statistical values

SOCIAL MEDICINE VS. SOCIALIZED MEDICINE

Topic	Social medicine	Socialized medicine
Definition	Social medicine is the study of man as a social being in his total environment comprising physical, biological and social environment	Socialized medicine is a term used to describe and discuss systems of universal health care that is, medical and hospital care for all at a nominal cost by means of government regulation of health care and subsidies derived from taxation

Contd...

Contd...

Topic	Social medicine	Socialized medicine
Term coined by	Jules Guérin	By advocates of the American Medical Association
Deals with	• Understanding how social and economic conditions impact on health, disease and the practice of medicine • Fostering conditions in which this understanding can lead to a healthier society	Medical and hospital services for the members of a class or population administered by an organized group (as a state agency) and paid from funds obtained usually by assessments, philanthropy, or taxation

COMMUNITY DIAGNOSIS VS. HOSPITAL MEDICINE

Topic	Community diagnosis	Hospital medicine
Service area	Provides health care of the people of defined geographical area	Draws patients from ill-defined catchment area
Operational strategy	Both active + passive operational strategies are applied, i.e. both provider + consumers are on the move	Only passive operational strategy is applied, i.e. responsibility lies on the patient to come to the hospital for treatment
Organizational framework	Consists of subcenter, PHC and CHC	Consists of a loose collection of primary, secondary and tertiary hospitals
Nature of care	Comprehensive care, i.e. preventive + promotive + curative + rehabilitative	Only curative care, i.e. deals with concerned disease only
Intersectoral coordination	Between the health department and health-related departments	Does not exist virtually
Program participation	Promotes active participation in active national health program	Limited scope of participation in national health program
Cost benefit analysis	More cost effective	Less cost effective
Focus on type of prevention	Primordial and primary	Secondary and tertiary

DISEASE CONTROL VS. DISEASE ELIMINATION VS. DISEASE ERADICATION

Topic	Disease control	Disease elimination	Disease eradication
Definition	Permitting the disease agent to persist in the community level where it ceases to be a public health problem according to local population (keeping the frequency of the disease in the accessible limits)	The interruption of transmission of disease from large geographical areas, with prevalence of disease reduced to very low levels	Termination of disease transmission by extermination of disease agent
Transmission of disease	At minimal but not interrupted	Interrupted	Terminated/"Tear out by roots"

Contd...

Contd...

Topic	Disease control	Disease elimination	Disease eradication
Disease prevalence	In all areas but under control	In some areas/ geographical areas	Disease ceases to exist
Prevalence rate	<1/1,000	<1/100,000	0
Example	Malaria, TB	Measles, diphtheria	Smallpox
	Describes ongoing operations aimed at reducing: • Incidence of disease • Duration of disease, and consequently the risk of transmission • The effects of infection including both the physical and psychological complications • Financial burden to the community	Regional elimination is now seen as an important precursor of eradication	• It is an absolute process • All or none phenomena • Signifies cessation of infection and disease from the whole world

IMPAIRMENT VS. DISABILITY VS. HANDICAP

Topic	Impairment	Disability	Handicap
Definition	Any loss of psychological, physiological or anatomical structure or function	Any restriction or lack of ability to perform an activity in the manner or within the range considered normal for a human being	A disadvantage for a given individual resulting from an impairment or a disability, that limits or prevents the fulfillment of a role that is normal (depending on age, sex, social and cultural factors) for that individual
Effect	It may be visible/ invisible, progressive/ regressive	Unable to carry out certain activities which are considered to be normal for his age, sex, etc.	The person experiences certain disadvantages in life and not able to discharge obligations required of him and play the role expected of him in the society
Example: **1. Vitamin-A deficiency**	Leading to corneal xerosis	Difficulty in vision	Blindness
2. Accident	Loss of foot	Inability to walk	Loss of job
3. Leprosy	Involvement of nerves	Inability to work because of claw hand	Unemployment
Sequence of events	Disease → Impairment → Disability → Handicap		

ISOLATION VS. QUARANTINE

Topic	Isolation	Quarantine
Definition	It is defined as separation for the period of communicability of infected persons or animals from others in such places and under such condition as to prevent or limit the direct or indirect transmission of the infectious agent from those infected to those who are susceptible or who may spread the agent to others	It is the separation and limitation of freedom of movements of such well persons or domestic animals exposed to communicable disease for period of time not longer than the longest usual incubation period of the disease in such a manner as to prevent effective contact with those not so exposed
Separation	It separates cases with nonexposed	Separates people who have been exposed to specific illness (yet not developed symptoms) with healthy contacts
Site of separation	Depends on degree of illness usually isolation ward of hospital	In his home
Beneficiary	Cases themselves	People around
Level of prevention	Secondary	Primary
Reason for separation	Prevents spread/transmission of disease	Some infections can be spread even before awareness of the patient/prior to development of sign-symptoms
Example	Cholera, chickenpox	Plague

DESCRIPTIVE EPIDEMIOLOGY VS. ANALYTICAL EPIDEMIOLOGY

Topic	Descriptive epidemiology	Analytical epidemiology
Basic description	Provides broad description of distribution of disease	Determines whether an association exists between two categories or events
Subject of interest	Entire population	Individual within the population
Questions to be answered	Who	Why
	Where	
	When	
Main objective	To formulate hypothesis	To test hypothesis

CROSS INFECTION VS. CROSS IMMUNITY

Topic	Cross infection	Cross immunity
Definition	It is a condition of acquiring a new infection by a person from another person where they are kept very close together	It is a condition when a person vaccinated or infected with certain disease also acquires immunity for some other related disease
Occurrence	Common in hospital admitted patients due to their staying together	Common among those vaccinated or infected with the particular disease
Condition of the patient	Occurs in people with low resistance	Occurs in the people with effective immunity
Transmission	Occurs due to quick transmission	Occurs due to antigenic sharing between the bacteria

Contd...

Contd...

Topic	Cross infection	Cross immunity
Advantage/ disadvantage	It is harmful	It is harmless

CASE CONTROL STUDY VS COHORT STUDY

Differences between Case Control and Cohort Studies

Features	Case control study	Cohort study
Purpose of the study	It is the first approach to test a hypothesis	It is the approach to test a precisely formulated hypothesis
Deals with	Study between the case and controls	It involves the study between the study cohort and control cohort
Direction	Effect to cause	Cause to effect
Starts with	The disease	Exposure
Time of exposure	Exposure and disease have already occurred at the time of initiation of study	Exposure has already occurred but the effect (disease) has not occurred at the initiation of the study
Number of subjects	Fewer	Large
Time needed	Quick results are obtained	Long follow-up results in delayed results
Expense yields	Inexpensive	Very much expensive
Calculates	Calculates Odds ratio, which is an indirect measure of relative risk	Relative risk as well as attributable risk and dose response ratio
Can evaluate	Multiple exposures	Multiple outcomes
Attrition	Attrition is not a problem due to the short duration of study	Attrition is a common problem due to the long follow-up time
Suitability of the study for rare diseases	Suitable	Not suitable
Information about diseases other than study	Cannot yield	Can yield
Ethical issue	Minimum	Ethical issue is there because when we accumulate evidence about an etiological factor, we become obliged to intervene and eliminate the factor as a doctor

LONGITUDINAL STUDIES VS. CROSS-SECTIONAL STUDIES

Topic	Longitudinal studies	Cross-sectional studies
Method	Repeated by means of follow-up examination in a population	Done only once in a population
Time period	Carried over a long period of time	Carried over a given point of time or period of time
Comparison with	Running cine film	Still photograph
Suitable for studying	Short lived diseases	Chronic diseases

Contd...

Contd...

Topic	Longitudinal studies	Cross-sectional studies
Finds out	Occurrence of new cases (incidence rate)	Existence of both old + new cases (prevalence rate)
Use	Helps to study the natural history of the disease and risk factors	Helps to study the distribution of a disease in a population rather than its etiology
Advantage/disadvantage	Time-consuming, difficult and costly	Not time-consuming, easier and cheap

INCUBATION PERIOD VS GENERATION TIME

Topic	Incubation period	Generation time
Definition	It is the time interval between invasion by an infectious agent and appearance of the first sign or symptom of the disease in question	It is the time interval between receipt of infection by the host and maximal infectivity to that host
Basis	Mainly based on onset of first sign/symptom	Mainly based on the time of maximum communicability
Example	In mumps, communicability (determinant of generation time) appears to reach its height about 48 hours before the onset of swelling of salivary glands (symptom → determinant of IP)	

INTRINSIC INCUBATION PERIOD VS EXTRINSIC INCUBATION PERIOD

Topic	Intrinsic incubation period	Extrinsic incubation period
Reference	To human being	To vector (usually arthropod)
Definition	It is the period between the entrance of the pathogen in a person and the appearance of the first sign and symptom	It is the period between the entrance of the pathogen/parasite inside the body of the vector till the agent reaches an optimum number/full development
Phenomena in this period	During this period the pathogen reaches the target organ, gets adopted, multiplies, causes damage to the target organ. During this period, the parasite undergoes biological transmission inside the vector (i.e. multiplication/development/both)	
Infectivity	Usually the person is not infective during this period, e.g. mumps, measles	Usually vector is never infective during this period and it becomes infective only after this period
Use	• Helps in making diagnosis • Finds out the source of infection • For immunization purposes and also • For assessing the prognosis	For control of vectors

POPULATION PYRAMID OF DEVELOPING COUNTRY VS. DEVELOPED COUNTRY

Topic	Developing country	Developed country
Base	Broad indicates → high birth rate	Narrow Indicates → low birth rate
Border	Concave concavity facing → outwards	Convex Convexity facing → outwards
Apex	Acute Indicates → less number of elderly people	Obtuse Indicates → more number of elderly people
Figure showing population pyramids of developing and developed countries (y-axis denotes age and X-axis denotes no. of people in that age group)	Expansive	Constrictive

HARD TICK VS. SOFT TICK

Topic	Hard tick	Soft tick
Anatomy:		
Capitulum (mouth)	Anterior, visible from above	Ventral, not visible from above
Scutum (dorsal shield)	Present	Absent
Sexual dimorphism	Dorsally present	Dorsally absent
Figure		

Topic	Hard tick	Soft tick
Habits: Blood meal	Requires continuous blood meal	Requires intermittent blood meal
Starvation resisting power	Absent, always search for body of host	Present, can resist for months
Location	Usually found on the body of the hosts	Crakes and crevices during day time
Diseases transmitted	• Tick typhus • African tick paralysis • Tularemia • Viral encephalitis • Hemorrhagic fever (KFD) • Rocky mountain spotted fever	Endemic relapsing fever (caused by *Borrelia duttoni*, a spirochete)

FOOD FORTIFICATION VS. FOOD ADULTERATION

Topic	Food fortification	Food adulteration
Definition	It is the process wherein nutrients are added in small quantities to the food, to maintain or to improve the quality of food aimed at prevention and control of some nutritional disorders as a long-term measure	It consists of large number of malpractices, such as mixing, substitution, removal, concealing the quality, selling decomposed products, misbranding (giving false labels), addition of toxicants, etc.
Criteria	Vehicle must be consumed consistently by the community as a part of regular diet. The amount of nutrient added must provide an effective supplement for low consumers of vehicle without causing hazardous excess to high consumers. Nutrients should not cause it to undergo noticeable change in taste, smell, appearance, or consistency. The cost of fortification should not be beyond the reach of the common people	It is a social evil This is done by the traders because of their greed for money
Effect	Advantageous as it improves the quality of food	Disadvantageous for the consumer, as: He is paying more money for foodstuff of low quality. He is at the risk of ill-health
Example	Milk/vanaspati: Vitamin A, vitamin D; Common salt: Na/K iodide	Cereal: Addition of stone grit; Milk: Water addition, removal of cream, addition of starch

KWASHIORKOR VS. MARASMUS

Topic	Kwashiorkor	Marasmus
Caused from deficiency of:	Protein	Protein + calories
General condition of the child	Dull, apathetic, disinterest in surroundings, hardly moves from the sitting position	Alert and irritable
Clinical features		
Facies	Bloated (moon-like facies)	Shriveled (monkey-like facies)
Growth failure	Less severe	More severe
Muscle wasting	Masked	Obvious
Edema	Always present	Absent
Hair changes	Lusterless hair, shows positive flag sign (alternate dark and pale bands in hair), sparse distribution, loss of curliness	Change in texture, thin and silky, does not show flag sign
Fat wasting	Often retained	Severely lost

Contd...

Contd...

Topic	Kwashiorkor	Marasmus
Skin changes	Paint-like patches present (flaky paint dermatoses)	Skin changes are absent
Mental changes	Present	Absent
Liver enlargement	Often present	Absent
Prognosis	Bad	Good
Biochemical investigations		
Serum total protein	Decreased	Normal
Serum cholesterol		Normal
Urinary nitrogen		Normal

Pictorial representation:

GROWTH MONITORING VS. NUTRITIONAL SURVEILLANCE

Topic	Growth monitoring	Nutritional surveillance
Strategy	Prevention + promotion of normal health	Detection of malnutrition
Purpose	Educational + motivational	Diagnostic + interventional
Subject	All growing children	All age group
Spectrum	To all individual child	Sample of all age group
Interval	Monthly	Periodically
Focus	On promoting health	On the nutritional status
Recorder	Mother guided by worker	Trained worker
Weight card	Simple	Precise
Mode of intervention	• Supplementary feeding • Immunization • Vitamin A syrup • Deworming • ORS	Nutrition programs, such as supplementary feeding
Response time	Shorter, till resumption of normal growth	Longer, till resumption of good community nutrition
Referral	Health system for checkup and possible brief food supplementation	Malnutrition rehabilitation center

OLD VS. NEW ICDS GROWTH CHART

Topic	Old ICDS growth chart	New ICDS growth chart
Standard	Developed based on National Center for Health Statistics (NCHS) standard	Based on WHO 2006 Child Growth Standard
Based on	It is based on a cross-sectional study on American children	It is based on a Multicenter Growth Reference Study (MGRS) organized over 6 countries (Brazil, Ghana, India, Norway, Oman, USA)
No. of reference curves	There are 4 reference curves present in the chart	There are 3 reference curves present in the chart
Position of the reference curves	Topmost: 80% of median, 2nd curve: 70% of median, 3rd curve: 60% of median, 4th curve: 50% of median	Topmost: Median, 2nd curve: M-2SD, 3rd curve: M-3SD Standard deviation (SD)
Categorization of nutritional basis (by measurement of weight)	≥80%: Normal, 70–80%: Mild (grade 1) 60–70%: Moderate (grade 2) 50–60%: Severe (grade 3) <50%: Severe (grade 4)	Above 2nd curve: Normal Below 2nd curve to 3rd curve: Moderately underweight Below 3rd curve: Severely underweight
Sex	It was valid for both sexes	Separate for boys and girls (pink for girls and blue for boys)
Plotting	Plotting was done at the middle of the boxes	Plotting is done on the line for each completed months
Differences in interpretation	Stunting will be greater throughout the childhood in the new growth chart Underweight will be greater during the first 6 months of delivery in the new growth chart Wasting will be higher during infancy in the new growth chart	

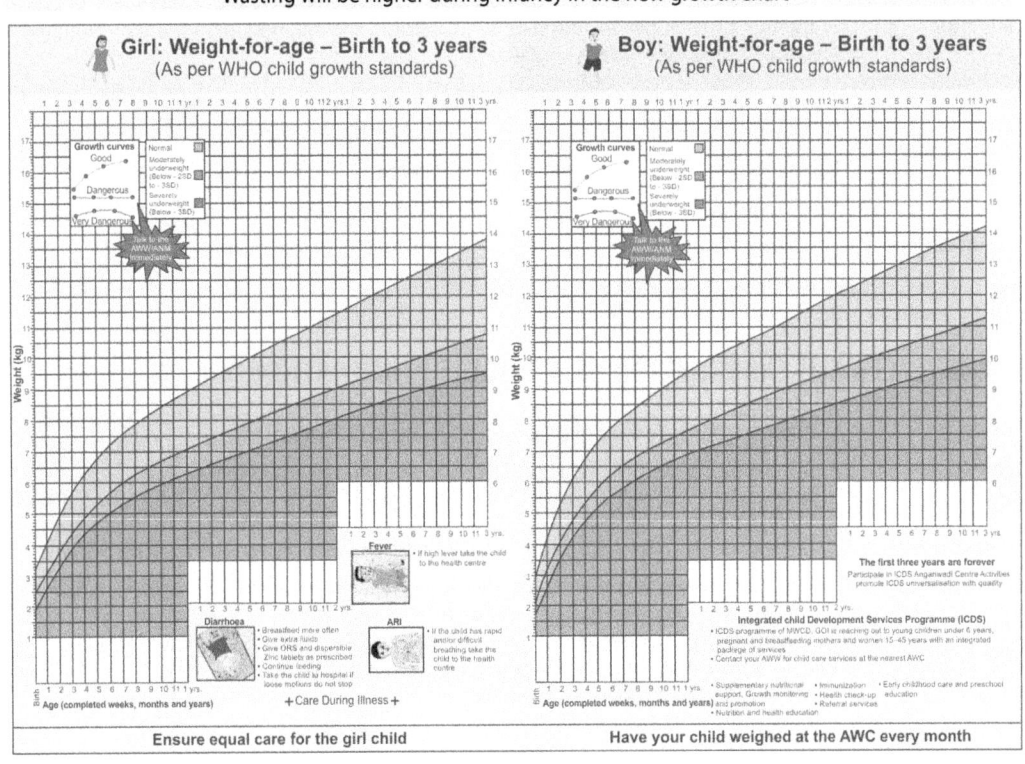

PASTEURIZATION VS. STERILIZATION

Topic	Pasteurization	Sterilization
Method	Milk is just heated and not boiled	Milk is only boiled
Procedure	• Holder process (65°C × 30 mins) • HTST*/flash process (72°C × 15 secs) • UHT** process (88°C × few secs → 125°C × few secs)	Boiling at 100°C × 20–30 minutes
Bacteriological profile	• 90% of pathogens + 90% of lactobacilli are destroyed • Remaining 10% of lactobacilli take time to multiply and cause fermentation (by lactose → lactic acid) • Then souring of milk is delayed/postponed • Spores are not destroyed	• 100% of pathogens + lactobacilli are destroyed • So no souring of milk • Spores are also destroyed
Chemical changes		
Proteins	Only 5% lactalbumin is lost	100% lactalbumin +100% lactoglobulin are lost
Carbohydrates	Lactose is not charred/caramelized (so no color change)	Lactose is completely charred/ caramelized
Fats	No scum/cream is formed and so calcium phosphorus are not taken up	Scum is formed and so calcium and phosphorus are taken up
Vitamins	Vitamin C is reduced	Vitamin C is lost
Minerals	Proportion of insoluble calcium salts is increased (other salts remain unaffected)	Calcium and magnesium salts are precipitated
Physical changes		
Color	No change	Slightly brownish
Taste	No change	Altered
Smell	No change	Slightly changed
Composition	No change	Affected (as described above)

*HTST= High temperature and short time process
**UHT= Ultra-high temperature

PREPLACEMENT EXAMINATION VS. PERIODIC EXAMINATION

Topic	Preplacement examination	Periodic examination
Timing	Before placing the worker to the job	After placement of the worker
No. of examination	Only once	Periodically
Detection	Helps to detect 'high-risk' group	Helps to detect who is going to be high-risk
Objectives	• To determine whether a person is physically and psychologically fit to perform a particular job • To ensure that his/her placement in this job will not represent a danger	• Identifying as early as possible any adverse health effects caused by work practices/exposures to potential hazards • Detecting the possible onset of an occupational disease
Level of prevention	Primary	Secondary

Contd...

Contd...

Topic	Preplacement examination	Periodic examination
Main activity	Ergonomics	Early diagnosis and treatment of health hazard
Purpose:	To ↑ the efficiency and production and ↑ the no. of accidents	To protect the individual from further complications

SOCIAL SECURITY VS SOCIAL ASSISTANCE

Topic	Social security	Social assistance
Contribution	Not only by the employees but also employers and organizations	No contribution system
Benefits	In terms of cash, not by sympathy but by a matter of right	Cash/a kind by sympathy/charity
Inferiority complex	Do not develop	May develop
Active involvement	Members are actively involved in economic planning for future	Not actively involved
Contribution	Suitable to the workers who can contribute	Suitable to the workers who cannot contribute
Dependency	May not arise permanently	May become permanently dependent on the scheme
Legislation	Many	Hardly any legislation
Beneficiary	Industrial worker, employees of State and Central Government	Unemployed, widows, orphans, handicapped, old age people
Example	ESI scheme, Public Provident Fund Scheme, LIC of India	Unemployment allowance, Sanjay Gandhi Niradhar Yojana, Workmen's Compensation Act, 1923

INCIDENCE VS. PREVALENCE

Topic	Incidence	Prevalence
Definition	Refers to occurrence of new cases in a given area during a given year	Refers to existence of both old and new cases in a given area during a given point/ period of time
Expression	Per 1000 population at risk	Per 100 population at risk
Estimation	From longitudinal studies	Cross-sectional studies
Knowledge of time of onset of the disease	Required for estimation	Not required
Incubation period	Refers to acute cases having short IP, e.g. rabies, measles	Refers to chronic cases having long IP, e.g. TB, leprosy
Duration of illness	Does not influence it	Prevalence = Incidence × duration of illness
Objective	An ideal measure to study the etiology of disease	To determine the magnitude of the problem
Importance	Helps to evaluate the control measures	Helps for health planning

SCREENING TEST VS. DIAGNOSTIC TEST

Topic	Screening test	Diagnostic test
Indication	Done on apparently healthy persons	Done on those with indications
Applied to	Groups	Patients
Results	Test results are arbitrary and final	Diagnosis is not final but modifiable according to evidences
Basis of evaluation	Single criterion or cut-off points	A number of symptoms, signs and laboratory findings
Basis of treatment	No	Yes
Accuracy	Less	More
Expense	Less	More
Initiative	Comes from the investigator or agency providing care	Comes from a patient with a complaint

HEALTH EDUCATION VS. HEALTH PROPAGANDA

Topic	Health education	Health propaganda
Acquisition of knowledge	Actively acquired	Passively acquired
Thought generation	People thinks before acting	It prevents thinking because of readymade information
Concern	It is mainly concerned with betterment of life	It is mainly concerned with the sale of products
Objective	To improve health	To derive profit
Aim	To change the attitude of the people	Does no aim at changing the attitude and behavior of the people
Basis	It is behavior-centerd	It is information centerd
Development of type of behavior	Reflective	Reflexive
Basis of the appeal	Reason	Emotion
Primitive desires	Disciplined	Allowed to stimulate

SHALLOW WELL VS. DEEP WELL

Topic	Shallow well	Deep well
Definition	Taps subsoil water (the water above the 1st impervious strata)	Taps water from below the 1st impervious strata
Chemical quality	Hard	Harder
Bacteriological quality	Grossly contaminated	Taps purer water
Yield	Usually goes dry in summer	Provides constant supply
Safety	Less safe	Safer
Cost of installation	Less	More

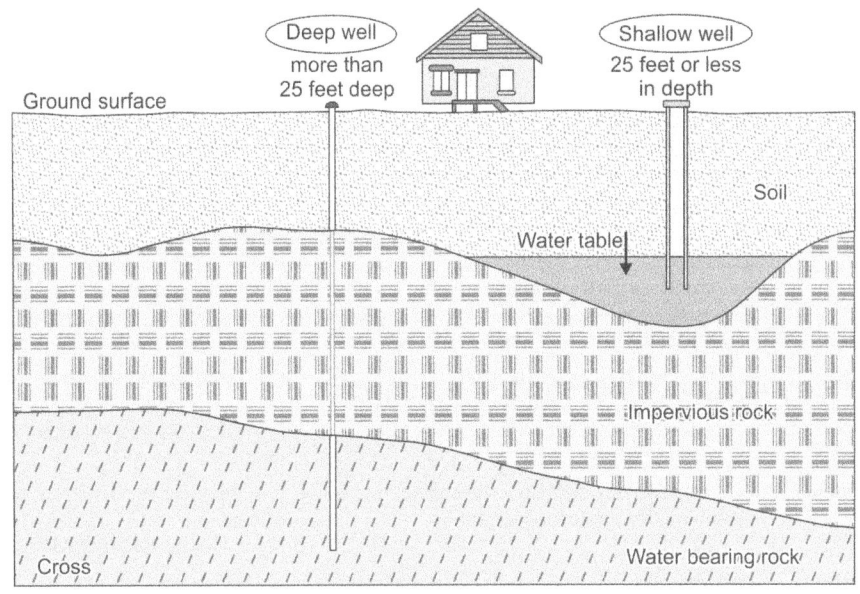

Shallow well vs Deep well

SLOW SAND FILTER VS. RAPID SAND FILTER

Topic	Slow sand filter	Rapid sand filter
Area requirement	Larger	Smaller
Sand bed height (in sqm)	1.2	1.0
Effective size of sand (mm)	0.15–0.3	0.6–2.0
Rate of filtration (in cu mt/sq mt/hr)	0.1–0.4	5–15
Loss of hydraulic load allowed (in ft)	2–4	8–10
Filter run	3 weeks–3 months	1–3 days
Mechanism of action	Mainly biological	Physical and chemical
Preliminary storage	Necessary	Unnecessary
Preliminary treatment	Unnecessary	Necessary
Suitability of turbid water	Not suitable	Suitable
Cleaning method	Scraping the sand bed	Backwashing
Removal of turbidity	By its vital layer	By alum coagulant
Removal of color	Fair	Good
Use of sludge	Sludge obtained after scraping is used as manure	Not obtained
Removal of bacteria (in %)	99.99	99
Posttreatment chlorination	Unnecessary	Must

PANEL DISCUSSION VS. GROUP DISCUSSION

Topic	Panel discussion	Group discussion
Definition	It is a setting where 4–8 qualified peoples talk about the topic, sit and discuss a given problem, or the topic in front of a large group/audience	A group is an aggregation of people interacting in face-to-face situation
Procedure	• A chairman/moderator opens the meeting welcomes the group and introduces panel speakers • He introduces the topic briefly • Then panel speakers express their view in front of the audience	A group leader initiates the subject, helps the discussion in proper manner involving all the members equally, by preventing side conversations, encouraging everyone to participate
Advantage	• Audience can be involved actively • Provides views from different speakers which helps to achieve a solution more easily	• Every individual/members can take part exchanging their views • Provides wider interaction among members
Disadvantage	• Success depends on efficiency of chairman as he determines the flow of conversation	• Shy people may not take part in the discussions • Some may dominate the discussion
Significance	• Very effective • Properly planned and guided	• Very effective • Helps in changing behaviors

SUPPLEMENTARY NUTRITION VS. THERAPEUTIC NUTRITION

Topic	Supplementary nutrition	Therapeutic nutrition
Prescribed to	• Pregnant and nursing mother • Adolescent girl • Children (<6 years) with grade I and II	Children suffering from grade III and IV malnutrition
Composition		
• Calorie	300 kcal	600 kcal
• Protein	10 g	20 g
Consistency	Normal (solid)	Semisolid for easy digestion and ingestion
Frequency	To be given at center	2 times in center and 2 times in home
Place of treatment	Domiciliary treatment	Institutional/hospital-based treatment

OBJECTIVE VS. TARGET VS. GOAL

Objective	Target	Goal
• It is the planned end point of all activities • It is precise and is concerned with problem itself	• It is a discrete activity which helps to measure the attainment of objectives • It is concerned with the factors involved in a problem	• Ultimate desired state towards which objective and resources are directed • It is NOT constrained with time and existing resources • It is not necessarily attainable

COST-EFFECTIVE ANALYSIS VS. COST BENEFIT ANALYSIS

Topic	Cost-effective analysis	Cost benefit analysis
Expression of results	In terms of natural units, i.e. no. of lives saved, no. of sickness free days gained, no. of heart attacks avoided, etc.	In monetary terms, i.e. cost of drug/hospitalization saved due to intervention and money earned in sickness free days

Contd...

Contd...

Topic	Cost-effective analysis	Cost benefit analysis
Type of study	Typically retrospective	Typically prospective
Types of technique	Economical and technical	Economical
Usefulness	Most appropriate for many health studies	Not suitable for many health studies
Application	For evaluating discrete interventions	For major capital investments

FAMILY PLANNING CONCEPT VS. FAMILY WELFARE CONCEPT

Topic	Family planning concept	Family welfare concept
Basis of the concept	Methods to control the child birth	Reveals to approaches that will affect the well-being of a population by taking intensive care of mother who gave birth to child will determine the health status of a population
Introduced in	1952	1977
Service	Only based on family planning methods	Based on full range of MCH services
Recipient	• Eligible couple • Target couple	• Pregnant and lactating mother • Children • Adolescent girls • Married women
Aim	To decrease fertility rate	Provide health services to ensure family welfare
Goal	Small family	Health for all
Services offered	• Marriage counseling • Contraceptive	• Family planning • Immunization
Approach	Top down, centralized	According to clients need

CHILD SURVIVAL AND SAFE MOTHERHOOD (CSSM) VS. REPRODUCTIVE AND CHILD HEALTH (RCH)

Topic	CSSM	RCH
Goal	2 child norm	Enable clients to meet their own goal
Approach	Top → down (centralized)	Bottom → up (decentralized)
Service	Mainly family planning	Full range maternal and child health care
Quality	Compromised	High quality
Attitude to client	To motivate and give them good reasons to take a choice	To listen, assess the need of the client, inform them and advice
Monitoring	Usually targets are monitored	Some of parameter that are monitored: • Quality of care • Coverage of services • Client satisfaction
Responsible to	An administrative system operated by large number of officials	Client and communities

ADMINISTRATION VS. MANAGEMENT

Topic	Administration	Management
Meaning	Broadly means "Getting the things done"	The purposeful and effective use of resources (manpower, material and finances) for fulfilling predetermined objective

Chapter

7

Immunization

Authors' Note

Immunization is one of the most important topics of community medicine. The students should know every details of this topic not only for the viva voce but also for theory and practical examinations. This part is also essential for clinical life of every budding doctor.

IMMUNIZATION

It is the process by which an individual's immune system becomes fortified against an immunogen.

A person is said to be immune when he possesses:

"Specific protective antibodies or cellular immunity as a result of previous infection or immunization, or is so conditioned by such previous experience as to respond adequately to prevent infection and/or clinical illness following exposure to specific infectious agent."

According to WHO

"Immunization is the process whereby a person is made immune or resistant to an infectious disease, typically by the administration of a vaccine."

TYPES

Active Immunity

It is the immunity which an individual develops as a result of infection or by specific immunization and is usually depends upon the humoral and cellular responses of the host.

Modes of Acquiring Active Immunity

❖ Clinical infection, e.g. rubella, chickenpox.
❖ Subclinical infection, e.g. polio, diphtheria.
❖ Immunization with an antigen, e.g. live attenuated vaccine, killed vaccine or toxoid.

Passive Immunity

Passive immunization is where presynthesized elements of the immune system are transferred to a person so that the body does not need to produce these elements itself.

Modes of Inducing Passive Immunity

❖ Physiological: When **antibodies** are transferred from mother to **fetus** during **pregnancy** across placenta (vertical transmission).

❖ Artificial:
  – By administration of an antibody containing preparation (immunoglobulin).
  – By transfer of lymphocytes to induce passive cellular immunity (still experimental).

Herd Immunity

Definition

Herd immunity (or community immunity) describes a form of **immunity** that occurs when the **vaccination** of a significant **portion** of a population (or herd) provides a measure of protection for individuals who have not developed immunity.

Mode of Action

❖ Herd immunity theory proposes that chains of infection are likely to be disrupted when large numbers of a population are immune or less susceptible to the disease (basically in case of contagious diseases)
❖ The greater the proportion of individuals who are resistant, the smaller the probability that a susceptible individual will come into contact with an infectious individual and become infected
❖ Herd immunity provides an *immunological barrier* to the spread of the disease in the human herd (population)
❖ Unvaccinated individuals are *indirectly protected by vaccinated individuals*, as the latter are less likely to contract and transmit the disease between infected and susceptible individuals.

Determinants of Herd Immunity

❖ Occurrence of clinical and subclinical immunity in the herd
❖ Immunization of the herd
❖ Herd structure:
  – Never constant
  – Depends on variation due to births and deaths and population mobility or migration
  – Includes not only host but also alternative animal hosts, insect carrier.

Herd Immunity Threshold

The proportion of immune individuals in a population above which a disease may no longer persist is the *herd immunity threshold*.

Its value varies with:
❖ The virulence of the disease
❖ The efficacy of the vaccine
❖ The contact parameter for the population.
Remember: No vaccine offers complete protection, but the spread of disease from person to person is much higher in those who remain unvaccinated.

Significance in Public Health

❖ A public health policy of herd immunity may be used to reduce spread of an illness and provide a level of protection to a vulnerable, unvaccinated subgroup.
❖ Especially, it is considered best for those who cannot safely receive vaccines because of a medical condition such as an **immune disorder**, transplant recipients, or people with **egg allergies**

❖ Herd immunity is compromised in some areas for some vaccine-preventable diseases, including **pertussis, measles and mumps**, in part because of parental refusal of vaccination.

Limitations

❖ Herd immunity generally applies only to contagious diseases
❖ It does not apply to diseases such as tetanus (which is infectious, but is not contagious), where the vaccine protects only the vaccinated person from disease
❖ Herd immunity does not apply to IPV because it protects only the individual from viremia and paralytic polio.

Difference between Immunization and Vaccination

Topic	Immunization	Vaccination
Definition	It is the process by which an individual's immune system becomes fortified against an immunogen	Vaccination is the process of immunization
Procedure	May be active or passive	Only active

Immunizing Agents

❖ *Vaccine:* Vaccine is an immunological substance designed to produce specific protection against a given disease and it stimulates the production of protective antibody and other immune substances.
❖ *Nomenclature:* The term "*vaccine:*" derives from **Edward Jenner's** 1796 use of *cowpox* (**Latin** *variola vaccinia*, adapted from the Latin *vaccīn-us*, from *vacca*, cow) to inoculate **humans**, providing them protection against **smallpox**.

Types

❖ Live attenuated
❖ Killed or inactivated
❖ Toxoids
❖ Subunit/cellular fragments
❖ Combined/mixed
❖ Experimental/future prospects.

Live Attenuated Vaccines

Definition: A live attenuated vaccine is a **vaccine** created by reducing the **virulence** of a **pathogen**, but still keeping it viable or "live".
❖ These organisms have lost their "antigenicity" (ability to produce full blown disease) but retain their immunogenicity.

Examples:
❖ **Viral**: Measles vaccine, mumps vaccine, rubella vaccine, live attenuated influenza vaccine (the seasonal flu nasal spray and the 2009 H1N1 flu nasal spray), chickenpox vaccine, oral polio vaccine, rotavirus vaccine, and yellow fever vaccine (Mnemonic—MMR I ROCY).
❖ **Bacterial**: BCG vaccine, typhoid vaccine and epidemic typhus vaccine.

Development:
Viruses may be attenuated via passage of the virus through a foreign host, such as:
❖ Tissue culture

❖ Embryonated eggs
❖ Live animals.

The initial virus population is applied to a foreign host. One or more of these will possess a mutation that enables it to infect the new host. These mutations will spread, as the mutations allow the virus to grow well in the new host.

Advantages:
❖ Activates all phases of the immune system (humoral + cellular immunity).
❖ Provides more durable immunity; boosters are required less frequently.
❖ Quick immunity.
❖ Easy to administer (for example, OPV for polio can be taken orally, rather than requiring a sterile injection by a trained health worker, as the inactivated form IPV does).
❖ Cost effective.
❖ Very few side effects in comparison to injected antibody vaccines (e.g. tetanus).
❖ Herd immunity may occur.

Disadvantages:
❖ Secondary mutation of attenuated virus can cause a reversion to virulence.
❖ Can cause severe complications in **immunocompromised** patients.
❖ Can be difficult to transport due to requirement to maintain conditions (e. g. temperature; as in OPV).

Killed Vaccines

These contain killed, but previously virulent, microorganisms that have been destroyed with chemicals, heat, radioactivity or antibiotics.

Examples:
Viral: IPV and killed influenza vaccine.
Bacterial: Typhoid vaccine, oral cholera vaccine, plague vaccine, and pertussis vaccine.

Development:
Virus particles are grown in culture and then killed using a method such as heat or formaldehyde.

Advantages:
❖ Less contraindication than that of live vaccines (except severe local or general reaction to a previous dose).
❖ More heat stable.
❖ No chance of reversion of virulence.
❖ Applicable to immunocompromised individual.

Disadvantages:
❖ Require multiple doses.
❖ Less effective.
❖ Difficult to administer.

1. **Explain why live vaccines are more potent than killed vaccines?**

OR

2. **Live vaccine requires single dose while killed vaccine require multiple doses.**

Because:
❖ Live organisms multiply in host and resulting antigenic dose is larger than what is injected
❖ Live vaccines have all major and minor antigenic components
❖ It engage certain tissues of the body, as for example, intestinal mucosa by OPV
❖ There may be other mechanisms, such as persistence of latent virus.

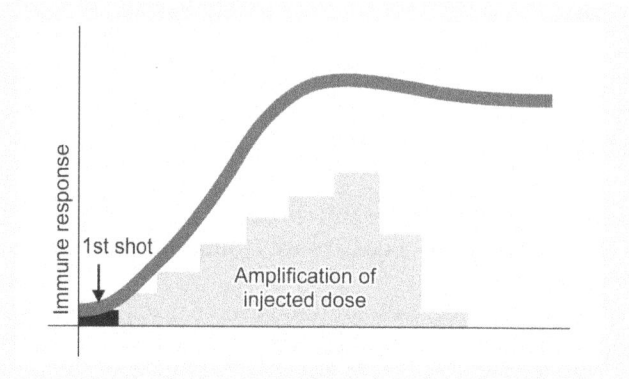

Immune response to replicating antigen (live vaccine)

In killed vaccine the virus particles are:
* Destroyed and
* Cannot replicate.

But the virus capsid proteins are intact enough to be recognized by the immune system and evoke a response. When manufactured correctly, the vaccine is not infectious. As the properly produced vaccine cannot reproduce within the host, so killed vaccines usually require primary series of 2–3 doses to produce an adequate antibody response, and thus in most cases booster doses are required.

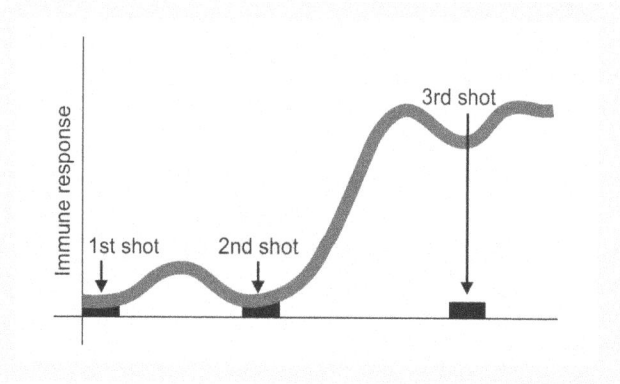

Immune response to three doses of nonreplicating native antigen vaccine (killed vaccine)

Thus, live vaccines require single dose, whereas killed vaccines require multiple doses.

TOXOID, SUBUNIT VACCINE, COMBINED VACCINE AND EXPERIMENTAL VACCINE

Toxoid

Toxoid vaccines are made from inactivated toxic compounds (usually exotoxins released by microorganisms).

Example: Toxoid-based vaccines like tetanus and diphtheria.

Advantages:
* Highly efficacious, and
* Safe.

Subunit/Cellular Fragment Vaccine

Without introducing an inactivated or attenuated microorganism to an immune system (which would constitute a "whole-agent" vaccine), a fragment (subunit) of it can create an immune response, it is called subunit/cellular fragment vaccine.

Example:
❖ Subunit vaccine against **hepatitis B virus** that is composed of only the surface proteins of the virus.
❖ Meningococcal and pneumococcal vaccine.
❖ Vaccine against influenza formed by hemagglutinin and neuraminidase subunits of the influenza virus.

Combined/Mixed Vaccine

If more than one kind of vaccine is included in the vaccine, it is called combined or cellular vaccine.

Example:
❖ DPT (diphtheria, pertussis and tetanus)
❖ DT (diphtheria-tetanus)
❖ DP (diphtheria, pertussis)
❖ MMR (Measles, mumps and rubella).

Advantages:
❖ Simplified administration for multiple vaccines through one bore of needle
❖ Cost effective
❖ Reduce number of contacts of the patient with the health system.

Experimental

Examples:
❖ **DNA vaccination:** Created from an infectious agent's DNA. It works by insertion of viral or bacterial DNA into human or animal cells (still experimental).
❖ **Recombinant vector:** By combining the physiology of one microorganism and **DNA** of the other, immunity can be created against diseases that have complex infection processes.

SOME OTHER DEFINITIONS

1. *Adjuvant:* A substance (e.g. aluminum salt) that is added during production of vaccine to increase the body's immune response.
   - Mechanism: Not well-understood. Probably due to formation of local granuloma which release antigen and from which antigen is slowly released.
   - Advantage: Greater immune response with lesser quantity of antigen (so lesser dose required).
   Example:
   - Bacterial products: Killed bacteria *Bordetella pertussis* (in DPT).
   - Nonbacterial agent: **Alum** (most commonly used) adjuvant. In DPT, HPV and hepatitis vaccines.
2. *Seroconversion:* Change from antibody negative state to antibody positive state.
3. *Seroprotection:* The state of protection (from disease) due to presence of humoral immunity or detectable antibody in serum.

ADVERSE EVENTS FOLLOWING IMMUNIZATION (AEFI)

Definition

WHO defines—*"An adverse event following immunization (AEFI) as a medical incident that takes place after an immunization, causes concern, and believed to be caused by immunization."*

Cause-specific Categorization of AEFI (CIOMS/WHO 2013)

Type	Definition	Example
Vaccine product-related reaction	An AEFI that is caused or precipitated by a vaccine due to one or more of the inherent properties of the vaccine product	Extensive limb swelling following DTP vaccination
Vaccine quality defect-related reaction	An AEFI that is caused or precipitated by a vaccine that is due to one or more quality defects of the vaccine product including its administration device as provided by the manufacturer	Failure by the manufacturer to completely inactivate a lot of IPV leads to cases of paralytic polio
Immunization error-related reaction (formerly "program error")	An AEFI that is caused by inappropriate vaccine handling, prescribing or administration and thus by its nature is preventable	Staphylococcal toxic shock syndrome after immunization with contaminated vaccine
Immunization anxiety-related reaction	An AEFI arising from anxiety about the immunization	Vasovagal syncope in an adolescent during/following vaccination
Coincidental event	An AEFI that is caused by something other than the vaccine product, immunization error or immunization anxiety	Pneumonia after OPV administration

Vaccine Product-related Reaction
❖ No vaccine that is 100% safe and without any risks
❖ Such events may range from mild side effects to life-threatening, but rare.

Mechanism:

Immune mediated local reactions
❖ Nongranulomatous inflammation ± regional lymphadenitis (Eg: Extensive limb swelling after DTP vaccination)
❖ Granulomatous inflammation ± regional lymphadenitis (most commonly related to BCG vaccine)

Immune mediated generalized reactions
❖ Systemic inflammatory response (resulting in fever)
❖ IgE mediated hypersensitivity (anaphylaxis) or nonIgE mediated hypersensitivity (anaphylactoid reactions)
❖ Disseminated granulomatous reaction (disseminated BCG in immunodeficient hosts)
❖ Immune complex mediated reaction (serum sickness reaction).

Autoimmune/undefined mechanism
❖ Demyelinating conditions, such as GB syndrome post-influenza vaccination
❖ Thrombocytopenia post-MMR vaccination.

Rare but Severe Reactions

Vaccine	Reaction	Onset interval	Rates per million doses
BCG	Suppurative lymphadenitis	2–6 months	100–1,000
	BCG osteitis	1–12 months	1–700
	Disseminated BCG	1–12 months	2
Hib	Anaphylaxis	0–1 hour	0–2
Hepatitis B	Guillain-Barre syndrome (plasma derived)	1–6 weeks	5
	Febrile seizures	5–12 days	333
	Thrombocytopenia	15–35 days	33
Measles/MMR	Anaphylaxis	0–1 hour	1–50
OPV	Vaccine associated paralytic polio (VAPP)	4–30 days	1.4–3.4
DTP	Persistent, inconsolable crying (>3 hours)	0–24 hours	1,000–6,0000
	Seizures	0–3 days	570
	Hypotonic, hyporesponsive episode	0–24 hours	570
	Anaphylaxis	0–1 hour	20
	Encephalopathy	0–3 days	0–1
Yellow fever	Postvaccination encephalitis	7–21 days	400–4,000 (in infants <6 m)
	Allergic/anaphylaxis	0–1 hour	5–20

Immunization error-related reaction (formerly "program error")

Cause:
* Faulty production of vaccine
* Improper immunization site/dose
* Wrong amount of diluents
* Incorrect diluents
* Contaminated vaccine
* Incorrect storage
* Contraindications ignored
* Incorrect sterile technique or inappropriate procedure.

Preventing immunization error-related AEFIs or program errors (Long Question may come as BMOH)

Immunization error-related reactions can be prevented by following the guidelines strictly:

1. Ensure storage temperatures of ILRs are within +2° and +8°C by checking and recording cabinet temperatures twice a day.
2. Follow the guidelines to store different vaccines at recommended order in the ILR with freeze sensitive vaccines and diluents always near the lid in the upper part of the ILR.
3. Never store any other drug in the ILR.
4. Read labels of vaccine vials and diluents properly to verify name, VVM, batch number and expiry date. In case of problems reading the fine print, please use magnifying lenses.
5. Always record batch details of diluents received with the vaccines in the stock register.

6. In the daily issue register, make sure that details of vaccines, diluents and syringes issued are entered in the morning and also details of those returned in the evening after the sessions. *This may take some effort but is important as this demonstrates you are careful with vaccines and logistics records and will be in your favor in case of any AEFIs.*

7. Issue one reconstitution syringe for each pair of vaccine vial and diluent requiring reconstitution. *Do not ask the vaccinator to reuse reconstitution syringes.*

8. Follow open vial policy guidelines strictly by checking VVM, condition of stopper, date and time of opening of vial, expiry date of each vial before receiving it at the end of a session and before issuing it in the morning of the session days.

9. If there is any suspicion on the sterility or storage of the syringes please check and report for testing.

10. Dispose of waste generated in the sessions properly to prevent reuse of vaccine vials, syringes and needles.

11. Ensure all vaccine carriers that go out in the morning of the session day and brought back to the cold chain point on the same day. If the vaccine carriers are not coming back the same day, take necessary actions.

    Note: It is possible that the unused, or partially used vaccines at the end of the session are being stored in the same vaccine carrier or in a domestic refrigerator, where the chances of cold chain breakage are high and vaccine safety and potency can be affected leading to AEFIs.

    (Handbook for Vaccine & Cold Chain Handlers, 2nd edition, Ministry of Health and Family Welfare, Government of India, 2016)

Immunization Anxiety-related Reaction

Individual reacts in anticipation to and as a result of injection of any kind, e.g. fainting is common. *Probable mechanisms:*

❖ Vasovagal mediated reactions
❖ Hyperventilation mediated reactions
❖ Stress-related psychiatric disorders.

Coincidental Events

Occurrence of disease/events totally unconnected with immunizing agent following immunization.

Example:

❖ Manifestation or complication of an underlying acquired disease condition that may or may not have been diagnosed prior to immunization.

Probable mechanism:

❖ The individual is harboring the infectious agent and administration of vaccine probably shortens the IP and produces the disease or what may have been otherwise a latent infection is converted to a clinical attack.

Importance of AEFI Monitoring

❖ Use sterile needle and syringe for every injection
❖ Reconstitute only with specific diluent
❖ Discard reconstituted vaccines after 6 hours
❖ Do not store drugs and other medicines in the same fridge containing vaccines and diluents

* Train and supervise health workers to ensure safe injection practices
* Monitor, investigate and act when AEFIs occur.

Steps in AEFI Surveillance

* Detection and reporting
* Investigation
* Data analysis
* Corrective and other actions
* Evaluation.

Mission Indradhanush

* Launched on 25th December 2014
* Cover children who are unvaccinated or partially vaccinated against seven vaccine preventable disease:
  1. Diphtheria
  2. Whooping cough
  3. Tetanus
  4. Polio
  5. Childhood TB
  6. Measles
  7. Hepatitis B.

Goal: To vaccinate all under 5-year-old by the year 2020.

* About 4 special vaccination campaigns will be conducted between January and June 2015
* About 201 high focus districts will be covered in first phase
* Mission supported by WHO, UNICEF and Rotary international.

National Immunization Schedule

National Immunization Schedule (NIS) for Infants, Children and Pregnant Women

Vaccine	When to give	Dose	Route	Site
For Pregnant Women				
TT-1	Early in pregnancy	0.5 mL	Intramuscular	Upper arm
TT-2	4 weeks after TT-1*	0.5 mL	Intramuscular	Upper arm
TT- Booster	If received 2 TT doses in a pregnancy within the last 3 years*	0.5 mL	Intramuscular	Upper arm
For Infants				
BCG	At birth or as early as possible till one year of age	0.1 mL (0.05 ml until 1 month age)	Intradermal	Left upper arm
Hepatitis B - Birth dose	At birth or as early as possible within 24 hours	0.5 mL	Intramuscular	Anterolateral side of mid-thigh
OPV-0	At birth or as early as possible within the first 15 days	2 drops	Oral	Oral
OPV 1, 2 and 3	At 6 weeks, 10 weeks and 14 weeks (OPV can be given till 5 years of age)	2 drops	Oral	Oral

Contd...

Contd...

Vaccine	When to give	Dose	Route	Site
Pentavalent 1, 2 and 3	At 6 weeks, 10 weeks and 14 weeks (can be given till one year of age)	0.5 mL	Intramuscular	Anterolateral side of mid-thigh
Rotavirus#	At 6 weeks, 10 weeks and 14 weeks (can be given till one year of age)	5 drops	Oral	Oral
IPV	Two fractional dose at 6 and 14 weeks of age	0.1 ml	Intradermal two fractional dose	Intradermal: Right upper arm
Measles/MR 1st Dose$	9 completed months–12 months. (can be given till 5 years of age)	0.5 ml	Subcutaneous	Right upper arm
JE - 1**	9 completed months–12 months.	0.5 ml	Subcutaneous	Left upper arm
Vitamin A (1st dose)	At 9 completed months with measles Rubella	1 ml (1 lakh IU)	Oral	Oral
For Children				
DPT booster-1	16–24 months	0.5 ml	Intramuscular	Anterolateral side of mid-thigh
Measles/MR 2nd dose$	16–24 months	0.5 ml	Subcutaneous	Right upper arm
OPV Booster	16–24 months	2 drops	Oral	Oral
JE-2	16–24 months	0.5 ml	Subcutaneous	Left upper arm
Vitamin A*** (2nd to 9th dose)	16–18 months. Then one dose every 6 months up to the age of 5 years	2 ml (2 lakh IU)	Oral	Oral
DPT Booster-2	5–6 years	0.5 ml	Intramuscular	Upper arm
TT	10 years and 16 years	0.5 ml	Intramuscular	Upper arm

*Give TT-2 or Booster doses before 36 weeks of pregnancy. However, give these even if more than 36 weeks have passed. Give TT to a woman in labor, if she has not previously received TT.

**JE Vaccine is introduced in select endemic districts after the campaign.

*** The 2nd to 9th doses of Vitamin A can be administered to children 1–5 years old during biannual rounds, in collaboration with ICDS.

#Phased introduction, at present in Andhra Pradesh, Haryana, Himachal Pradesh and Odisha from 2016 and expanded in Madhya Pradesh, Assam, Rajasthan, and Tripura in February 2017 and planned in Tamil Nadu and Uttar Pradesh in 2017.

$Phased introduction, at present in five states namely Karnataka, Tamil Nadu, Goa, Lakshadweep and Puducherry (As of Feb 2017).

Recent Updates on Universal Immunization Program

1. **Rotavirus vaccine:** Rotavirus is one of the leading causes of severe diarrhea and death among children less than 5 years of age.

   The introduction of rotavirus vaccine will enable to directly address the problem of diarrheal deaths.

   The rotavirus vaccine has been developed indigenously, under a public-private partnership by the Ministry of Science and Ministry of Health and Family Welfare.

   Vaccine type: Live attenuated vaccine

   Dosing schedule: 3 doses: 6–10–14 weeks

   Dose: 5 drops per dose orally (2 mL)

   Vaccine name: Rotavac

2. **Pentavalent vaccine:** The pentavalent vaccine is a combination of DPT, hepatitis B and Hib vaccines. DPT and hepatitis B vaccines are already a part of the immunization program. They are being replaced by liquid pentavalent vaccine (LPV) in a phased manner in the country.

3. **Inactivated polio vaccine:** Injectable inactivated polio vaccine (IPV) was introduced in the ongoing Universal Immunization Program simultaneously with the existing OPV from 30.11.2015. It was initially introduced in 6 states with expansion in a phased manner later on.

   Note: *Until polio is eradicated globally, OPV is still the main preventive measure against polio. Thus, IPV is recommended in addition to OPV and does not replace OPV.*

4. **Pneumococcal conjugate vaccine:** The Health Ministry has approved the introduction of pneumococcal conjugate vaccine (PCV) under Universal Immunization Program. PCV was initially introduced in 4 states in 2017 with expansion in a phased manner later on.

5. **National vaccine reminder:** It is a free reminder for every vaccination of child.
   Child's name and date of birth is to be registered.
   Reminder is sent to registered contact number via SMS 2 days in advance.
   This reminder is sent till 12 years age of the child.

6. **Electronic vaccine intelligence network:** Electronic vaccine intelligence network (eVIN) is designed and implemented to enable real time information on cold chain temperatures and vaccine stocks and flows in all the 160 districts of Madhya Pradesh, Rajasthan and Uttar Pradesh.

SITES OF ADMINISTRATION OF DIFFERENT VACCINES

BCG Vaccine

Stands for Bacillus Calmette–Guérin.

Types
- ❖ Live attenuated vaccine
- ❖ Liquid (fresh) vaccine
- ❖ Freeze dried lyophilized (more stable than liquid vaccine)
- ❖ Light sensitive, so kept in amber colored vial.

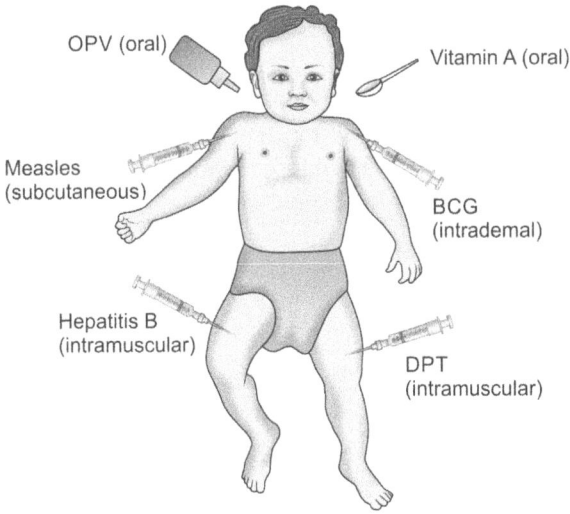

WHO recommended strain
❖ Danish 1331
❖ Derived from *Mycobacterium bovis*
❖ Prepared by BCG laboratory, Guindy, Chennai.

Reconstituent
❖ Normal saline
❖ Distilled water can cause irritation
❖ Reconstituted vaccine must be used within 3 hours
❖ Left over vaccine should be discarded.

Dosage
❖ Strength: 0.1 mg in 0.1 mL
❖ <4 weeks— 0.05 mL
❖ >4 weeks— 0.1 mL.
   As skin of newborn is thin, hence might penetrate into deeper tissue and give rise to local abscess, enlarged axillary lymph nodes.

Indications
❖ Active immunization against TB.
❖ Can be given in tuberculin negative patients.

Storage: 2°–8°C.

Administration
❖ Route: Intradermal (if given subcutaneously chance of abscess formation is more).
❖ Syringe: Tuberculin syringe (omega microstat syringe fitted with a 1 cm steel 26 gauge intradermal needle).
❖ Site: Just above the insertion of LEFT deltoid (if proper positioning is not done adjacent lymph nodes may be affected).
❖ Alcohol should not be used to swab skin and vaccine must not be contaminated with antiseptic or detergent.

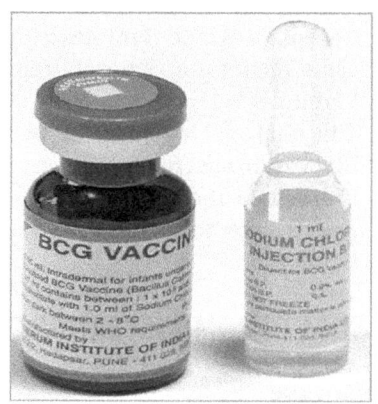

BCG vaccine
(Freeze dried)—20 doses
(*Courtesy:* Serum Institute of India Ltd, India)

Age for vaccination
❖ At birth (for institutional deliveries)
❖ At 6 weeks (with other vaccines like OPV, DPT)
   – Direct BCG: It is administered up to 1 year of age, without Mantoux test.
   – Indirect BCG: Beyond age of 1 year, it is recommended after prior Mantoux test.

Phenomena after vaccination

Sequel	Associated phenomena
Immediately	Small swelling persists for 6–8 hours, then disappears
2–3 weeks	Papule formation
5 weeks	4–8 mm diameter of papule
6–8 weeks	Breaks into shallow ulcer, seen covered with crust
6–12 weeks	Permanent tiny, round scar, typically 4–8 mm diameter
8–14 weeks	Mantoux test becomes positive

Sometimes, this process of ulceration and healing recurs 2–3 times. The ultimate typical puckered scar is formed which remains for lifetime. If ulceration occurs within 7 days of injection (usually takes 6–8 weeks), one must report to the doctor, as it may be a sign of tuberculosis in the child.

Protective efficacy
- For pulmonary TB: 0%
- For severe forms of TB: 0–80%
- For leprosy: 20–40%

Protection duration
- Starts from 15 days
- Lasts for 15-20 years.

Complications
- *Local:* Prolong severe inflammation (ulcer, abscess, keloid at the site of vaccination) maximum in 28 days
- *Regional:* Axillary lymphadenitis
- *General:* Disseminated BCG infection (<1 per million vaccinations), osteomyelitis.

Uses
- Protection from severe form of TB in children (however, it does not protect child from adult form of TB).

It also protects from:
  - TB meningitis
  - Miliary TB.
- In treatment of carcinoma bladder.

Contraindications
- Patient suffering from generalized eczema
- Infective dermatosis
- Hypogammaglobulinemia
- Patients with history of deficient immunity (symptomatic HIV, leukemia, other congenital immune deficiency disorders)
- Patient undergone immunosuppressive treatment (corticosteroid, anticancer drugs)
- Pregnancy.

WHO recommended policy on BCG vaccination in HIV
- Asymptomatic HIV (+) infants in:
  - High endemic areas: BCG can be given
  - Low endemic areas: BCG need not be given.

Additional Questions and Answers Regarding BCG

1. What is a BCG vaccine?

BCG vaccine is a live bacterial vaccine given for protection against tuberculosis, mainly severe forms of childhood tuberculosis.

2. How is BCG vaccine given?

BCG vaccine is given over the left arm. A wheal or swelling of 6 mm is raised above the surface. No spirit or antiseptic should be applied over the site before injection because spirit may kill attenuated vaccine virus. Good bath with soap and water is enough to clean the local injection site. At the most one can use normal saline to clean the area.

3. What if BCG is not given at birth?

BCG should be given as early as possible in life, before child comes in contact with tuberculosis. It can be given up to 20 years of age. If it is given beyond 1 year it is preferable to do a prior Mantoux test to see if the patient is already sensitized to tuberculosis. If patient is already sensitized as shown by positive MT, BCG is not necessary.

4. When is a booster dose of BCG vaccine given?

Neither Govt. of India nor Indian Academy of Pediatrics recommends a booster dose of BCG in India. Some countries like in Gulf recommend one or more booster doses.

5. Why is BCG not recommended in developed countries like USA?

In developed countries like USA, very few cases of **tuberculosis** occur. As **BCG** does not prevent primary TB or the adult type of tuberculosis no benefit will be derived by routine BCG vaccination in such countries. Hence, BCG is not recommended in USA routinely.

6. What local care should we take at injection site?

Injection site should not be pressed or rubbed. It should not be fomented. Nothing needs to be applied locally. In fact, bath with soap and water should be done even when it has ulcerated.

7. What if the child develops fever?

BCG does not lead to **fever**. Hence search for another cause and treat accordingly.

8. Can BCG be given over thigh from beauty point of view so that scar is hidden?

By convention BCG scars are looked for over the left arm to maintain uniformity and for helping surveyors in verifying the receipt of the vaccine. Hence, BCG should only be given over left arm and nowhere else.

9. What if scar is not seen after BCG vaccination?

Formation of scar is neither necessary nor is the only indication of success of **BCG vaccine**. However, it is the only simple and convenient way of determining success of BCG vaccine. It may take 3–6 months for the scar to form. If no scar is visible revaccination is not required.

10. Can BCG be given with other vaccines?

BCG can be given with other vaccines except **Measles** and **MMR**.

11. Why do we give 0.05 mL dose of BCG to newborns (below 1 month of age)?

This is because the skin of newborns is thin and an intradermal injection of 0.1 mL may break the skin or penetrate into the deeper tissue and cause local abscess and enlarged axillary lymph nodes.

12. Why is BCG given only up to 1 year of age?

Most children acquire natural clinical/subclinical TB infection by the age of 1 year. This too protects against severe forms of childhood tuberculosis, e.g. TB meningitis and miliary disease.

DPT VACCINE

❖ **Nature of vaccine**
  – Combined triple vaccine for diphtheria, pertussis and tetanus
  – 'D' and 'T' are toxoids
  – 'P' is whole cell killed pertussis bacilli.
❖ **Dose:** 0.5 mL.
❖ **Route:** Deep intramuscular.
❖ **Site:** Anterolateral aspect of thigh (middle 1/3rd).
❖ **Types:**
  – Plain
  – Absorbed (on a mineral carrier like aluminium phosphate/hydroxide)—WHO recommended
  – Aluminium salts act as adjuvant.
❖ **Composition:**

Contents	Amount per dose (0.5 mL) (Glaxo)
Diphtheria toxoid	25 Lf
Tetanus toxoid	5 Lf
Pertussis killed acellular bacilli	20,000 million
Aluminium phosphate	2.5 mg
Thimerosal (as preservative)	0.01%

❖ **Storage:**
  – $+2°-8°C$
  – DPT is supplied as liquid, store refrigerated
  – If DPT vaccine gets frozen accidentally: Discard the vaccine
  – Aluminium adjuvanated vaccines should not be frozen
  – When issued on subcenter the vaccine should be used within a week.
❖ **Dosing schedule:**

Dose	Age
DPT1	6 weeks of age
DPT2	10 weeks of age
DPT3	14 weeks of age
DPT booster	16–24 months of age
DPT booster	5 years of age

2 months gap between 2 successive doses of DPT do not offer any advantage over 1 month interval.
❖ **Indication:** For active immunization of infants against diphtheria, pertussis and tetanus simultaneously.
❖ **Efficacy:**
  – Diphtheria and tetanus components are highly immunogenic and antibodies to them are almost completely protective
  – Pertussis enhances potency of diphtheria toxoid, but its efficacy is 70–80% only.
❖ **Reactions:**
  – Minor reaction:
    - Fever of $\geq 39°C$ (2–6% cases)

- Swelling, induration (5–10% cases)
- Pain for >2 days.
  - Severe reactions:
    - Anaphylactic shock
    - Neurological complications (encephalitis/encephalopathy, prolonged convulsions, infantile spasms and Reye's syndrome).
- ❖ **Contraindications:**
  - Absolute contraindications:
    - Severe hypersensitivity reaction to previous dose (shock like state, persistent screaming, fever >40°C, convulsions, neurological manifestations and anaphylactic shock)
    - Progressive neurological diseases (e.g. active epilepsy) (though DPT can be used in cerebral palsy and seizures controlled on antiepileptics).
  - Relative contraindications:
    - Acute febrile illness
    - History of convulsion.
- ❖ **Precautions:**
  - Vial should be shaken before use and if turbidity or floccules are seen, then vial should be discarded
  - Vaccine should be used before date of expiry
  - Exposure to direct sunlight should be prevented
  - Half used vial should not be put back into the cold chain after session.

Additional Questions and Answers Regarding DPT

1. What are the types of diphtheria immunization?

Types:
- ❖ Combined/mixed vaccine:
  - DPT
  - DPwT, (w = whole cell pertussis) contains entire killed form of pertussis bacteria
  - DPaT (a = acellular pertussis) contains only few proteins of the pertussis germ
  - DT (diphtheria–tetanus toxoid)
  - dT (diphtheria–tetanus, adult type) useful to boost **immunity** in adults and prevent side effects due to minimal strength of the vaccine.
    Both DPwT, DPaT vaccines are very effective, but DPaT has lesser side effect.
- ❖ Single vaccine:
  - FT (Formal toxoid)
  - APT (Alum-precipitated toxoid)
  - PTAP (Purified toxoid aluminium phosphate)
  - PTAH (Purified toxoid aluminium hydroxide)
  - TAH (Toxoid-antitoxin flocculus).
- ❖ Antisera:
  - Diphtheria antitoxin.

2. Why DPT vaccine is not given in the gluteal region?

Presence of fat in the buttocks breaks the adjuvant and reduces absorption of DPT vaccine.

3. What is the treatment of side effects following DPT?

❖ Paracetamol or ibuprofen can be used to treat pain, swelling, redness, difficulty in walking and fever. It takes 2–3 days for the symptoms to disappear
❖ In case abscess has formed, treat with **antibiotics** and drainage
❖ Applying ice wrapped in handkerchief over the injection site helps to reduce swelling and pain to some extent
❖ Persistent nodule should be left alone, as it does not lead to any other symptoms.

4. When is DT used?

It is used in patients where pertussis component is contraindicated.

5. What is DT vaccine?

DT vaccine has 1/10th dose of diphtheria toxoid than present in DT/DPT. If full dose of diphtheria toxoid is given as present in DT/DPT in children above 10 years of age, it can lead to serious side effects like heart toxicity, serum sickness like reactions, etc. One needs to give booster of diphtheria at 10 years and maybe every 10 years thereafter to maintain protective titres. DT is useful in such cases as a booster at 10 years (instead of TT).

6. What is acellular pertussis DPT vaccine?

As seen before, the severe adverse side effects seen with DPT are due to *pertussis component*. It was realized that the reactions were due to components of cell wall of pertussis organism, which are not required for efficacy of vaccine. An acellular pertussis vaccine that does not have whole cell wall of pertussis has been developed that can be routinely used for immunization.

7. What should one do if the child is found allergic to DPT or develops encephalopathy after DPT?

A child who is allergic to DPT or develops encephalopathy after DPT should be given the DT vaccine instead of DPT for the remaining doses, as it is usually the P (whole cell pertussis) component of the vaccine which causes the allergy/encephalopathy.

8. How do you know that the DPT vial has not been frozen?

By "Shake Test"

Procedure

❖ Test vial:
   – Take a vaccine vial you suspect that may have been frozen.
   – This is "TEST" vial.
❖ Control vial:
   – Take a vaccine vial of the same antigen, same manufacturer, and same batch number as the suspect vaccine vial you want to test.
   – Freeze solid this vial at (-) 20°C overnight in the deep freezer, and this is the 'CONTROL' vial and label accordingly to avoid its usage.
❖ Let it thaw. Do not heat it.

RECENT UPDATES: PENTAVALENT VACCINE

Introduction

Pentavalent vaccine provides protection to a child from 5 life-threatening diseases—diphtheria, pertussis, tetanus, hepatitis B and Hib. DPT and Hep B are already part of routine immunization in India; Hib vaccine is a new addition. Together, the combination is called pentavalent.

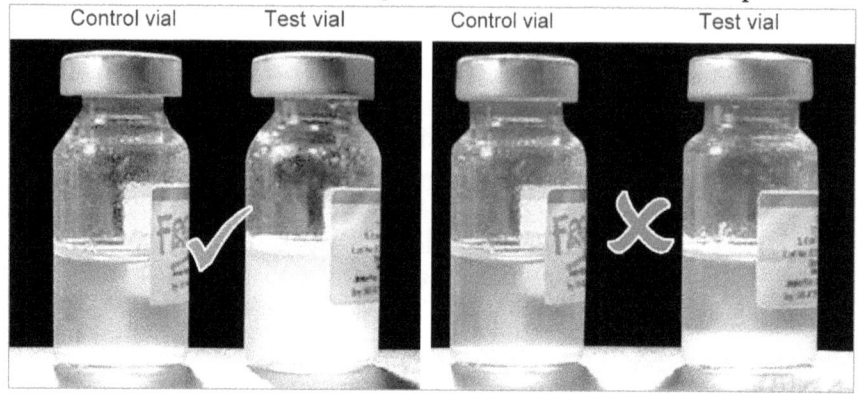

Dose: 0.5 mL

Route: Intramuscular.

Site: Anterolateral aspect of the mid-thigh (left).

Form:
❖ The pentavalent vaccine is available in various forms of liquid and lyophilized.
❖ However, under the UIP in India, the vaccine is available as a liquid formulation only. So, it is also called liquid pentavalent vaccine.
❖ In UIP, pentavalent vaccine comes in a liquid form in a vial which contains 10 doses.

Storage and transport:
❖ Pentavalent vaccine should be stored at temperature of 2–8°C in the basket of ice-lined refrigerator (ILR) and should never be frozen
❖ Conditioned ice packs should be used during transportation to prevent freezing.

Indication:

In addition to DPT and hepatitis B, the Hib component can prevent serious diseases caused by *Haemophilus influenzae* type B like pneumonia, meningitis, bacteremia, epiglottitis, septic arthritis, etc.

Efficacy: 85–95% protection after completion of the schedule.

Long-term protection:

Current scientific evidence suggests that protection is life-long. A booster dose is not recommended in India.

Dosing schedule:
❖ The pentavalent vaccine has replaced the previous hepatitis B and DPT primary vaccination schedule in the immunization program.
❖ Additionally, hepatitis B birth dose will continue as before, in institutional birth within 24 hours of birth. DPT boosters at 16–24 months and 5–6 years will continue as before.

❖ The revised immunization schedule is as:

Timing	Vaccine
At birth	BCG, Hep B birth dose, OPV-0
6 weeks	Pentavalent 1 , OPV 1
10 weeks	Pentavalent 2 , OPV 2
14 weeks	Pentavalent 3 , OPV 3
9 months	Measles 1 with vitamin A
16–24 months	Measles 2, DPT booster 1, OPV booster
5–6 years	DPT booster 2

❖ Pentavalent vaccine can be given to any child aged more than 6 weeks and up to 1 year of age.

Side effects:
❖ Pentavalent vaccine has not been associated with any serious side effects. However, redness, swelling, and pain may occur at the limb site where the injection was given. These symptoms usually appear the day after the injection has been given and last from 1 to 3 days. Less commonly, children may develop fever for a short time after immunization.

Contraindications:
❖ Severe allergic reactions
❖ Children with moderate or severe acute illness should not be administered pentavalent vaccine until their condition improves. The minor illnesses, however, such as upper respiratory infections (URI) is not a contraindication to vaccination.

Additional Questions and Answers Regarding Pentavalent Vaccine

1. **A child who is 10 months old has not received any immunization. What are the vaccines that can be given to her?**

❖ The child should receive BCG, measles, first dose of pentavalent vaccines with OPV1 and vitamin A syrup.
❖ If pentavalent vaccine is not available, give DPT 1 and Hep B1.

2. **If a child comes unimmunized at completing 12 months of age, what vaccines would you give?**

Give three doses of DPT and OPV at intervals of 4 weeks and a booster dose of DPT after 6 months. Also give measles vaccine and vitamin A solution with the first dose of DPT.

ORAL POLIO VACCINE

Introduction
Oral polio vaccine (OPV) is a live attenuated vaccine used for active immunization against poliomyelitis, the dreaded childhood disease leading to paralysis of various groups of muscles for under-5 children.

Recent Updates
❖ Previously trivalent OPV (containing type 1, type 2 and type 3 strains) was administered under UIP.
❖ But from April 25, 2016 onwards, Govt. of India started switching from trivalent OPV to bivalent (containing only types 1 and 3) OPV. This date is also called "National switch date".

❖ Rationale of switch/OPV 2 withdrawal:
  – Since 1999, type 2 wild poliovirus has not been detected.
  – The type 2 component of trivalent OPV:
    - Caused >90% of vaccine derived polioviruses (VDPV)
    - Caused ~40% of vaccine associated paralytic polio (VAPP) cases
    - Interfered with the immune response to poliovirus type 1 and type 3.

Discovered by: Albert Sabin.

Nature of vaccine: Live attenuated 'bivalent' vaccine containing 2 strains of polio virus.

Composition

1. Live attenuated Sabin strain: Type 1
2. Live attenuated Sabin strain: Type 3
3. Stabilizer: $MgCl_2$

Mechanism of Action

❖ *Primary multiplication*: In intestinal epithelium cells (results in the formation of duodenal IgA)
❖ *Secondary multiplication*: Peyer's patches where subsequent viremia occurs. Then virus spreads to the other areas of the body resulting in the formation of circulating antibody (serum IgM, IgG, IgA).

Dosing Schedule

Dose	Age
OPV 0	At birth
OPV 1	6 weeks
OPV 2	10 weeks
OPV 3	14 weeks
OPV B (booster dose)	16–24 months

Dose: 1 dose = 2 drops = 0.1 mL.

Mode of Administration

Head of the child is tilted backward → mouth is forced to open by gently squeezing the cheeks or pinching the nose → 2 drops are dropped onto the tongue by dropper.

Mother is advised not to administer food, hot liquid, breast milk an hour prior to and after vaccination as these may interact with vaccine viruses.

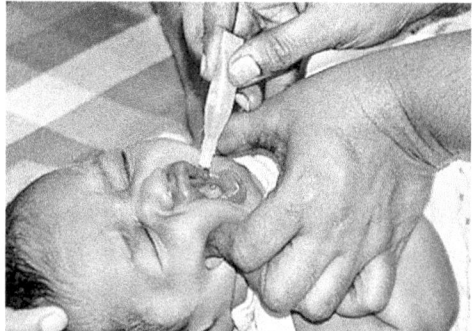

OPV administration to a child

Indication

For active immunization against polio for under-5 children.

Storage

❖ +2–+8°C (–20 to –40°C only for long-term use)

❖ During transportation OPV should be kept on:
  – Dry ice (solidified CO_2) or
  – Freezing mixture wet ice + ammonium chloride)
❖ Shelf-life: 24 months at –20°C.
❖ The vaccine is approved for use for up to 28 days after opening the vial.

Adverse Effects

Vaccine associated paralytic poliomyelitis (VAPP):
❖ OPV is remarkably free from complications.
❖ VAPP is the most important of the rare adverse events associated with OPV.
❖ Cases of VAPP are clinically indistinguishable from poliomyelitis caused by WPV.
❖ It is most frequently associated with Sabin 3 strains (60% of cases) followed by Sabin 2 and Sabin 1.
❖ The risk of VAPP is higher particularly for persons with B-lymphocyte disorders (e.g. agammaglobulinemia and hypogammaglobulinemia).

Contraindications

Nothing as per National Pulse Polio Program. But it should be avoided in:
❖ Diarrheal disease (OPV not counted)
❖ Malignancy (like leukemia, etc.)
❖ Steroid or immunosuppressive drugs therapy.
Such children should be administered inactivated polio vaccine.

Efficacy

No. of doses (OPV)	% of protection offered
3	85%
4	90%
5	95%

Advantages

❖ Painless, easy to administer
❖ Highly trained staff not required
❖ Induces both humoral and cellular immunity
❖ Quick production of large dose of antibody in single dose only provides herd immunity
❖ Useful in controlling epidemics
❖ Even a single dose can produce substantial immunity (except in tropical countries)
❖ Cheaper
❖ Easy to manufacture.

Disadvantages

❖ Required to be stored and transported in sub-zero temperature (unless stabilized)
❖ Frequent vaccine failure reported
❖ May revert to its wild form and cause neurovirulence.

Additional Questions Regarding Polio Vaccine

1. What are the types of polio vaccine?

There are two types of polio vaccines, one is live oral polio vaccine and the other is **injectable killed polio vaccine**. Both these vaccines contain all the 3 types of polioviruses.

2. Can polio vaccine be given along with other vaccines?

Both OPV/IPV can be given along with other vaccines.

3. What is pulse polio immunization?

It is a strategy of mass **immunization** to eradicate poliomyelitis. Extra doses (pulses) of OPV are given to all children below 5 years of age in an area (like country, state, city) at a time on a given day. Such pulses are repeated every year. The aim is to achieve 100% coverage.

4. How does pulse immunization work?

Wild poliovirus can survive either in the intestines of a susceptible host (usually children <5 years of age) or in the sewage water. In the sewage water it can survive only for 48–72 hours and hence it has to find shelter into another susceptible host for it to survive and to continue cycle of transmission. When you give pulse OPV to all the children of <5 years of age, the intestines of these children are flooded by vaccine virus and hence wild poliovirus cannot get entry into it. As wild poliovirus cannot survive for more than 48–72 hours in environment, its circulation will drastically fall. When such pulse is repeated after 6 weeks it still further reduces transmission. Such pulses done every year will ultimately eradicate the wild poliovirus from nature.

5. Do you need to give regular OPV doses when pulse OPV is taken?

The answer is an emphatic yes.

6. A patient survived from polio should he be receive polio vaccine again?

Attack by one strain provides immunity against that strain but other strains can infect. So vaccination required.

INACTIVATED POLIO VACCINE

Introduction: Inactivated polio vaccine is a type of killed vaccine.

Discovery: It is the first effective polio vaccine was developed in 1952 by Jonas Salk.

Nature of vaccine: It is a killed vaccine produced from formaldehyde. Killed polio virus grown in monkey kidney or human diploid cell.

Composition

Components (polio virus strain)	Strength
Type 1	20 D antigen units
Type 2	2 D antigen units
Type 3	4 D antigen units

Composition of Improved IPV

Components (polio virus strain)	Strength
Type 1	40 D antigen units
Type 2	8 D antigen units
Type 3	32 D antigen units

Mechanism of action: It induces humoral immunity (with the formation of IgM, IgG, and IgA).

Schedule: Two fractional dose at 6 and 14 weeks of age.

Dose: 0.1 mL.

Mode of administration: Intradermal: Right upper arm.

Indication: For active immunization against polio for under-5 children.

Storage
❖ IPV should not be frozen. It should be stored at 0°C to +8°C.
❖ Shelf life at this temperature: 12–18 months
❖ It can withstand 4 weeks at 37°C.

Adverse effects
❖ Minor local erythema
❖ Induration
❖ Tenderness.

Contraindication
In epidemics.

Advantages
❖ Safe in immunodeficient disorders
❖ Safe in persons with immunosuppressive/corticosteroid therapy
❖ Useful >50 years of age
❖ Safe in pregnancy
❖ No risk of VAPP.

Disadvantages
❖ IPV is unsuitable in epidemics; because:
  – Immunity is not achieved immediately by single dose, multiple doses are required
  – Injections can precipitate paralysis during epidemics
  – Costly as its virus content is 10,000 times than OPV
  – Trained personnel required.

Difference between OPV and IPV

Topic	OPV	IPV
Type	Live attenuated vaccine	Killed formolized vaccine
Discovery	Albert Sabin (1962 got license)	Jonas Salk (1952)
Route of administration	Oral	Intradermal (right upper arm)

Contd...

Contd...

Topic	OPV	IPV
Dose	2 drops	0.1 mL
Contents	2 strains of poliovirus (type 1 and type 3)	All 3 strains of poliovirus
Immunity	Induces humoral + cellular immunity	Only humoral
Epidemics control	Useful in controlling epidemics	Not useful
Prevention of	Paralysis intestinal reinfection	Prevents paralysis only, cannot prevent intestinal reinfection by wild polio viruses
Cost effectiveness	Cheaper	Expensive
Storage and transport	Require sub-zero temperature	Less stringent conditions
Shelf life	Short	Longer
VAPP	<1/11 million vaccine	Zero

MEASLES VACCINE

Type: Live attenuated lyophilized (freeze dried) vaccine (tissue culture vaccine-chick-embryo/human diploid cell line vaccine).

Strain used
❖ Edmonston-Zagreb (EZ)strain—most commonly used
[Each dose (0.5 mL) contains ≥1,000 TCID—50 live attenuated EZ strain of measles virus grown on human diploid cells]
❖ Schwartz strain
❖ Moraten strain.

Diluent: Pyrogen free double distilled water.

Administration
❖ Schedule: 9 months of age (1st dose) → at 16–24 months (2nd dose, along with the booster dose of DPT)
    Though measles vaccination can be done at 6 months of age; in case of:
    – Outbreak in the refugee camp/in epidemics
    – Severely malnourished child as measles can occur earlier (here reimmunization done after 4 months).

Site: Right upper arm

Route: Subcutaneous

Dose: 0.5 ml in a dose

No. of doses/vial: 5 doses

Amount of diluent: 5 doses are kept in 1 vial
❖ Diluent required/dose = 0.5 mL
❖ Total diluent required per vial = (5 × 0.5) mL = 2.5 mL.

Indications
❖ For active immunization against measles
❖ For contact measles case (provides protective effects within 7 days).

Contraindications

- ❖ Immunocompromised patient/patients undergone immunosuppressive therapy
- ❖ Convulsion, CNS disorders
- ❖ Pregnancy
- ❖ Allergy to neomycin/gelatin.

Time limit for use after reconstitution: 4 hours.

Storage

- ❖ To be kept dried in + 2 to + 8°C in small ILR (in PHC).
- ❖ The diluent can be kept in room temperature. But prior to vaccination it should be kept at + 2 to + 8°C before 24 hours.
- ❖ It is both thermolabile and thermostable.

Immunity: Life-long, develops after 11–12 days after vaccination.

Efficacy

- ❖ Infants vaccinated at 9 months show seroconversion rate of about 90%
- ❖ One dose at 11–12 months of age appears to be 99% effective.

Ideal gap between 2 successive doses of measles vaccine: 6 months.

Adverse effects:

- ❖ Pseudomeasles/minimeasles:
  - – Sometimes when the vaccine injected into the body the attenuated virus multiplies and induces a "mild measles illness" (associated with fever and rash) in 15–20% vaccine after 5–10 days of vaccination. Fever subsides in 1–2 days and rash in 1–3 days.
- ❖ Toxic shock syndrome:
  - – Occurs when:
    - - Measles vaccine is contaminated
    - - Same vial is used for more than 4 hours/next day.
- ❖ Encephalitis (1 in 1 million)
- ❖ **Thrombocytopenia**
- ❖ Guillain–Barré syndrome
- ❖ **Subacute sclerosing panencephalitis (SSPE).**

Measles vaccine in HIV(+) infant:

In case of asymptomatic/symptomatic HIV(+) infant (unless severely immunocompromised): Should be routinely administered.

Combined vaccine: MR, MMR, mumps, measles, rubella, varicella (MMRV).

Age: Up to 5 years of age, it can be done. If the child has already been suffered from measles before immunization there is NO need for measles immunization.

Passive immunization:

- ❖ Type: Human normal immunoglobulin
- ❖ Dose (WHO recommended): 0.25 mL/kg body weight (BW)/ im (within 3–4 days of exposure)
- ❖ Revaccination: After 8–12 weeks.

Additional Questions and Answers Regarding Measles Vaccine

1. **Why measles vaccine is given at 9 months of age?**

Because immunization for measles:
* ❖ *Before 9 months*: Will render the vaccine ineffective by interaction with maternal antibodies present in body of the infant.
* ❖ *After 9 months*: Will not be very effective. Because, after 6 months a level of maternal antibody starts declining and after 9 months antibody level declines to such an extent that the newborn becomes susceptible to measles. So, vaccination for measles should be done as close as possible in 9 months.

Though measles vaccination can be done at 6 months of age; in case of:
* ❖ Outbreak in the refugee camp/in epidemics
* ❖ Severely malnourished child as measles can occur earlier.

2. Measles vaccine should be administered within 4 hours of reconstitution. Explain.

Because:
* ❖ Reconstituted vaccine loses 50% of its potency after 1 hour at 20°C.
* ❖ It loses almost all its potency after 1 hour at 37°C. As it is also a sunlight sensitive vaccine, after reconstitution vaccine should be stored in colored glass vials in dark at 2–8°C and administered within 4 hours of reconstitution.

TETANUS TOXOID

Beneficiary
* ❖ Pregnant women
* ❖ Children at 10 years and 16 years.

Type
* ❖ Toxoid
* ❖ Toxins produced by tetanus bacilli is detoxicated and used in the preparation of vaccines.

Administration
Schedule:

Situation	Preferable dosing schedule
Antenatal period	• 2 doses of TT to be given, 1 month apart (preferably in 4th and 5th month of period of gestation) • If not given at 5th month, 2nd dose should be given at least <3 weeks prior to delivery, so that there is enough time for good antibody titres to develop in mother and for it to be passed on to the fetus to prevent tetanus in newborn • 2 doses provide protection for subsequent pregnancies in next 5 years (only 1 booster dose is sufficient)
Pregnant woman comes at 8th month of gestation for the first time	• 2 TT doses are given irrespective of delivery time (i.e. second dose is given at the time of delivery) • This results in complete immunization of mother for subsequent 5 years, but infants remain unimmunized • In this case 750 IU heterologous serum should be administered within 6 hours of birth
Pregnant woman in labor	• Give TT to a woman in labor, if she has not previously received TT
Children up to 1 year of age	• As a part of DPT or pentavalent vaccine at 6, 10 and 14 weeks
Older children and adults	• Booster doses are given to children of 10 and 16 years of age who have received their primary doses/boosters of DPT/DT before (as they do not need both diphtheria and pertussis components). It can be then taken every 5–10 years to maintain protection life-long

Site: Upper arm.

Dose: 0.5 mL.

Route: Intramuscular.

No. of doses: 2.

Interval between 2 doses: 4 weeks.

Timing: Booster doses/2nd dose before 9 months of pregnancy.

Types of immunity produced
- ❖ For mother: Active immunity
- ❖ For child: Passive immunity
- ❖ But NO herd immunity is produced.
- ❖ The antibiotics produced neutralize the toxic moiety produced during infection rather than act upon the organisms.

Storage temperature: 4–10°C in ILR.
- ❖ It must not be frozen, because freezing will dissociate the Ag from adjuvant interfering with the immunogenicity of vaccine.

Adverse effects following immunization:
- ❖ Fever, redness, swelling around the injections
- ❖ Soreness or tenderness around the injection
- ❖ Malaise and nonspecific symptoms (up to 25%).

Additional Questions and Answers Regarding Tetanus Toxoid

1. A patient recovered from tetanus does he need vaccine? Why?

Yes. Because the lethal infective dose is not sufficient to produce much protective antibody.

2. When is TT given to an adult with injury?

- ❖ An adult who has never received or has received incomplete course of TT before in life should be given 3 doses of tetanus toxoid (TT) at 4 weeks interval followed by a booster after 1 year and then every 5 years. If he then develops any injury or requires any surgery there is no need to take anymore TT as he is protected in between the doses.
- ❖ If such an adult has taken the last TT beyond 4–5 years in past, he can be given one dose of TT which acts as a booster. It is neither required nor desirable or safe to give TT for each and every injury every now and then in such a protected person.

3. What if the child gets injured, should he receive TT?

A child who has received 3 primary doses of DPT/DT is protected till 15 months of age and does not need TT. If he is 15–18 months of age he should receive his first booster of OPV + DPT which will also boost up antitetanus immunity. Such a child is protected till 4 years and does not need a TT till that age. If he is between 4–6 years he should receive his 2nd booster of DT or OPV + DPT which will boost up his antitetanus immunity too. Such a child is now protected till 10 years of age. After this a booster of TT is given at 10 years, 16 years and every 5 years thereafter. In between such doses there is no need to give TT for injury.

4. What harm is done if one gives TT frequently?

If TT is given frequently, it will hyperimmunize the patient. Such a patient can develop arthus like phenomenon with development of fever, rash, joint pain, joint swelling, etc. Hence, it is not desirable to give frequent injections of TT in an otherwise immunized patient.

HEPATITIS B VACCINE

Type: Recombinant (subunit) HBV vaccine.

Composition: (HbsAg produced in yeast or mammalian cells by recombination + alum + thiomersal) may be monovalent (or in fixed combination with DPT, Hib, Hep-A, IPV).

Administration:
❖ Schedule:

Topic	Infants and children <2 years	Adult and older children
Schedule	Birth dose <24 hours Then at 6th, 10th,14th weeks of age	0, 1, 6 months
Route	Deep IM	Deep IM
Site	Anterolateral aspect of mid-thigh	Upper arm (at the insertion of deltoid)
Dose	0.5 mL	1.0 mL

Time limit for birth dose: 24 hours

In adults and older children:
❖ 3 doses schedule on 0, 1st, 6th months (alone or as a part of pentavalent vaccine)
❖ Vaccine dose:
   – Adult dose: 10–20 µg
   – Children <10 years: 5–10 µg.

Indications:
❖ Pre-exposure prophylaxis:
   – At risk individual:
      - IV drug user
      - Persons requiring several blood/blood products
      - People with high-risk sexual behavior
      - Recipient of solid organ transplantation
      - International travelers to HBV endemic countries.
❖ Postexposure prophylaxis: It is indicated in newborn to carrier mothers and individuals exposed parenterally to HBV infection within 12 hours but not later than 48 hours.

Contraindications
❖ Individuals with history of allergic reactions
❖ Pregnancy/lactation are NOT contraindications for vaccination.

Adverse effects
❖ Local reaction (pain, swelling, redness) (up to 50%)
❖ Anaphylaxis.

Vaccine efficacy
❖ About 95% in infants, children and young adults, after 40 years of age efficacy decreases.
❖ Reduced immunogenicity due to associated diseases:
   – Advanced HIV infection
   – Chronic liver disease
   – Chronic renal failure
   – Diabetes.

Duration of protection: Life-long.

Shelf life: 36 months in 2°–8°C

Storage: 2°–8°C at ILR
It must not be frozen. Because freezing dissociates Ag from alum adjuvant and precipitates. This alters the potency of the vaccine.

Passive Immunization

Indication
* Surgeon
* Nurses/laboratory workers
* Newborn infant of carrier mother
* Sexual contacts of acute Hep B patients.

Timing: As soon as possible (ideally within 6 hours, should be <48 hours)

Dose: 0.05–0.07 mL/kg of BW (2 doses 1 month apart)

Protection for: 30 days.

Passive Active Immunization

Indications:
* As prophylaxis of accidental exposure to Hep B containing blood
* Newborn infant of carrier mother.

Vaccines:
* Both HIBG + Hep-B vaccine given together
* Better than HIBG alone.

Doses:
* 0.05–0.07 mL/kg of BW, as soon as possible within 24 hours
* Hep B virus vaccine 1 mL (20 µg/mL) im within 7 days (2nd and 3rd dose at 1, 6 months).

Additional Questions and Answers regarding Hep B

1. Why birth dose of Hep B is given?
To prevent vertical transmission of infection.

2. What if the child comes late for subsequent doses?
There is no need to restart the course. Instead just complete the remaining doses as per original schedule.

If the primary series are interrupted after the 1st dose, 2nd dose should be given as early as possible, 3rd dose minimum after 4 weeks of 2nd dose.

However, such delays are not desirable as the child remains unprotected till the course of 3 doses is completed.

3. Should hepatitis B vaccine be given to a carrier or to a patient who has recovered from HBV infection?
Neither the carrier nor the patient who has recovered needs hepatitis B vaccine. In fact, a patient of HBV infection develops protective antibodies to surface antigen (anti-HBs) on recovery. There is no risk associated with vaccination, but it is a total waste of such an expensive vaccine.

4.   Can hepatitis B vaccine be mixed in the same syringe with DPT and given as one injection?

No, DPT and hepatitis B vaccine (if supplied separately) cannot be mixed or administered through the same syringe.

5.   Why in case of adults and older children vaccines are injected in the upper arm (at the insertion of deltoid) NOT in gluteal region?

Because, gluteal injection often cause deposition of vaccine in fat rather than in muscle with fewer serological conversion.

6.   What will be Hep B vaccination status for premature, LBW (<2 kg) baby?

Sometimes, in such cases Hep B birth dose do not respond well. Here vaccine given at birth should not be counted towards in primary series and additional 3 doses should be given according to the NIS.

VITAMIN A IN OIL

❖ Vehicle used for vitamin A solution: Arachis oil, as it is fat-soluble vitamin. Water-soluble vitamin A can be used in patient suffering from fat malabsorption disease.
❖ **Dose and schedule:**
  – Prophylactic:
    - 1st dose—1 lakh IU at 9 months
    - Subsequent doses—2 lac IU each up to 5 years in every 6 months
    - Total 17 lac IU is given
    - Given 6 monthly as liver can store vitamin A in the form of retinol palmitate for 6 to 9 months. Thus 1 mega dose fulfills requirements for 6 months.
  – Therapeutic:
    - 2 massive doses of vitamin A (0–28 days as per age of the child)

Age	Quantity (in IU)
<6 months	50,000
6–12 months	100,000
>1 year	200,000

  – Oral dose of retinol palmitate, where 55 mg = 100,000 IU
    Special condition for administration:

Disease	Dosing schedule
Measles	2 doses of vitamin A successively in 2 days
Complicated measles	2 doses of vitamin A successively in 2 days → another dose after 4 weeks
Severe acute malnutrition	One extra dose of vitamin A
Diarrhea	One extra dose of vitamin A

Vitamin A spoon: "2 mL spoon"
❖ Inner marking measures: 100,000 IU
❖ Filled to brim: 200,000 IU

Strength of vitamin A: 1 lac IU/mL

Bottle of vitamin A to be used after opening: Within 6–8 weeks (write the date of opening the bottle).

Source of vitamin A:
- ❖ Vegetable source:
  - – Green leafy vegetables, like spinach, amaranths, etc.
  - – Green and yellow fruits like papaya, mango, etc.
  - – Carrot
  - – Tomato
  - – Pumpkin.
- ❖ Animal source:
  - – Cod liver oil
  - – Halibut liver oil
  - – Butter
  - – Egg
  - – Cheese
  - – Meat
  - – Cow milk.

Daily intake of vitamin A recommended by ICMR (2010):

	Group	RDA of Vitamin A (retinol) by ICMR (in µg)
Adult	Man	600
	Woman	600
	Pregnancy	800
	Lactation	950
Infant	0–12 months	350
Children	1–6 years	400
	7–9 years	600
Adolescent	10–17 years	600*

* To get these values in β-carotene (mcg), multiply the values with 8.

- ❖ Vitamin A deficiency was dealt in:
  - – 1970—Under National Program for Prevention of Nutritional Blindness
  - – 1976—Under National Program for Control of Blindness (NPCB)
  - – 1992—Under Child Survival and Safe Motherhood (CSSM)
  - – 1997—Under Reproductive and Child Health (RCH)
  - – 2006—Under National Rural Health Mission (NRHM).
- ❖ ***Xerophthalmia:*** *(Greek word; means dry eye)*
  - – **Definition**: Abnormal dryness of the conjunctiva and cornea of the eye with inflammation and ridge formation typically associated with vitamin A deficiency.
  - – **First clinical sign**: *Conjunctival xerosis*
  - – **First clinical symptom**: *Night blindness* [due to lack of production of rhodopsin, responsible for sensing low light situations. Rhodopsin is composed of retinal (an active form of vitamin A) and opsin (a protein). Because the body cannot create retinal in sufficient amounts, a diet low in vitamin A will lead to a decreased amount of rhodopsin in the eye, as there is inadequate retinal to bind with opsin. Night blindness results.]

- **Age group:** Most commonly 1–3 years.
- **WHO grading:**
  - XN = Night blindness
  - X1 = Conjunctival xerosis (X1A) with Bitot,s spots (X1B)
  - X2 = Corneal xerosis
  - X3 = Corneal ulceration/keratomalacia
  - Involving:
    * < One-third (X3A)
    * > One-third (X3B)
  - XS = Corneal scar
  - XF = Xerophthalmic fundus.

Prevalence criteria for determining the xerophthalmia problem (Important for MCQ)

Criteria	Prevalence in population at risk (6 months – 6 years)
Night blindness	>1%
Bitot's spots	>0.5%
Corneal xerosis/corneal ulceration/ keratomalacia	>0.01%
Corneal ulcer	>0.05%
Serum retinol (<10 µg/dL)	>5%

- **Prevention strategy:**
  - Short-term: Vitamin A prophylaxis to vulnerable group
  - Medium-term: Fortification of certain food with vitamin A
  - Long-term:
    * Promotion of consumption of green leafy vegetables
    * Promotion of breastfeeding as long as possible
    * Immediate treatment against diarrhea
    * Immunization against measles
    * Improvement of environmental health
    * Social and health education.
❖ *Extraocular manifestation of vitamin A deficiency:*
  - Follicular hyperkeratosis
  - Growth retardation
  - Anorexia
  - Recurrent respiratory tract infections
  - Reproductive problems like sterility in males
  - Dry and rough skin
  - Hyperkeratinization of epithelium of respiratory tract, urinary tract and gastrointestinal tract.

MAXIMUM AGE OF VACCINATION

Vaccine	Maximum age of administration	Comment
BCG	1 year	>1 year recommended after prior to Mantoux test (but unnecessary for Indian scenario)
OPV	5 years	Pulse polio immunization is over and above routine immunization

Contd...

Contd...

Vaccine	Maximum age of administration	Comment
DPT	7 years	For adults, if need arises, DT vaccine is given (2 doses, 1 month apart and booster dose after 1 year)
Hep B & Pentavalent	1 year	—
Measles	5 years	If the child has already suffered from measles disease before immunization there is no need for measles immunization
Vitamin A	5 years	Xerophthalmia cases are most common <5 years

DELAYED IMMUNIZATION

Delayed Dose

Definition of delayed dose in vaccination

Vaccine doses	Timing
Starting dose	For institutional deliveries: • Hep B Birth dose → after 24 hours • BCG, OPV-0 dose → after 24 hours For home deliveries: • BCG, OPV-0 dose → after 24 hours
Subsequent doses	After 2 weeks

Vaccines to be given in case of delayed immunization

Age of 1st attendance for vaccination	Vaccines to be given
9 months	• BCG • OPV1 (next 2 doses 1 month apart each and booster dose after 1 year of 3rd dose) • Pentavalent 1 (next 2 doses 1 month apart each) • Measles vaccination • Vitamin A (1 lakh IU)
18 months	• DPT 1, OPV 1 (next 2 doses 1 month apart each and booster dose after 1 year of 3rd dose) • HepB1 (next 2 doses 1 month apart each) • Measles vaccination (if not suffer from measles disease previously) • Vitamin A (2 lakh IU)
30 months	• DPT1, OPV1 (next 2 doses 1 month apart each and booster dose after 1 year of 3rd dose) • Measles vaccination (if not suffer from measles disease previously) • Vitamin A (2 lakh IU)
4 years	• DPT1, OPV1 (next 2 doses 1 month apart each and booster dose after 1 year of 3rd dose) • Measles vaccination (if not suffer from measles disease previously) • Vitamin A (2 lac IU)

Some Points to Remember

❖ Any no. of killed or live vaccines are given together
❖ Dosage and schedule remain same even if baby is premature and/or underweight
❖ Minor fever, diarrhea, ARI or other minor illness is not contraindication for any vaccine
❖ Indian Academy of Pediatrics (IAP) guidelines are some different from NIS guidelines.

Vaccine contraindications:

Case	Contraindicated vaccines
Pregnancy	All live attenuated vaccine (LAV) except yellow fever vaccine
Asymptomatic HIV	None
Symptomatic HIV	All LAV except BCG
Immunosuppression	All LAV
Corticosteroid therapy	All LAV
Contraindicated together	Yellow fever vaccine and cholera vaccine
Preterm and premature babies <2 kg	Hepatitis B
Severe general reactions with previous dose	Only contraindication for killed vaccine
Progressive neurological disease	Pertussis vaccine

VACCINE VIAL MONITOR

❖ *Definition*: It is a label containing heat-sensitive material which is placed on the vaccine vial to register cumulative heat exposure between the time period of exit from the manufacturing site till the time of use.

   They are the only temperature monitoring devices throughout the entire cold chain.

❖ *Principle*: The combined effects of time and temperature causes the inner square of the vaccine vial monitor (VVM) to darken gradually and irreversibly. Before opening a vial, check the status of the VVM.

   Remember:
   – Only the inner square changes color, whereas outer circle always remain blue.
   – At the starting point inner square is approximately 10% of the outer circle color.
   – There is direct relationship exists between the rate of color change and temperature, it means the lower the temperature, the slower the color change and vice versa.

❖ **Content:**
   – An outer circle
   – An inner square (made of heat sensitive material of secret composition).

❖ Measurement of validation of VVM: Can be done by optical densitometer (for color density measurement).

❖ **Vaccines with VVM:**
   – OPV
   – Hepatitis-B vaccine.

❖ **Stages:**

Symbol	Explanation	Stage
	The inner square is lighter than the outer circle. If the expiry date has not passed USE the vaccine	I
	As time passes the inner square is still lighter than the outer circle. If the expiry date has not passed USE the vaccine	II

Contd...

Contd...

Symbol	Explanation	Stage
✖	**Discard point:** The color of the inner square matches that of the outer circle DO NOT USE the vaccine	III
✖	Beyond the discard point: Inner square is darker than the outer circle. DO NOT USE the vaccine	IV

Source: Adapted from WHO

❖ **Advantages:**
  – Simple tool to identify the heat damaged vaccine
  – Avoid unnecessary discarding of vaccine because suspected heat exposure
  – Can identify cold chain problem.
❖ **Disadvantage:** Does not directly measure the potency of vaccine but gives information about potency.

AD SYRINGE

❖ AD: Automatic disable, autodisable.
❖ **Advantages:**
  – No need to dispose separately
  – As it of one time use and disabled by its own.
❖ **Disadvantage:** Once it drawn the syringe cannot be withdrawn back inside.
❖ How disposed: As per solid sharp waste management.

Mode of injection	Given at an angle of
Intramuscular (im)	90°
Intradermal (ID)	15°
Subcutaneous (sc)	45°

COLD CHAIN

❖ *Definition*: System of storage and transport of vaccines at low temperature from the manufacturer to the actual vaccination site for ensuring safety, potency and quality of vaccine.
❖ *Vaccines never allowed to freeze:*
  – DPT, TT, IPV, pentavalent, Hep B and diluents should never be kept directly on the floor of the refrigerator as they can freeze and get damaged.
  (MNEMONIC: Do not freeze "T": Look for letter "T" containing vaccines, e.g. DP**T**, **TT**, HEPATITIS B, PENTAVALEN**T**, INACTIVA**T**ED POLIO VACCINE, DILUEN**T**S).

Vaccine vials not to be kept in the cold chain:
1. That have crossed expiry date
2. That are frozen
3. That failed "Shake test"
4. VVM status beyond the discard point
5. That crossed 28 days since the date of opening.

Thermostability of vaccines:

❖ According to sensitivity to heat: **Reconstituted BCG>Yellow fever vaccine>OPV>Measles and reconstituted measles>Hep-B>DPT>DT>BCG>TT (Do not confuse thermostability with freeze sensitivity)**
❖ Most thermostable vaccine: TT
❖ Most thermolabile vaccine: Reconstituted BCG vaccine.

STORAGE OF VACCINE AT DIFFERENT LEVELS

Level	Cold chain equipment	Temperature (°C)
State/regional level	Walk-in-cold rooms (WIC)	+2 to +8
	Walk-in-freezer (WIF)	– 15 to –25
District level	Large ILRs	+2 to +8
	Large DF	– 15 to – 25
PHC level	Small ILRs	+2 to +8
	Small DFs	– 15 to – 25
Subcenter level	Vaccine carrier	+2 to +8
	Day carrier	+2 to +8
Subcenter level	Fully frozen carrier	
Private setup	Domestic refrigerator	+2 to +8

VACCINE STORAGE AND TRANSPORTATION EQUIPMENT

Special Note: Hold over Time of Equipment

Definition: In the event of power failure, "Hold over time" is defined as the time taken by the equipment to raise the inside cabinet temperature from its temperature at the time of powercut to maximum temperature limit of its recommended range."

Example: In case of an ILR, if the cabinet temperature is 4°C at the time of power cut, then the time taken to reach 8°C from 4°C will be the "holdover time "for that ILR.

Determinants:

Hold over time depends on the following factors:
❖ Ambient temperature: More the ambient temperature less will be the hold over time
❖ Frequency of opening of lid and use of basket
❖ Quantity of vaccines kept inside with adequate space between the containers (equipment empty/loaded)
❖ Condition of ice pack lining (frozen/partially frozen/melted).

Ice-Lined Refrigerator (ILR)

Introduction

It is one of the most important component of cold chain in India. It is a top opening because they can hold the cold air inside better than a front opening refrigerator.

Mechanism

❖ Inside the ice-lined refrigerator there is a lining of water containers (ice packs or tubes) fitted all around the walls and held in place by a frame.

❖ When the refrigerator is functioning the water in the containers freezes and cools the cabinet. When the electricity supply fails, then the ice lining maintains the inside temperature of the refrigerator at a safe level for vaccines.

❖ Therefore the temperature is maintained in ILR for much longer duration than in the deep freezers and domestic refrigerator. Thus *ILR is an ideal option for safe storage of vaccines*.

Principle

❖ ILR maintains a cabinet temperature in the range of +2° to +8°C. However within the range there are various temperature zones.

❖ Based on the temperature zone, inside of the ILR can be divided into 2 parts, upper part and lower part.

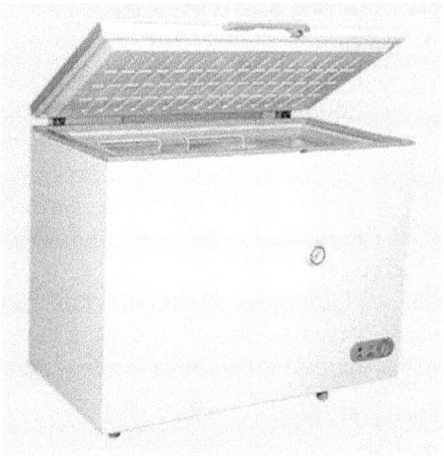

Ice lined refrigerator

❖ In most of the ILR models, the lower part is cooler, compared to the upper part, as the cooler air is heavier and settles down at the bottom of ILR. Hence upper part is preferred location for storing the freeze sensitive vaccines.

Arrangement of vaccines inside ILR from above to bottom (2016 Guidelines by Govt. of India):

Diluents		Diluents		T H	Diluents		Diluents	
Hep B	Hep B	Hep B	Hep B	E R	Hep B	Hep B	Hep B	Hep B
Pentavalent		Pentavalent		M	Pentavalent		Pentavalent	
DPT	DPT	DPT	IPV	O M	IPV	IPV	IPV	IPV
TT	TT	TT	TT	E	TT	TT	TT	TT
BCG	BCG	BCG	BCG	T E	JE	JE	JE	JE
Measles		Measles		R	Measles		Measles	
OPV	OPV	OPV	OPV		OPV	OPV	OPV	OPV

Empty ice packs

Empty ice packs

Note:

❖ Arrange 2 layers of empty ice packs at the bottom of ILR.

❖ Keep OPV and measles vaccines first on top of the empty ice packs.

❖ Then store other vaccines as described above.

Temperature: +2° to +8°C

Monitored by:

❖ Dial thermometer (acts by thermocouple principle)

❖ Stem thermometer (contains alcohol)

❖ Recorded twice a day (in morning and evening) by PHN

❖ Alarm indicates temperature <+2°C and > +8°C.

❖ It can keep vaccine safe with minimum 8 hours continuous electricity supply in a 24 hour period.

Do's and Don'ts of ILR/Freezer:

❖ **Do's:**
  - Equipment should be kept 10 cm away from wall and also away from direct sunlight
  - Equipment should be fixed through voltage stabilizer
  - Space should be kept between vaccines for circulation of air
  - Equipment should be locked properly and opened only when necessary
  - If vaccines are kept in the carton holes should be kept for air circulation
  - Periodical defrostation should be done.

❖ **Don'ts:**
  - Nothing except vaccines and diluents (e.g. drugs, foods, drinking water, even outdated vaccines) should be kept in the equipment
  - Requirements of vaccines >1 month should not be kept in it.

Deep Freezer

❖ *Use:*
  - *District level:* Storage of vaccines + preparation of ice packs
  - *PHC level:* Preparation of ice packs only.

Temperature: -15°C to -25°C

Can withstand temperature for: 18–22 hours in case of power cut

Special note: Unlike the ILR, the deep freezer (DF) has got little or limited holdover time which is dependent on the number of frozen ice packs in it and the frequency of opening.

Domestic Refrigerators (Front Load Refrigerators)

Use:

Domestic refrigerators can be used for storage of vaccine at private clinics and nursing homes, provided continuous power supply is ensured and they are dedicated for only storage of vaccines.

Temperature: +2° to +8°C

Placementm of vaccines:

Chiller tray	OPV, rota, measles
1st shelf	BCG, TT
2nd shelf	DPT, IPV
3rd shelf	Hep B, pentavalent
	Diluents next to the vaccine with which they were supplied

Do's:

❖ Freeze and store ice packs in the freezer compartment.
❖ All the vaccines and diluents have to be stored in the refrigerator compartment.
❖ Arrange the boxes of vaccine in stacks so air can move between them.
❖ Keep boxes of freeze-sensitive vaccine away from the freezing compartment.
❖ Keep ice packs filled with water on the bottom shelf and in the door of the refrigerator.

Don'ts:

❖ Do not store other supplies, such as drugs, ointment, serum, samples, food articles, drinks, etc.
❖ Do not put vaccines on the door shelves. The temperature in door shelves is too warm to store vaccines, and when the door is opened shelves are instantly exposed to room temperature.
❖ Do not place vaccines in the freezer, chiller or baskets.

Cold Box

Introduction

A cold box is an insulated container that can be lined with ice packs to keep vaccines and diluents within recommended temperatures during *transportation and emergency storage* of vaccines/ice packs for short period (as per the holdover time).

Holdover Time (at +43°C ambient temperature, if the cold box is not opened at all):

❖ Small cold box (5–8 L): More than 90 hours
❖ Large cold box (20–22 L): 6 days.

Uses:

❖ Collect and transport large quantities of vaccines
❖ Store vaccines for transfer up to 5 days, if necessary for outreach sessions or when there is a power cut
❖ As a contingency measure store vaccine in case of breakdown of ILR
❖ Also used for storing frozen ice packs, e.g. in emergency and before campaigns, etc.

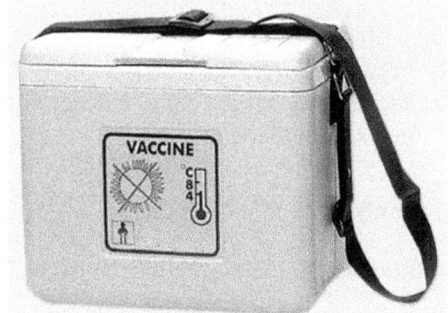

Cold box

Special note:

Ice packs are frozen in between –15°C to – 25°C and therefore *need to be conditioned* before laying out in the cold boxes to prevent freezing of vaccines. To condition the hard frozen ice packs keep them out of deep freezer to allow them to 'sweat' and a cracking sound of water would be heard on shaking the ice packs. This will protect freeze sensitive vaccines from getting frozen.

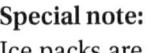

Vaccine Carrier

Vaccine carrier

Use: To carry small no. of vaccine vials (16–20 vials)

No. of ice packs in vaccine carrier: 4, only used for lining the sides.

Do's and Don'ts:

❖ Should be closed tightly
❖ Not to place anything upon it.

Vials of DPT, DT, TT and diluents not to be placed in direct contact with frozen ice packs.

Day Carriers

Use: To carry small no. of vaccine vials (6–8 vials).

No. of ice packs in vaccine carrier: 2
Only for use in nearby session of short duration.

Ice Pack

Preparation: By keeping in deep freezer.

Contents: Water, nothing should be added to water

❖ Water *filled up to the level horizontally marked* on each side for carrying the vaccine from ILR, deep freezer to PHC subcenter level/during use (as water expands on freezing).

Before Use to be done: "Conditioning" of Ice Packs

❖ At the time of immunization the vial of vaccines are kept in the ice packs, but before this the frozen ice packs has to be brought back to 0°C to avoid freeze damage of vaccines like DPT, Hep B and TT.

❖ This is done by keeping the ice packs at room temperature for a few seconds and wait for appearance of water droplets (by condensation) on its surface. After this vaccine can be used. This is known as *"conditioning" of ice packs.*

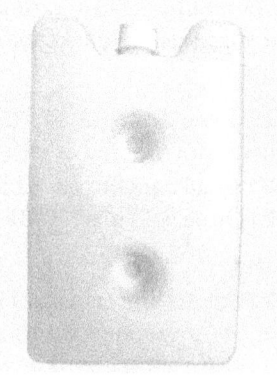

Ice pack

Use:

For temperature maintenance of vaccine content during:

❖ Immunization session

❖ Transportation in vaccine carrier.

Use of holes: To fill with vaccine vials.

Capacity: 320–340 mL

❖ In case any *leakage,* ice packs should be immediately *discarded.*

❖ Highest risk of cold chain failure: At subcenter and village level, so supplied vaccine must be used on that day only.

OPEN VIAL POLICY (2015)

Introduction

Implementation of open vial policy allows reuse of partially used multidose vials of applicable vaccines under UIP in subsequent session (both fixed and outreach) up to 4 weeks (28 days) subject to meeting certain conditions and thus reduces vaccine wastage.

Applicable to only: DPT, TT, Hep B, OPV, IPV and pentavalent vaccine.

Guidelines:

Any vial of the applicable vaccines opened/used in a session can be used at more than one immunization session up to four weeks (28 days) provided that:	Discard vaccine vial in case any one of the following conditions is met:
• The expiry date has not passed	• Expiry date has passed
• The vaccines are stored under appropriate cold chain conditions both during transportation and storage in cold chain storage point	• VVM reached/crossed discard point or vaccine vials without VVM or disfigured VVM
• The vaccine vial septum has not been submerged in water or contaminated in any way	• No label/partially torn label and/or writing on label not legible
• Aseptic technique has been used to withdraw vaccine doses	• Any vial thought to be exposed to nonsterile procedure for withdrawal
• The VVM has not reached the discard point	• Open vials that have been under water or vials removed from a vaccine carrier that has water
	• If vaccine vial is frozen or contains floccules or any foreign body
	• If there is breakage in the continuity of the vials (crack/leaks)
	• If there is any reported AEFI following use of any of the vaccine vial

Chapter
8
Family Planning

Authors' Note

The population of India is rising rapidly in 21st century and it has been remarked as one of the most dreadful national problems presently. For this reason, the importance of this chapter is increasing day by day. So, every student must know every detail of this chapter, not only for mere examination purpose (it may be asked in theory or viva-voce) but also its social point of view.

DEFINITIONS

Definition of Family Planning (FP): (Expert Committee—1971)

A way of thinking and living that is adopted voluntarily based on knowledge, attitude and responsible decision by individuals and couples, in order to promote the health and welfare of family group and thus contribute effectively to the social development of a country.

Definition of Contraception

Contraception refers specifically to mechanisms are intended to reduce the likelihood of the fertilization of an ovum by a spermatozoon.

Definition of Birth Control Method

It is a regimen of one or more actions, devices, or medications followed in order to deliberately prevent or reduce the likelihood of pregnancy or childbirth.

OBJECTIVES

Family planning refers to practices that help individuals and couples in:
- ❖ Avoiding unwanted births
- ❖ Bringing about wanted births
- ❖ Regulating pregnancy intervals
- ❖ Ages of the parent
- ❖ Number of the children in family.

Scopes of Family Planning: WHO (1970)
- ❖ The proper spacing and limitation of births
- ❖ Advice on sterility
- ❖ Education for parenthood
- ❖ Sex education

❖ Screening for pathological conditions related to the reproductive system (e.g. cervical cancer)
❖ Genetic counseling
❖ Premarital consultation and examination
❖ Carrying out pregnancy tests
❖ Marriage counseling
❖ Preparation of couples for the arrival of their first child
❖ Providing services for unmarried mothers
❖ Teaching home economics and nutrition
❖ Providing adoption services.
❖ **Small family norm**
It is very important because small differences in the family size will make big differences in the birth rate.
❖ **Family planning to family welfare concept**
 – Change of name since 1977–1978
 – Here no place of compulsion
 – Shift of focus from demography to health, welfare, development and quality of life
 – The concept of welfare is very comprehensive and is basically related to quality of life.

New punch line for family planning adopted by Govt. of India—"Plan Banate Hain" (let's make a plan) in place of "Hum Do Humare Do".

Other Important Definitions

❖ **Eligible couple:**
 – All currently married couple living together with wife in reproductive age group.
 – Terminology: 'Currently married' means their current marital status is 'married'
 – Age group or 15–44 years or 49 years
 – Number: 150–180/1000 population
 – *Importance of selection of eligible couples*:
  - Target group for providing education about benefit of FP and knowledge about contraceptives
  - Easy accessibility to eligible couples
  - Information regarding availability of contraceptives to them.
❖ **Target couples:** Referred to eligible for family planning methods.
❖ **Couple protection rate:**
 – *Definition*: It is defined as number of eligible couples effectively protected against childbirth by one or the other "Approved methods of family planning"(viz. sterilization, IUD, condom or OCP) (*mnemonic*: SICO) taking into account their effectivity
 – Current CPR (couple protection rate): 52.5%
 – Contraceptive prevalence rate: Percentage of currently married women (age 15–49 years) using any method of contraceptive (including natural methods)
 – National goal: Goal for CPR (contraceptive prevalence rate) in RCH-II (2004–2009): >65%
 – Importance: CPR is an indicator of prevalence of contraceptive practice in a community.

❖ **Effective couple protection rate:**
- Effectivity of approved contraceptive methods:

Contraceptive method	Effectivity (in %)
Conventional contraceptives (condoms)	50
IUDs	95
OCPs	100
Sterilization (vasectomy/tubectomy)	100

- Contraceptive methods providing maximum couple protection in the community— Tubectomy
- Most cost effective contraceptive method—Vasectomy.

❖ **Total fertility rate (TFR):**
- TFR represents the average number of children, a woman would have, if she passed through her reproductive years bearing children at the same rates as the women now in each age group.
- Target TFR: 2.1.

❖ **Net reproduction rate (NRR):**
- Definition: NRR is defined as the number of daughters, a newborn girl will bear during her lifetime assuming fixed age-specific fertility and mortality rates.
- Characteristics:
  - The NRR is particularly relevant where sex ratios at birth are significantly affected by the use of reproductive technologies, or where life expectancy is low.
- Significance of NRR value:

NRR	Significance
=1	Each generation of mothers is having exactly enough daughters to replace themselves in the population
<1	The reproductive performance of the population is below replacement level

NRR = 1 can be achieved if CPR > 60%.

It is equivalent to cutting off almost all third or higher order of births, leaving 2 or less surviving children per couple.

- *Points to remember:*
  - Time of birth: 20–30 years
  - Spacing of birth: minimum 3 years
  - Limiting of birth: 2 size family norm
  - Avoidance of unwanted pregnancy: safe abortion
  - The recommended interval before attempting the next pregnancy after an abortion is at least 6 months.

❖ **Cafeteria choice:**
Offer all methods from which one can choose according to needs, wishes, and preferences.
- *Principle of cafeteria choice/informed choice:*
  - Clients have the right and ability to make their own decisions
  - Clients are individuals with different needs and circumstances
  - Clients need reliable, timely, clear, accurate, specific and understandable information, including risks and benefits of methods

- Clients have the right to a choice of methods, whether through clinics, pharmacies or community distributors spacing and limiting, are available.
- Clients must be able to decide freely—without stress, pressure, coercion, or incentives.

❖ **Mode of intervention of family planning**: Health promotion (primary prevention).

Benefits of FP Services

Beneficiary	Benefits
Women	• Reduce health risk • Less worry about unplanned pregnancy • More time for herself • Greater educational employment/career opportunity • Increase social participation • Improved quality of life
Child	• Prevents LBW • Reduce congenital anomaly • More time to breastfeed and childcare • Reduce incidence of infectious diseases • Promote child growth, development and nutrition • Reduce neonatal, infant and child mortality
Family	• Higher health, nutrition, educational expenditure • Greater attention and parenteral care
Community	• Increase productivity • Greater savings and investment • Reduce burden and natural resources
Country	• Population control/stabilization • Link with sustainable development • Reduce poverty, reduce hunger, helps in maintaining gender equality • Ultimately helps in achieving national and international goals • Cost effective

Unmet Need of Family Planning

❖ *Definition*: Many women who are sexually active would prefer to avoid becoming pregnant although they are not using any methods of contraception (including use by their partner). These women are considered to have an "unmet need" for family planning.

❖ *Limitation of use*:
- Although the concept of "unmet need" may be applied to married women and sexually active unmarried women; *its measurement has been limited to married women only.*

❖ *Reasons of unmet need*:
- Inconvenience of unsatisfactory services
- Lack of information
- Fears about contraceptive side effects
- Opposition from husband/relatives.

Methods of Contraception

❖ **Spacing methods:**
- Barrier methods:
  - Physical methods: Male condom, female condom, diaphragm, vaginal sponge
  - Chemical methods: Spermicidal foams, creams, jellies and pastes, suppositories
  - Combined methods: Physical + chemical methods (e.g. condom + spermicidal jelly).

- Intrauterine devices:
  - 1st generation (non-medicated), e.g. Lippes loop
  - 2nd generation (medicated), containing metallic ions (Cu), e.g. CuT 220 B, CuT 380 A or Ag
  - 3rd generation (bio-active IUDs), e.g. progestasert, LNG-20.
- Hormonal methods:
  - Oral pills (*mnemonic:* CP POM)
    * Combined pill
    * Progestogen only pill (POP):
      ◊ Post-coital pill
      ◊ Once a month pill
  - Depot formulations
    * Injectables
      ◊ Progesterone only injectables (DMPA, NET-EN)
      ◊ Combined injectables
    * Subcutaneous: e.g. Norplant
    * Vaginal rings
- Post-conceptional methods:
  - Abortion
- Miscellaneous
  - Abstinence
  - Withdrawal
  - Safe period (rhythm method)
  - Custodial separation
  - Natural family planning methods:
    * Basal body temperature method (BBT)
    * Cervical mucus method
    * Symptothermic method.
❖ **Terminal methods:**
  - Male sterilization:
    - Vasectomy
    - No scalpel vasectomy.
  - Female sterilization:
    - Laparoscopic
    - Mini-lap operation.
❖ **Recent updates in family planning:**
  - Tagline: "Acchi Aadat Hai" (It is a Good Habit)
  - New package for Mala D
  - Max. contraceptive usage in India: Sterilization (2015).

CONVENTIONAL CONTRACEPTIVES

1. Barrier Methods

Physical methods:
❖ Condoms: Male condoms and female condoms
❖ Diaphragm
❖ Vaginal sponge.

Condoms

Male condoms and female condom.

Male Condoms

❖ **Nomenclature**:

(Latin *'condus'* = receptacle)

It is named after the inventor Dr. Condum, who recommended it to King Charles II to prevent illegal offspring.

❖ **Characteristics**:
  - Made up of latex, a kind of plastic
  - Shape: Cylindrical
  - Length: 15–20 cm
  - Diameter: 3 cm
  - Thickness: 0.003 cm
  - Used by the male partner to cover erect penis during coitus
  - Closed at one end with a teat-end and open at other end, with an integral ring.

❖ **Steps for proper use of condom (according to NACP)**:

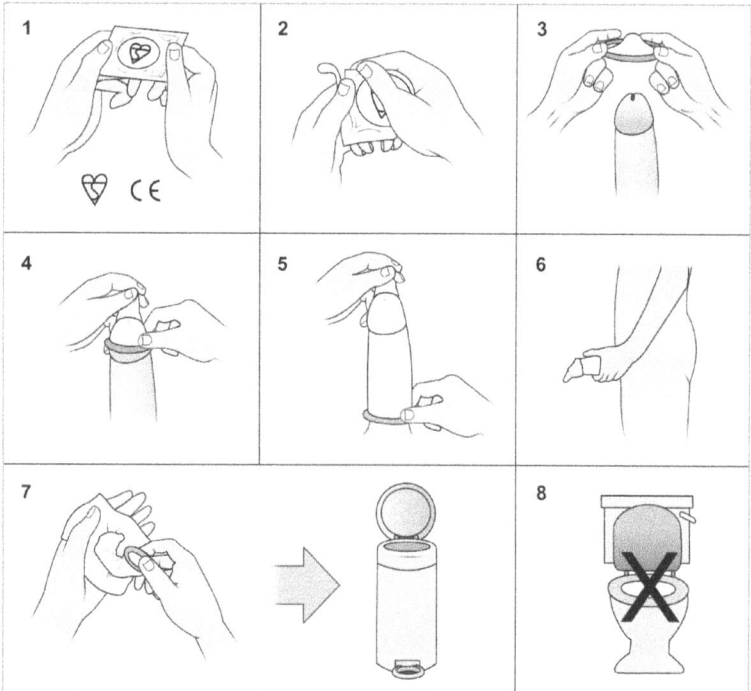

1. Open the pack carefully without damaging the condom. Wear the condom only after penis becomes fully erect.
2. Press the tip of the condom to expel air from the teat-end making room for the collection of the semen and fix it on the erect penis.
3. Hold the tip of the condom and slowly unroll it to full length so that the penis is completely covered
4. Ensure that condom is in position before commencement of sexual intercourse

5. After ejaculation hold the condom and gently withdraw the penis.
6. Remove the condom carefully without spilling the semen
7. Dispose the used condom wrapping in a piece of paper into the garbage bin, but not in dustbin or commode of latrine. Do not reuse.
8. One condom should be used for each sexual act.

❖ **Sterilization:** It is electronically pretested and pre-sterilized by gamma-radiation and make available in packs.
❖ **Storage**: > 3 years can weaken latex and increase chances of breakage.
❖ **Types of male condom:**
   – Dry type/non-lubricated: Nirodh (Sanskrit means prevention), it had already been phased out.
   – Deluxe types/lubricated: Lubricants used: spermicide, glycerine, etc., but oil based lubricants should not be used, as they weaken the rubber very quickly
   – Super deluxe: Colored, thinner, lubricated variety.

Non-contraceptive use of condom
   i. As tourniquet
  ii. For collection of urine
 iii. Helps in prevention of STD, carcinoma cervix, PID.

Female Condom
Also called 'Femidom'.
❖ **Characteristics**:
   – Made up of thin transparent, soft plastic, closed at smaller end and opened at wider end
   – Stiff flexible rings at both ends
   – Before sex woman places the closed end of the sheath high up in the vagina and larger open end stays outside the vulva.
   – **Velvet:**
      - 1st indigenous female condom
      - 1st contraceptive method which provides protection against STDs and serves as contraception.

Diaphragm
(or vaginal diaphragm, Dutch diaphragm).

Also called Dutch cap (named after German physician Dutch neo-Malthusians).
❖ **Characteristics**:
   – Size: 5-10 cm diameter
   – Soft latex/silicone dome with spring molded into the rim
   – Diaphragm is not in national program.
❖ **Method of insertion:**
   – Hold the diaphragm with dome down, like a cup, with a tablespoon (5 mL) of jelly into the cup
   – Press the opposite sides of the rim together
   – Push the diaphragm into the vagina as far as it goes
   – Make sure that it covers the cervix with her fingers
      - When it is inserted, it lies snugly between the sacrum and pubic symphysis.
      - It is held in position partly by the tone of vaginal muscles.

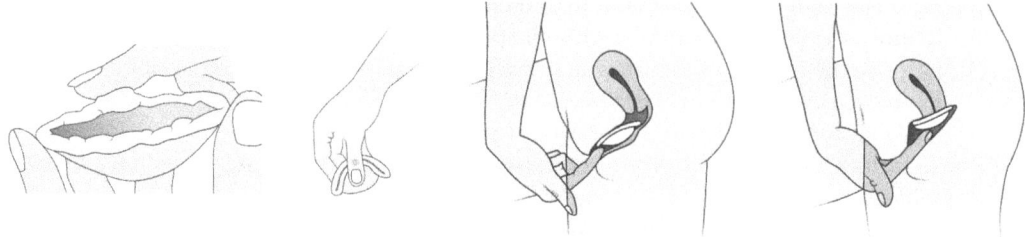

- ❖ **Time of insertion**: Just before the intercourse
- ❖ **Time of removal**: At least 6 hours of act of intercourse. It should not be retained for > 24 hours (toxic shock syndrome may occur in that case).
- ❖ **Method of removal**: She should hook the rim behind the pubic symphysis and pull out carefully. After removal it should be thoroughly washed with soap and water.

Vaginal Sponge

- ❖ **Brand name**: TODAY

Combines barrier+ spermicidal methods

- ❖ **Characteristics:**
  - – Small poly urethane sponge
  - – Size: 5 cm × 2.5 cm
  - – Saturated with 1 g of spermicide 'Non-oxynol-9'.
- ❖ **Mode of use**:
  - – Vaginal sponge must run under water till thoroughly wet before insertion
  - – Inserted vaginally prior to intercourse and must be placed over the cervix to be effective
  - – Must be left in place for hours after ejaculation and removed within specified time limits according to the manufacturer.

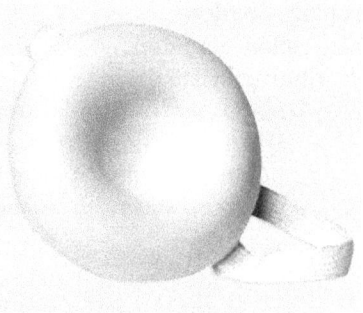

Vaginal sponge

2. Chemical Methods

- ❖ Categories:
  - – Spermicidal foams
  - – Creams
  - – Jellies and pastes
  - – Suppositories.
- ❖ Mechanism of action:
  - – Spermicides contains a base into which a spermicide is incorporated.
  - – Commonly used spermicides are surface active agents which attach themselves to spermatozoa and inhibit oxygen uptake and kill sperms.

3. Combined Methods

Both physical + chemical methods used at a time, e.g. condom + spermicidal jelly; diaphragm + jelly. Effectivity much better than physical/chemical methods are used alone.

INTRAUTERINE DEVICES (IUDs)

These are the devices when placed inside the uterus, prevent the birth of child, by acting as a foreign body.

❖ Historical backgrounds:
  - Arabs used this principle to control conceptions in camels by introducing a small spherical stone into each horn of uterus
  - 1st person successfully used IUD in woman was Mr. Ota in Japan

❖ Parts: It consists of:
  i. Copper T
  ii. Inserter and plunger with blue depth gauge/ flange
    - Blue gauze: for measurement of length (flange).
    - Horizontal stem: 3.2 cm; placed in between 2 cornu of uterus
    - Vertical stem: 3.6 cm
    - Strings:
      * For easy removal of IUD
      * Woman can feel that it is in position.

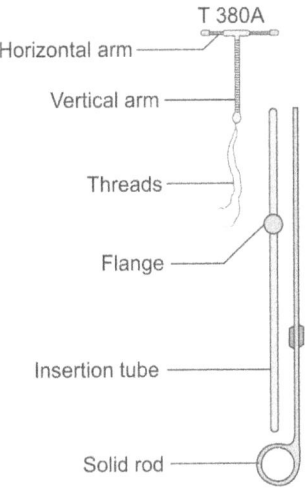

Parts of Cu T

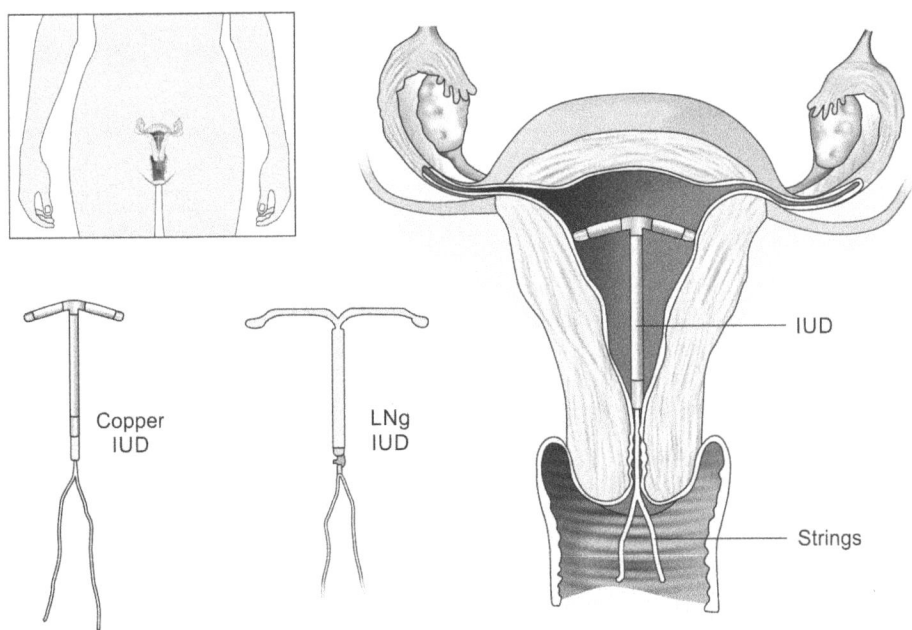

❖ Classification of IUDs:

Types of IUD	Non-medicated IUDs	Medicated IUDs	Bioactive IUDs
Generations	1st generation	2nd generation	3rd generation
Material used	Polyethylene and impregnated with barium sulfate for radio-opacity	Inert IUDs Polyethylene and reinforced with copper metal and barium sulfate	Made from vinyl co-polymer which contains the requisite quantity of progesterone hormone and also contains barium sulfate for radio-opacity
Shape	Open serpentine, open spiral, configuration of 8, etc.	'T' or modified 'T' shaped Some also have surrogate fins, e.g. multiload devices	Mostly 'T' shaped devices that releases a fixed quantity of progesterone hormones
Mode of actions	• Cellular/biochemical changes in endometrium/uterine fluids • Impair viability of gamete • Reduces chance of fertilization, rather than implantation	Acts primarily by releasing Cu ions which: • Enhances cellular response in endometrium • Affects enzymes in uterus • Alter cervical mucus thus affecting sperm motility, capacitation and survival	• Increase viscosity of cervical mucus • Prevent sperm from entering cervix • Hinders the maturation of endometrium as well as making it unfavorable for implantation (high progesterone and low estrogen)
Major disadvantages	• Increased complication • Increased menstrual bleeding • High rate of expulsion • Increase chance of ectopic pregnancy • Higher pregnancy rate	• Increased menstrual bleeding, but less than 1st generation devices	• Expensive
Advantages	Safe while breastfeeding	• Failure rates of <1%/year • Can be used as an emergency contra-ceptive (3–5 days of unprotected intercourse) • Better tolerated and easier to fit in nullipara • Low expulsion rate • Less side effects	• No menorrhagia (applicable in high prevalence of anemic countries) • Less chance of expulsion • Less incidence of side effects
Examples	• Lippes loop • Grafenberg's ring	Earlier devices: • Cu -7 • Cu-T 200 Newer: • CuT 220 B, • CuT 380 A or Ag • Multiload devices	Progestasert (not used nowadays), LNG-20

❖ **Some points to remember:**

In CuT 220 B, CuT 380 A or Ag
  – Numbers (220, 380) represent surface area of copper (in sq. mm) on the device
  – 'B' in CuT 220 B represent: size of IUD (different sizes A, B, C and D; D is the largest).
    [Larger sized IUD has:

- Greater anti-fertility effect and lower expulsion rate
- But a higher removal rate due to increased side effects (e.g. pain, bleeding, etc.)
- Suitable for multiparous women]
  - A or Ag in CuT 220B represent: *Silver (with Cu)* to give strength to CuT.

Progestasert

❖ T-shaped device filled with 38 mg of progesterone
❖ Reservoir: Silicon oil
❖ Rate of hormone release: 65 µg/day
❖ Shelf life: 1–1.5 years
❖ Disadvantage of progestasert:
- Expensive
- Highest no. of ectopic pregnancies
- Not used nowadays.

LNG-20

(Levonorgestrel-20 IUD)
❖ Rate of hormone release: 20 µg/day
❖ Effective life: 10 years

Advantage

Less menstrual bleeding and fewer days of bleeding than the Cu devices.

Disadvantage

Expensive.

Points to Remember

Parameters	Highest	Lowest
Expulsion rate	Lippes loop	Progestasert
Removal rate	LNG-20 IUD	Progestasert
Pregnancy rate	Lippes loop	LNG-20 IUD

Ideal Candidate for IUD

According to Planned Parenthood Federation of America (PPFA), the ideal candidate for IUD are:
❖ Who has borne at least one child
❖ Has no history of pelvic disease
❖ Has normal menstrual periods
❖ Is willing to check the IUD tail
❖ Has access to follow up and treatment of potential problems, and
❖ Is in a monogamous relationship.

According to American College of Obstetricians and Gynecologists (ACOG), IUDs are "not recommended for women who have not had children or who have or who have multiple partners, because of risk of PID and possible infertility".

Timing of Insertion of IUD

Loop insertion at any time during women's reproductive years (except during pregnancy):

Timing	Comment

During/within 10 days of beginning of menstrual period (counting from 1st day)	• Easy insertion
	• Because:
	  – Cervical canal diameter more
	  – Uterus relaxed + myometrial contractions lead to less expulsion
	  – Less chance of pregnancy

Immediate postpartum insertion (during 1st week after delivery before woman leaves hospital)	• High chance of perforation • High chance of expulsion
Post-puerperal insertion (during 6–8 weeks after delivery)	• Convenient • Can be combined with follow-up visit for mother and child • Not recommended after 2nd trimester abortion
Post abortal	Within 1st trimester
Emergency	Within 5 days of unprotected intercourse

Non-contraceptive Benefits of IUD

❖ Synechiolysis in Asherman's syndrome (uterine synechiae)
❖ Reduction of risk of endometrial cancer
❖ Hormone replacement therapy (HRT)
❖ Adjuvant therapy to tamoxifen (LNG IUD).

Follow up

❖ Objective:
  – To provide motivation + emotional support
  – Confirmation of presence of IUD
  – Diagnose and treat any side effects/complications.
❖ Timing:
After 1st menstrual period → 3rd menstrual period → 6 month or 1 year.

Follow up	Objective
After 1st menstrual period	Chances of loop expulsion high in this period
After 3rd menstrual period	To evaluate the problems of pain
After 6 months/1 year	Depending upon the facilities and conveniences of the patient

❖ Side effects:

Side effects	Manifestations	Treatment	Special notes

Bleeding (Most common complication)	• Menstrual bleeding:
	  – amount
	  – duration
	• Midcycle bleeding usually disappear by 3 months
		• Reassurance (Don't remove IUD)
		• Ferrous sulfate tab. 100 mg daily × 100 days
		• Heavy persistent bleeding: remove IUD
			• Can lead to iron deficiency anemia
			• MC side effect of IUD insertion
			• Leads to 10–20% of all IUD removal

Pain (most common complication which entails removal of IUD)	Causes of severe pain in IUD insertion: • Incorrect placement • Disparity of size (most common) • Uterine perforation and infection	• Usually disappears by 3 months • Slight pain: ibuprofen+ PPI • Intolerable pain: removal of IUD	• 2nd MC side effect of IUD insertion • MCC of IUD removal (15–40%)

Contd...

Contd...

Side effects	Manifestations	Treatment	Special notes
	Common in: • Nullipara and • Women not having child for many years		

Pelvic infection (pelvic inflammatory disease)
Organisms (*Gardnerella*, Anaerobic strep., Bacteroides)
	• Vaginal discharge
	• Pelvic pain and tenderness
	• Abnormal bleeding
	• Chill sand fever
	• Ultimately may lead to infertility
		• Prompt treatment with broad spectrum antibiotic
		• If no response to antibiotics in 24–48 hours: remove IUDs
			• IUD ↑ risk of PID in woman—2–8 times
			• Higher risk in:
			  – Women with greater no. of sexual partners
			  – In few months after insertion

Uterine perforation	More common in: IUD inserted in 2 days–6 weeks of postpartum	Diagnosis : By pelvic X-ray Treatment: Removal of IUD	Incidence: 1:150–1:9000 insertions
Pregnancy with in-situ	Outcomes : Spontaneous abortion: 50% Successful pregnancy: 25%	• If woman requests: MTP • If she wants to continue pregnancy and threads are visible: Remove IUD gently by pulling the threads • If she wants to continue pregnancy and threads are NOT visible: do careful examination for complication; if any infective sign (+ve) → give broad spectrum antibiotic	Actual failure rate in 1st year: 3%.
Ectopic pregnancy IUD-in-situ	• Lower abdominal pain • Dark and scanty vaginal bleeding or amenorrhea	Woman with IUDs be taught to recognize symptoms	Woman with high risk of ectopic pregnancy: should not use IUDs
Spontaneous expulsion	Usually occurs in: first few weeks following insertion or during menstruation		Expulsion rate: 12–20% High risk group: • Young, nulliparous women • Postpartum insertion • Inert (non-medicated IUDs)
Mortality associated with IUD use	Very low 1 death/1 lac woman-years of use		Safer than OCP

❖ Contraindications of IUD insertion:

Absolute	Relative
• Suspected pregnancy	• Anemia
• Pelvic inflammatory disease	• Menorrhagia
• Vaginal bleeding of undiagnosed etiology	• History of PID since last pregnancy
• Cancer of the cervix, uterus or adnexa and other pelvic tumors	• Purulent cervical discharge
• Previous ectopic pregnancy	• Distortions of uterine cavity due to congenital malformations, fibroids
	• Unmotivated person

❖ WHO medical eligibility criteria for contraceptive use:
 Category-I: Can use
 Category-II: Can use, but have any contraindication
 Category-III: Cannot use; but can be used with permission in special condition CuT not recommended
 Category-IV: Cannot use; CuT contraindicated.
❖ Warning signs for IUD according to PPFA (Planned Parenthood Federation of America): (Mnemonic: PAINS)
  – P—Period late (pregnancy), abnormal spotting or bleeding
  – A—Abdominal pain, pain during intercourse
  – I—Infection (any STI), abnormal discharge
  – N—Not feeling well, fever, chills
  – S—Strings missing, shorter or longer.
❖ IUD come out technique/insertion/IUD loading technique:
  – Nowadays pull/withdrawal technique.
 Uterine length measured by uterine sound method
 (Normal uterine length: 6.5 cm)
 IUD insertion can be done by trained ANMs.
❖ Method of insertion of IUDs (CuT 200/CuT 380A):
 Preliminary steps:
  – History taking and examinations (general and pelvic) to exclude any contraindication of insertions.
  – Patient is informed about various problems, the device is shown to her and consent is obtained
  – Insertion is done in OPD taking aseptic precaution without sedation or anesthesia.
  – To reduce cramping pain Ibuprofen (200–400 mg) 30 minutes before insertion
  – Placement of the device inside the inserter— the device is taken out from the sealed packet. The thread and the vertical stem are introduced through the distal end of the inserter. The device is now ready for introduction. "No touch" insertion method is preferred.

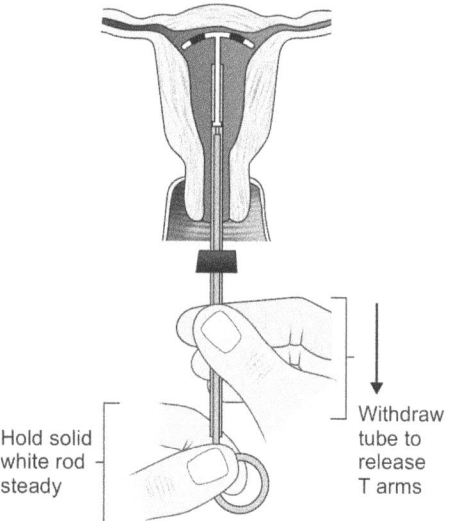

Hold solid white rod steady

Withdraw tube to release T arms

 Prerequisites:
  – The patient empties her bladder
  – Position: lithotomy
 "No touch" insertion technique includes:
  – Loading the IUD in the inserter without opening the sterile package. The loaded inserter is now taken out of the package without touching the distal end
  – Not to touch the vaginal wall and the speculum while introducing the loaded IUD inserter through the cervical end.
 Multiload 375:
 The applicator with the device is just to be taken out of the sealed packet in a 'no-touch' method and the same is pushed through the cervical canal up to the fundus of the uterus. The applicator is then withdrawn.

Instructions to the patient:
– The possible symptoms of pain and slight vaginal bleeding should be explained.
– Patient should be advised to feel the thread periodically by the finger.

Complication during insertion and treatment:
Perforation:
– Major perforation : Rest
– Minor perforation: Hysterectomy/laparotomy.

Restoration of fertility after removal:
– Fertility is not impaired after removal of IUD (provided there is no episode of PID)
– 70% of IUD users conceive within 1 year of removal.

HORMONAL METHODS

Also called steroidal contraceptives (not synonymous to "steroid" usually used to refer adrenocortical hormones).
❖ Synthetic estrogen, e.g. ethinyl estradiol and mestranol
❖ Synthetic progesterone, e.g. medroxyprogesterone acetate, norethisterone acetate, etc.

Oral Pills

Combined pill: Contains both synthetic estrogen and progestogen in low dose (so called as "Low dose oral contraceptive") as to be safe and effective
❖ Estrogen–Ethynyl estradiol → 30–35 µg
❖ Progesterone–Norethisterone → 0.5–1.0 mg
❖ FDA approves Lo-Loestrin 10 mg (minimum possible dose).

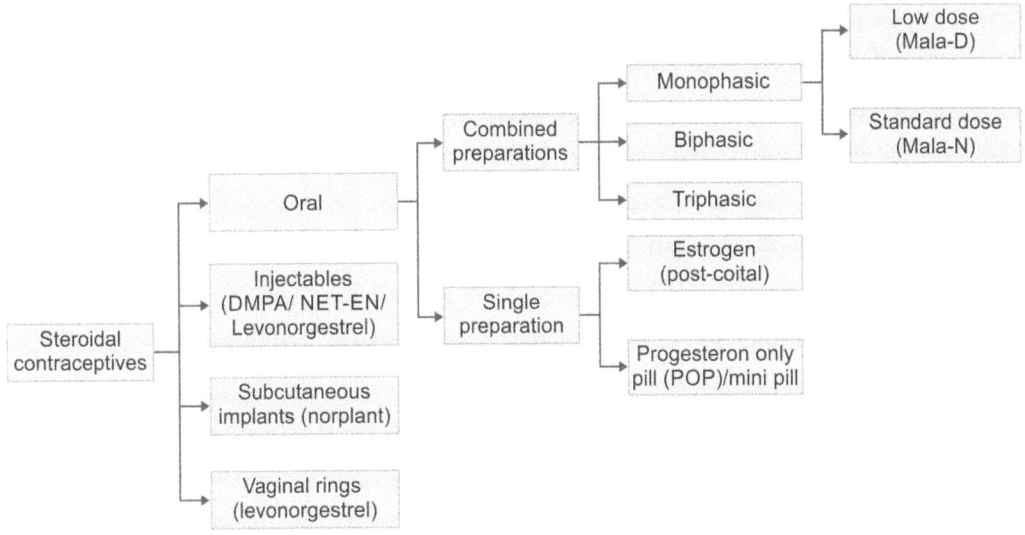

Mechanism of Action
❖ Suppresses ovulation by suppression of hypothalamo-pituitary-gonadotropin axis.
❖ Progesterone component: increases thickness of cervical mucosa.
❖ Increases tubal motility.

Different types of pills:

❖ **Monophasic pill**
- Monophasic pills are oral contraceptives that have the same amount of estrogen and progestin in each active pill in a pack.
- Due to the consistent hormone level in each pill, monophasic pills are less likely to cause side effects that may stem from fluctuating hormones.
- Monophasic pills are classified by their estrogen level:
  - Low dose pills have the least amount of estrogen (20 μg)
  - Regular dose pills contain 30–35 μg estrogen
  - High dose pills have about 50 μg of estrogen
- Remember:
  - Mala-**N** → under **N**ational program
  - Mala –D → under social marketing.

❖ **Biphasic pill**
- Biphasic birth control pills alter the level of hormones once during the menstrual cycle.
- Biphasic pills deliver the same amount of estrogen each day, but the level of progestin is increased about halfway through the cycle.
- Although the estrogen level remains the same, during the first half of the cycle, the progestin/estrogen ratio is lower to allow the endometrium to thicken as it normally does. During the second half of the cycle, the progestin/estrogen ratio is higher to allow for the normal shedding of the lining of the uterus.
- The first 7 to 10 days are one strength (and usually one color), and the next 11 to 14 pills are another strength (and another color).
- The last 7 tablets (if included) are placebo pills and contain no hormones.

❖ **Triphasic pill**
- Triphasic combination pills contain 3 different doses of hormones in the 3 weeks of active pills, so the hormone combination changes approximately every 7 days throughout the pill pack.
- Depending on the brand, the amount of estrogen may change as well as the amount of progestin. In a single month's supply, triphasic pills may have a gradual estrogen increase and/or some pills may also increase the dose of progestin.
- Therefore, since there are 3 different strength combinations in each pack, the first third pills consist of one strength (and one color).
- The next 5, 7 or 9 pills are another strength (and another color). The final phase of pills are a different color.
- The last 7 pills (if included) are placebo pills and contain no hormones.

Instructions:
- The pill is given orally for 21 consecutive days beginning on the 5th day of the menstrual cycle
- Preferably at bed-time
- In the direction of the arrow over the packet
- Followed by break for 7 days in case of 21 pills packet or continue one placebo daily in case of 28 pills (during this time period the woman will have menstruation)
- Usually bleeding occurs 2–3 days after the last menstrual period
- When bleeding occurs it is considered to be the 1st day of the next cycle
- She must take pills as long as she does not want to continue her pregnancy.

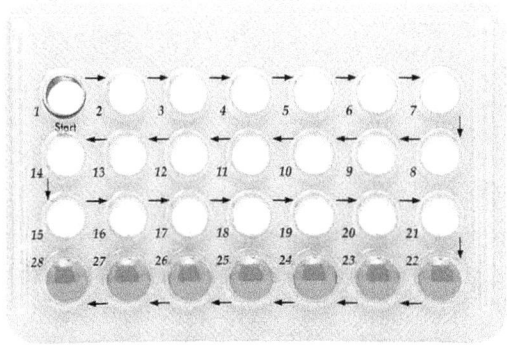

❖ **Missed pills:**

Missed 1 pill in any row?
- Take it as soon as she remembers
- Take rest as usual.

Missed 2 or more pills in first 14 pills?
- Take 1 now.
- Take all the rest as usual.
- Also use condoms or spermicide for 7 days.

Missed 2 or more of pills in 3rd row (15th to 21st pill)?
- Take 1 now.
- Take rest of this row, on each day.
- Start a new pack on the next day.
- Throw the last row of this pack away.
- Also use condoms or spermicide for 7 days.

Missed array of 7 pills of 4th row (22nd to 28th pill)?
- Throw the missed pills away.
- Take the rest usual.

Never take 3 pills in a day.

Benefits of Contraceptive Pills

a. *Contraceptive benefits*: Single most benefit of the pill is it's almost 100% effectiveness in preventing pregnancy and thereby removing anxiety and risk of unplanned pregnancy.
b. *Non-contraceptive benefits*:
   - Regularization of irregular menstrual cycles especially in Stein Levinthal syndrome (polycystic ovarian disease).
   - Reduced incidence and improvement in:
     - Benign breast disorders (fibrocystic disease, fibroadenoma)
     - Benign ovarian disease (ovarian cysts)
     - Malignant ovarian disease (ovarian cancer)
     - Pelvic inflammatory disease
     - Ectopic pregnancy
     - Iron deficiency anemia (anemia related to menstruation)
     - Dysmenorrhea
     - Mild to moderate acne
     - Hirsutism

- Endometriosis
- Adenomyosis
- Endometrial cancer
- Colorectal cancer
- Osteopenia, osteoporosis.

Adverse Effects of Combined OCP

❖ Cardiovascular disease (due to estrogenic effects):
  – MI
  – Cerebral thrombosis
  – Venous thrombosis
  – Hypertension.
❖ Carcinogenesis:
  – Cervical cancer
  – Breast cancer.
❖ Metabolic effects:
  – Hypertension
  – Altered lipid profile ($\downarrow$ HDL)
  – Blood clotting
  – Hyperglycemia and $\uparrow$ Plasma insulin.
❖ Other adverse effects:
  – Liver disorders
    - Hepatocellular adenoma
    - Gallbladder disease
    - Cholestatic jaundice
  – Lactation (due to estrogenic effect): Alter quality, quantity and frequency of breast milk
  – Subsequent fertility: Slight delay in returning conception upon discontinuation
  – Ectopic pregnancy: More common in women taking POPs
  – Fetal development: Birth defects of fetus.
❖ Common unwanted effects:
  – Breast tenderness
  – Weight gain
  – Headache and migraine
  – Bleeding disturbances.

Contraindications

Absolute contraindications	Special problems requiring medical surveillance
◆ Cancer of breast and genitals	◆ Age >40 years
◆ Liver disease	◆ Smoking and age >35 years
◆ History of thromboembolism	◆ Mild hypertension
◆ Cardiac abnormalities	◆ Chronic renal disease
◆ Congenital hyperlipidemia	◆ Epilepsy
◆ Undiagnosed abnormal uterine bleeding	◆ Migraine
	◆ Nursing mothers (0–6 months)
	◆ Diabetes mellitus
	◆ Gallbladder disease
	◆ History of infrequent bleeding
	◆ Amenorrhea

Duration of Use

❖ Usually recommended for young women
❖ >35 years should go for other modes of contraception
❖ >40 years usually not prescribed (↑ incidence of cardiovascular complications).

Medical Supervision

Checklist for prescription of oral contraceptives:
❖ >40 years of age
❖ >35 years of age + heavy smoker
❖ Seizures
❖ Severe pain in the calves/thighs
❖ Severe chest pain
❖ Symptomatic varicose veins in the legs
❖ Severe headache and/or visual disturbances
❖ Lactating <6 months
❖ Inter-menstrual bleeding and/or bleeding after sexual intercourse
❖ Amenorrhea
❖ Abnormally yellow skin and eyes
❖ SBP >140 and/or DBP >90 mm Hg
❖ Mass in the breast
❖ Swollen legs (edema).

Instruction: If all the above is found (–) → The woman may be given OCPs. If any are (+) → She must be first seen by the doctor.

Progestogen Only Pill (POP)

❖ Also called: 'Minipill'/'Micropill'
❖ Contains progesterone (Norethisterone and Levonorgestrel) in small amount
❖ It makes cervical mucus viscid.

Indications

❖ Good for lactating mother
❖ Young woman with risk of neoplasia
❖ Older woman with cardiovascular risks
❖ When estrogen is contraindicated → ectopic pregnancy.

Mechanism of Action

❖ Thickens the cervical mucosa, affects penetrability of sperms
❖ It induces a thin, unfavorable, atrophic endometrium.

Instructions

❖ Can start any time after childbirth/miscarriage.
❖ No need to wait for menstrual periods to return ensuring that she is not pregnant
❖ The 1st day of bleeding is the best time to start (if periods have returned)
❖ When she finishes 1 pack next pack immediately should be started
❖ No wait between the packs
❖ Each pill should be taken at same time everyday
❖ Delay between 2 pills should increase the risk of pregnancy.

Missed Pills

❖ If forgot to take ≥1 pill(s) she should take 1 pill as soon she remembers and then keep taking 1 pill each day as usual.
❖ In case of delay for >3 hours in woman (with returned menses) barrier methods should be used for 2 days and take the missed pill as soon as she remembers and then keep taking 1 pill each day as usual.

Effectiveness

For breastfeeding women effectiveness is >99%.

Advantages

❖ Good choice for lactating mother as it do not suppress breastfeeding
❖ Free from estrogen-induced side effect
❖ May help to prevent benign breast disease, PID, endometrial and ovarian cancer
❖ Lengthen the period of lactational amenorrhea.

Disadvantages

❖ Poor cycle control
❖ ↑ Pregnancy rate.

Postcoital Pill

Emergency contraception (= Postcoital contraception).

Definition

Emergency contraceptive methods are the backup methods for contraceptive emergencies, which women can use within the first few days of an unprotected coitus to prevent an unwanted pregnancy.

It is not a regular family planning method.

Aims of Emergency Contraception

❖ Reduce maternal mortality
❖ Reduce the fertility levels.

[The Government of India introduced Emergency Contraceptive Pills (ECP) in the National Family Welfare Programmes (in 2003) as one of the strategies to prevent unwanted pregnancies].

Indications

❖ After voluntary sexual act without contraceptive protection
❖ Incorrect/inconsistent use of regular contraceptive method.
  – Failure to take OCPs for > 3 days
  – Starting a new pack > 3 days later
  – Being late for contraceptive injection.
❖ Contraceptive failure/mishaps:
  – Slippage/leakage/breakage of condoms
  – Miscalculation of safe period
  – Failed coitus interruptus.

Different Methods

- ❖ Non-hormonal method: Cu-IUD
- ❖ Hormonal pills:
    - Also called morning after pills.

Regimen	Dosing	Timing of dose after intercourse	Reported efficacy	Remarks
Levonorgestrel	0.75 mg/1.5 mg	0–72 hrs	75–85%	Single dose
Combined pills (EE* -0.1 mg + NG*- 1 mg/NE*-2 mg) (Yuzpe method)	One stat dose and the dose is to be repeated after 12 hrs	0–75 hrs	75%	2 pills (containing EE—50 µg) stat and 2 pills after 12 hrs 4 pills (containing EE—30/35 µg) stat and 4 pills after 12 hrs

*Ethinyl estradiol (EE), Norgestrel (NG), Norethisterone (NE)

- ❖ Mifepristone not an EC pill—Abortifacient
- ❖ Under RCH LNG 1.5 mg tabs are the dedicated product for EC.

Mechanism of Action

- ❖ Depends on the phase of the menstrual cycle
- ❖ Inhibits ovulation/fertilization/implantation
- ❖ Not effective once the implantation has occurred
- ❖ 72 hours should be calculated from the first unprotected coital act of the cycle
- ❖ Effectiveness: 85% within 72 hours.

Advantages

- ❖ Safe and effective
- ❖ Widely available
- ❖ Does not require physical examination
- ❖ Does not require the prescription of RMP
- ❖ Can be given to a woman in whom hormonal pills are contraindicated
- ❖ Can be taken as many times as possible during a cycle
- ❖ Does not cause fetal malformations
- ❖ Not an abortifacient
- ❖ No delay in return of fertility.

Side Effects

Bleeding
- ❖ 10–15% women complain regarding the amount, duration and timing of the menstruation
- ❖ Irregular bleeding—LMP may start earlier or later.

Management
- ❖ Counsel that these are normal
- ❖ If menstruation delayed for > 7days: Suspicion of pregnancy.

Nausea and vomiting
- ❖ Vomiting within 2 hours of taking the EC pills, the dose is to be repeated
- ❖ Anti-emetics if required.

Abdominal pain, fatigue, dizziness, headache, breast tenderness
- ❖ Analgesics.

Limitations
- ❖ Closer a woman is to the ovulation time, less effective are the pills
- ❖ Inability to render protection beyond the 72–120 hours
- ❖ Does not protect against STI.

Role of a Service Provider
- ❖ Never be denied to clients of the reproductive age irrespective of age and marital status
- ❖ Clients should be informed regarding availability
- ❖ Provide EC pills as back up methods in case of contraceptive failure
- ❖ Encourage users of emergency contraceptive pills to accept a regular contraceptive method (through informed choice) or return to the method that was being used earlier, or switch to a different method that is more suitable.

Who are the service providers?
- ❖ EC pills:
  - Trained ASHAs, ANMs, LHVs, SNs and doctors-village level.
- ❖ IUD:
  - Trained and certified ANMs (Auxiliary nurse midwifes), LHVs (Lady health visitors), SNs and doctors
  - Subcentre and higher levels.
- ❖ Request for EC:
  - LMP (last menstrual period)
  - Length of the menstrual cycle
  - All unprotected coitus that had taken place during that cycle
  - The hours/days elapsed since the first unprotected intercourse
  - E.C fails → Client pregnant → Counsel for MTP.

Centchroman
- ❖ Synthetic non-steroidal oral contraceptive.
- ❖ *Brand name*: Saheli.
- ❖ *Component*: Ormeloxifene.
- ❖ *Mechanism of action*:
  - Act as SERM (Selective estrogen receptor modulator)
  - Works as weakly estrogenic and potent anti-estrogenic properties.
- ❖ *Dosage*: 1 tab. (30 mg) twice a week × 3 months → then 1 tab. (30 mg) once a week.
- ❖ *Use*:
  - As a contraceptive
  - As a treatment of dysfunctional uterine bleeding.
- ❖ *Contraindications*:
  - Polycystic ovarian disease (PCOD)
  - Cervical hyperplasia
  - Recent history of jaundice
  - Severe allergic disease.

Once a Month Pill

❖ Long acting estrogen + short acting progesterone
❖ Unacceptable for high pregnancy rate and irregular bleeding
❖ Example: Quinesterol.

Male Pill

Principle of action:
❖ To prevent spermatogenesis
❖ To interfere with storage and maturation of sperms
❖ To prevent transportation of sperms in the vas
❖ To change the composition of the seminal fluid so as to affect viability of sperms, example: Gossypol.

Depot Formulations

❖ Injectables:
  Progesterone only injectables:
  – DMPA = Depot Medroxy Progesterone Acetate
    Dose: 150 mg IM → 3 months
  – Good choice for multi-parae >35 years who have completed their family.
  – NET-EN = Norethindrone enantate
    Dose: 200 mg every 60 days.
  Combined injectables:
  Estrogen + progesterone
  Given at monthly intervals ± 3 days.
❖ Subcutaneous:
  Implanted beneath the skin of forearm/upper arm
  Norplant:
  Consists of 6 silastic capsules containing 35 mg (each) LNG
  Norplant (R) -2: Easier to insert and remove
❖ Vaginal rings:
  Rings containing LNG inserted in the vagina.
  It is worn for 3 weeks of the cycle and removed during 4th week.
❖ **Recent updates of injectable contraceptives under National Program:**
  Pilot project tested in Haryana
  (Program: SALAMATI all PHCs, CHCs, SDH and DH will be provided free of cost).

THE MEDICAL TERMINATION OF PREGNANCY (MTP) ACT, 1971

It extends to the whole of India except the State of Jammu and Kashmir.

Features

MTP Act—an enabling act which aims to improve the maternal health scenario by preventing large number of unsafe abortions and consequent high incidence of maternal mortality and morbidity.

❖ Legalizes abortion services
❖ Promotes access to safe abortion services to women
❖ De-criminalizes the abortion seeker
❖ Offers protection to medical practitioners who otherwise would be penalized under the Indian Penal Code (Sections 315–316).

Indications

Mnemonic: THES
❖ *Therapeutic*: Continuation of pregnancy constitutes risk to the life or grave injury to the physical or mental health of woman
❖ *Humanitarian*: Pregnancy caused by rape (presumed grave injury to mental health)
❖ *Eugenic*: Substantial risk of physical or mental abnormalities in the fetus as to render it seriously handicapped
❖ *Social:* Contraceptive failure in married couple (presumed grave injury to mental health).

Place Where Pregnancy may be Terminated?

A hospital established or maintained by Government.

Or

A place approved for the purpose of this Act by a District-level Committee constituted by the government with the CMHO as Chairperson.

Who can Terminate Pregnancies?

❖ For termination up to 12 weeks:
  – A practitioner who has assisted a registered medical practitioner in performing 25 cases of MTP of which at least 5 were performed independently in a hospital established or maintained or a training institute approved for this purpose by the government.
❖ For termination up to 20 weeks:
  – A practitioner who holds a postgraduate degree or diploma in obstetrics and gynecology.
  – A practitioner who has completed 6 months housestaffship in obstetrics and gynecology.
  – A practitioner who has at least one-year experience in practice of obstetrics and gynecology at a hospital which has all facilities.
  – A practitioner registered in state medical register immediately before commencement of the Act, (1971) experience in practice of obstetrics and gynecology for a period not less than three years.

When the Pregnancies can be Terminated

❖ Up to 20 weeks gestation
❖ With the consent of the woman. If the woman is below 18 years or is mentally ill, then with consent of a guardian
❖ With the opinion of a registered medical practitioner, formed in good faith, under certain circumstances
❖ Opinion of two RMPs required for termination of pregnancy between 12 and 20 weeks (up to 12 weeks –single opinion).

MTP Rules 2003

Persons who have carry out MTP should be having 3 years experiences in gynecology and obstetrics, or has obtained a PG degree.

NATURAL FAMILY PLANNING METHODS

Basal Body Temperature (BBT)

Definition

Basal body temperature is the lowest temperature attained by the body during rest (usually during sleep).

Depends on: Rise of temperature [(0.3–0.5°C (or 0.5–1°F) after ovulation]

Phase	BBT	Hormonal basis
Before ovulation	Low	Since the higher levels of estrogen present during the preovulatory (follicular) phase of the menstrual cycle lower BBTs
After ovulation	Rises slightly to about 0.3–0.5°C	Because the higher levels of progesterone released by the corpus luteum after ovulation raise BBTs

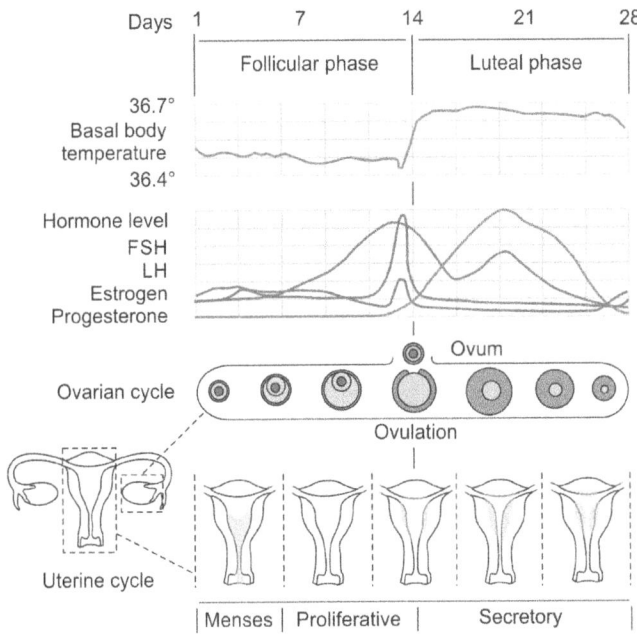

Role in Birth Control

Couples who wish to avoid a pregnancy abstain from intercourse from the onset of menses until three days after the woman's basal body temperature has risen, to about 0.3–0.5°C (or 0.5–1°F) signifying the end of the fertile phase.

Disadvantages

- ❖ Abstinence necessary for entire preovulatory period
- ❖ Cough, cold, fever, infective conditions may alter BBT
- ❖ No protection for STD
- ❖ Technical errors like:
  - – Recording failure
  - – Instrumental error.

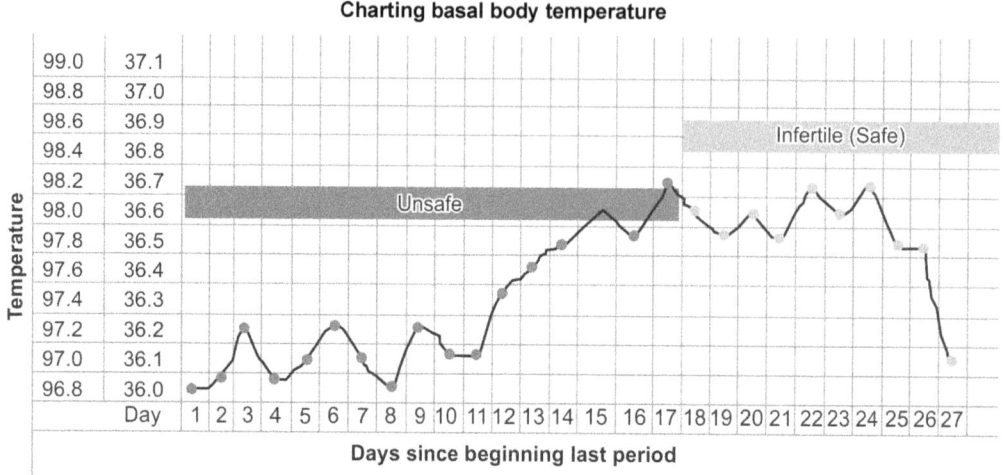

Charting basal body temperature

Cervical Mucus Methods

Also called: Billing's method/Ovulation method.

Method:

Slippery cervical mucus   No slippery cervical mucus
(avoid sexual intercourse)   (have sexual intercourse)

It is recommended that the women uses a tissue paper to wipe the inside of vagina to assess the quantity and characteristics of mucus.

Based on: Timing	Changes in the characteristics of cervical mucus
At ovulation	Watery, clear, smooth, slippery, profuse (like egg white)
After ovulation	Thickens and lessens in quantity (due to effect of progesterone)

OTHER METHODS OF CONTRACEPTION

Lactational Amenorrhea Method (LAM)

Lactational amenorrhea is the temporary **postnatal** infertility that occurs when a woman is **amenorrheic** (not menstruating) and fully **breastfeeding**.

Criteria to Achieve 98% Effectiveness of LAM during 1st 6 months of Postpartum

❖ Breastfeeding must be the infant's only (or almost only) source of nutrition. Feeding formula, pumping instead of nursing, and feeding solids all reduce the effectiveness of LAM.

❖ The infant must breastfeed at least every four hours during the day and at least every six hours at night.

❖ The infant must be less than six months old.

❖ The mother must not have had a period after 56 days postpartum (when determining fertility, bleeding prior to 56 days postpartum can be ignored).

Return of Fertility

❖ Widely variable

❖ Average return of menses for women following all the criteria is 14 months after childbirth (may vary from 2 months–14 months).

Calendar Method

❖ The Calendar Rhythm Method is a natural form of contraception based on abstaining from sex (or using barrier methods of contraception) during the time that a female is likely to be fertile.

❖ The calendar method helps to estimate the time of ovulation after a woman has charted the lengths of her menstrual cycles for several months.

Method of using the Calendar Method

❖ A woman should keep track of the lengths of her menstrual cycles for 6–12 months. Day 1 is considered as the first day of menstrual bleeding.

❖ After six or twelve months of data collection, the length of the shortest and longest menstrual cycle to be assessed.

Prediction first fertile day of current cycle

❖ It is = (the length of shortest cycle – 18).

❖ For example, if the shortest cycle was 24 days long, then the first fertile day would be day 6 (as 24–18 = 6) of the current cycle.

Prediction last fertile day of current cycle

❖ It is = (the length of longest cycle – 11).

❖ For example, if the shortest cycle was 32 days long, then the last fertile day would be day 21 (as 32–9 = 21) of the current cycle.

During this fertile period (e.g. Day 6 through Day 21) one must abstain from having unprotected intercourse.

"Fertile" Period

❖ As described above—if the longest cycle was 32 days, and the shortest was 24, a woman would potentially be fertile from day 6 of her cycle through day 21 of her cycle.

❖ The length of potential fertility is greater as the distance between her longest and shortest menstrual cycles increases.

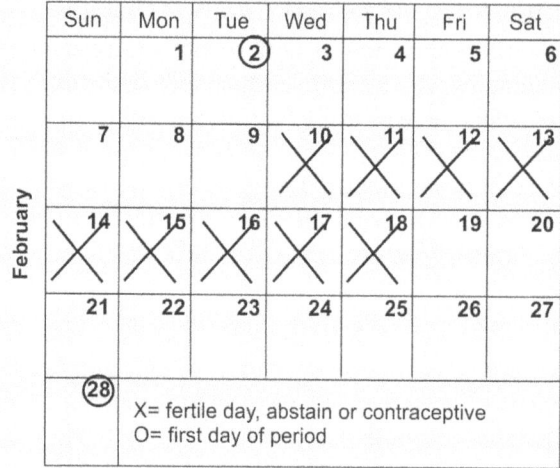

Standard Days Method (SDM)

❖ It is a calendar based method.
❖ This method works for women with menstrual cycles from 26–32 days long.
❖ If a woman has >1 cycle/year that is shorter than 26 days or longer than 32 days method effectiveness decreases significantly.

Days of menstrual cycle	Considerations in this methods
1–7	Infertile
8–19	Considered unsafe for unprotected intercourse
20–end of cycle	Infertile

Symptothermal Method

❖ Combines temperature + cervical mucus methods + calendar methods
❖ *Aim*: To identify fertile period
❖ *Advantage*: More effective than "Billing's method".

TERMINAL METHODS (= STERILIZATION METHODS)

These are permanent methods:
❖ Vasectomy
❖ Tubectomy.

Guidelines for sterilization:
❖ Age limit for sterilization:

Spouse	Minimum age for sterilization
Husband	25–50 years
Wife	20–45 years

❖ Couple must have 2 living children at the time of operation.
❖ If couple has >3 living children, lower limit for age of husband/wife may be relaxed at the discretion of operating surgeon.
❖ If couple has one child and they want a permanent method, age of the child should be >1 year.

❖ It is sufficient if:
  - Acceptor declares having obtained by consent of spouse not under any pressure, inducement, warning.
    (Consent should be given in sound state of mind, if beneficiary is psychiatric patient, to be consulted with psychiatrist).
  - Acceptor knows that procedure is practically irreversible.
  - Spouse has not been sterilized earlier.

Male Sterilization

Types

❖ Conventional vasectomy
❖ No scalpel vasectomy (NSV).

Features of Vasectomy

❖ Vasectomy is the most cost effective FP method
❖ Cost wise ratio is 5 vasectomies to 1 tubectomy
❖ No scalpel vasectomy was invented by Shung Quang Li (1974)
❖ It is not castration, so sexual ability remains unaffected (as testicular hormone release unaffected).

Procedure

Conventional Vasectomy
❖ A small incision is made in the scrotum on the either side above the testes under local anesthesia, and aseptic precautions.
❖ Vas deferens tubes are lifted and minimum 1 cm of vas deferens is cut.
❖ Ends are ligated and folded back to themselves.
❖ Incisions are closed with stitches.
❖ Then bandage is put.
❖ Person is NOT sterile until after 30 post-vasectomy ejaculations.

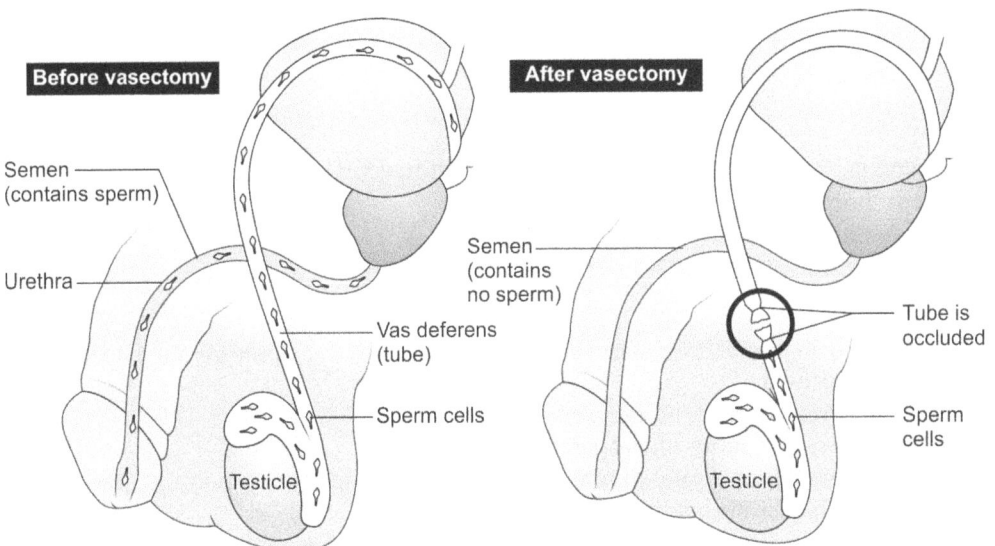

No Scalpel Vasectomy

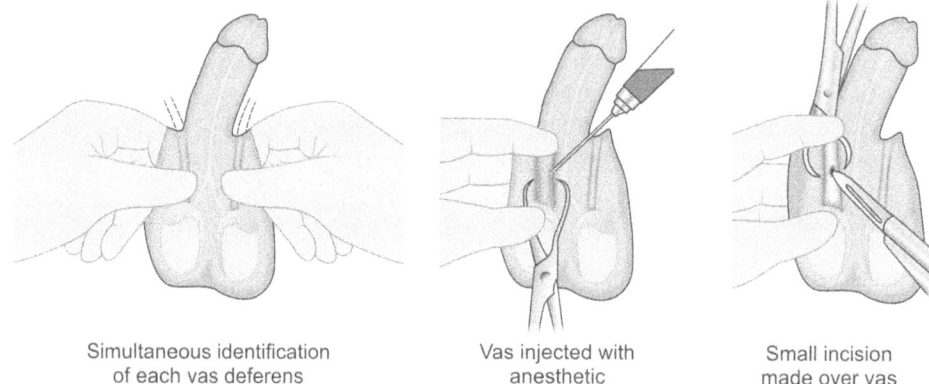

| Simultaneous identification of each vas deferens | Vas injected with anesthetic | Small incision made over vas |

❖ One sided vas deferens is palpated over scrotal skin to hold it by ring fixation clamp
❖ Puncture hole is made by dissecting forceps near median raphe
❖ Vas is delivered by the hole, and after making a loop it is ligated
❖ Minimum 1 cm of vas deferens is cut
❖ Cut ends are cauterized
❖ At the end it is not sutured just bandage is sufficient.

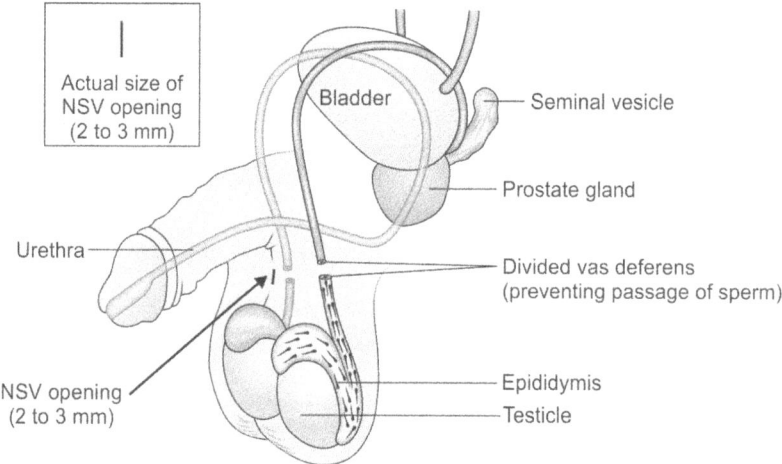

Advantages of No Scalpel Vasectomy over Conventional Vasectomy
❖ It takes shorter duration
❖ Less painful and bruising
❖ Shorter recovery time.

Postoperative Advice
❖ Patient need 30 ejaculations after vasectomy, before turning sterile (seminal examination becomes negative)
❖ To use of barrier methods till aspermia
❖ To avoid bath for 24 hours after operation
❖ To wear T bandage or scrotal support for 15 days, keep site dry
❖ To avoid cycling, lifting heavy weights for 15 days
❖ Stitch removal on 5th day of operation (for conventional vasectomy).

Complications of Vasectomy

Operative:
- ❖ Pain, scrotal hematoma and local infection
- ❖ Proper hemostasis and antibiotic may reduce such complications.

Sperm granules:
- ❖ 7 mm painful mass produced by sperm accumulation
- ❖ Appear after 10–14 days of vasectomy
- ❖ Can cause reanastomosis of vas
- ❖ Using metal clips may reduce this problem.

Spontaneous recanalization:
- ❖ Seen in 0–6% cases
- ❖ Require regular follow-up for 3 years.

Autoimmune response:
- ❖ Normally 2% fertile men have circulating antibodies against their own sperm.
- ❖ But it is seen in 54% of vasectomized patients
  (Blocking of the vas causes reabsorption of spermatozoa and subsequent development of autoantibodies against sperm in the blood)
- ❖ Require regular follow-up for 3 years.

Psychological:
↓ Sexual vigor, impotence, headache, fatigue, etc.

Postvasectomy pain syndrome:
- ❖ Primary long-term complication.

Failure of Vasectomy
Most common cause in India: Wrong identification of vas.

Other causes:
- ❖ Spontaneous recanalization
- ❖ Multiple vas in one side
- ❖ Sexual intercourse before establishment of post-vasectomy aspermia.

Follow-up visit:
1st visit (after 48 hours) → 2nd visit (after 7th day) → 3rd visit (after 3 months).

Female Sterilization
Also known as voluntary surgical contraception.

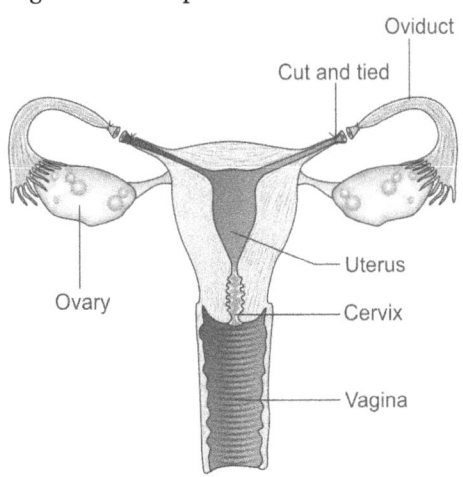

Approaches

❖ Mini-laparoscopic (Pomeroy technique/Interval procedure)
❖ Laparoscopic.

Procedure

a. **Mini-laparoscopic** (Pomeroy technique/Interval procedure):
   – A small (2.5–3 cm) transverse incision is applied just above the pubic hair line, under aseptic precaution and local anesthesia with mild sedation.
   – Finger passed through the incision.
   – Uterus is identified, raised and turned with the elevator to bring each of the fallopian tubes under the incision.
   – Each tube is tied and cut or else closed with a clip or ring.
   – Incision is closed with stitches and bandage is put.
   – She can leave hospital in few hours.
      More suitable than laparoscopy for immediate post-partum period, i.e. 6 weeks after childbirth.

b. **Laparoscopic:**
   – Under local anesthesia, a special needle is put into her abdomen and inflated with gas or air, so as to raise the wall of abdomen away from the organ inside.
   – Laparoscope is inserted through a small incision of about 2 cm.
   – Another instrument is inserted through the laparoscope to close off the tubes with a clip or ring or by electrocoagulation.
   – Instrument with laparoscope is removed.
   – The gas/air is let out of the abdomen.
   – Incision is closed with stitches and covered with abdomen.

Complications

❖ Dysfunction and uterine bleeding
❖ Psychological: Regret and depression.

Follow-up visit

1st visit (after 48 hours) → 2nd visit (after 7 days) → 3rd visit (after 1 month/1st menstrual period after operation) → Next visit if complication arises.

Use of Methods According to RMNCH Guidelines

Delaying the first child	◆ Condoms ◆ Oral contraceptive pills ◆ Intrauterine contraceptive devices (IUCDs) ◆ Emergency contraceptive pills (not to be used routinely).
Healthy spacing between two deliveries	◆ Condoms ◆ IUCDs ◆ OCPs (need to be related to breastfeeding) ◆ Lactational amenorrhea method (need to be followed-up by other methods 6 months after delivery)
Limiting methods	◆ Female sterilization ◆ Male sterilization/vasectomy

Availability of Different Family Planning Services at Different Levels

Subcenter	PHC	CHC	District hospital
Services			
Counseling	All the services available at subcenter +	All the services available at PHC +	All the services available at CHC/FRU on daily basis
IUD insertion			
OCP distribution			
Condom distribution			
ECP distribution			
Follow up of acceptors			
	Minilap sterilization including PPS (fixed day basis/camps)		
	NSV (fixed day basis/camps)		
	Referral linkages		
		Laparotomy/sterilization (fixed day basis/camps)	
		Management of complications	
		PPIUCD insertion	

PPS: Postpartum sterilization; NSV: No scalpel vasectomy; PPIUCD: Postpartum IUCD

Counseling

New clients with no method in mind	New clients with a method in mind
• Discuss the client's situation, plans, and what is important to the client about a method	• Check that the client's understanding of the method is accurate. Support the client's choice, if the client is medically eligible for the method
• Help the client consider methods that might suit the client. If needed, help the client reach a decision	• Help the client choose another method, if needed
• Support the client's choice, give key instructions on use and discuss how to cope with any side effects	• Discuss how to use the method
• Mention that methods switching is possible and allowed.	• Tell the client about possible side effects and how to cope with them
• Schedule a return visit	• Schedule a return visit

Returning clients with no problems or concerns	Returning clients who are experiencing problems/ have concerns
Ask friendly questions about how the client is doing with the method	Explore and understand the problem
	Help the client resolve the problem: Is the problem side effects, or difficulty using the method?
Answer all questions of the client	If needed, help the client change method
Provide more supplies or routine follow-up. Schedule a return visit	If needed, help the client understand and manage side effects

Evaluation of Contraceptive Methods

❖ Pearl index
❖ Life table method
❖ Method failure
❖ User failure.

Pearl Index

The Pearl index/Pearl rate is the most common technique used in **clinical trials** for reporting the effectiveness of a **birth control** method.

❖ Definition: Pearl index is defined as the number of "failures per 100 woman-years of exposure".

$$\text{Failure rate per HWY} = \frac{\text{Total accidental pregnancies}}{\text{Total months of exposure}} \times 1200$$

- The factor 1200 signifies the number of months in 100 years
- Denominator is obtained by deducing from the period of follow-up (observation) in number of months (during which contraception was not possible, by convention 10 months are deducted for a full-term pregnancy and 4 months for an abortion)
- Minimum 600 months of exposure to a method of contraception is essential for designing a use effectiveness trial and interpret the results.

❖ Information needed to calculate a Pearl Index for a particular study:
- The total number of months or cycles of exposure by women in the study
- The number of pregnancies
- The reason for leaving the study (pregnancy or other reason).

❖ Types:
- Actual use Pearl Index: Includes all pregnancies in a study and all months (or cycles) of exposure.
- Perfect use or Method Pearl Index: Includes only pregnancies that resulted *from correct and consistent use of the method.*

Life Table Method

This is expressed as the percentage of women who continue to use method at the end of one year unless they become pregnant.

Effectiveness of Different Contraceptive Methods

Method*	Perfect use	Typical use
Top tier: Most effective		
♦ Intrauterine devices		
– Levonorgestrel system	0.2	0.2
– T 380A copper	0.6	0.8
♦ Levonorgestrel implants	0.05	0.05
♦ Female sterilization	0.5	0.5
♦ Male sterilization	0.1	0.15

Contd...

Contd...

Method*	Perfect use	Typical use
Second tier: Very effective		9
◆ Combination pill	0.3	9
◆ Vaginal ring	0.3	9
◆ Patch	0.3	9
◆ DMPA	0.2	6
◆ Progestin-only pill	0.3	9
Third tier: Effective		
◆ Condom		
– Male	2	18
– Female	5	21
◆ Diaphragm with spermicides	6	12
◆ Fertility-awareness		
– Standard days	5	24
– Two days	4	
– Ovulation	3	
– Symptothermal	0.4	
Fourth tier: Least effective		
◆ Spermicides	18	28
◆ Sponge		
– Parous women	20	24
– Nulliparous women	9	12
No WHO category		
◆ Withdrawal	4	22
◆ No contraception	85	85

* Methods organized according to tiers of efficacy by World Health Organization (WHO), Johns Hopkins Bloomberg School of Publich Health, 2007.
DMPA (depot medroxyprogesterone acetate)
Data from Trussell, 2011a

Method Failure

This is expressed as the percentage of women becoming pregnant in the first year of use of a contraceptive excluding user failure.

User Failure

This is expressed as the percentage of women becoming pregnant in the first year of use of a contraceptive method including user failure.

PROBLEM-BASED QUESTIONS

1. Ranu, 23-year-old lady, comes to UTC for family planning advices. She is married before 2 months and the couple planned to have 1st child after 2 years. No menstrual abnormality and general examination reveals everything normal.

   A. What is your suggestion?
   B. What methods are not suggested? And why not suggested?

A. My suggestions:
   – Conventional contraceptives:
      - Barrier method (male condom).

B. Methods not to be suggested:

Methods	Why not suggested
IUDs	• Due to increase chance of pelvic inflammatory diseases leading to infertility in nulliparous uterus • More chance of ectopic pregnancy • Nulliparous uterus has increased chance of minor side effects
Terminal methods	• Couple must have 2 living children at the time of operation, but she is nulliparous

2. **Kalyani, 30-year-old lady, with a daughter of 8 months age comes to UTC for family planning advices. Her husband is alcoholic and refuses to come to subcenter. She has suffered from jaundice and menstrual history is normal.**

    A. What is your suggestion?

    B. What methods are not suggested?

A. My suggestions will be:

IUDs (because she had already 1 child and no help of her alcoholic husband is required). Ideally IUDs to be inserted after 7–10 days of LMP, because:
    –   Least chance of pregnancy and expulsion
    –   Genital tract is much dilated.

B. Methods not to be suggested:

Methods	Why not suggested
OCPs	History of jaundice
Conventional methods	Husband uncooperative and alcoholic
Terminal methods	Couple must have 2 living children at the time of operation for undergoing terminal methods

3. **A couple has come to the post-partum unit of your hospital. Husband is 32 years and wife is 26 years old with 2 female children aged 6 years and 14 months respectively. History of ectopic pregnancy 3 years ago. Little child is still on breastfeeding.**

    A.   What is your suggestion?

    B.   What methods are not suggested?

A. My suggestions will be:
    –   Terminal methods
    –   OCPs
    –   Conventional methods (barrier methods + natural methods).

B. Methods not to be suggested:

Methods	Why not suggested
IUDs	Contraindication for IUD insertion. (Remember ectopic pregnancy if followed by a full-term pregnancy → IUD is not absolute contraindication, rather a relative contraindication)

(As per Handbook for Reproductive, Maternal, Neonatal, and Child Health (RMNCH) Counsellors; Family planning division, Ministry of Health and Family Welfare, Govt. of India.)

Advantages and Disadvantages of Contraceptive Methods

Methods	Advantages	Disadvantages
Condom	• Moderately effective • Effective immediately • Only method that prevents STIs, including HIV/AIDS, as well as pregnancy (dual protection), when used correctly during intercourse • No effect on breast milk production • No hormonal side effects • Can be stopped at any time • Easy to keep stock handy, can be used by men of any age • Can be used without initially seeing a health care provider • Enables a man to take responsibility for preventing pregnancy and disease • Condoms are readily available free of cost at the government health facilities or home delivered by ASHA at a nominal cost	• Condoms should not be reused and should be discarded after every act of intercourse • Supplies must be readily available before intercourse begins • Some men or women may feel that it interferes with their sexual pleasure • Latex condoms may cause itching for a few people who are allergic to latex
Diaphragm	• Absence of risks • Absence of medical contraindications	• Initially a physician/trained person is needed to demonstrate the technique of insertion of the diaphragm into the vagina • Risk of toxic shock syndrome if left in the vagina for an extended period • Use of it requires privacy for insertion and facilities for washing and storing it properly
Spermicides	If used along with diaphragm, it is a good contraceptive	• They have a high failure rate when used alone • They must be introduced into those regions of vagina where sperms are likely to be deposited • They must be used almost immediately before intercourse • There are risks of burning and irritation
Intrauterine device (IUD)	• Highly effective, reversible FP method • Can be used for spacing or limiting with pregnancy rates of <1% • Available free of cost at government health facilities • Independent of sexual activity • Does not interfere with sexual intercourse • Immediately reversible with no delay in return to fertility • Does not interfere with breastfeeding • No interactions with any medicines • Initial follow-up visit required after next periods or 6 weeks of postpartum insertion followed by visits at 3 and 6 months (to ensure retention as this is the period of	Possibility of minor side effects which decrease after initial few months: • Longer and heavier menstrual periods • Bleeding or spotting between periods • More cramps or pain during periods • Does not protect against STIs and HIV • Requires a trained health care provider to insert and remove the IUD • May be expelled spontaneously, in a few cases

Contd...

Contd...

Methods	Advantages	Disadvantages
	maximum spontaneous expulsion) then the woman needs to return to the clinic only if she has a problem • Women do not need to purchase any supplies • Can act as emergency contraceptive method when inserted within 5 days of unprotected sex	
Hormonal contraceptives	• Effective (almost 100%) if used according to directions • Highly effective, reversible, easy to use • Effective within first 2 weeks • Safe for most women • Regulate the menstrual cycle • Reduce menstrual flow (which may be useful to anemic women) • Decrease the risk of ovarian and uterine cancer, benign breast disease, and incidence of acne • Do not interfere with sexual intercourse • Pelvic examination not required before use • Can be provided by trained non-medical staff • Immediate return of fertility on discontinuation	• Must be taken everyday • Require regular/dependable supply • Pills may cause side effects in some women, such as nausea/headache/ bleeding between menses or mid-cycle bleeding/weight gain • Do not protect against STIs and HIV • Risk of developing cardiovascular disease in women >35 years of age and who smoke
Depot formulations (DMPA and NET-EN)	Highly effective Long lasting Reversible contraceptive (Women continue being pregnant after 5.5 months of discontinuation)	Disruption of normal menstrual cycle (with symptom of unpredictable and excessive bleeding)
Safe period method		• If a woman's menstrual cycle is irregular, then it is difficult to predict the safe period • High failure rates • Compulsory abstinence of sexual intercourse for a period of 1 week • Requires a high degree of motivation, cooperation and education • Risk of ectopic pregnancy and embryonic abnormalities
Male sterilization/ Vasectomy	• Very effective, permanent procedure • Not effective immediately after the procedure. The couple needs to use a backup method such as condom for the first 3 months after the procedure for the semen to be sperm free • Does not interfere with sexual intercourse/ sexual pleasure • Simple surgery performed under local anesthesia by trained providers • No known long-term side effects	• Permanent • Delayed effectiveness (requires at least 3 months or 20 ejaculations for procedure to be effective) • Does not protect against STIs and HIV • Scrotal support to be maintained for the initial few days to prevent pain at the operation site

Contd...

Contd...

Methods	Advantages	Disadvantages
	◆ No repeat clinic visits required, no supplies needed, except the use of backup method/ condoms for the first 3 months ◆ Easier to perform than female sterilization. ◆ No change in sexual function ◆ No effect on hormone production	
Female sterilization/ ligation	◆ Very effective and simple surgery performed on women under local anesthesia ◆ Permanent procedure ◆ Effective immediately ◆ Nothing to remember, no supplies needed, no repeat clinic visits required after initial follow-up visits on 7th day to remove the stitches ◆ Does not interfere with sexual intercourse ◆ No effect on breast milk production ◆ No known long-term side effects or health risks ◆ Can be performed any time during the menstrual cycle when it is reasonably sure that the woman is not pregnant/within 7 days of delivery/post abortion, after ruling out infection	◆ Short-term discomfort/pain following procedure ◆ Uncommon complications of surgery include: 　– Bleeding from surgical site 　– Infection 　– Injury to internal organs 　– Requires a trained provider and health facility providing the service 　– Does not protect against STIs and HIV
Lactational amenorrhea method (LAM)	◆ Effective (1–2 pregnancies per 100 women during first six months of use) ◆ Immediate breastfeeding provides additional protection against infections for the newborn ◆ Exclusive breastfeeding (EBF) promotes health benefits to the infant and increases survival ◆ Promotes mother and infant bonding ◆ Helps mother's uterus return to normal size quicker than non-breastfeeding women ◆ Effective immediately ◆ Does not interfere with intercourse ◆ No systemic side effects ◆ No medical supervision necessary ◆ No supplies required ◆ No cost ◆ Helps reduce the amount of bleeding after delivery by keeping the uterus contracted	All 3 criteria need to be met for effectiveness: 1. The woman exclusively breastfeeds her baby including night feeds 2. Less than six months passed after delivery 3. The woman's menses have not returned: 　– May be difficult to practice due to social circumstances like lack of privacy for breastfeeding in a joint family/working woman 　– Does not protect against STIs and HIV 　– Women who are infected with HIV or who have AIDS or taking antiretroviral drugs can use LAM, however, there is a chance that some percentage of infants will get HIV through breast milk

Chapter
9

Specimens

IRON AND FOLIC ACID TABLETS

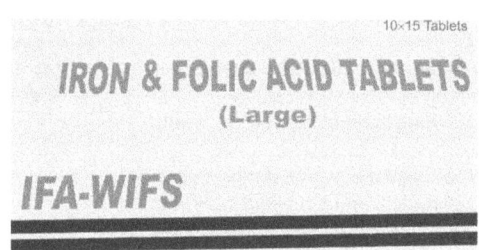

10×15 Tablets

IRON & FOLIC ACID TABLETS
(Large)

IFA-WIFS

Iron and folic acid tablets

1. Under which national program iron and folic acid (IFA) tablets are given?

❖ Previously: Through National Nutritional Anemia Control Programme (NNACP)
❖ From 2018 onwards: Intensified National Iron Plus Initiative (i-NIPI).

2. What do you mean by nutritional anemia?

Nutritional anemia is defined as the condition that results from the inability of the erythropoietic tissue to maintain a normal hemoglobin concentration *on account of an inadequate supply of one or more essential nutrients* (WHO).

3. What are the cut-off values for different groups below which anemia is said to be present?

Hemoglobin levels to diagnose anemia (g/dL):

Age groups	No anemia	Mild	Moderate	Severe
Children 6–59 months of age	≥11	10–10.9	7–9.9	<7
Children 5–11 years of age	≥11.5	11–11.4	8–10.9	<8
Children 12–14 years of age	≥12	11–11.9	8–10.9	<8
Nonpregnant women (15 years of age and above)	≥12	11–11.9	8–10.9	<8
Pregnant women	≥11	10–10.9	7–9.9	<7
Men	≥13	11–12.9	8–10.9	<8

Source: Hemoglobin concentration for the diagnosis of anemia and assessment of severity. WHO

4. **What do you mean by I-NIPI? Who are its beneficiaries? What are the age specific interventions with IFA supplementation in I-NIPI?**

Introduction

Intensified National Iron Plus Initiative (I-NIPI) of the Anemia Mukt Bharat campaign launched by Ministry of Health and Family Welfare, Government of India in April, 2018 under POSHAN (PM's overarching scheme for holistic nourishment) abhiyaan.

6×6×6 Strategy

* 6 interventions
* 6 beneficiaries
* 6 institutional mechanisms.

Vision: Anemia Mukt Bharat.

Objective: Reduction of anemia prevalence by 18% in all target age groups by 2022.

6 Beneficiaries

1. Children (6–59 months)
2. Children (5–9 years)
3. Adolescents males and females (10–19 years)
4. Pregnant women
5. Lactating women
6. Women of reproductive age (20–49 years)—nonpregnant and nonlactating (NPNL).

6 Interventions

1. Prophylactic IFA supplementation
2. Periodic deworming
3. Intensified year round behavior change communication (BCC) campaign
4. Testing of anemia using digital methods and point of care treatment
5. Mandatory provision of IFA fortified foods in public health program
6. Addressing nonnutritional causes of anemia (malaria, fluorosis, sickle cell anemia).

6 Institutional Mechanisms

1. Intraministerial coordination
2. National Anemia Mukt Bharat unit
3. National centre of excellence and advanced research on anemia control
4. Convergence with other ministries
5. Strengthening supply chain and logistics
6. Anemia Mukt Bharat dashboard and digital portal.

Age group	Dose of IFA	Frequency	Color
Children (6–59 months)	1 mL of IFA syrup containing 20 mg of elemental iron and 100 µg of folic acid	Biweekly	Red syrup
Children (5–9 years)	45 mg elemental iron and 400 µg of folic acid	Weekly	Pink tab
Adolescents (10–19 years)	60 mg elemental iron and 500 µg of folic acid	Weekly	Blue tab

Contd...

Contd...

Age group	Dose of IFA	Frequency	Color
Women in reproductive age group (NPNL)	60 mg elemental iron and 500 µg of folic acid	Weekly	Red tab
Pregnant and lactating women	60 mg elemental iron and 500 µg of folic acid starting from 14th week of gestation, continued throughout pregnancy (minimum 180 days during pregnancy) and to be continued for 180 days postpartum: a total of 1 year	Daily	Red tab

DISPOSABLE DELIVERY KIT

❖ *Disposable delivery kit (DDK)* is given to mother to observe 7 Cs at the time of the last antenatal checkup by health worker female with an instruction to be opened only by the trained birth attendant at the time of delivery.
❖ *Aim:* To reduce incidence of neonatal tetanus by prevention of wound contamination due to birth of a neonate with tetanus spore.
❖ *Contents of DDK:*

Contents	Amount
Gauze piece (7.5 cm × 1 mt)	1 no.
Ligature	2 nos.
Razor blade (ISI)	1 no.
Soap (10 g)	1 no.
Antiseptic lotion	10 mL
Cotton	10 g
Chloramphenicol applicap	2 nos.

❖ *Sterilization:* Available in presterilized packet by gamma radiation

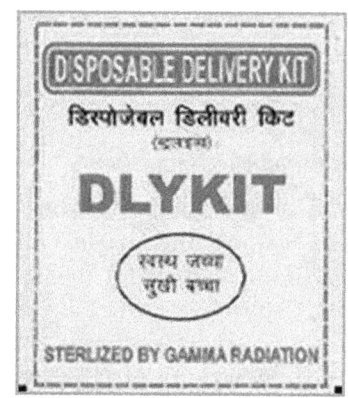

Disposable delivery kit

– **3 Cs:**
Clean:
  - Delivery surface
  - Hands
  - Cord care.
– **5 Cs:**
Clean:
  - Delivery surface: Plastic sheet
  - Hands: Soap and clean water of birth attendant
  - Cord cut: A new razor blade
  - Cord tie: A clean piece of thread
  - Cord stump: Nothing applied to cord.
– **7 Cs:**
5 Cs + clean:
  - Water
  - Towel for handwashing.

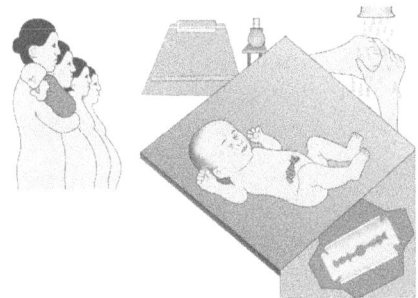

7 Cs

ORS

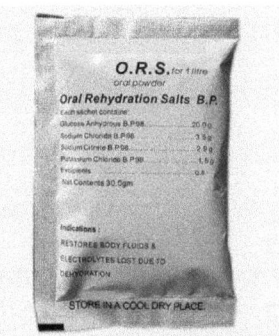

Oral rehydration solution

Full name: Oral rehydration solution.

Introduction

ORS is a very important tool for *fluid replacement* used for the treatment of dehydration.

ORS is considered as the "most important discovery of 20th century".

Composition

Composition	Gram	In low osmolarity ORS (gram)
Sodium chloride	3.5	2.6
Potassium chloride	1.5	1.5
Sodium bicarbonate/citrate	2.5/2.9	2.9 (sodium citrate)
Glucose	20	13.5
Total	27.5/27.9	20.5

Composition of ORS in Osmolar Concentration

Composition	Gram	In low osmolarity ORS (gram)
Sodium	90	75
Potassium	20	20
Chloride	80	65
Bicarbonate/citrate	30/10	10
Glucose	111	75
Total	331/311	245

Physiological Basis of ORS Administration

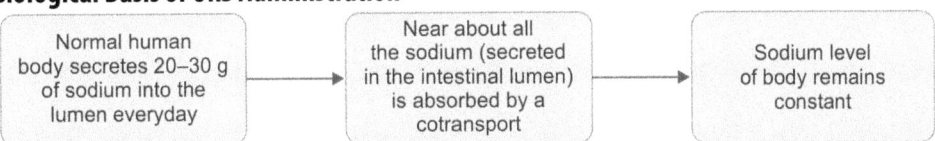

Normal human body secretes 20–30 g of sodium into the lumen everyday → Near about all the sodium (secreted in the intestinal lumen) is absorbed by a cotransport → Sodium level of body remains constant

Maintenance of sodium balance in the body

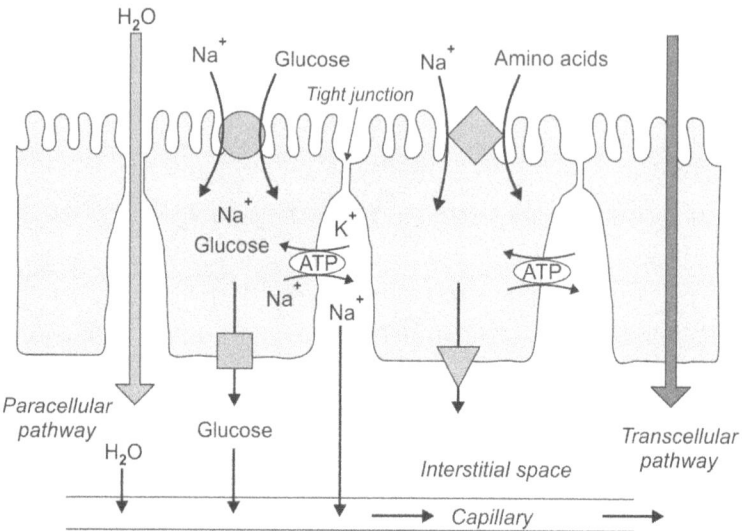

Physiological basis of ion absorption during ORS administration

But in case of diarrheal diseases, this physiological process hampers and Na-rich intestinal secretions are lost before they can be reabsorbed. So life-threatening hypovolemia occurs within hours.

Mechanism of Action of ORS

❖ Even in severe diarrheal diseases, *Na-glucose co-transporter (SGLT1)* remains intact and this pathway is used to combat diarrhea by replenishing the water loss.

❖ **2 Na+ ions** and **1 molecule of glucose** are transported together across the cell membrane via this transporter.

❖ As SGLT1 is cotransporter; both Na+ and glucose are required to get absorbed by intestinal epithelial cells.

That is why ORS includes both sodium and glucose.

1. ORS is the best treatment for diarrhea.

Because:

❖ Composition of ORS (WHO) is very effective and scientific in controlling dehydration state (it has been experienced that as many as 90–95% of cholera and diarrhea can be treated by oral fluids alone)

❖ Cost effective

❖ Easy to administer, do not need medical personnel

❖ Can be undertaken at home for management of diarrhea by the mother

❖ It also ensures proper utilization of *appropriate technology* under PHC.

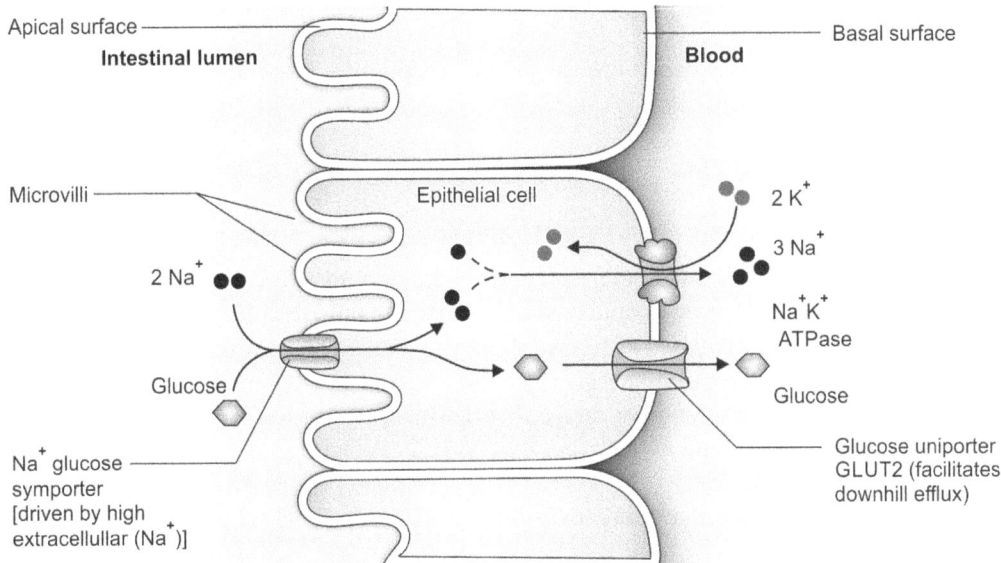

Mechanism of action of ORS at molecular level via SGLT1 cotransporter

2. ORS is considered as an example of appropriate technology.

Criteria for "appropriate technology"	Reason
Scientifically sound	• ORS can be safely and scientifically used in treating acute diarrhea due to all etiology in all age group, in all country • 90–95% of all cases of diarrhea can be completely treated by ORS
Acceptable to those who apply it	• Easy to prepare • Easy to administer • Can be prepared at home • No boiling/sterilization needed
Acceptable to those on whom it is applied	• Orally administrated • Self-administrated • Less expensive • Minimum side effects

❖ Low osmolarity ORS:
   – In 2003, clinical trials and comparisons with rice water led to a reduction in the recommended osmolarity of ORS by joint activity of WHO and UNICEF.
   – The guidelines were updated in 2006.
   – The recommended osmolarity of ORS was reduced from 311 mmol/L to 245 mmol/L.
   – The concentration of glucose and NaCl were reduced, while that of K⁺ and citrate remained the same.

   Basic advantages of low osmolarity ORS in diarrhea over previous one:
   – It decreases vomiting
   – It decreases stool volume by about 25%
   – It reduces the need for IV therapy by about 30%.

❖ Common homemade ORS: These are used when the WHO mixture of salts is not available. These include:
  – Table salt (1 level teaspoon) + Sugar (6 level teaspoon) + 1 liter of water.
  – Rice water
  – Unsalted soup
  – Yoghurt drinks
  – Green coconut water
  – Weak tea, etc.
❖ Recommendations to be read before preparing a homemade ORS:
  – Wherever possible these should contain at least one fluid that contains salt.
  – Fluids which are sweetened with sugar should be avoided because they can cause osmotic diarrhea and hypernatremia, e.g.
    - Commercial carbonated beverages (cold drinks)
    - Commercial fruit juices
    - Sweetened tea
  – Fluids that have stimulant purgative/diuretic effect should also be avoided like coffee.

Zinc Therapy in Diarrhea

❖ Advantages of associated zinc therapy is beneficial in management of diarrhea:
  – It reduces the episodes' *duration* and *severity*
  – When given for 10–14 days lowers the *incidence* and *risk* of diarrhea in the following 2–3 months.
❖ Dosing schedule: WHO and UNICEF recommendation of zinc supplement:
  – <6 months: 10 mg daily ⎫
  – >6 months: 20 mg daily ⎭ for 10–14 days
❖ Mechanism of action of zinc in diarrhea:
  – Zinc inhibits cAMP induced, chlorine-dependent fluid secretion
  – Zinc inhibits basolateral K^+ channels.

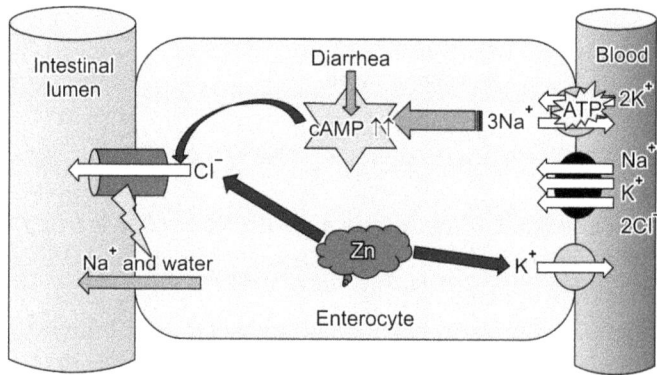

Mechanism of action of zinc in diarrhea at molecular level

❖ Role of zinc in diarrhea (UNICEF):
  – Zinc reduces the fluid and salt loss in stools by improving mucosal permeability
  – Accelerated regeneration of mucosa
  – Increased levels of brush-border enzymes

- Enhanced cellular immunity
- Higher levels of secretory antibodies
- Zinc improves absorption of ORS
- Reduces the severity and duration of illness
- Reduces need for antibiotics
- Reduces the chances of complications
- Full dose for 14 days protects against diarrhea and pneumonia for next 3 months
- Acts as a general tonic, improves appetite and promotes growth.

❖ Effectiveness of ORS: As many as 90–95% of all cases of cholera and acute diarrhea can be treated with oral fluid only.
❖ Between 1980 and 2006, the introduction of ORT is estimated to have decreased the number of deaths worldwide from 5 to 3 million per year.
❖ Some intravenous rehydration solution:
- Ringer's lactate solution/Hartman's solution—best. It corrects both hypovolemia and metabolic acidosis (*Note*: Lactate is metabolized into bicarbonate in the liver).
- Diarrhea treatment solution (DTS).
- Normal saline—poorest.

Chapter
10
Definitions

CONCEPT OF HEALTH AND DISEASE

1. *Health****: "Health is a state of complete physical, mental and social well-being and not merely an absence of disease or infirmity."
   Source: WHO (1948).
2. *Operational definition of health***: "Health is a condition or quality of the human organism expressing the adequate functioning of the organism in given conditions, genetic or environmental."
   Source: WHO (1957).
3. *Standard of living*: Income and occupation, standards of housing, sanitation and nutrition, the level of provision of health, educational, recreational and other services may all be used individually as measures of socioeconomic status, and collectively as an index of the "standard of living".
   Source: WHO (1975).
4. *Quality of life*: "WHO defines Quality of Life as individuals' perception of their position in life in the context of the culture and value systems in which they live and in relation to their goals, expectations, standards and concerns."
   Source: WHO (1997).
5. *Indicators of health: A measurable characteristic that describes*:
   - The health of a population (e.g. life expectancy, mortality, disease incidence or prevalence or other health states).
   - Determinants of health (e.g. health behaviors, health risk factors, physical environments and socioeconomic environments).
   - Health care access, cost, quality and use.
   Source: CDC.
6. *PQLI (Physical quality of life index)**: "The PQLI measure consolidates three indicators—infant mortality, life expectancy at age one, and literacy—into a single composite index having a minimum of zero and a maximum of 100."
   Source: WHO (1981).

7. *Human development index (HDI)**: "The Human Development Index is a composite statistic of life expectancy, education, and income indices used to rank countries into four tiers of human development."
Source: United Nations Development Programme (UNDP).

8. *Disability adjusted life years (DALY)*: "The sum of years of potential life lost due to premature mortality and the years of productive life lost due to disability."
Source: WHO.

9. *Epidemiological triad*: The epidemiologic triad is a model that scientists have developed for studying health problems. It can help to understand infectious diseases and how they spread.

The triad has three vertices:

a. *Agent*: Microbe that causes the disease.
b. *Host*: Organism harboring the disease.
c. *Environment*: Those external factors that cause or allow disease transmission.

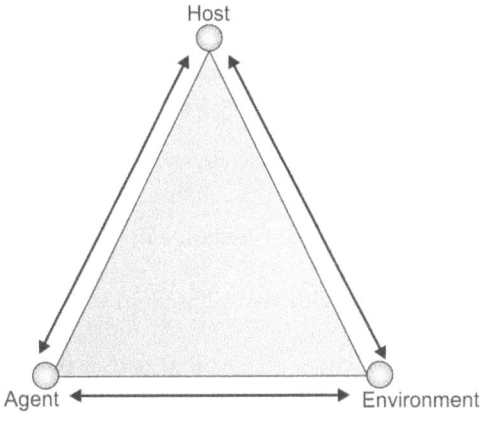

Epidemiological triad
Source: CDC.

10. *Natural history of disease**: Natural history of disease refers to the progression of a disease process in an individual over time in the absence of treatment.

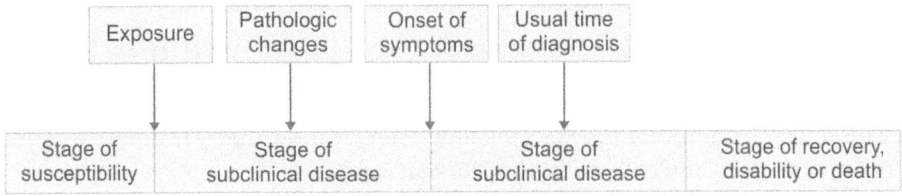

Natural history of disease
Source: CDC.

11. *Disease control**: The reduction of disease incidence, prevalence, morbidity or mortality to a locally acceptable level as a result of deliberate efforts; continued intervention measures are required to maintain the reduction.

Example: Control of diarrheal diseases.

Source: CDC.

12. *Disease elimination**: Reduction to zero of the incidence of a specified disease in a defined geographical area as a result of deliberate efforts; continued intervention measures are required.

 Example: Elimination of measles, polio, diphtheria, neonatal tetanus, etc. from a defined geographic area.

 Source: CDC.

13. *Disease eradication**: Permanent reduction to zero of the worldwide incidence of infection caused by a specific agent as a result of deliberate efforts; intervention measures are no longer needed.

 Example: Smallpox eradication.

 Source: CDC.

14. *Monitoring**: "Monitoring refers to the routine and continuous tracking of the implementation of planned surveillance activities and of the overall performance of surveillance and response systems."

 Source: WHO (2006).

15. *Surveillance**: "Surveillance is the ongoing, systematic collection, analysis and interpretation of outcome-specific data for use in planning, implementing and evaluating public health policies and practices."

 Source: WHO (2006).

16. *Types of surveillance*:

 a. *Active surveillance*: Public health surveillance in which the health agency solicits reports.

 b. *Passive surveillance*: Public health surveillance in which data are sent to the health agency without prompting.

 c. *Sentinel surveillance*: Surveillance system that uses a prearranged sample of sources (e.g. physicians, hospitals or clinics) who have agreed to report all cases of one or more notifiable diseases.

 Source: CDC.

17. *Impairment*: "Impairment is any loss or abnormality of psychological, physiological, or anatomical structure or function."

 Source: WHO (1980).

18. *Disability*: "A disability is any restriction or lack (resulting from an impairment) of ability to perform an activity in the manner or within the range considered normal for a human being."

 Source: WHO (1980).

19. *Handicap*: "A handicap is a disadvantage for a given individual resulting from an impairment or a disability that limits or prevents the fulfillment of a role that is normal (depending on age, sex, and social and cultural factors) for that individual."

 Source: WHO (1980).

20. *Rehabilitation*: "Rehabilitation of people with disabilities is a process aimed at enabling them to reach and maintain their optimal physical, sensory, intellectual, psychological and social functional levels. Rehabilitation provides disabled people with the tools they need to attain independence and self-determination."

 Source: WHO.

21. *Hygiene*: "Hygiene is defined as the science of health and it embraces all factors which contribute to healthful living."

22. *Public health**: "Public health refers to all organized measures (whether public or private) to prevent disease, promote health, and prolong life among the population as a whole."
Source: WHO.

23. *Preventive medicine*: "Preventive medicine is defined as that specialty of medical practice which focuses on the health of individuals and defined populations in order to protect, promote, and maintain health and well-being and prevent disease, disability, and premature death."
Source: American Board of Preventive Medicine.

24. *Social medicine*: "Social medicine is a medicine that seeks to understand the impact of socioeconomic conditions on human health and diseases in order to improve the health of a society and its individuals."
Source: PubMed.

25. *Community medicine***: "Community medicine is the field concerned with the study of health and disease in the defined community or group. Its goal is to identify the health problems and needs of people (community diagnosis) and to plan, implement and evaluate the effectiveness of healthcare system."
WHO has suggested that every country should have its own definition of community medicine.

26. *Community diagnosis*: "It is a quantitative and qualitative description of the health of citizens and the factors which influence their health. It identifies problems, proposes areas for improvement and stimulates action."
Source: WHO.

27. *Community treatment*: "It is the sum of steps decided upon to meet the health needs of the community taking into account the resources available and the wishes of the people, as revealed by community diagnosis."

EPIDEMIOLOGY

1. *Epidemiology****: "The study of the distribution and determinants of health-related states or events in specified populations, and the application of this study to control the health problems."
Source: John M Last (1988).

2. *Infection*: The entry and development or multiplication of an infectious agent in the body of man or animals.

3. *Contamination*: The presence of an infectious agent on a body surface or/in any other inanimate articles/substances.

4. *Infestation*: Lodgement, development and reproduction of arthropods on the surface of the body/in the clothing.

5. *Host*: A person or other living animal including birds and arthropods that afford subsistence or lodgement to an infectious agent under natural conditions.

6. *Types of hosts*:
   a. *Obligatory host*: The only host existing for a parasite, e.g. man in measles.
   b. *Primary/definitive host*: Host in which the parasite attains maturity or passes its sexual stage are primary or definitive hosts, e.g. mosquito in malaria/man in taeniasis.
   c. *Secondary/intermediate host*: Host in which the parasite is in a larval or asexual state are secondary or intermediate hosts, e.g. man in malaria/pig in taeniasis.

    d. *Transport host*: A transport host is a carrier in which the organism remains alive but does not undergo development, e.g. pseudophyllidean tapeworm larvae in fish.

7. *Infectious disease*: A clinically manifest disease of man/animals resulting from an infection.

8. *Contagious disease*: A disease that is transmitted through contact, e.g. STD, scabies, etc.

9. *Epidemic*: "Epidemic refers to an increase, often sudden, in the number of cases of a disease above what is normally expected in that population in that area."
   Source: CDC.

10. *Endemic*: "Endemic refers to the constant presence and/or usual prevalence of a disease or infectious agent in a population within a geographic area."
    Source: CDC.

11. *Hyperendemic*: "Hyperendemic refers to persistent, high levels of disease occurrence."
    Source: CDC.

12. *Pandemic*: "An epidemic occurring worldwide or over a very wide area, crossing boundaries of several countries, and usually affecting a large number of people."
    Source: WHO.

13. *Sporadic*: "Sporadic refers to a disease that occurs infrequently and irregularly."
    Source: CDC.

14. Zoonoses: "Zoonoses is defined as diseases and infections that are naturally transmitted between vertebrate animals and humans."
    Source: WHO.

15. *Epizootic*: "An outbreak/epidemic of disease occurring in an animal population."

16. *Epornithic*: "An outbreak/epidemic of disease occurring in a bird population."

17. *Enzootic*: "An endemic of disease occurring in an animal population."

SCREENING

1. *Screening****: "Screening is the process of using tests on a large scale to identify the presence of disease in apparently healthy people. Screening tests do not usually establish a diagnosis, but rather the presence or absence of an identified risk factor, and thus require individual follow-up and treatment."
   Source: WHO (2006)

2. *Lead time*: "It refers to the interval between the time when the disease can be first diagnosed by screening and when it is usually diagnosed in patients presenting with symptoms."
   Note: A short lead time implies a rapidly progressing disease, and treatment initiated after screening is unlikely to be more effective than that begun after the more usual diagnostic procedures, e.g. noise-induced hearing loss has a very long lead time; pancreatic cancer usually has a short one.
   Source: WHO (2006).

3. *Sensitivity*: "Sensitivity is the proportion of people with the disease in the screened population who are identified as ill by the screening test."
   (It implies, "When the disease is present, how often does the test detect it?")
   Source: WHO (2006).

4. Specificity: "Specificity is the proportion of disease-free people who are so identified by the screening test."
   (It implies, "When the disease is absent, how often does the test provide a negative result?")
   Source: WHO (2006).

5. *Yield*: "Yield is the amount of previously unrecognized disease that is diagnosed as a result of the screening effort."

For example: If high-risk population is selected for screening, the yield increases.

Simple formulas for sensitivity, specificity, positive predictive value and negative predictive value:

		Disease	
		Present	Absent
Screening test	Positive result	a	b
	Negative result	c	d
		a+c	b+d

$$Sensitivity = \frac{True\ posititve}{Disease\ positive} = \frac{a}{a+c}$$

$$Specificity = \frac{True\ negative}{Disease\ negative} = \frac{d}{b+d}$$

$$PPV = \frac{True\ positive}{Test\ positive} = \frac{a}{a+b}$$

$$NPV = \frac{True\ negative}{Test\ negative} = \frac{d}{c+d}$$

COMMUNICABLE DISEASES

1. *Communicable disease*: "An illness due to a specific infectious agent/its toxic products capable of being directly/indirectly transmitted from man to man, animal to animal or from the environment to man or animal."
2. *Incubation period***: "The incubation period is defined as the time from exposure to onset of disease. When limited to infectious diseases, it corresponds to the time from infection with a microorganism to symptom development."
3. *Pulse polio*: "Pulse polio is an immunization campaign established by Government of India in 1995–1996 to eradicate poliomyelitis in India by sudden, simultaneous and mass administration of OPV on a single day to all children 0–5 years of age, regardless to previous immunization status."
4. *Definitions regarding tuberculosis:*
   Case definitions:
   I. *Microbiologically confirmed TB* case refers to a presumptive TB patient with biological specimen positive for acid-fast bacilli, or positive for *Mycobacterium tuberculosis* on culture, or positive for tuberculosis through quality assured rapid diagnostic molecular test.
   II. *Clinically diagnosed TB* case refers to a presumptive TB patient who is not microbiologically confirmed, but has been diagnosed with active TB by a clinician on the basis of X-ray abnormalities, histopathology or clinical signs with a decision to treat the patient with a full course of anti-TB treatment.

   Classification based on anatomical site of disease:
   a. *Pulmonary tuberculosis (PTB)* refers to any microbiologically confirmed or clinically diagnosed case of TB involving the lung parenchyma or the tracheobronchial tree.

b. *Extrapulmonary tuberculosis (EPTB)* refers to any microbiologically confirmed or clinically diagnosed case of TB involving organs other than the lungs, such as pleura, lymph nodes, intestine, genitourinary tract, joint and bones, meninges of the brain, etc.

Note: A patient with both pulmonary and extrapulmonary TB should be classified as a case of PTB.

Classification based on history of TB treatment:
a. *New case*: A TB patient who has never had treatment for TB or has taken anti-TB drugs for less than one month is considered as a new case.
b. *Previously treated* patients have received 1 month or more of anti-TB drugs in the past.
   i. *Recurrent TB case*: A TB Patient previously declared as successfully treated (cured/treatment completed) and is subsequently found to be microbiologically confirmed TB case is a recurrent TB case.
   ii. *Treatment after failure patients* are those who have previously been treated for TB and whose treatment failed at the end of their most recent course of treatment.
   iii. *Treatment after loss to follow-up:* A TB patient previously treated for TB for 1 month or more and was declared lost to follow-up in his most recent course of treatment and subsequently found microbiologically confirmed TB case
   iv. *Other previously treated patients* are those who have previously been treated for TB but whose outcome after their most recent course of treatment is unknown or undocumented.
c. *Transferred in:* A TB patient who is received for treatment in a tuberculosis unit, after registered for treatment in another TB unit is considered as a case of transferred in.

Classification based on drug resistance:
a. *Mono-resistance (MR)*: A TB patient, whose biological specimen is resistant to one first-line anti-TB drug only.
b. *Polydrug Resistance (PDR)*: A TB patient, whose biological specimen is resistant to more than one first-line anti-TB drug, other than both INH and Rifampicin.
c. *Multidrug resistance (MDR)*: A TB patient, whose biological specimen is *resistant to both isoniazid and rifampicin* with or without resistance to other first line drugs, based on the results from a quality assured laboratory.
   Note: Patients, who have any Rifampicin resistance, should also be managed as if they are an MDR-TB case.
d. *Extensive drug resistance (XDR):* An MDR-TB case whose biological specimen is additionally resistant to a fluoroquinolone (ofloxacin, levofloxacin, or moxifloxacin) and a second-line injectable anti-TB drug (kanamycin, amikacin, or capreomycin) from a quality assured laboratory.

Classification based on treatment outcomes for drug-susceptible TB patients:
a. *Cured*: Microbiologically confirmed TB patients at the beginning of treatment who were smear or culture negative at the end of the complete treatment.
b. *Treatment completed*: A TB patient who completed treatment without evidence of failure or clinical deterioration but with no record to show that the smear or culture results of biological specimen in the last month of treatment was negative, either because test was not done or because result is unavailable.
c. *Treatment success*: TB patients either cured or treatment completed are accounted in treatment success.

d. *Failure*: A TB patient whose biological specimen is positive by smear or culture at end of treatment.

e. *Failure to respond*: A case of pediatric TB who fails to have microbiological conversion to negative status or fails to respond clinically/or deteriorates after 12 weeks of compliant intensive phase shall be deemed to have failed response provided alternative diagnoses/reasons for non-response have been ruled out.

f. *Lost to follow up*: A TB patient whose treatment was interrupted for 1 consecutive month or more.

g. *Not evaluated*: A TB patient for whom no treatment outcome is assigned. This includes former "transfer-out".

h. *Treatment regimen changed*: A TB patient who is on first line regimen and has been diagnosed as having DRTB and switched to drug-resistant TB regimen prior to being declared as failed.

i. *Died*: A patient who has died during the course of anti-TB treatment.

Source: Technical and Operational Guidelines for Tuberculosis control in India (2016).

5. *Leprosy case:* A case of leprosy is diagnosed by eliciting cardinal signs of leprosy through systematic clinical (and wherever required bacteriological) examination. At least one of the following signs must be present to diagnose leprosy:

   1. Hypopigmented or reddish skin lesion(s) with definite sensory deficit
   2. Involvement of the peripheral nerves, as demonstrated by definite thickening with loss of sensation and weakness/paralysis of the corresponding muscles of the hands, feet or eyes
   3. Demonstration of *Mycobacterium leprae in the lesions.*
      Source: WHO Guidelines (2017).

6. *HIV case*: HIV infection in adults is diagnosed based on:
   - Positive HIV antibody testing (rapid or laboratory-based enzyme immunoassay). This is usually confirmed by a second HIV antibody test (rapid or laboratory-based enzyme immunoassay) relying on different antigens or of different operating characteristics and/or,
   - *A positive virological test for HIV or its components* (HIV-RNA/HIV-DNA/ultrasensitive HIV p24 antigen) confirmed by a second virological test obtained from a separate determination.
   Source: WHO (2006).

NONCOMMUNICABLE DISEASES

1. Classification of blood pressure in adults:
   ACC/AHA 2017 Hypertension Guidelines:

Designation	SBP (mm Hg)		DBP (mm Hg)
Normal BP	<120	AND	<80
Elevated BP	120–129	AND	<80
Stage 1 hypertension	130–139	OR	80–89
Stage 2 hypertension	≥140	OR	≥90

Recommendations for treatment and follow up:
- Normal BP:
  - Promote optimal lifestyle habits
  - Reassess in 1 year.
- Elevated BP:
  - Nonpharmacological therapy
  - Reassess in 3–6 months.
- Stage 1 hypertension:
  - Estimated 10 years cardiovascular disease risk <10%:
    * Nonpharmacological therapy
    * Reassess in 3–6 months.
  - Estimated 10 year cardiovascular disease risk ≥10%:
    * Nonpharmacological therapy + BP-lowering medications*
    * Reassess in 1 month.
- Stage 2 hypertension:
  - Nonpharmacological therapy + BP-lowering medications*
  - Consider initiation of pharmacological therapy with 2 antihypertensive agents of different classes
  - Reassess in 1 month.
    *If BP goals are met: Reassess in 3–6 months
    If BP goals are not met: Consider intensification of therapy.
2. *Blindness*: "Blindness is defined as a presenting visual acuity of worse than 3/60 or a corresponding visual field loss to less than 10° in the better eye."
   Source: WHO (2012).

DEMOGRAPHY AND FAMILY PLANNING

1. *Demography*: "Demography is the study of the size, territorial distribution, and composition of population, changes therein, and the components of such changes."
   Source: Hauser and Duncan (1959).
2. *Census*: Total process of collecting, compiling and publishing demographic, economic and social data pertaining at a specified time or times to all persons in a contrary or delimited.
3. *Sex ratio*: "Sex ratio is defined as the number of female per 1,000 males."
4. *Dependency ratio*: "The proportion of persons above 65 years of age and children below 15 years of age are considered to be dependent on the economically productive age group (15–64 years). This ratio is called total dependency ratio (TDR)." It is expressed in terms of percentage.

$$TDR = \frac{\text{Children} <15 \text{ years of age} + \text{Persons} >65 \text{ years of age}}{\text{Population (15–64 years of age)}} \times 100$$

5. *Life expectancy*: "Life expectancy is the average number of years a person can expect to live, if in the future they experience the current age-specific mortality rates in the population."
   Source: WHO (2014).
6. *Net reproduction rate (NRR)*: "NRR is defined as the number of daughters a newborn girl will bear during her lifetime assuming fixed age specific fertility and mortality rates."
   Source: World Bank (1987).

PREVENTIVE MEDICINE IN OBSTETRICS, GYNECOLOGY AND PEDIATRICS

1. *Infant, Pre-school age, School age*:

Designation	Age
Infant	Up to 1 year of age
Pre-school age	1–4 years
School age	5–14 years

2. *At-risk infant*: The basic criteria for identifying "at-risk" infants are:
   - Birth weight <2.5 kg
   - Twins
   - Birth order ≥5
   - Artificial feeding
   - Weight <70% of expected weight
   - Failure to gain weight during 3 successive months
   - Children with protein-energy malnutrition/diarrhea
   - Working mother/one parent.
3. *Low birth weight (LBW)*: "Low birth weight has been defined as weight at birth less than 2500 g."
   Source: WHO.
4. *Preterm, term and post-term baby*: According to the previous definitions, which are still being followed in our country (It should be told first at viva table):

Designations	Description
Preterm	Birth before 37 weeks of pregnancy
Term	Birth anytime from 37 to 42 weeks of pregnancy
Post-term	Birth after 42 weeks of pregnancy

   Note: According to "The American College of Obstetricians and Gynecologists—ACOG" November 2013 recommendations, the designation "Preterm" has been eliminated and "Term" has been replaced by "Early term, Full term, Late term" with "Post term" remains as it was before.
   - Early term: Between 37 weeks 0 days and 38 weeks 6 days
   - Full term: Between 39 weeks 0 days and 40 weeks 6 days
   - Late term: Between 41 weeks 0 days and 41 weeks 6 days
   - Post-term: Between 42 weeks 0 days and beyond
   (New definitions as proposed by ACOG).
5. *Juvenile delinquency*:
   Juvenile: "A boy who has not attained the age of 16 years and a girl who has not attained the age of 18 years."
   Delinquent: *"A child who has committed an offence."*
   Source: The Children Act, 1960.
   Note: In a broader sense, juvenile delinquency includes not only juvenile crime, but all aspects of deviations from normal behavior like habitual disobedience, interaction with immoral people and antisocial activities.

6. *Battered baby syndrome*: "The term 'battered baby syndrome' is defined as a clinical condition, usually in children under 3 years of age, who have suffered nonaccidental injury, on one or more occasions, by an adult in the position of trust usually a parent, a guardian or a foster parent."
   Source: Cameron JM (1972).

NUTRITION

1. *Balanced diet*: A balanced diet is defined as one which contains a variety of foods in such quantities and proportions that need for energy, amino acids, vitamins, minerals, fats, carbohydrate and other nutrients is adequately met for maintaining health, vitality and general well-being and also makes a small provision for extra nutrients to withstand short duration of leanness.

2. *Dietary goals*:

Dietary factors	Goals (% of total energy, unless otherwise stated)
Total fat	15–30%
◆ Saturated fatty acids	◆ <10%
◆ PUFA	◆ 6–10%
◆ n-6 PUFA	◆ 5–8%
◆ n-3 PUFA	◆ 1–2%
◆ Transfatty acid	◆ <1%
Total carbohydrate	55–75%
◆ Free sugars	◆ <10%
Protein	10–15%
Cholesterol	<300 mg/day
Salt (NaCl)	<5 g/day
Fruits and vegetables	≥400 g/day

   Source: WHO (2003).

3. *Nutritional surveillance*: "Keeping watch over nutrition, in order to make decisions that will lead to improvement in nutrition in population."
   Source: WHO (1986).

4. *Food safety/Food hygiene*: "All conditions and measures that are necessary during the production, processing, storage, distribution and preparation of food to ensure that it is safe, sound, wholesome and fit for human consumption."
   Source: WHO (1984).

5. *Pasteurization**: "It is defined as heating of milk to such temperatures and for such periods of time as are required to destroy any pathogens that may be present while causing minimal changes in the composition, flavor and nutritive value."
   Source: WHO (1970).

6. *Food fortification/enrichment*: "Fortification or enrichment means the addition of one or more essential nutrients to a food whether or not it is normally contained in the food for the purpose of preventing or correcting a demonstrated deficiency of one or more nutrients in the population or specific population groups."
   Source: WHO/FAO International Food Standards Codex 61 (1987).

HOSPITAL WASTE MANAGEMENT

1. *Biomedical waste****: "Biomedical waste means any waste, which is generated during the diagnosis, treatment or immunization of human beings or animals or in research activities pertaining thereto or in the production or testing of biologicals, and including categories mentioned in Schedule I."
   Source: Bio-Medical Waste (Management and Handling) Rules, 1998.
2. *Sewage**: Sewage is waste water from a community containing solid and liquid excreta derived from houses, street and yard washing, factories and industries.

DISASTER MANAGEMENT

1. *Disaster****: "Any occurrence that causes damage, ecological disruption, loss of human life or deterioration of health and health services on a scale sufficient to warrant an extraordinary response from outside the affected community or area."
   Source: WHO (1999).
2. *Hazard*: "Any phenomenon that has the potential to cause disruption or damage to people and their environment."
   Source: WHO (2004).
3. *Triage**: "Triage is the process of categorising patients according to the severity of their injuries or illness, and prioritising treatment according to the availability of resources and the patients' chances of survival. The underlying principle of triage is allocating limited resources in a manner that provides the greatest health benefit to the greatest number."
   Source: WHO and Sphere Project.
4. *Disaster preparedness/Emergency preparedness***: "It is a program of long-term activities whose goals are to strengthen the overall capacity and capability of a country or a community to manage efficiently all types of emergencies and bring about an orderly transition from relief through recovery, and back to sustained development."
   Source: WHO (2007).

OCCUPATIONAL HEALTH

1. *Ergonomics*: "Ergonomics is the scientific discipline concerned with the understanding of interactions among humans and other elements of a system, and the profession that applies theory, principles, data and methods to design in order to optimize human well-being and overall system performance."
   Source: International Ergonomics Association (2014).
2. *Pneumoconiosis*: "Pneumoconiosis is the accumulation of dust in the lungs and the tissue reactions to its presence. For the purpose of this definition, 'dust' is meant to be an aerosol composed of solid inanimate particles."
   Source: Fourth International Conference on Pneumoconiosis, 1971.
3. *Sickness absenteeism*: "Work non-attendance for which access to sick leave is sought, i.e. absence attributed to sickness."
   Source: Royal Australasian College of Physicians (1999).

HEALTH STATISTICS

1. *Sampling*: "Sampling is the process by which inference is made to the whole by examining a part."
2. *Sample*: "A portion drawn from a population, the study of which is intended to lead to statistical estimates of the attributes of the whole population."
3. *Mean*: "The mean is defined as sample average."
4. *Median*: "The median is defined as the middle after all the measurements have been put in order according to their values."
5. *Mode*: "The mode is the value of the measurement in the sample that occurs most frequently."

OTHER IMPORTANT DEFINITIONS

1. *Health education****: According to WHO: "Health education is any combination of learning experiences designed to help individuals and communities improve their health, by increasing their knowledge or influencing their attitudes."

   According to Alma-Ata declaration (1978):
   "A process aimed at encouraging people to want to be healthy, to know how to stay healthy, to do what they can individually and collectively to maintain health, and to seek help when needed."

   According to John M Last:
   "The process by which individuals and groups of people learn to behave in a manner conducive to the promotion, maintenance or restoration of health."
2. *Primary health care****: "Primary health care is essential health care made universally accessible to individuals and acceptable to them, through their full participation and at a cost the community and country can afford."
   Source: Declaration of Alma-Ata (1978).
3. *Intersectoral coordination/Intersectoral action for health*: "It is defined as a recognized relationship between part or parts of the health sector with parts of another sector which has been formed to take action on an issue to achieve health outcomes in a way that is more effective, efficient or sustainable than could be achieved by the health sector acting alone."
   Source: WHO (1997).
4. *Health for all*: It can be defined as "attainment of a level of health that will enable every individual to lead a socially and economically productive life".

Chapter
11

Statistical and Epidemiological Exercises

Numerical Problems

MORTALITY RATES

1. In a village of 5000 population, 3000 are males and 2000 females. 100 had died in that year. It was estimated that 1000 persons belong to the age group of 20–40 years and 50 persons of that age group died that year. Among males, 75 males died that year. Calculate the:
   A. Crude death rate.
   B. Age specific death rate for 20–40 years.
   C. Sex specific death rate for males.

$$\text{Crude death rate (CDR)} = \frac{\text{Total number of death during that year}}{\text{Mid-year population of that year}} \times 1000$$

So, putting the above values,

$$\text{CDR} = \frac{100}{5000} \times 1000 = 20$$

So, CDR in the given year is 20 per 1000 population.

Age specific death rate for 20–40 years

$$= \frac{\text{Number of deaths of persons aged 20–40 years during the given year}}{\text{Mid-year population of persons aged 20-40 years during the given year}} \times 1000$$

So, putting the above values,

$$\text{Age specific death rate for 20–40 years} = \frac{50}{1000} \times 1000 = 50$$

So, Age specific death rate for 20–40 years age group in the given year is 50 per 1000 population.

Sex specific death rate for males

$$= \frac{\text{Number of deaths among males during the given year}}{\text{Mid-year population of males in the given year}} \times 1000$$

So, putting the above values,

$$\text{Sex specific death rate for males} = \frac{75}{3000} \times 1000 = 25$$

So, sex specific death rate for males in the given year is 25 per 1000 males.

2. In a town, there are 10,000 residents. Among them, 200 persons suffered from tuberculosis and 10 died from tuberculosis in the year 2016. Overall 80 persons died in that year. Calculate the:
   A. Case fatality rate for TB.
   B. Proportional mortality rate for TB.
   C. Specific death rate for TB.

$$\text{Case fatality rate} = \frac{\text{Total no. of deaths due to a disease}}{\text{Total no. of cases of the disease}} \times 100$$

So, putting the above values,

$$\text{Case fatality rate} = \frac{10}{200} \times 100 = 5\%$$

So, Case fatality rate for TB in 2016 is 5%.

Proportional mortality rate

$$= \frac{\text{Total no. of deaths from a disease in a year}}{\text{Total no. of deaths from all cases in that year}} \times 100$$

So, putting the above values,

$$\text{Proportional mortality rate} = \frac{10}{80} \times 100 = 12.5\%$$

So, Proportional mortality rate of TB in the year 2016 is 12.5%.

Specific death rate for a disease

$$= \frac{\text{No. of deaths from the disease during that year}}{\text{Mid-year population of that year}} \times 1000$$

So, putting the above values,

$$\text{Specific death rate for TB in 2011} = \frac{10}{10,000} \times 1000 = 1$$

So, Specific death rate for TB in the year 2016 is 1 per 1000.

MORBIDITY AND FERTILITY INDICATORS

1. In a community with a population of 60,000; there were 120 cases of pulmonary TB on 1st January, 2016. 90 new cases were detected by repeat survey on 31st December, 2016. Calculate:
   A. Incidence.
   B. Point prevalence on 1st January and 31st December.
   C. Period prevalence of pulmonary TB in the year 2016.

$$\text{Incidence} = \frac{\text{No. of new cases of a disease during a given time period}}{\text{Population at risk during that period of time}} \times 1000$$

So, putting the above values,

$$\text{Incidence} = \frac{90}{60,000} \times 1000 = 1.5$$

So, the incidence of TB in the year 2016 is 1.5 per 1000 population at risk.

Point prevalence

$$= \frac{\text{No. of all (new + old) cases of a disease at a given point of time}}{\text{Estimated population at risk the same point of time}} \times 100$$

So, putting the above values,

Point prevalence on 1st January $= \dfrac{120}{60,000} \times 100 = 0.2$

Point prevalence on 31st December $= \dfrac{(120 + 90)}{60,000} \times 100 = \dfrac{210}{60,000} \times 100 = 0.35$

So, point prevalence of TB on 1st January and 31st December are 0.2% and 0.35% respectively.

Period prevalence

$$= \frac{\begin{array}{c}\text{No. of existing (new + old) cases of a specific disease}\\ \text{during a given period of time interval}\end{array}}{\text{Estimated mid-interval population at risk}} \times 100$$

So, putting the above values,

Period prevalence of pulmonary TB in 2016 $= \dfrac{(120 + 90)}{60,000} \times 100 = 0.35$

So, period prevalence of pulmonary TB in the year 2016 is 0.35%.

2. **In a community with a population of 60,000; 10% children are <5 years of age. No. of episodes of ARI and diarrhea are 200 and 100 respectively. Calculate incidence spells of ARI and diarrhea.**

No. of <5 years children = 60,000 × 10% = 6,000

Incidence spells of a disease,

$$= \frac{\text{No. of episodes of that disease in a given period of time}}{\text{Mean no. of persons exposed to that disease in that time}} \times 1000$$

So, putting the above values,

Incidence spells of ARI $= \dfrac{200}{6,000} \times 1000 = 33.33$

Incidence spells of diarrhea $= \dfrac{100}{6,000} \times 1000 = 16.66$

So, incidence spells of ARI and diarrhea are 33.33 per 1000 population at risk and 16.66 per 1000 population at risk, respectively.

3. **There were 101 residents in a hostel. 40 cases of chickenpox were reported following 1 primary case within 2 weeks. On investigation, it was found that 52 individuals had previous history of chickenpox. Calculate secondary attack rate.**

Secondary attack rate (SAR)

$$= \frac{\begin{array}{c}\text{No. of exposed persons developing the disease within the range}\\ \text{of 1 incubation period following exposure to primary case}\end{array}}{\text{Total no. of exposed persons}} \times 100$$

Here,

Total no. of exposed persons

= [Total no. of residents – No. of primary case (s) –
No. of previously immunized persons] = (101 – 1– 52)
= 48

So, putting the above values,

$$SAR = \frac{40}{48} \times 100 = 83.33\%$$

So, the secondary attack rate of chicken pox is 83.33%.

4. **In an area with an estimated mid-year population of 100,000; 1500 live births occur in a year. Women in reproductive age group comprise 20% of the population. Calculate the general fertility rate (GFR).**

General fertility rate

$$= \frac{\text{Total no. of live births in a year}}{\text{No. of women in reproductive age group (15 – 49 years)}} \times 1000$$

No. of women in reproductive age group = 100,000 × 20% = 20,000

So, putting the above values,

$$GFR = \frac{1500}{20,000} \times 1000 = 75$$

So, general fertility rate is 75 per 1000 mid-year population in the given year.

5. **In an area, mid-year population is 70,000. 1050 live births occur in a year. Calculate the crude birth rate (CBR).**

$$\text{Crude birth rate (CBR)} = \frac{\text{Total no. of live births in a year}}{\text{Mid-year population}} \times 1000$$

So, putting the above values,

$$CBR = \frac{1050}{70,000} \times 1000 = 15$$

So, CBR is 15 per 1000 population.

NEONATAL, POSTNATAL AND INFANT MORTALITY RATES

1. **In a block of West Bengal, population is 100,000. In the year 2016, there were 3100 total births, in which 100 stillbirths and 1000 deaths occurred. 30 children died between 0–7 days and another 15 died between 8–28 days of age. There were 120 infant deaths in the year. Calculate:**

   A. **Neonatal mortality rate**   B. **Early neonatal mortality rate**
   C. **Late neonatal mortality rate**   D. **Post-neonatal mortality rate**
   E. **Infant mortality rate.**

Neonatal mortality rate (NMR)

$$= \frac{\text{No. of deaths of children up to 28 days of life}}{\text{Total no. of live births}} \times 1000$$

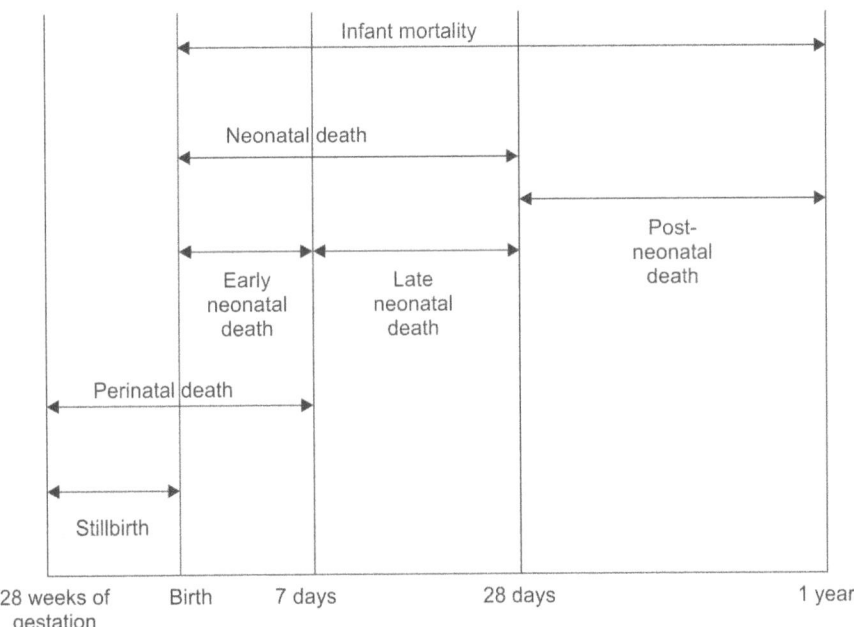

Neonatal, postnatal and infant mortality according to specific time period

No. of deaths of children up to 28 days of life= (No. of child death between 0–7 days + No. of child death between 8–28 days) = (30 + 15) = 45

Total no. of live births = (Total birth – Stillbirths) = (3100 – 100) = 3000

So, putting the above values,

$$\text{NMR} = \frac{45}{3000} \times 1000 = 15$$

So, Neonatal mortality rate is 15 per 1000 live births in the year 2016.

$$\text{Early NMR} = \frac{\text{No. of deaths of children up to 7 days of life}}{\text{Total no. of live births}} \times 1000$$

So, putting the above values,

$$\text{Early NMR} = \frac{30}{3000} \times 1000 = 10$$

So, Early neonatal mortality rate is 10 per 1000 live births in the year 2016.

$$\text{Late NMR} = \frac{\text{No. of deaths of children between 8–28 days of life}}{\text{Total no. of live births}} \times 1000$$

So, putting the above values,

$$\text{Late NMR} = \frac{15}{3000} \times 1000 = 5$$

So, Late neonatal mortality rate is 5 per 1000 live births in the year 2016.

$$\text{Post-NMR} = \frac{\text{No. of deaths of children aged} >28 \text{ days but} <1 \text{ year}}{\text{Total no. of live births}} \times 1000$$

Post-neonatal deaths

= Infant deaths – Early neonatal deaths – Late neonatal deaths

= 120 – 15 – 30 = 75

So, putting the above values,

$$\text{Post - NMR} = \frac{75}{3000} \times 1000 = 25$$

So, post-neonatal mortality rate is 25 per 1000 live births in the year 2016.

Infant mortality rate (IMR)

$$= \frac{\text{No. of deaths of children up to 1 year of age}}{\text{Total no. of live births}} \times 1000$$

So, putting the above values,

$$\text{IMR} = \frac{120}{3000} \times 1000 = 40$$

So, Infant mortality rate is 40 per 1000 live births in the year 2016.

2. In 2009, in a block of UP with a population of 200,000; 9000 live births and 900 infant deaths occurred. Similarly, in another block of MP with a population of 150,000; 5500 live births and 660 infant deaths occurred. Compare the IMRs of the blocks with the national goal.

Infant mortality rate (IMR)

$$= \frac{\text{No. of deaths of children up to 1 year of age}}{\text{Total no. of live births}} \times 1000$$

Putting the above values,

$$\text{IMR in the block of UP} = \frac{900}{9000} \times 1000$$

= 100 per 1000 live births in 2009

$$\text{IMR in the block of MP} = \frac{660}{5500} \times 1000$$

= 120 per 1000 live births in 2009

According to the RCH 2010, the national goal for IMR is to keep it below 28 per 1000 live births.

While comparing the national goal with the scenario of the two blocks of UP and MP, we find that the IMRs of both the blocks far exceeds the national goal.

PERINATAL, UNDER FIVE AND CHILD MORTALITY RATES

1. In a rural PHC of Bihar with a population of 30,000; there were 800 live births and 80 infant deaths in the year 2010. Of these, 50 infants died in the 1st 28 days of life and within them, 25 died in the 1st week of life. There were 15 stillbirths in the same year. Calculate the perinatal mortality rate and comment.

[National average of PMR in 2010 was 32]

No. of perinatal deaths

= No. of stillbirths + No. of early neonatal deaths

= 15 + 25 = 40

Perinatal mortality rate (PMR)

$$= \frac{\text{Total no. of perinatal deaths}}{\text{Total no. of live births}} \times 1000$$

So, putting the above values

$$\text{PMR} = \frac{40}{800} \times 1000 = 50$$

So, the perinatal mortality rate in the PHC in the year 2010 was 50 per 1000 live births, which was much greater than the national average of 32 per 1000 live births. So, interventional measures to control perinatal mortality should have to be implemented.

2. In a rural block with a population of 40,000; 1800 live births and 200 stillbirths occurred in the year 2010. In the same year, 100 infants died in that block along with 20 children aged 1–4 years. Calculate:

   A. Child death rate and
   B. Under 5 mortality rate.

(<5 years age group constitutes 13% of the population and 1–4 years age group constitutes 10% of the population)

Child death rate

$$= \frac{\text{No. of deaths of children aged 1-4 years}}{\text{Mid-year population of children aged 1-4 years}} \times 1000$$

Mid-year population of children aged 1–4 years

$$= 10\% \text{ of the population} = 40{,}000 \times 10\% = 4000$$

So, putting the above values

$$\text{Child death rate} = \frac{20}{4000} \times 1000 = 5$$

So, child death rate in the year 2010 was 5 per 1000 mid-year population in 1–4 years of age group.

Under 5 mortality rate

$$= \frac{\text{No. of deaths in} < 5 \text{ years age group in a year}}{\text{Total no. of live births in the given year}} \times 1000$$

No. of deaths in <5 years are group in 2010
= Infant deaths + Deaths in age group of 1–4 years
= 100 + 20 = 120

So, putting the above values,

$$\text{Under 5 mortality rate} = \frac{120}{1800} \times 1000 = 66.66$$

So, under 5 mortality rate in the year 2010 was 66.66 per 1000 live births.

3. The crude birth rate (CBR) in a block with a population of 100,000 is 20 per 1000 in the year 2011. Calculate:

   A. Perinatal mortality rate
   B. Child death rate
   C. Under 5 mortality rate.

(Given that early and late neonatal deaths are 75 and 65 respectively; still births 40, 190 under-5 deaths and 175 child deaths. Total no. of under-5 children is 120 and children in age group of 1–4 years constitute 10% of the population.)

$$\text{Perinatal deaths} = \text{Stillbirths} + \text{Early neonatal deaths}$$
$$= 40 + 75 = 115$$

We know that,

$$\text{Crude birth rate} = \frac{\text{Total no. of live births}}{\text{Mid-year population}} \times 1000$$

$$\text{Total no. of live births} = \frac{\text{Mid-year population} \times \text{CBR}}{1000}$$

Putting the above values, we get,

$$\text{Total no. of live births} = \frac{100,000 \times 20}{1000} = 2000$$

$$\text{Perinatal mortality rate} = \frac{\text{Total no. of perinatal deaths}}{\text{Total no. of live births}} \times 1000$$

So, putting the above values,

$$\text{Perinatal mortality rate} = \frac{115}{2000} \times 1000 = 57.50$$

So, perinatal mortality rate is 57.50 per 1000 live births in the year 2011.

Child death rate

$$= \frac{\text{No. of deaths of children ages 1–4 years in a year}}{\text{Mid-year population of children aged 1–4 years in that year}} \times 1000$$

Mid-year population of children aged 1–4 years in 2011
$$= 10\% \text{ of the population} = 10\% \text{ of } 100,000 = 10,000$$

So, putting the above values,

$$\text{Child death rate} = \frac{175}{10,000} \times 1000 = 17.50$$

So, child death rate is 17.50 per 1000 mid-year population in the year 2011 in the age group 1–4 years.

Under 5 mortality rate

$$= \frac{\text{No. of deaths in under 5 age group in a year}}{\text{Total no. of live births in that year}} \times 1000$$

So, putting the above values,

Under 5 mortality rate

$$= \frac{190}{2000} \times 1000 = 95$$

So, under 5 mortality rate is 95 per 1000 live births in the year 2011.

MATERNAL MORTALITY RATIO

1. In a city, total number of live births registered in 2011 was 369,800 and stillbirths were 28,965. Deaths due to the following causes were:

    - Eclampsia: 200
    - Accidents: 350
    - Unsafe abortion: 25
    - Cholera: 15
    - Puerperal sepsis: 12
    - Anemia: 250
    - Obstructed labor: 200
    - Antepartum hemorrhage: 150
    - Postpartum hemorrhage: 450

Calculate the maternal mortality ratio (MMR) and comment.

Definition of Maternal Death According to WHO

Maternal death is defined as, "the death of a woman while pregnant or within 42 days of termination of pregnancy, irrespective of the duration and site of pregnancy, from *any cause related to or aggravated by the pregnancy or its management* but not from accidental or incidental causes."

According to this definition, actual number of maternal deaths in 2011 was:

Cause	No. of deaths
Eclampsia	200
Unsafe abortion	25
Puerperal sepsis	12
Anemia	250
Obstructed labor	200
Antepartum hemorrhage	150
Postpartum hemorrhage	450
Total	**1287**

(Deaths due to accidents and cholera have not been taken as they are incidental/accidental causes).

Maternal mortality ratio

$$= \frac{\text{Total no. of maternal deaths in an area in a year}}{\text{Total no. of live births in same area in that year}} \times 100,000$$

So, putting the above values,

$$\text{MMR} = \frac{1287}{369,800} \times 100,000 = 348.02$$

The MMR in the city was 348.02 per 100,000 live births in the year 2011, which is much greater than the national goal set by MDG (109 per 100,000 live births by the year 2015). So, interventional measures must be implemented to control the MMR of the city.

2. **In a PHC with a population of 36,000; there were 9000 total births and 460 stillbirths. Maternal deaths from all causes included:**
   - Postpartum hemorrhage: 6
   - Heart disease: 2
   - Breast cancer: 2
   - Eclampsia: 2
   - Ruptured uterus: 1
   - Obstructed labor: 1
   - Accidents: 10
   - Suicidal deaths: 3
   - Puerperal sepsis: 4
   - Abortion: 2
   - Anemia: 4
   - Malaria: 2

Calculate the maternal mortality ratio (MMR) and comment.

Definition of Maternal Death According to WHO

Maternal death is defined as, "the death of a woman while pregnant or within 42 days of termination of pregnancy, irrespective of the duration and site of pregnancy, from any cause related to or aggravated by the pregnancy or its management but not from accidental or incidental causes."

According to this definition, actual number of maternal deaths in 2010 in the PHC was:

Causes	No. of deaths
Postpartum hemorrhage	6
Heart disease	2
Eclampsia	2
Ruptured uterus	1
Obstructed labor	1
Puerperal sepsis	4
Abortion	2
Anemia	4
Malaria	2
Total	**24**

(Deaths due to breast cancer/accidents/suicidal deaths have not been taken as they are incidental/accidental causes).

Maternal mortality ratio

$$= \frac{\text{Total no. of maternal deaths in an area in a year}}{\text{Total no. of live births in same area in that year}} \times 100,000$$

Total no. of live births = Total births – Stillbirths
$$= 9000 - 460 = 8540$$

So, putting the above values,

$$\text{MMR} = \frac{24}{8540} \times 100,000 = 281.03$$

The MMR of the PHC in 2010 was 281.03 per 100,000 live births; which is much greater than the national goal set by MDG (109 per 100,000 live births by the year 2015). So, interventional measures must be implemented to control the MMR of the PHC.

3. **From a survey, in a community health centre (CHC) with a total population of 160,000 in 2010, the following data were obtained:**
   - **Total births: 4900**
   - **Stillbirths: 400**

   Maternal deaths from all causes included:
   - **Eclampsia: 4**
   - **Postpartum hemorrhage: 8**
   - **Obstructed labor: 3**
   - **Anemia: 5**
   - **Road traffic accident: 4**
   - **Asthma: 1**
   - **Suicide: 2**
   - **Domestic violence: 2**

Calculate the maternal mortality ratio (MMR) and comment.

Definition of Maternal Death According to WHO

Maternal death is defined as, "the death of a woman while pregnant or within 42 days of termination of pregnancy, irrespective of the duration and site of pregnancy, from any cause related to or aggravated by the pregnancy or its management but not from accidental or incidental causes."

According to this definition, actual number of maternal deaths in 2010 in the CHC was:

Causes	No. of deaths
Eclampsia	4
Postpartum hemorrhage	8
Obstructed labor	3
Anemia	5
Total	**20**

(Deaths due to Road traffic accidents/Asthma/Suicide/Domestic violence have not been taken as they are incidental/accidental causes and not aggravated/ precipitated by pregnancy).

Maternal mortality ratio

$$= \frac{\text{Total no. of maternal deaths in an area in a year}}{\text{Total no. of live births in same area in that year}} \times 100,000$$

Total no. of live births = Total births – Stillbirths
   = 4900 – 400 = 4500

So, putting the above values,

$$\text{MMR} = \frac{20}{4500} \times 100,000 = 444.44$$

The MMR of the CHC in 2010 was 444.44 per 100,000 live births; which is much greater than the national goal set by MDG (109 per 100,000 live births by the year 2015). So, interventional measures must be implemented to control the MMR of the CHC.

RISK ASSESSMENT

1. **A healthy cohort of 18000 was followed for 25 years. 12500 of them had a sedentary lifestyle and within them, 150 developed CHD and 7 of those with active lifestyle developed CHD. Find the relative risk of sedentary lifestyle for development of CHD.**

In this question, sedentary lifestyle constitutes the exposure and CHD is the disease:

	CHD	No CHD	Total
Sedentary lifestyle	150	12350	12500
Active lifestyle	7	5493	5500
Total	**157**	**17843**	**18000**

$$\text{Relative risk} = \frac{\text{Incidence of disease among exposed}}{\text{Incidence of disease among non-exposed}}$$

So,

Relative risk of sedentary lifestyle for development of CHD

$$= \frac{\text{incidence of CHD among those with sedentary lifestyle}}{\text{Incidence of CHD among those with active lifestyle}}$$

Incidence of CHD among those with sedentary lifestyle

$$= \frac{150}{12500} \times 1000 = 12 \text{ per } 1000$$

Incidence of CHD among those with active lifestyle

$$= \frac{7}{5500} \times 1000 = 1.27 \text{ per } 1000$$

So,

Relative risk of sedentary lifestyle for development of CHD

$$= \frac{12 \text{ per } 1000}{1.27 \text{ per } 1000} = 9.45$$

So, the relative risk of sedentary lifestyle for development of CHD is 9.45.

2. **3000 smokers and 5000 non-smokers were followed up for 20 years. 84 smokers and 87 non-smokers developed CHD. Calculate relative risk (RR) and attributable risk (AR) of smoking for development of CHD.**

In this question, smoking constitutes the exposure and CHD is the disease:

	CHD	No CHD	Total
Smokers	84	2916	3000
Non-smokers	87	4913	5000
Total	**171**	**7829**	**8000**

$$\text{Relative risk} = \frac{\text{Incidence of disease among exposed}}{\text{Incidence of disease among non-exposed}}$$

So,
Relative risk of smoking for development of CHD

$$= \frac{\text{Incidence of CHD among smokers}}{\text{Incidence of CHD among non-smokers}}$$

Incidence of CHD among smokers

$$= \frac{84}{3000} \times 1000 = 28 \text{ per 1000 persons}$$

Incidence of CHD among non-smokers

$$= \frac{87}{5000} \times 1000 = 17.40 \text{ per 1000 persons}$$

So,
Relative risk of smoking for development of CHD

$$= \frac{28 \text{ per 1000 persons}}{17.40 \text{ per 1000 persons}} = 1.61$$

Attributable risk

$$= \frac{\text{Incidence of disease among exposed} - \text{Incidence of disease among non-exposed}}{\text{Incidence of disease among exposed}} \times 100$$

So,
Attributable risk of smoking for the development of CHD

$$= \frac{28 - 17.40}{28} \times 100 = \frac{10.60}{28} \times 100 = 37.85\%.$$

Relative risk of smoking for development of CHD is 1.61. Attributable risk of smoking for development of CHD is 37.85%.

3. **A total 50 cases of cerebral palsy and 95 controls were surveyed; out of which 47 cases and 62 controls gave history of forceps delivery. Calculate the Odds ratio as a risk for cerebral palsy.**

In this question, forceps delivery constitutes the exposure and cerebral palsy is the disease.

	Cases of cerebral palsy	Controls	Total
History of forceps delivery	47 (a)	62 (b)	109
No forceps delivery	3 (c)	33 (d)	36
Total	**50**	**95**	**145**

(The numbers in bold are given in the question).

$$\text{Odds ratio} = \frac{\text{Odds of cases being exposed}}{\text{Odds of controls being exposed}}$$

$$\text{Odds of cases being exposed} \frac{a}{c} = \frac{47}{3}$$

$$\text{Odds of controls being exposed} \frac{b}{d} = \frac{62}{33}$$

So,

$$\text{Odds ratio} = \frac{\dfrac{47}{3}}{\dfrac{62}{33}} = \frac{15.67}{1.88} = 8.34$$

So, Odds ratio as a risk for cerebral palsy is 8.34. It implies that babies delivered by forceps delivery are at 8.34 times more risk of developing cerebral palsy than babies delivered otherwise.

SENSITIVITY, SPECIFICITY, POSITIVE AND NEGATIVE PREDICTIVE VALUE

General Concepts and Formulas

There are three inherent properties of a screening test; which together determines the 'validity' of a screening test; that is, the extent to which the test accurately measures which it purports to measure.

A. Sensitivity
B. Specificity
C. Predictive accuracy: Positive and negative predictive value.

❖ *Sensitivity*: Ability of a test to identify correctly all those who actually have the disease (true-positive).
❖ *Specificity*: Ability of a test to identify correctly all those who actually don't have the disease (true-negative).
❖ *Positive predictive value (PPV)*: Probability of the person actually having the disease when the test is positive.
❖ *Negative predictive value (NPV)*: Probability of the person not having the disease when the test is negative.

Note: *Relation between predictive value and prevalence of a disease*: A crucial point to note is that prevalence affects the predictive value of any test. The more prevalent a disease is in the population, the more accurate the predictive value will be (for a positive screening test).

Mathematical Representation

In the table below:
❖ **a**: Persons who actually have the disease and tested positive for the disease (true-positive)
❖ **b**: Persons who actually do not have the disease and tested positive for the disease (false-positive)
❖ **c**: Persons who actually have the disease and tested negative for the disease (false-negative)
❖ **d**: Persons who actually do not have the disease and tested negative for the disease (true-negative).

Screening test results	Diagnosis		Row total
	Diseased	*Not diseased*	
Positive	a (TP)	b (FP)	a + b
Negative	c (FN)	d (TN)	c + d
Column total	a + c	b + d	a + b + c + d

In this case, the following formula can be worked out:

$$\text{Sensitivity} = \frac{\text{True positive}}{\text{True positive} + \text{False negative}} = \frac{a}{a+c}$$

$$\text{Specificity} = \frac{\text{True negative}}{\text{True negative} + \text{False positive}} = \frac{d}{d+b}$$

$$\text{Positive predictive value (PPV)} = \frac{\text{True positive}}{\text{True positive} + \text{False positive}}$$

$$= \frac{a}{a+b}$$

$$\text{Negative predictive value} = \frac{\text{True negative}}{\text{True negative} + \text{False negative}}$$

$$= \frac{d}{d+c}$$

RELEVANT QUESTIONS

1. A medical research team identified breast CA promoting factor (BCPF) in explant culture of breast tumor. A pilot study reveals that plasma level of BCPF was elevated in confirmed breast CA patients. The investigators conducted a clinical trial to determine whether the measurement of plasma BRPF level would be used to diagnose breast CA or not. 600 patients were demonstrated to have breast CA by breast biopsy (Gold standard) and 1000 were found to be disease free. 570 of breast CA patients and 150 of patients not suffering from breast CA had a +Ve BCPF test. Calculate sensitivity, specificity and predictive accuracy of the test.

Screening test (serum BCPF) results	Diagnosis		Row total
	Diseased	Not diseased	
Positive	570	150	720
Negative	30	850	880
Column total	600	1000	1600

Sensitivity = Ability of the test to detect true positives

$$= \frac{TP}{TP + FN} = \frac{570}{570 + 30} = \frac{570}{600} \times 100\% = 95\%$$

Specificity = Ability of the test to detect true negatives

$$= \frac{TN}{TN + FP} = \frac{850}{850 + 150} = \frac{850}{1000} \times 100\% = 85\%$$

Positive predictive value (PPV)

= Probability of a person actually having the disease when the test is positive

$$= \frac{TP}{TP + FP} = \frac{570}{570 + 150} = \frac{570}{720} \times 100\% = 79\%$$

Negative predictive value

= Probability of a person not having the disease when the test is negative

$$= \frac{TN}{TN + FN} = \frac{850}{850 + 30} = \frac{850}{880} \times 100\% = 96.6\%.$$

2. **A test for hepatitis C is performed for 200 patients with biopsy-proven disease and 200 patients known to be free of the disease. The test shows positive results on 180 of the patients with the disease and negative results on 150 patients without the disease. Calculate the sensitivity, specificity and predictive accuracy of the test.**

Screening test results	Diagnosis		Row total
	Diseased	Not diseased	
Positive	180	50	230
Negative	20	150	170
Column total	**200**	**200**	400

Sensitivity = Ability of the test to detect true positives

$$= \frac{TP}{TP + FN} = \frac{180}{180 + 20} = \frac{180}{200} \times 100\% = 90\%$$

Specificity = Ability of the test to detect true negatives

$$= \frac{TN}{TN + FP} = \frac{150}{150 + 50} = \frac{150}{200} \times 100\% = 75\%$$

Positive predictive value (PPV)

= Probability of a person actually having the disease when the test is positive

$$= \frac{TP}{TP + FP} = \frac{180}{180 + 50} = \frac{180}{230} \times 100\% = 78.26\%$$

Negative predictive value

= Probability of a person not having the disease when the test is negative

$$= \frac{TN}{TN + FN} = \frac{150}{150 + 20} = \frac{150}{170} \times 100\% = 88.24\%$$

3. **The findings of a test using a screening level of 130 mg/dL of random blood glucose are shown in the following table:**

Test	Diabetic	Non-diabetic	Total
Positive	66	98	164
Negative	84	9782	9836
Total	150	9850	10000

Calculate the sensitivity and specificity.

Sensitivity = Ability of the test to detect true positives

$$= \frac{TP}{TP + FN} = \frac{66}{66 + 84} = \frac{66}{150} \times 100\% = 44\%$$

Specificity = Ability of the test to detect true negatives

$$= \frac{TN}{TN + FP} = \frac{9782}{9782 + 98} = \frac{9782}{9880} \times 100\% = 99\%$$

4. **In a population of 10000 people, the prevalence of a disease is 20%. The sensitivity of a screening test is 95% and specificity is 80%. Calculate the positive predictive value (PPV) of the test.**

Persons actually having the disease = 10000 × 20% = 2000

Persons actually not having the disease = (10000 – 2000) = 8000

$$\text{Sensitivity} = \frac{\text{True positive}}{\text{Persons actually having the disease}}$$

So,

True positive

= Persons actually having the disease × Sensitivity

= 2000 × 95% = 1900

$$\text{Specificity} = \frac{\text{True negative}}{\text{Persons actually not having the disease}}$$

So,

True negative

= Persons actually not having the disease × Specificity

= 8000 × 80% = 6400

Now, if we construct the table

Screening test results	Diagnosis		Row total
	Diseased	Not diseased	
Positive	1900	1600	3500
Negative	100	6400	6500
Column total	2000	8000	10000

Positive predictive value (PPV)

= Probability of a person actually having the disease when the test is positive

$$= \frac{\text{TP}}{\text{TP + FP}} = \frac{1900}{1900 + 1600} = \frac{1900}{3500} \times 100\% = 54.29\%$$

MEDICAL STATISTICS

1. **In a secondary school, number of students present in the mid-day meal in a week was as follows:**

    – Monday: 70
    – Tuesday: 56
    – Wednesday: 60
    – Thursday: 65
    – Friday: 51
    – Saturday: 70

Calculate: The mean, the median, the mode.

$$\text{Mean} = \frac{\text{Sum of individual values}}{\text{Total no. of observations}} = \frac{\Sigma n}{n}$$

Putting the above values,

$$\text{Mean} = \frac{70 + 56 + 60 + 65 + 51 + 70}{6} = \frac{372}{6} = 62$$

The mean no. of students is 62.

Median is depicted by the middle value in order of magnitude.

No. of students
70
56
60
65
51
70

Data unarranged

No. of students
51
56
60
65
70
70

Data arranged in order of magnitude

As the number of observations (n) is even (6), so

$$\text{Median} = \frac{\frac{n}{2}\text{th observation} + \left(\frac{n}{2} + 1\right)\text{the observation}}{2}$$

$$= \frac{\frac{6}{2}\text{th observation} + \left(\frac{6}{2} + 1\right)\text{the observation}}{2}$$

$$= \frac{\text{3rd observation} + \text{4th observation}}{2} = \frac{60 + 65}{2} = \frac{125}{2}$$

$$= 62.50$$

Note: If the number of observations (n) would be odd, then

$$\text{Median} = \left(\frac{n + 1}{2}\right)\text{th observation}$$

The median no. of students is 62.5.

Mode is depicted by the value with highest frequency.

Data: **70**, 56, 60, 65, 51, **70.**

Hence, mode value is 70 students.

The mode value is 70.

Frequency Distribution

Relevant information needed to deal with this type of questions:

❖ **Frequency (f)**: The frequency of a particular observation is the number of times, the observation occurs in the data.

❖ **Distribution**: The distribution of a variable is the pattern of frequencies of the observation.

❖ **Frequency distribution**: It can show either the actual number of observations falling in each range or the percentage of observations.

❖ **Class interval**: If a variable has a large number of values, it is easier to present the data by grouping the values into class intervals, e.g. age of the population presented as age groups (years): 0–4, 5–9, 10–14, 15–19, etc.

❖ Methods to graphically represent a frequency distribution:

– **Frequency table**: A table presenting statistical data by putting together the values of a characteristic along with the number of times each value appears in the data set.

Example: Frequency table to show the distribution of the number of cars in a car park according to the colors:

Color of car	Tally	Frequency
Red	JHT JHT I	11
Blue	JHT	5
Green	JHT III	8
Black	IIII	4
White	I	1
Other	JHT II	7
Total		**36**

– **Frequency histogram**: A graph that consists of a series of columns, each having a class interval as its base and frequency of occurrence as its height.

Example:

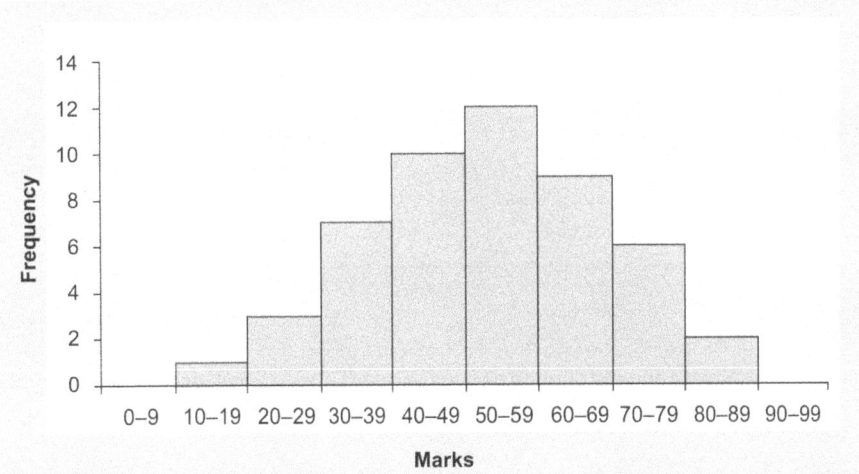

Frequency histogram to show the distribution of marks achieved by the students in an examination

– **Frequency polygon**: A graph formed by joining the midpoints of histogram column tops.

Example:

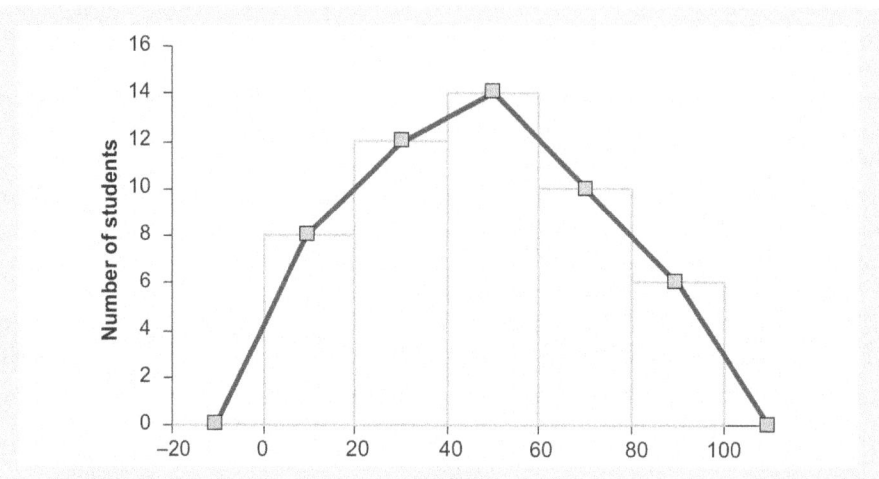

Frequency polygon to show the distribution of marks achieved by the students in an examination

- **Bar diagram**: A separate horizontal/vertical bar is drawn for each category. The length of the bars is proportional to the frequency in that category. The bars are separated by small gaps to indicate that the data are categorical and separate from each other.

   Example:

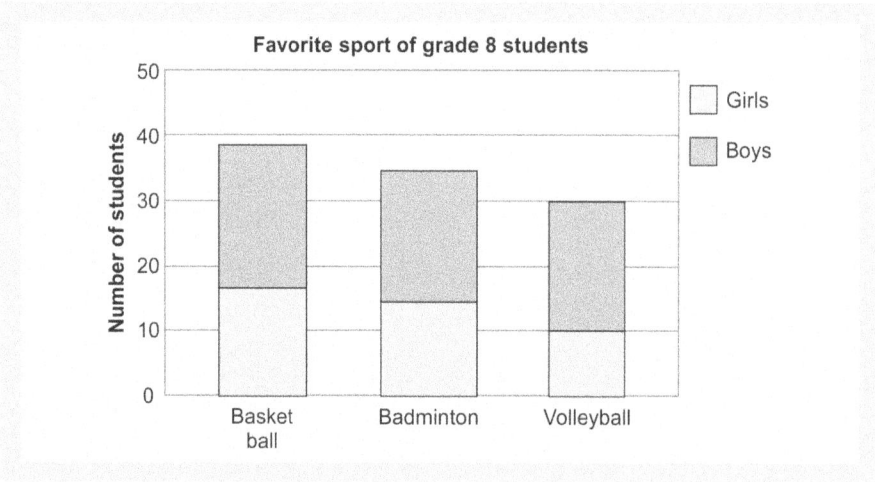

Bar diagram showing the distribution of favorite sports (basket ball, badminton, volleyball) in grade 8 students of a school

- **Pie chart**: A circular 'pie' is split into sectors, one for each category, so that the area of each sector is proportional to the frequency in that category (Here 360 degree is equivalent to 100%).

Example:

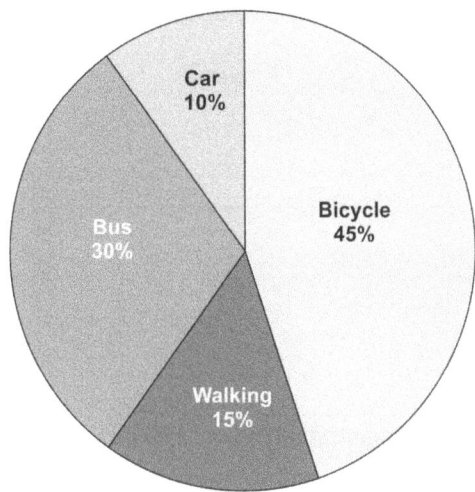

Pie chart showing the distribution of route of transportation in a group of students for attending school

RELEVANT QUESTIONS

1. In June 2012, 15 patients were admitted in pediatrics department of a medical college. Their age in years was as follows: 1, 5, 12, 3, 3, 8, 2, 1, 1, 9, 3, 11, 7, 1, 2.

Draw a frequency distribution table with the given data.

Class interval (in years)	Tally bar	Frequency (f)	Percentage (%)
1–2	ЖІ	6	$\frac{6}{15} \times 100 = 40$
3–4	|||	3	$\frac{3}{15} \times 100 = 20$
5–6			1	$\frac{1}{15} \times 100 = 6.7$
7–8	||	2	$\frac{2}{15} \times 100 = 13.3$
9–10			1	$\frac{1}{15} \times 100 = 6.7$
11–12	||	2	$\frac{2}{15} \times 100 = 13.3$
Total		**15**	**100**

Special note: Do not make too much class intervals; try to keep it around 5.

Frequency distribution table showing the distribution of age of patients (in years) admitted to the pediatrics department

Age in years	Frequency	Percentage
1–2	6	40%
3–4	3	20%
5–6	1	6.7%
7–8	2	13.3%
9–10	1	6.7%
11–12	2	13.3%
Total	**15**	**100%**

2. Number of infants attending immunization clinic of a medical college in the first 3 days of the last week was as follows:

Day	No. of infants
Monday	10
Tuesday	15
Wednesday	10

Represent the Data with a Bar diagram

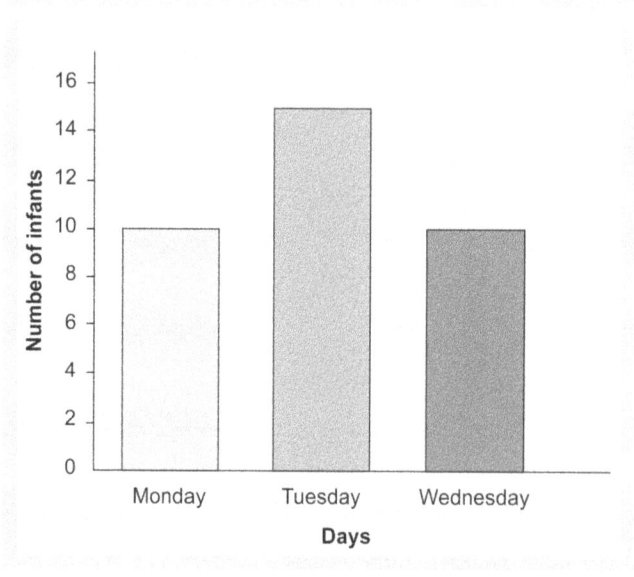

Bar diagram showing the number of infants attending immunization clinic of a medical college in the first 3 days of last week

3. **Distribution of blood groups in a group of students are as follows:**

Blood group	No. of students
A	50
B	20
O	20
AB	10

Construct a pie diagram with the above data.

Blood group	No. of students	Percentage	Angle in pie chart (°)
A	50	50%	$\dfrac{50}{100} \times 360 = 180°$
B	20	20%	$\dfrac{20}{100} \times 360 = 72°$
O	20	20%	$\dfrac{20}{100} \times 360 = 72°$
AB	10	10%	$\dfrac{10}{100} \times 360 = 36°$
Total	**100**	**100%**	**360°**

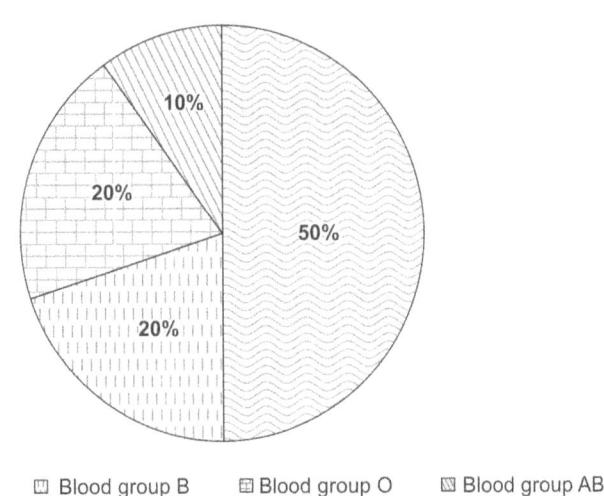

Blood group A   Blood group B   Blood group O   Blood group AB

Pie chart showing distribution of blood groups in students

Chapter
12
Family

1. What type of family you got?

Answer accordingly.

2. Define family.

Family is a group of people related by blood or marriage or adoption, living together under the same roof and eating from a common kitchen.

3. What are the types of family?

Family can be classified from different aspects:

According to structure of family:
- ❖ Nuclear family:
  - – It consists of the married couple and their children (till they are regarded as dependents).
  - – In the nuclear family, husband usually plays the dominant role in the household.
- ❖ Joint family:
  - – It consists of a number of married couples and their children who live together in the same household.
  - – All the men are related by blood and all the women are their wives/unmarried girls/widows.
- ❖ Three generation family:
  - – Here, three generations related to each other (young couples with their children and parents) live together due to unavailability of a separate house.

According to pattern of marriage:
- ❖ *Monogamous:* Monogamy is the practice of being married to only one person at any one time. Therefore, a monogamous family is one in which the husband and wife are in a monogamous relationship. In other words, they are married to one another exclusively.
- ❖ *Polygamous:* Polygamy is the practice of having more than one spouse—usually, it refers to a situation in which a husband has more than one wife.
- ❖ *Polyandrous:* Polyandry is practice whereby a woman takes two or more husbands at the same time.

According to sanction of marriage:
- ❖ Exogenous family
- ❖ Endogenous family.

According to dependency:
- ❖ *Patriarchal family:* Here males are the primary authority figures central to social organization, occupying roles of political leadership, moral authority, and control of property and where fathers hold authority over women and children.

❖ *Matriarchal family*: Here mother/female plays the central role in the family.

Abnormal family:
❖ *Broken family:*
   − A broken family is one where the parents have separated/where death of one/both of the parents has occurred.
   − This separation may be of two types:
     - *Paternal separation:* Separation of the child from its father.
     - *Dual parental separation:* Separation of the child from both of its parents.
❖ *Problem family:*
   Problem families are those which *lag behind the rest of the community, where the standards of life are far below the accepted minimum and where parents are unable to meet the physical and emotional needs of their children.*

4. What are the advantages and disadvantages of joint and nuclear family?

Type	Advantages	Disadvantages
Nuclear family	• Here husband-wife relationship is likely to be more intimate • Family relationship is principally focused inwardly and ties to extended kin are voluntary and based on emotional bonds, rather than duties and obligations	Does not provide sharing of responsibilities of greater economic and social security
Joint family	• Responsibilities are shared giving family greater economic and social security • Old, helpless, unemployed and children are provided security socially and economically • Family relations enjoy primary over marital relations • Merit of joint family is based on the motto of "union is strength"	Intimacy of husband and wife is sometimes compromised

5. What are the stages of family cycle?

Stages of family cycle and their characteristics are as follows:

Phases of family cycle	Beginning	End
Formation	Marriage	Birth of 1st child
Extension	Birth of 1st child	Birth of last child
Complete extension	Birth of last child	1st child leaves home
Contraction	1st child leaves home	Last child leaves home of parents
Complete contraction	Last child leaves home of parents	1st spouse dies
Dissolution	1st spouse dies	Death of survivor (extinction)

6. What are the functions of family?

❖ Residence
❖ Division of labor
❖ Reproduction and bringing up of children

❖ Socialization
❖ Economic function
❖ Social care
❖ Education
❖ Emotional support
❖ Bridging up the generation gap.

7. What are the importance of religion, language and caste in the family?

	Importance
Religion	• Some religion practices such behaviors that affect health or disease pattern in the community
Language	• For making IEC material • For communication with health care provider individual
Caste	• For providing different scheme under national health policy (SC, ST, OBC)

8. Who is HOF/head of family?

HOF is the principal decision maker/principal earning member of the family.

9. What are the important social problems?

❖ School drop outs
❖ Child labor
❖ Unemployment
❖ Poverty
❖ Illiteracy
❖ Drug addiction
❖ Alcohol abuse
❖ Unmarried mother
❖ Prostitution
❖ Delinquency
❖ Handicapped/chronically ill individual.

10. What social problems did you encounter in the family?

Answer accordingly.

11. How will you determine socioeconomic status?

By modified Kuppuswami scale (used for urban families).
❖ Parameter of modified Kuppuswami scale:
   – Education of HOF
   – Occupation of HOF
   – Income of the family per month.

Scoring System

Score	Socioeconomic class
26–29	Upper
16–25	Upper middle
11–15	Lower middle
5–10	Upper lower
<5	Lower

Other socioeconomic scales (also important for MCQs)

Socioeconomic scales	Example(s)
Urban socioeconomic scale	• Modified Kuppuswami scale • Kulshrestha scale • Srivastava scale
Rural socioeconomic scale	• Udai Pareek scale • Modified BG Prasad scale
Both rural + urban socioeconomic scale	• Prasad scale
Student's socioeconomic scale	• Bharadwaj scale
Non-Indian socioeconomic scale	• Holligsheed scale • Henderson scale

12. How will you determine age of the child?

By:
❖ Documentary evidence, e.g. birth certificate, immunization card, etc.
❖ Oral evidence, e.g. local events calendar.

13. Who is a literate?

Literate is a person who can read and write understanding any language above 7 years of age.

14. What are the different educational qualifications?

Educational qualification	Class
Primary	Up to class IV
Middle	Class V–VIII
Secondary	Class IX–X
Higher secondary	Class XI–XII

15. Who is a skilled worker?

A person who has trained a particular trade, e.g. carpenter, driver, manson, tailor, etc.

16. Who is an unskilled worker?

A person not trained in a particular occupation, e.g. daily wager, rickshaw puller, maid servant, etc.

17. What are the energy requirements of adult Indians?

Age group	Category	Body weight (kg)	Energy requirement (kcal)
Man	• Sedentary work • Moderate work • Heavy work	60 60 60	2320 2730 3490
Woman	• Sedentary work • Moderate work • Heavy work	55 55 55	1900 2230 2850
Pregnant woman		55 + GWG	+ 350
Lactational woman		55 + WG	+ 600 (0–6 months) + 520 (6–12 months)

(GWG: Gestational weight gain; WG: Gestational weight gain remaining after delivery)

18. Who are reference Indian adult man and woman?

Criteria	Reference man	Reference woman
Age (years)	18–29	18–29 (NPNL)
Weight (kg)	60	55
Height (meter)	1.73	1.61
BMI	20.3	21.2

Other criteria	• On each working day he/she involves moderate activity
	 • While when not at work he/she:
	   – Spends 8 hours in bed
	   – 4–6 hours in sitting
	   – Moving about 2 hours in walking, active recreation or house-hold activities	

(NPNL: Non-pregnant, non-lactating; BMI: Body mass index)

19. Define child labor, school dropout and consumption unit.

❖ ***Child labor***: Below 14 years of age if a child is engaged in a work inside or outside the family.

❖ ***School dropout***: 5–14 years old children not going to school for >3 months without major illness or vacation.

❖ ***Consumption unit***: The energy consumption of an average male *doing sedentary work* is taken as 1 CU.

20. What are the criteria for the following?

i. Sanitary latrine
ii. Overcrowding
iii. Ventilation
iv. Housing.

Sanitary Latrine

A sanitary latrine should fulfill the following criteria:

Excreta should not:

❖ Contaminate the ground or surface water

❖ Pollute the soil

❖ Be accessible to flies, rodents, animals (pigs, dogs, cattle, etc.) and other vehicles of transmission.

❖ Create nuisance due to odor/unsightly appearance.

Overcrowding

Definition

Overcrowding refers to the situation, in which more people are living within a single dwelling than there is space for, so that:

❖ Movement is restricted

❖ Privacy secluded

❖ Hygiene impossible

❖ Rest and sleep difficult.

Accepted Standards with Respect to Overcrowding

1. **Person per room:** Accepted standards

Room	Person
1	2
2	3
3	5
4	7
5	10
>5	Add 2 per room

2. **Floor space:** Accepted standards

Floor space (sq ft)	Persons
≥110	2
90–100	1.5*
70–90	1
50–70	0.5*
<50	0

(* Children aged <12 months are not counted. Children aged 1–10 years are counted as 0.5.)

3. **Sex separation:** Overcrowding is considered to be present if 2 persons aged >9 years, who are not husband and wife and of opposite sexes are obliged to sleep in the same room.

Ventilation

Cubic Space

Standards for minimal fresh air supply → 300–3000 cu ft/hr/person.

(Fresh air supply: 3000 cu ft/hr/person; when:
CO_2 concentration due to respiration <2/10,000 parts in air)

Air Change

Type of room	Air changes/hr
Living room	2–3
Work room/assemblies	4–6

(If air changes >6/hr → may cause drought)

Floor Space

Optimum floor space: 50–100 sq ft
Height >10–12 ft are ineffective from the view point of ventilation.

Housing

Parameters	Criteria
Site	• Elevated from surroundings • Away from nuisance • Subsoil water below loft

Contd..

Contd..

Parameters	Criteria
Set back	Built up to 2/3 of total area
Floor	Pucca, height of plinth 2–3 ft
Walls	9 inch brick, well plastered, low heat capacity
Rooms	Should be depending on family size
Roof	• >10 ft (in absence of AC) • Low heat transmittance co-efficient
Floor area	50–100 sq ft/person
Cubic space	>500 cu ft per capita
Windows	• 1/5 of floor space • Doors + windows → 2/5 of floor space • Placed at height of not >3 ft from floor
Lighting	Day light factor >1% over ½ of floor area
Kitchen	• Separate • Impervious floor • Adequately lightened, provided with water supply and drainage
Privy	Sanitary privy in each house
Garbage and refuse	Sanitary disposal method
Bathing and washing	Exclusive facilities
Water supply	Safe + adequate water supply

Rural housing standards in India

Parameters	Criteria
Living room	Minimum—2
Verandah space	Ample
Set back	Built up area up to 1/3 of total area
Kitchen	Separate kitchen with paved sink/platform
Sanitary latrine	Discussed earlier
Windows area	>10% of floor space
Cattle shed	>25 ft away from dwelling
Distance from nearest sanitary well/tube well	<¼ mile
Disposal of waste water, refuse and garbage	Adequate arrangement

21. What are the advantages and disadvantages of intermittent and continuous water supply?

Points	Advantages	Disadvantages
Intermittent water supply	• Less wastage of water • Less energy consumption • Less expenditure	• Inconvenient for users • Stored water may be contaminated • Sometimes intermittent water supply creates (-ve) suction pressure which can cause contamination by various organisms, soil, etc.
Continuous water supply	• 24 × 7 hours water supply is very convenient for users • Less chance of contamination	• More water wastage • More energy consumption • More expenditure

22. What is exclusive breastfeeding (EBF)?

EBF is defined as feeding only breast milk and giving no food or drinking water or anything other than breast milk; except medication when indicated.

23. Define other types of breastfeeding.

Type of feeding	Description
Predominant feeding	Breast milk + water/water-based product
Mixed feeding	Breast milk + milk/milk-based product
Token feeding	Mainly artificial feeding + occasionally breastfeeding

24. What is good positioning and good attachment?

Good Position/Correct Position

❖ The baby's whole body should face the mother and be close to her
❖ The baby's head and neck should be supported, in a straight line with his body, to face the breast
❖ Baby's abdomen should touch mother's abdomen, to be as close as possible to his mother.

Signs of a Good/Correct Attachment

❖ The baby's mouth is wide open
❖ The baby's chin touches the breast
❖ The baby's lower lip is curled outward
❖ Usually the lower portion of the areola is not visible.

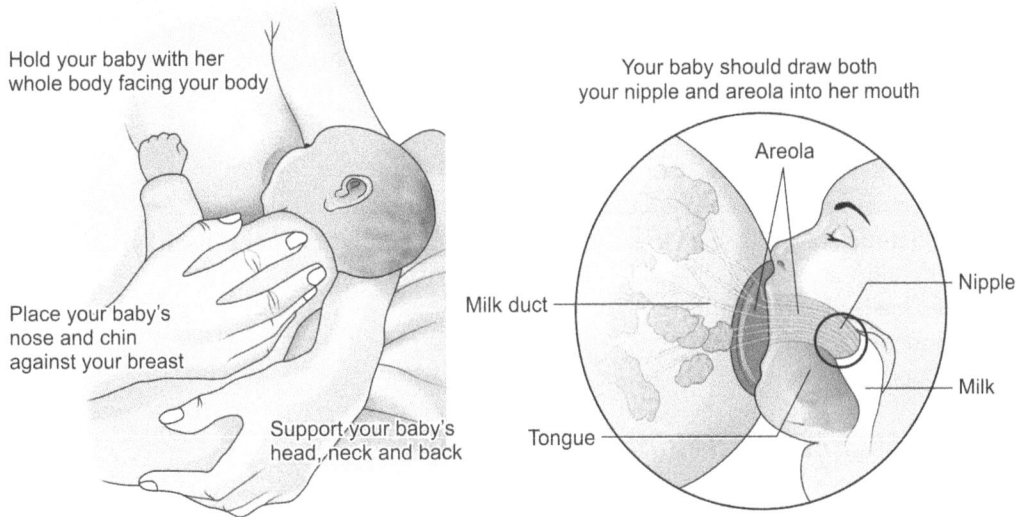

Proper breastfeeding position and latch-on

Chapter
13

Project

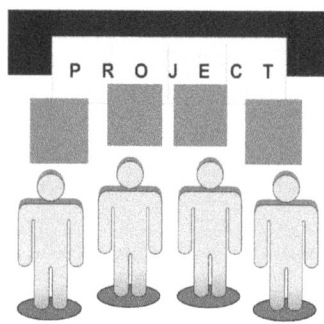

DEFINITION

Project is a set of activity carried out by a single person or in groups either to gain new knowledge or to test hypothesis or to find out empirical solutions of problems and give some recommendations.

VARIABLE

It is the measurable characteristic of a person or a thing that can vary.

TYPES

A. On the basis of measurability:
- Qualitative (can be measured and counted), e.g. height and weight.
- Quantitative (cannot be measured but can be counted), e.g. sex, healthy/unhealthy, literate/illiterate.

B. On the basis of dependence:
- Independent/input
- Dependent/output.

DIFFERENCE BETWEEN PROJECT AND PROGRAM

Topic	Project	Program
Time	Limited	Not such
Resource	Limited	Not limited
Orientation	Objective oriented	Goal oriented

CENSUS

Primary data collected from every member of target population.

DATA

When a variable is counted, measured and recorded it is called data (singular: *Datum*).

Types

A. On the basis of mode of collection:
- *Primary*: Collected by the investigator himself or under his supervision for the purpose of his concerned research.
- *Secondary*: Collected by somebody else for a different purpose and the investigator uses those data for his/her concerned purpose.

B. On the basis of ability to measure:
- *Quantitative data*: Obtained by measurement.

  Continuous data:
  - Measurements are in precise value and fractions are possible, e.g. height, weight, Hb, etc.

  Discrete data:
  - Measurements are in whole number (range is given), fractions are not possible, e.g. red blood cell (RBC) count, blood pressure (BP) estimation, etc.

- *Qualitative data*:
  - Obtained by enumeration or counting
  - Data only in full numbers not in fractions, e.g. sex, occupation, etc.

Population

A population can be defined as including all people or items with the characteristic one wishes to understand.

Because there is very rarely enough time or money to gather information from everyone or everything in a population, the goal becomes finding a representative sample (or subset) of that population.

Study Population

Population for which the research is being done, i.e. on whom the findings of the research or the benefit of the research will be implemented/recommended/generalized/established.

Study Type and Design

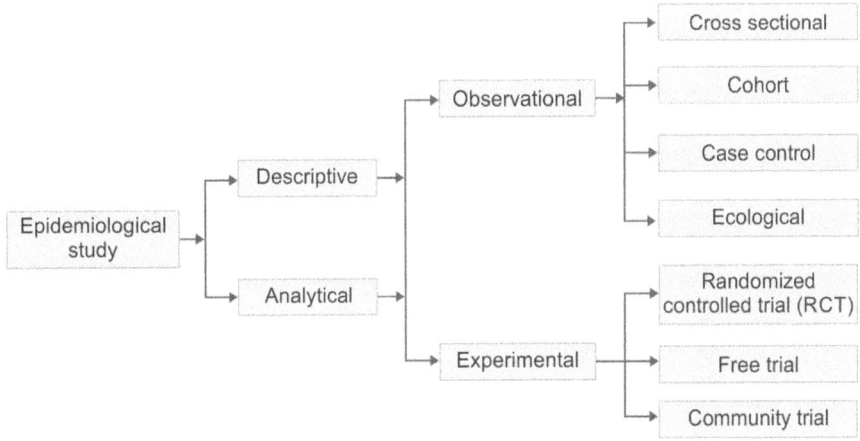

Sampling

See sampling Short Note Page No. 235.

Procedures of Data Collection

A. Questionnaire:
❖ Open
❖ Closed
❖ Mixed.

B. Schedule:
❖ Structured
❖ Semi-structured
❖ Unstructured.

Pretesting is done on the similar group of persons as in the study population but not within it. Done on 5% of total study population.

Give special stress on the following points of your project work in the viva table:
❖ Title
❖ Objective
❖ Methodology
  - Type of study
  - Design of study
  - Study area/study setting
  - Duration of study
  - Study population
  - Study variables
    - Outcome/dependent variable
    - Independent
  - Technique of data collection
  - Tool for data collection
  - Data collection
❖ Summary
❖ Recommendation
❖ Limitation of the study.

Chapter
14

Problem Cards

Authors' Note

Importance of this chapter in examination

For theory purpose

Frequently comes as long questions

For practical purpose

It contains 10 marks in practical examination as "Problem solving exercises"

DISEASE RELATED

1. A 28-year-old male patient presents with history of a discharge from penis. On examination, you find presence of urethral discharge, but no genital ulcer.
    A. What is the most probable cause of this condition?
    B. Outline the management components of this patient according to syndromic approach.

Most Probable Cause of this Condition

❖ Gonorrhea
❖ Nongonococcal urethritis (Chlamydia, Trichomoniasis).

Management Components of this Patient

Diagnosis

History:
❖ Increased frequency of urination
❖ Pain along with burning sensation while passing urine
❖ High-risk sexual behavior, e.g. multiple sexual partners.

Symptoms:
❖ Urethral discharge/vaginal discharge (usually pus/mucopurulent)
❖ Genital swelling/ulcer/wart
❖ Scrotal swelling
❖ Lower abdominal pain.

Laboratory investigation: If possible.

Treatment:
❖ General consideration
❖ Specific treatment.

Specific Treatment

❖ Provide KIT-1 (gray color) under supervision:
  – Tablet cefixime 400 mg OD stat and
  – Tablet azithromycin 1 g OD stat
  – Advice the patient to return after 7 days
❖ If patient is allergic to azithromycin, tablet erythromycin 400 mg 4 times daily for 7 days is preferred.
❖ If discharge persists: Give secnidazole 2 g orally single dose.
❖ If still discharge persists: Refer the patient to higher center.

Note: In case of female patient, KIT-1 is administered only after rule out pregnancy and history of allergy.

2. **A 28-year-old lady complains of excessive vaginal discharge. On examination, there is mucopurulent cervical discharge and tenderness on bimanual pelvic examination. She tells that her husband is a truck driver and has a 2nd wife.**

   A. **What is your provisional diagnosis?**

   B. **How will you manage this case?**

My provisional diagnosis is pelvic inflammatory disease (PID).

Management of the Case

Diagnosis

History:
❖ Lower abdominal pain
❖ Vaginal discharge
❖ Fever
❖ Menstrual irregularities like heavy, irregular, painful bleeding
❖ Dysmenorrhea: Pain during menstruation that interferes with daily activity
❖ Dyspareunia: Pain during intercourse
❖ Dysuria: Painful urination
❖ Lower backache.

Examination:
❖ *It may reveal cervical motion tenderness.*
❖ *Laboratory investigation (if possible):*
  – Wet smear
  – Gram stain
  – Preg-color test
  – Urine examination.

Treatment:
❖ General consideration
❖ Specific treatment.

Specific Treatment

❖ Provide KIT-6 (yellow color) under supervision:
  – Tablet cefixime 400 mg OD stat

    – Tablet metronidazole 400 mg BD × 14 days and
    – Tablet doxycycline 100 mg BD × 14 days.
❖ Follow up at 3rd, 7th and 14th days
❖ If the patient is an IUD user, remove the IUD under cover of antibiotics for 24–48 hours
❖ If there are no signs of improvement in the serial follow-up visits, the patient should be referred to higher centers
❖ If there is severe pain, a potent analgesic may be prescribed along with KIT-6 (ibuprofen with ranitidine).

Reproductive Tract Infection (RTI)/Sexually Transmitted Infection (STI) Syndromic Case Management

Advantages of syndromic management:
❖ The aim of STI/RTI syndromic case management is to identify the syndrome correctly and manage them accordingly.
❖ While clinical diagnosis is based on identifying the specific causative agent, syndromic diagnosis leads to immediate treatment for all of the most important possible causative agents. This is important because mixed infections occur frequently in STI/RTI.
❖ Besides, syndromic management of STI/RTI can effectively treat cases in settings with limited or no laboratory facilities. This means syndromic treatment can quickly render the patient non-infectious.

Primary symptom	Urethral discharge	Cervical discharge	Painful scrotal swelling
Associated symptoms	• Urethral discharge (pus or mucopurulent) • Pain or burning while passing urine • Increased frequency of urination • Systemic symptoms like malaise, fever	• Nature and type of discharge (quantity, color and odor) • Burning while passing urine, increased frequency • Genital complaints by sexual partners • Low backache (take menstrual history to rule out pregnancy)	• Swelling and pain in the scrotal region • Pain or burning while passing urine • Systemic symptoms like malaise, fever • History of urethral discharge
Kit		Kit 1 (gray)	
Contents		Tablet azithromycin 1 gm OD stat + Tablet cefixime 400 mg OD stat	
Partner management	Treat all recent partners	Treat partners when symptomatic	Treat all recent partners

Primary symptom	Vaginal discharge	Genital ulcer—nonherpetic
Associated symptoms	• Nature and type of discharge (quantity, color and odor) • Burning while passing urine, increased frequency • Genital complaints by sexual partners • Low backache (take menstrual history to rule out pregnancy)	• Genital ulcer, single or multiple, painful or painless • Burning sensation in the genital area • Enlarged lymph nodes

Contd...

Contd...

Primary symptom	Vaginal discharge	Genital ulcer—nonherpetic	
Kit	Kit 2 (Green)	Kit 3 (White)	Kit 4 (Blue)
Contents	• Tablet secnidazole 2 g OD stat + • Capsule fluconazole 150 mg OD stat	• Injection benzathine penicillin (2.4 MU)— 1 vial + • Tablet azithromycin (1 g) single dose	• If allergic to Injection penicillin: Doxycycline 100 mg (BD for 15 days) + Azithromycin 1 g (single dose)
Partner management	Treat partners when symptomatic	Treat all sexual partners for past 3 months	

Primary symptom	Genital ulcer—herpetic	Lower abdominal pain (LAP)	Inguinal bubo (IB)
Associated symptoms	• Genital ulcer or vesicles, single or multiple, painful, recurrent • Burning sensation in the genital area	• Lower abdominal pain • Fever • Vaginal discharge • Menstrual irregularities like heavy, irregular vaginal bleeding, dysmenorrhea, dyspareunia, dysuria, tenesmus • Lower backache • Cervical motion tenderness	• Swelling in inguinal region which may be painful • Preceding history of genital ulcer or discharge • Systemic symptoms like malaise, fever, etc.
Kit	• Kit 5 (Red)	• Kit 6 (Yellow)	• Kit 7 (Black)
Contents	• Tablet acyclovir 400 mg TDS for 7 days	• Tablet cefixime 400 mg OD stat+ • Tablet metronidazole 400 mg BD × 14 days+ • Tablet doxycycline 100 mg BD × 14 days	• Tablet azithromycin 1 g OD stat + • Tablet doxycycline 100 mg BD × 21 days
Partner management	• No partner treatment	• Treat male partners with Kit 1	• Treat all sexual partners for past 3 weeks

Important considerations for management of all STI/RTI

• Educate and counsel client and sexual partner/s regarding STI/RTI, safer sex practices and importance of taking complete treatment
• Treat partner(s)
• Advise sexual abstinence or condom use during the course of treatment
• Provide condoms, educate about correct and consistent use
• Refer all patients to ICTC
• Follow up after 7 days for all STI, 3rd, 7th, and 14th day for LAP and 7th, 14th, and 21st day for IB
• If symptoms persist, assess whether it is due to re-infection and advise prompt referral
• Consider immunization against hepatitis B

3. **A 42-year-old daily laborer comes to OPD because he developed 2 hypopigmented patches on his left arm over the last 1 year. The patches are well circumscribed with loss of sensation. On examination, his ulnar nerve shows thickening.**

   A. **What is your provisional diagnosis? Support it.**

   B. **Mention the treatment of the case as per national guidelines.**

   C. **Should the patient be allowed to continue his work?**

My provisional diagnosis is paucibacillary leprosy (PBL).

There are three cardinal features of leprosy, all of which are present in the patient:
a. Hypopigmented patches.
b. Loss of sensation (anesthesia)
c. Nerve thickening.

   Leprosy is classified as paucibacillary or multibacillary, based on the number of skin lesions, presence of nerve involvement and identification of bacilli on slit-skin smear.

Characteristics	PBL	MBL
Skin lesion	1–5	>5
Peripheral nerve involvement	0–1	>1
Skin smear	Negative at all sites	Positive at any site

MDT for PBL in Adults [NLEP Guidelines 2019]:

Drug	Dosage	Frequency	Duration
Dapsone	100 mg	Once daily	6 months
Rifampicin	600 mg	Once monthly	

The patient should be allowed to continue his work because:
❖ As the patient has PBL, he is not likely to transmit the disease to community
❖ Treatment with rifampicin will render him noninfectious within 3 weeks
❖ Continuing the work will help him/his family to be financially stable as the patient needs to earn daily to support his family.

4. **A 19-year-old lady noticed hypopigmented patches on his left leg. She went to nearby subcenter and undergo thorough examination, which reveals four macular anesthetic skin patches with well-defined margins. Two thickened nerve trunks were also found on her leg.**

   A. **What is your provisional diagnosis? Support it.**

   B. **Name the two most common nerve trunks that might be thickened in this case.**

   C. **Outline the treatment.**

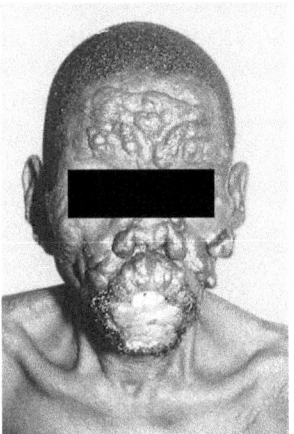

My provisional diagnosis is multibacillary leprosy (MBL).

   Although the number of characteristic skin patches is 4 (<5), the patient is diagnosed as MBL because the number of nerve trunk involved is 2 (>1).

The two most probable nerves that may be involved in this case are:
1. Posterior tibial nerve
2. Common peroneal nerve.

Note that, in upper extremity, the most common nerves involved are ulnar and radial nerves.

MDT for MBL in Adults [NLEP Guidelines 2019]:

Drug	Dosage	Frequency	Duration
Dapsone	100 mg	Once daily	
Rifampicin	600 mg	Once monthly	12 months
Clofazimine	50 mg	Once daily	
Clofazimine	300 mg	Once monthly	

5. **A child of 14 months has come to OPD with fever and rash. He also has cough and running nose. On examination, conjunctival congestion is detected.**

    A. **What is the probable diagnosis?**

    B. **How you manage this case?**

    C. **What are the complications of this case?**

Diagnosis

The probable diagnosis is measles.

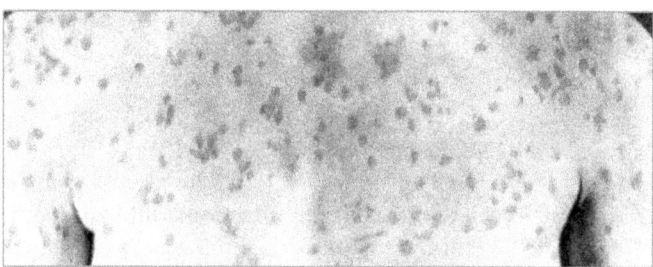

Management of the Case

❖ Vitamin A administration:
   – 1st dose (2 lakh IU): On diagnosis
   – 2nd dose (2 lakh IU): After 24 hours
   – If there is any symptoms of complication another dose should be given at 28th day.
❖ Advice to the mother:
   – To let her child to take rest
   – To continue normal feeding
   – About the symptoms and signs suggestive of complications.
❖ Antipyretic therapy: Paracetamol administration in proper dose, if fever persists
❖ Provide information to nodal officer and DIO/DMCHO/SMO (since measles is on the verge of eradication)
❖ Initiate epidemic investigation (in consultation) if required, when:
   – Occurrence of >5 clinical case in a block in a week, or
   – Occurrence of a death due to measles, or
   – Occurrence of a case of measles in the area bordering >1 adjacent block

❖ Shipment blood sample for IgM ELISA (enzyme-linked immunosorbent assay)
❖ Necessary feedback to community, family, health center
❖ Ask the mother about the child's vaccination status and remind mother about the next dose
❖ Measles eradication strategy.

Complications of Measles

❖ Respiratory complications (cause of >90% measles-related deaths)
  – Croup
  – Pneumonia:
    - Most common life-threatening complication
    - Mostly viral cause
    - Occurrence rate <10% in developed countries and <20–80% in developing countries.
  – Tuberculosis (TB)
  – Otitis media:
    - Most common complication in children
    - 5–15% cases.
❖ Gastrointestinal complications:
  – Acute gastroenteritis (+ severe dehydration + malnutrition)
❖ Neurological complications:
  – Most severe complications
  – Febrile convulsion
  – Encephalitis (1 in 1,000 cases)
  – Subacute sclerosing panencephalitis (SSPE):
    - Also called Dawson's encephalitis/Dawson's disease
    - Rare (1:300,000 cases of measles)
    - Characterized by progressive mental deterioration followed by paralysis
    - Measles vaccination provides huge protection for such neurological and other complications.
❖ Ophthalmological complications:
  – Conjunctivitis
  – Corneal ulcer.

6. **A 2-year-old child comes to the OPD with symptoms like malaise, fever, sore throat, bluish white membranous patch over tonsils.**

   A. **What is the probable diagnosis?**

   B. **How you manage this case?**

❖ Probable diagnosis: Diphtheria.

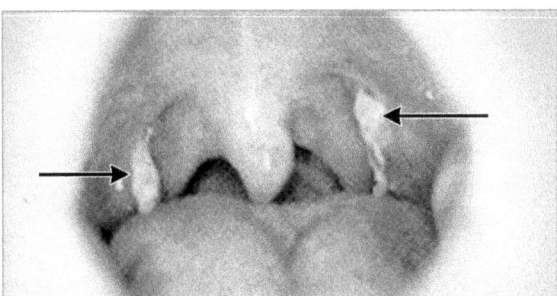

White membranous patch over tonsils (arrows)

Management

❖ Administration of antitoxin:
  – Dose: 20,000-100,000 IU depending upon severity
  – Route: IM/IV

Type	Dose (IU)
Mild/early pharyngeal or laryngeal/faucial (<2 days)	20,000–40,000
Moderate nasopharyngeal disease	40,000–60,000
Severe/extensive/late (≥3 days)	80,000–100,000

  – Sensitivity test:
    - Prior sensitivity test is very important to detect sensitization to horse serum
    - Preliminary test dose: 0.2 mL
    - Route: Subcutaneous (SC)
    - Tests: Skin test, scratch test
    - In case of allergy prior desensitization is important.
  – Antibiotic therapy:
    - Procaine penicillin G
    - Dose:
      * <10 kg—3 lakh IU
      * ≥10 kg—6 lakh IU
          Or
      * Erythromycin (40 mg/kg × 14 days)
  – Culture of nasal and throat swabs:
    - Two samples at least 24 hours apart after completion of therapy
    - Result: If (+ve) continue antibiotic for another 10 days and culture again.
  – Start active immunization during convalescence, if nonimmunized.
  – Advice for contacts:
    - According to immunization status:

Immunization status	Advice	
Last dose <2 years earlier	Nothing to do	
Last dose >2 years earlier	1 booster dose	
Unknown vaccination status/unvaccinated	Antibiotic administration + active and passive immunization	
	Antibiotic:	Immunization:
	Benzathine penicillin: (<6 years 6 lakh IU ≥6 kg 1.2 million IU)	Active immunization: By DPT vaccine Passive immunization: By 1,000–2,000 unit diphtheria antitoxin

    - Bacteriological surveillance of close contacts should be continued for several weeks by repeated swabbing at approximately weekly intervals.

7. **A 19-year-old boy presented with low-grade fever preceding skin manifestations (such as pleomorphic rash, usually starting on the head and trunk and spreading to the rest of the body) by 1–2 days with typical complaint of intense pruritus, headache, malaise, cough, etc. Later on he was clinically diagnosed as having chickenpox. Describe management protocol.**

Treatment of chickenpox involves keeping the person as comfortable as possible.

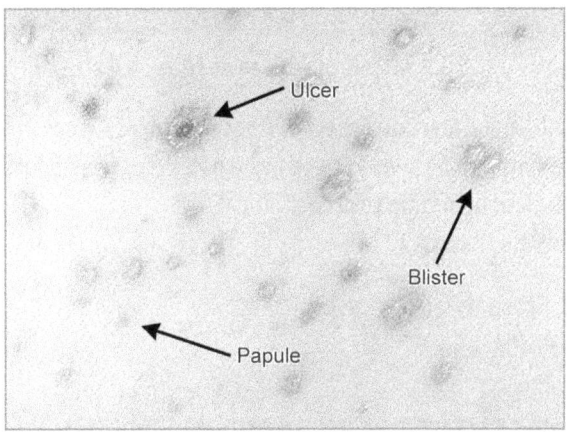

❖ **I will advise the following:**
  – Avoid scratching or rubbing the itchy areas. Keep fingernails short to avoid damaging the skin from scratching
  – Wear cool, light, loose clothes. Avoid wearing rough clothing, particularly wool, over an itchy area
  – Take lukewarm baths using little soap and rinse thoroughly. Try a skin-soothing oatmeal or cornstarch bath
  – Apply a soothing moisturizer after bathing to soften and cool the skin
  – Avoid prolonged exposure to excessive heat and humidity
  – A child with chickenpox should not return to school or play with other children, until all chickenpox sores have crusted over or dried out. Adults should follow this same rule when considering when to return to work or be around others.

❖ **Medications:**
  Some do's and don'ts about medications
  – Not to give everyone
  – To work well, medications usually must be started within the first 24 hours of the rash
  – Antiviral medication is not usually prescribed to otherwise healthy children who do not have severe symptoms. Adults and teens, who are at risk for more severe symptoms, may benefit from antiviral medication, if it is given early
  – May be very important in those who have skin conditions (such as eczema or recent sunburn), lung conditions (such as asthma), or who have recently taken steroids.

❖ **Drugs:**
  – Antiviral drug used: Acyclovir 800 mg 5 times a day × 5–7 days
  – Aspirin or ibuprofen like drugs **MUST NOT BE GIVEN** to someone who may have chickenpox as use of aspirin has been associated with a serious condition called **Reye's**

syndrome. Ibuprofen has been associated with more severe secondary infections. Acetaminophen may be used.

- Oral antihistamines such as diphenhydramine, cetirizine can be given.

❖ **For contacts:**
- Passive immunization: Within 96 hours of exposure (for contacts)
- Dose: 125 U/10 kg.

❖ **For prevention:**
- Vaccination may be done
- Live attenuated vaccine 0.5 mL SC (1st dose at 15th month → next at 5–6 years).

8. Ramesh, a 66-year-old male, attended chest OPD with cough of 3 weeks. Two sputum smears were examined and 1 was found to be +ve. Previously he had never been diagnosed to be a case of TB.
   A. Categorize the patient according to proper guidelines.
   B. How will you manage the case?

Tuberculosis Category: Category-I (New cases)

Please see Chapter 18 for further details.

INTEGRATED MANAGEMENT OF CHILDHOOD ILLNESS (IMCI) RELATED

1. A mother has come to the immunization clinic of your medical college with her 4-month-old boy for 3rd dose of OPV, DPT and Hep-B. She complains that the child is having cough for last 2 days. On examination of the baby, the following were found:
   - Respiratory rate = 46/min.
   - Axillary temperature = Normal.
   - The child is alert, without any wheeze or stridor.
   - No chest indrawing.
   - Nutritional status = Normal.
   A. What is he suffering from? How will you classify?
   B. Would you recommend the 3rd dose immunization on that day?
   C. What advice will you give the mother regarding management of the illness?

2. The mother of Jaya, a 6-year-old girl, said that she has difficulty in breathing and has cough for 3 days. Although she is not eating well, she is able to drink. On examination, the following were found:
   - Respiratory rate = 54/min.
   - Axillary temperature = 39.4°C.
   - No chest indrawing, wheeze or stridor.
   - Nutritional status = Normal.
   - The girl is alert.

A. What is she suffering from? Give reasons.

B. Outline the management.

C. What advices you will give the mother regarding the illness?

Please see Chapter 15 "ICMR Guidelines".

OBSTETRIC CARE RELATED

1. A 24-year-old 2nd gravida gave birth to a baby boy at home. An untrained dai delivered the baby who weighed 2.6 kg and appeared normal at birth. The mother did not receive any antenatal checkup (ANC) during this pregnancy. 5 days later, the baby stopped sucking, developed trismus, had few episodes of convulsions and ultimately died after 2 days.

A. What is the possible cause of death?

B. How this death could have been prevented?

The most probable cause of death is Neonatal Tetanus (NNT).

Prevention of NNT

a. **Administration of tetanus toxoid:** Administration of 2 doses of tetanus toxoid (TT) injection to a pregnant woman is an important step in the prevention of neonatal tetanus.
   - The first dose of TT should be given after the 1st trimester, or as soon as the woman registers for ANC
   - The second dose of TT is to be given 1 month after the 1st dose, but preferably at least 1 month before the expected date of delivery (EDD), because if the gap between the 2nd dose of TT and the EDD is <4 weeks, the efficacy of the vaccine will be reduced
   - *Dose*: Injection TT is to be given as 0.5 mL per dose
   - *Route of administration*: Deep intramuscular in the upper arm
   - If the woman has already received 2 doses of injection TT in a previous pregnancy, a single dose of TT is sufficient
   - However, in any case of doubt, 2 injections should be given
   - Inform the woman that there may be slight swelling/pain/redness at the injection site for 1–2 days.

b. **Ensuring the 7Cs at the time of delivery:** Training should be given to traditional birth attendants to practice the rule of 7Cs, because this measure alone can reduce the incidence of deaths due to NNT by 90%:
   1. Clean hands
   2. Clean fingernails
   3. Clean delivery surface
   4. Clean blade for cutting the cord
   5. Clean tie for the cord
   6. No application on the cord stump
   7. Keeping birth canal clean by avoiding harmful practices.

c. **Institutional delivery should be promoted and infrastructure should be available for this purpose.**

2. **A 19-year-old female patient gave birth to a baby girl 2 days back, who is her 3rd child. She was married at 15 years of age. The girl child weighs 2.3 kg at birth.**

   A. **Comment on the birth weight of the child.**

   B. **Enumerate four points that ASHA should discuss with the mother.**

   C. **Specify biological causes of such a birth weight.**

   D. **Enumerate health problems arising from such a condition.**

   The baby is a low birth weight (LBW) baby.

   LBW has been defined by WHO, as weight at birth less than 2,500 grams (irrespective of the gestational age).

Four points that ASHA should discuss with the mother:

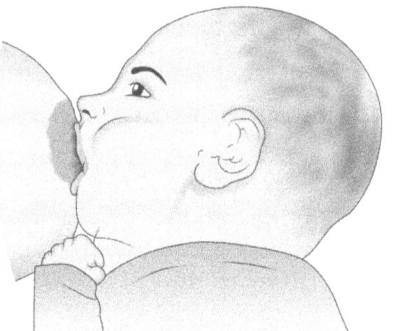

1. The mother should continue exclusive breastfeeding up to 6 months of age of the baby. The ASHA worker should show the correct position and attachment that should be followed at the time of breastfeeding.

   Correct position:
   - The baby's whole body should face the mother and be close to her
   - The baby's head and neck should be supported, in a straight line with his body, to face the breast
   - Baby's abdomen should touch mother's abdomen, to be as close as possible to his mother.

   Signs of a correct attachment:
   - The baby's mouth is wide open
   - The baby's chin touches the breast
   - The baby's lower lip is curled outward
   - Usually the lower portion of the areola is not visible.

2. Prevention of hypothermia:
   Maintain "*warm chain*" by:
   - Appropriate clothing.
   - Skin-to-skin contact.
   - First bath of the baby should be delayed till the cord falls/till the weight of the baby comes to ≥2.5 kg.

3. Mother should be instructed to immunize the baby at appropriate ages.

4. The mother and her husband should be counseled thoroughly for adoption of a proper family planning method (in this case, a terminal method like tubectomy/vasectomy is preferred and if the couple refuses, then barrier/IUD should be advocated) as the 2 child norm is already exceeded by this family.

Biological causes of low birth weight:

- ❖ Too early child birth (prematurity).
- ❖ Too many child births (lack of counseling).
- ❖ Too frequent child births (lack of family planning practices).

Health problems/risks which may arise in a LBW baby:

- Birth asphyxia
- Hypothermia
- Feeding difficulties
- Infections
- Hyperbilirubinemia
- Respiratory distress
- Retinopathy of prematurity
- Apneic spells
- Intraventricular hemorrhage
- Hypoglycemia
- Metabolic acidosis.

3. A 32-year-old female patient visited UTC with history of amenorrhea for 2 months and urinary pregnancy test (UPT) was positive. On examination, no abnormality was found, except pale palpebral conjunctiva.

   A. What routine investigation has to be done?

   B. Should she be registered early?

   C. Why early registration is necessary?

   D. How many antenatal visits are recommended?

Routine investigations to be done:
- Blood for—Hb + Blood grouping + VDRL + Malaria + Hepatitis B + HIV
- Urine for albumin and sugar.

Yes, she should be registered early (within 12 weeks of pregnancy).

Early registration is necessary because:
- It helps to detect high-risk pregnancies (anemia/teenage/bad obstetric history).
- It helps to screen the high-risk pregnancies throughout the period of gestation.
- It helps in early referral of complications arising out of pregnancy.

At least 4 antenatal visits (including registration) are recommended at 12, 20, 32, 36 weeks.

Note: Under the Pradhan Mantri Surakshit Matritva Abhiyan campaign, a minimum package of antenatal care services would be provided to the beneficiaries on the 9th day of every month at the PMSM clinics to ensure that every pregnant woman receives at least one checkup in the 2nd and 3rd trimester of pregnancy.

For the lady in question (high-risk pregnancy), the following antenatal checkup schedule is recommended:
- First 7 months: Monthly visits
- 8th month: 2 visits monthly
- After 8th month: Weekly visits.

4. An 18-year-old female delivered her 2nd daughter normally on 18.9.11 at a Gramin hospital. The birth weight of the child noted by the ANM was 2200 g. The child was given to the mother after 40 minutes. They were discharged on 19.9.11.

A. Comment on birth weight of the baby and state the probable causes.
B. Schedule of postnatal visits in this case.
C. Were they discharged at ideal time?

The baby is a low birth weight (LBW) baby.

Probable causes of LBW:

❖ Too early/too many/too frequent births
❖ Antepartum hemorrhage and other antenatal complications
❖ Malnourishment of mother
❖ Poor access to the healthcare facility
❖ Poverty/illiteracy.

Schedule of postnatal visits:

❖ For home delivery: 7 visits—day 1, 3, 7, 14, 21, 28, 42.
❖ For institutional delivery: 6 visits—day 3, 7, 14, 21, 28, 42.

Comment: The mother and the baby were not discharged at ideal time because there should be special care in every healthcare facility for LBW babies. They should not ideally be discharged before they gain a weight 2.5 kg.

Special care needed for LBW babies are:

❖ Prevention of hypothermia
❖ Skilled person needed for effective resuscitation
❖ Early detection of complications and early intervention
❖ Special feeding schedule of LBW infants, e.g. Gavage feeding/Katori spoon feeding
❖ Vitamin and iron supplements
    For all these special care, it is recommended to treat a LBW baby in a hospital setup. So, the baby was not discharged at time.

5. **Neeta, a 26-year-old 2nd gravida comes to PHC for antenatal registration. She also complains of reeling of head and swelling of her feet. After taking history, the MO comes to know that she had her LMP (last menstrual period) 1 month before.**

    A. What are the routine investigations to be done?
    B. What measures will you take as MO for pallor?

At first BP is to be measured as swelling of feet may be due to hypertensive disorders of pregnancy (Pre-eclampsia/eclampsia).

Then the following routine investigations are to be done:
❖ Blood for—Hb + Blood grouping + VDRL + Malaria + Hepatitis B + HIV
❖ Urine for albumin and sugar.

Measures to be taken as a MO for pallor:
❖ Iron-folic acid (IFA) tablets for adults BD for 100 days (as therapeutic dosage)
❖ Dietary changes:
    – Liver/meat/poultry/fish (contain mainly heme iron)
    – Cereals/green leafy vegetables/legumes/nuts, etc. (contains mainly non-heme iron)
    – To increase bioavailability of vegetable non-heme iron: Advice to eat fresh fruits that contain vitamin C (amla/guava/cabbage/amaranth/cauliflower/orange, etc.)

- One extra meal on evening with at least 350 Kcal extra and 18 grams protein
- Advice to cook in iron (Fe) vessels.
❖ Use of antihelminthic drugs (single dose albendazole) and promote use of chappals at times of walking
❖ Promote use of sanitary latrines.

IMMUNIZATION RELATED

1. **An 11-month-old boy presents at OPD with bilateral pearly white foamy triangular spots on the bulbar conjunctiva.**

   A. **What is this sign called?**
   B. **Name the earliest ocular symptom and sign which result from this condition.**
   C. **What is the line of management according to national program?**

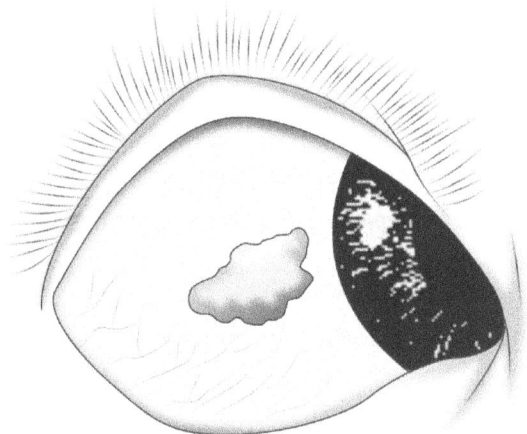

This sign is called "Bitot's spot". It is a sign of vitamin A deficiency. The earliest ocular symptom of vitamin A deficiency is night blindness and the earliest ocular sign of vitamin A deficiency is conjunctival xerosis.

Management
Therapeutic dose of vitamin A (1 lakh IU) has to be given orally. After 4 weeks, a second dose (2 lakh IU) is given orally.

Advice to the Mother
❖ Continue prophylactic doses up to 5 years of age (a total of 9 megadoses—at intervals of 6 months)
❖ Breastfeeding should be continued up to 2 years of age
❖ Immediate measles immunization, if not taken already
❖ Vitamin A rich foods should be given to the baby, which should include green leafy vegetables and fruits.

2. **The ice pack in a vaccine carrier melted within 2 hours.**

    A. **Identify the possible causes.**

    B. **How many ice packs should be kept?**

    C. **Which vaccine vials should not be kept in direct contact with the ice pack?**

Possible causes of melting of ice pack in a vaccine carrier:
- ❖ Improper closure of the lid of vaccine carrier
- ❖ Improper preparation of the ice packs
- ❖ Repeated opening and closure of the lid
- ❖ Crack/leakage/damage of the vaccine carrier
- ❖ Putting the carrier in direct sunlight/hot source for a long time.

Four ice packs should be kept in a single vaccine carrier.

Remember: The "T series" vaccines (Hepatitis B, DPT, DT, TT, diluents) should NEVER BE KEPT in direct contact with the ice packs because on freezing, the adjuvant is detached from the vaccine.

3. **You are a medical officer in a PHC. You have made an indent for the universal immunization program (UIP) vaccines.**

    A. **Where will you keep the vaccines?**

    B. **How should you arrange the vaccines in the equipment?**

    C. **In which equipment will he prepare ice packs and how are these placed?**

I will prefer an ice lined refrigerator (ILR) for keeping the vaccines, where a core temperature of 2–8°C can be maintained continuously.

Arrangement of vaccines inside ILR from above to bottom (2016 Guidelines by Govt. of India):

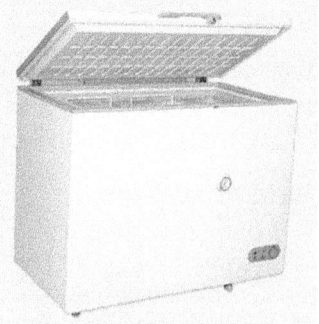

Diluents		*Diluents*		T	*Diluents*		*Diluents*	
Hep-B Hep-B		Hep-B Hep-B		H	Hep-B Hep-B		Hep-B Hep-B	
Pentavalent		Pentavalent		E R	Pentavalent		Pentavalent	
DPT DPT		DPT IPV		M O	IPV IPV		IPV IPV	
TT TT		TT TT		M	TT TT		TT TT	
BCG BCG		BCG BCG		E T	JE JE		JE JE	
Measles		Measles		E R	Measles		Measles	
OPV OPV		OPV OPV			OPV OPV		OPV OPV	
Empty ice packs								
Empty ice packs								

(Hep-B: Hepatitis B; DPT: Diphtheria-tetanus-pertussis; TT: Tetanus toxoid; BCG: Bacillus Calmette-Guerin; JE: Japanese encephalitis; OPV: Oral polio vaccine)

Note:
- Arrange 2 layers of empty ice packs at the bottom of ILR.
- Keep OPV and measles vaccines first on top the empty ice packs.
- Then store other vaccines as described above.

Temperature: +2° to +8°C

Monitored by:

❖ Dial thermometer (acts by thermocouple principle)

❖ Stem thermometer (contains alcohol)

❖ Recorded twice a day (at morning and evening) by PHN

❖ Alarm indicates temperature <+2°C and > +8°C.

❖ It can keep vaccine safe with minimum 8 hours continuous electricity supply in a 24-hour period.

The principle of **"FIRST IN FIRST OUT"** (FIFO) should be followed, that is, if the vaccine remains unused after 1st day, a rubber band is encircled to the vaccine, if it remains unused after 2nd day, another rubber band is encircled to the vaccine and after 3 consecutive days of no use, the vaccine is discarded.

The principle of **"EARLY EXPIRY FIRST OUT"** (EEFO) is also followed, that is, the vaccines which are already expired should be discarded first.

4. **An ILR in a PHC is showing a temperature of 8°C for several days. You have to allow repairing the equipment. Where will you keep the vaccines at the time of repair?**

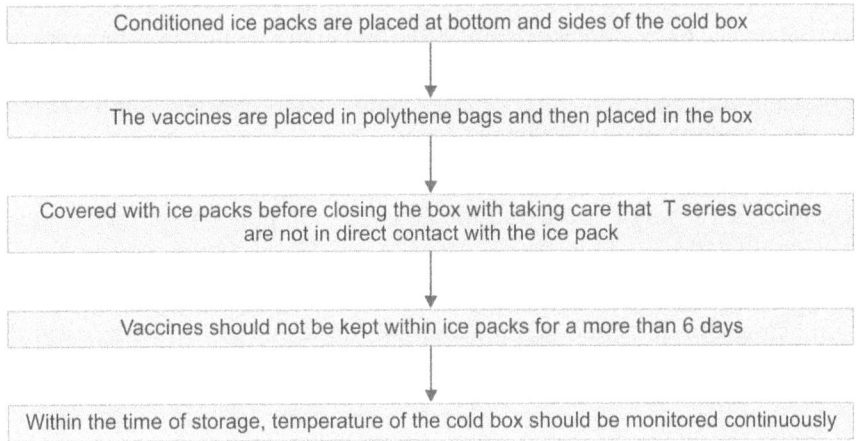

Conditioned ice packs are placed at bottom and sides of the cold box

↓

The vaccines are placed in polythene bags and then placed in the box

↓

Covered with ice packs before closing the box with taking care that T series vaccines are not in direct contact with the ice pack

↓

Vaccines should not be kept within ice packs for a more than 6 days

↓

Within the time of storage, temperature of the cold box should be monitored continuously

5. **ANM is carrying vaccines to a subcenter from the PHC on the immunization day.**

   A. **What precautions should she take while carrying them?**

   B. **How will she handle waste sharps in the subcenter?**

The ANM should take the following precautions while carrying the vaccines:

❖ Before carrying the vaccines:
   – Check for 4 conditioned ice packs in the vaccine carrier
   – Check for vaccines in plastic zipper bags
   – Freeze sensitive vaccines should not be in contact with ice packs
   – Check for any crack/holes in the carrier
   – Check whether the lid is tightly closed or not
   – Check that nothing other than vaccines is in the carrier.

❖ While carrying the vaccines, ensure that:
   – The lid is not repeatedly opened and closed
   – The carrier is not put under direct sunlight for long time

- No one sit over the carrier
- The carrier reaches the subcenter on the shortest route.

Handling of sharps in subcenter:

Step 1:
Remove needles from auto-disk (AD) syringe immediately after administering injection at the site using a suitable *syringe cutter* that cuts *plastic hub* of syringe and not the metal part of needle.

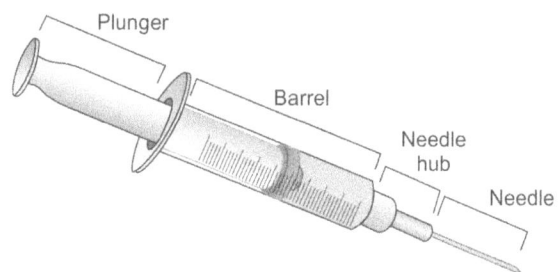

The removed needle having the detached plastic hub of the syringe shall be made to fall in an attached white translucent sturdy and puncture proof container having a capacity to store at least 45 needles and designed to ensure no spillage of stored needles while handling the syringe cutter or carrying the same while travelling.

Step 2:
Store *broken vials* in a separate white translucent sturdy and puncture proof container or in the container mentioned at Step 1 in case its capacity is able to accommodate broken vials.

Step 3:
Segregate and store the detached syringe and the discarded unbroken vials in the *red container*.

Step 4:
Label the red and white translucent containers with *Biohazard symbol*.

Step 5:
Carry and handover these containers to the District Hospitals/CHC/PHC, etc. while *unused remaining vaccines* are carried to the District Hospitals/CHC/PHC, etc. for *cold storage* and to do other documentation work.

Step 6:
Maintain a proper record at the District Hospitals/CHC/PHC, etc. in order to assess that waste (needles/syringes/vials) reported back to District Hospital/CHC/PHC matches with the stock issued to ANM/HV in the morning. *Such matching is to be done by weighing, but not by counting in order to avoid occupational and safety hazards.*

6. **A 9-month-old unimmunized child has come to the immunization clinic of the hospital.**

    A. **Plan the vaccination schedule.**

    B. **Mention four things that you must tell the mother regarding immunization.**

Vaccination schedule in an unimmunized child of 9 months of age:

- ❖ BCG
- ❖ OPV-1 (next 2 doses 1 month apart each and booster dose after 1 year of 3rd dose)
- ❖ Pentavalent-1 (next 2 doses 1 month apart each)
- ❖ Measles vaccination
- ❖ Vitamin A (1 lakh IU).

Four advices to the mother regarding immunization:

- ❖ What vaccines are given and which diseases they prevent.
- ❖ Common side effects of the vaccine and how to manage them.
- ❖ To keep the immunization card safely and to bring it on subsequent visits.
- ❖ When she has the next visit.

FAMILY PLANNING RELATED

1. A couple has come to OPD of your medical college for family planning advices. Age of husband and wife is 32 years and 26 years, respectively. They have 2 girl children aged 6 years and 14 months, respectively. The younger child is still on breastfeeding. Mother has history of ectopic pregnancy 3 years back.

   A. Mention contraceptive method(s) contraindicated for this couple. Why these methods are contraindicated?

   B. Mention other absolute contraindication for the said method(s).

   C. Define eligible couple and couple protection rate (CPR).

Intrauterine device (IUD) is absolutely contraindicated just after ectopic pregnancy.

IUD is relatively contraindicated in case of ectopic pregnancy followed by term pregnancy. So, IUD cannot be used in this case.

Other absolute contraindications of IUD:

- ❖ Pregnancy
- ❖ Nulliparity
- ❖ Ectopic pregnancy
- ❖ PID/RTI
- ❖ Undiagnosed bleeding
- ❖ Reproductive tract anomaly
- ❖ Malignant growth in the reproductive tract.

Eligible Couple

An eligible couple refers to a currently married couple wherein the wife is in the reproductive age, which is generally assumed to lie between the ages of 15 and 45 years.

Couple Protection Rate

CPR is defined as the percentage of eligible couple effectively protected against childbirths by one or the other approved methods of family planning (sterilization/IUD/condom/oral pills).

2. A 23-year-old lady comes to UTC for family planning advices. She is married for 2 months. The couple has planned to have their first child at least after 2 years. Her menstrual history is normal and so is general examination.

   A. Which family planning method(s) is best for her?

   B. Which family planning method(s) is not appropriate for her?

Best methods for this couple are:
- ❖ Barrier method
- ❖ Oral contraceptive pill (OCP).

Methods not appropriate for her:
- ❖ IUD (increased risk of expulsion, PID and ectopic pregnancy)
- ❖ Permanent sterilization methods.

3. A 30-year-old female has come to your subcenter for family planning advices. She has a daughter of 8 months age. Her husband is an alcoholic, beats her regularly and refuses to come to subcenter. She has suffered from jaundice twice in last year, but she has normal menstrual periods.

   A. Which family planning (FP) methods are not appropriate for her?

   B. What will be your suggestion regarding FP?

   C. What is the ideal time for adoption of this method?

Family planning (FP) methods not appropriate for the female:
- ❖ Barrier method (the husband is alcoholic and non-compliant)
- ❖ OCP (history of jaundice is a contraindication of OCP).

My suggestion to her will be to adopt IUD as FP method.

Ideal time for IUD insertion: During menstrual period/within 10 days of beginning of a menstrual period because, at that time:
- ❖ Chance of pregnancy is least
- ❖ Cervical canal is more dilated
- ❖ Uterus is relaxed
- ❖ Myometrial contractions are least at that time.

So, insertion of IUD is technically easier.

Note: Another convenient time for IUD insertion is 6–8 weeks after delivery. This is called ***postpuerperal insertion***, which has the advantage of combining it with the postnatal follow-up visits.

GROWTH CHART RELATED

1. Priya was born on 8th March 2014 by an untrained dai. Her birth weight was not recorded. Subsequently, her mother attended the local AWC. The weights recorded by the AWW were:

14th May: 3.5 kg.

15th June: 4.1 kg.

14th July: 5.4 kg.

17th August: 5.9 kg.

A. Draw a growth curve and comment on it.

B. Discuss four points you would like to discuss with the mother.

Systemically arranging the given data, we get:

Dates	Completed months	Weight (kg)
8th March to 8th May	2	3.5
8th May to 8th June	3	4.1
8th June to 8th July	4	5.4
8th July to 8th August	5	5.9

Accordingly, the growth chart has to be drawn (see the next page for drawn growth chart and comment).

Four points I would like to discuss with the mother:

1. Complementary feeding:
   - Gradual introduction of semisolid foods along with breastfeeding at 6 months of age
   - The food introduced should be cheap, locally available, hygienically prepared and easily digestible
   - Choice of complementary food (according to national guidelines):
     - The staple cereal of the family should be used to make the first food for an infant
     - The breakfast can be made with suji, broken wheat, atta, ground rice, ragi, millet, etc. by using a little water or milk, if available
     - Roasted flour of any cereal can be mixed with boiled water and sugar to make the first complementary food for the baby and could be started on the day the child becomes 6 months of age. Adding sugar/jiggery/ghee/oil increases the energy value of the food
     - Fresh seasonal fruits (e.g. papaya, mango, banana, etc.) and green leafy vegetables should be added as protective foods
     - Once the child is eating breakfast well, mixed foods including cooked cereal, pulse and vegetables could be given to the child, e.g. *khichidi, dalia, suji kheer, upma, idli, dhokla, bhaat-bhaji,* etc.
     - Modified family's food is one of the most effective ways of ensuring complementary feeding of infants.
2. Advice the mother to regularly monitor the growth of the child herself/take the child to nearby health facility at a regular interval.
3. Aware the mother about benefits of immunization and tell her to come at specific dates for scheduled immunization of the child and keep the immunization card at a safe place.
4. Counsel the mother for adopting an appropriate family planning method for a birth spacing of at least 3 years.

   Comment on growth chart:
   ❖ As the child is now in the green color band of the growth chart, her growth is normal
   ❖ As the direction of the child's growth curve is directed upwards, it indicates that the child is gaining weight adequately. So she is growing well and healthy.

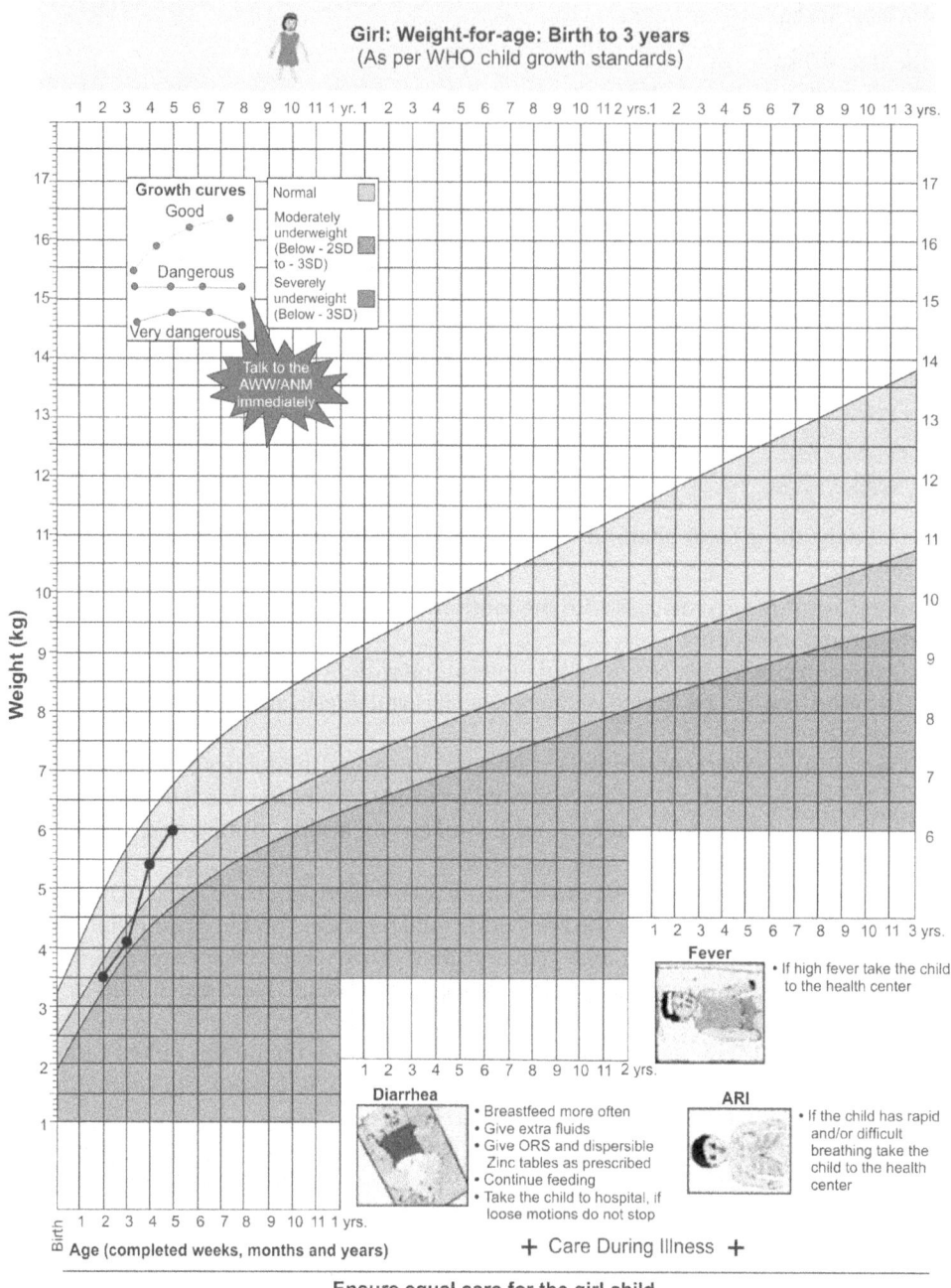

Girl: Weight-for-age: Birth to 3 years
(As per WHO child growth standards)

Growth curves
Good
Dangerous
Very dangerous

Normal
Moderately underweight (Below - 2SD to - 3SD)
Severely underweight (Below - 3SD)

Talk to the AWW/ANM immediately

Weight (kg)

Age (completed weeks, months and years)

Fever
• If high fever take the child to the health center

Diarrhea
• Breastfeed more often
• Give extra fluids
• Give ORS and dispersible Zinc tables as prescribed
• Continue feeding
• Take the child to hospital, if loose motions do not stop

ARI
• If the child has rapid and/or difficult breathing take the child to the health center

+ Care During Illness +

Ensure equal care for the girl child

2. **Rahim was born on 14th July 2003. The birth weight was 3.5 kg. The weights recorded at nearby AWC were as followed:**

17th August 2003: 4 kg.

19th September 2003: 4.3 kg.

A. **Plot the weight on growth chart.**

B. **What is the direction of growth curve? Comment on it.**

C. **What advices would you like to give the mother?**

Systemically arranging the given data, we get:

Dates	Completed months	Weight (kg)
Birth weight		3.5
14th July to 14th August	1	4
14th August to 14th September	2	4.3

Accordingly, the growth chart has to be drawn (see the next page for drawn growth chart and comment).

Advices to the Mother

a. Continue exclusive breastfeeding. Show the mother the correct position and attachment at times of breastfeeding.
   Correct position (see Fig. on page 486):
   - The baby's whole body should face the mother and be close to her
   - The baby's head and neck should be supported in a straight line with his body to face the breast
   - Baby's abdomen should touch mother's abdomen, to be as close as possible to his mother.
   Signs of a correct attachment:
   - The baby's mouth is wide open
   - The baby's chin touches the breast
   - The baby's lower lip is curled outward
   - Usually the lower portion of the areola is not visible.
b. Advice the mother to regularly monitor the growth of the child herself/take the child to nearby health facility at a regular interval.
c. Aware the mother about benefits of immunization and tell her to come at specific dates for scheduled immunization of the child and keep the immunization card at a safe place.

Comment on growth chart:

The direction of growth curve is upward but not satisfactory as there is no significant weight gain between 1st and 2nd month. If this trend continues, there might be a flattening of curve which is dangerous for the health of the child.

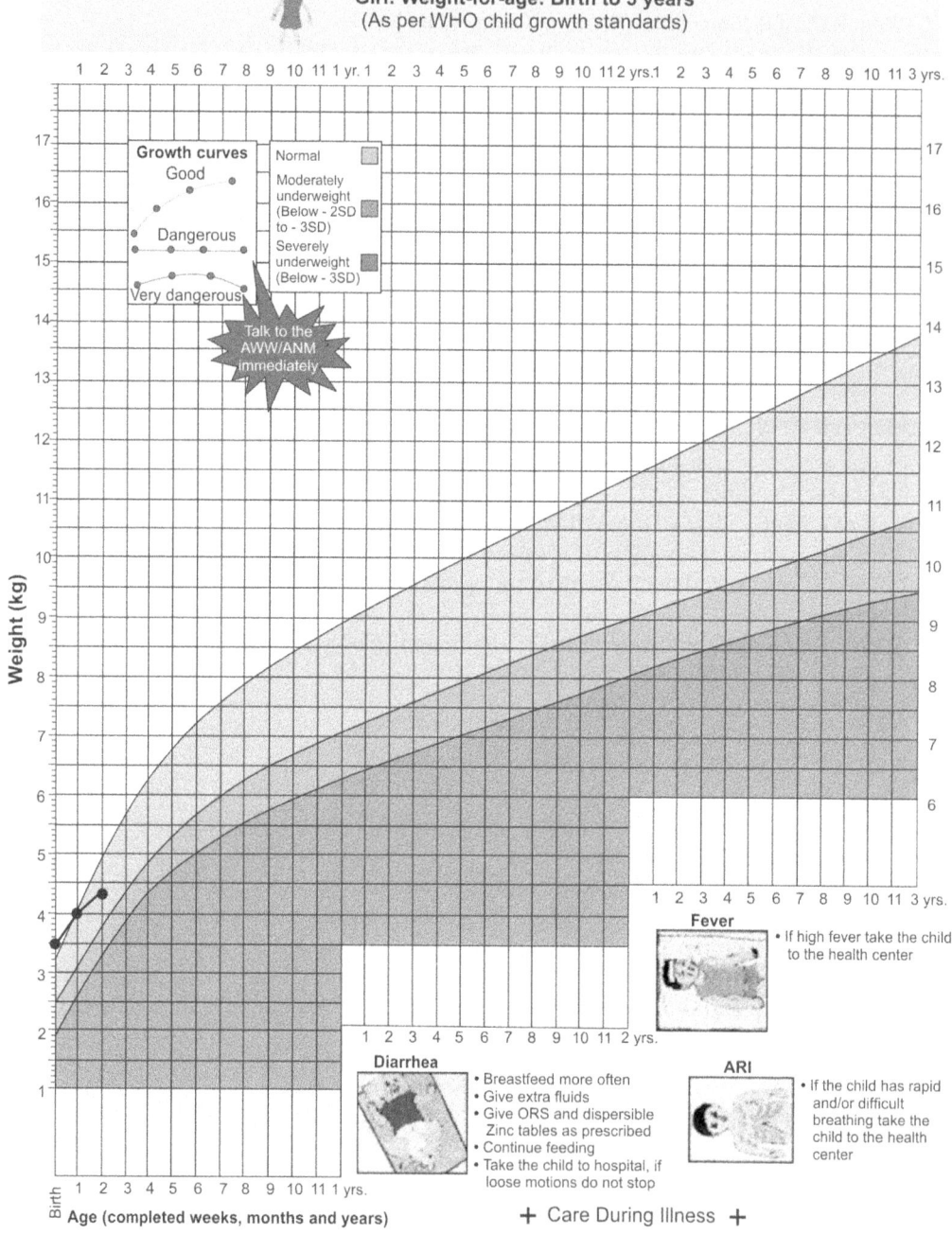

Girl: Weight-for-age: Birth to 3 years
(As per WHO child growth standards)

Growth curves

Good

Dangerous

Very dangerous

Normal

Moderately underweight (Below - 2SD to - 3SD)

Severely underweight (Below - 3SD)

Talk to the AWW/ANM immediately

Weight (kg)

Birth

Age (completed weeks, months and years)

Fever
• If high fever take the child to the health center

Diarrhea
• Breastfeed more often
• Give extra fluids
• Give ORS and dispersible Zinc tables as prescribed
• Continue feeding
• Take the child to hospital, if loose motions do not stop

ARI
• If the child has rapid and/or difficult breathing take the child to the health center

✚ Care During Illness ✚

Ensure equal care for the girl child

Chapter

15

COVID-19

Authors' Note

At the very beginning of this chapter, we pay tribute to all healthcare workers including but not limited to doctors, nurses, internees, paramedical stuffs, laboratory technicians, ambulance stuffs, scientists and all others who had contributed in any extent to help our planet fight this deadly disease for the whole of 2020 and in the years to come. Most of us had lost one or more of our loved ones in fighting COVID-19. Let's take a promise for them, we will never, in any ways, let their sacrifices go in vain. We will keep fighting against COVID-19 and any other upcoming disease that will come in the path of the great journey of humanity with all our tears, sweats and blood.

1. What is COVID-19/COV-19?

COVID-19 is the disease caused by a new coronavirus called SARS-CoV-2. WHO first learned of this new virus on 31 December 2019, following a report of a cluster of cases of 'viral pneumonia' in Wuhan, People's Republic of China.

2. What is the type/genre of CoVs?

CoVs are enveloped, positive-stranded RNA viruses with nucleocapsid.

3. What is the unique about the structure of CoVs?

In CoVs, the genomic structure is organized in a +ssRNA of approximately 30 kb in length—the largest known in any RNA viruses.

4. How the SARS-CoV-2 enter the cells of respiratory passage/ lung?

The spike RBD (receptor-binding domain) allows the binding to the ACE2 receptor in the lungs and other tissues.

5. Is there any increased risk of getting infected/ having a severe SARS-CoV-2 infection in persons taking ACE-inhibitor drugs?

Although initially assumed, inhibitors of the renin-angiotensin-aldosterone system do not increase the risk of hospitalization for COVID-19 and severe disease.

6. What are the different modes of transmission of SARS-CoV-2?

Modes of transmission:
  i. Droplet infection (most important mode): The virus can spread from an infected person's mouth or nose through respiratory droplets' when they cough, sneeze, speak, sing or breathe heavily. The risk is more when people are in direct or close contact (less than 1 meter apart) with an infected person.

ii. Droplet nuclei: Aerosol transmission can occur in specific settings, particularly in indoor, crowded and inadequately ventilated spaces, where infected person(s) spend long periods of time with others, such as medical facilities where specific aerosol generating procedures, are conducted, restaurants, choir practices, fitness classes, nightclubs, offices and/or places of worship.

iii. Fomites: The virus can also spread after infected people sneeze, cough on, or touch surfaces, or objects, such as tables, doorknobs and handrails. Other people may become infected by touching these contaminated surfaces, then touching their eyes, noses or mouths without having cleaned their hands first.

Environmental contamination leading to SARS-CoV-2 transmission is unlikely to occur in real-life conditions, provided that standard cleaning procedures and precautions are enforced.

7. What is the period of communicability of SARS-CoV-2?

Whether or not they have symptoms, infected people can be contagious and the virus can spread from them to other people. Infected people appear to be most infectious just before they develop symptoms (namely 2 days before they develop symptoms) and early in their illness. People who develop severe disease can be infectious for longer.

8. What is the currently accepted theory of pathogenesis of SARS-CoV-2 induced pneumonia?

The data so far available seem to indicate that the viral infection is capable of producing an excessive immune reaction in the host. In some cases, a reaction takes place which as a whole is labeled a *'cytokine storm'*. The effect is extensive tissue damage with dysfunctional coagulation.

9. What are the risk factors for severe illness from COVID-19?

Risk factors for severe illness from COVID-19 (WHO, CDC):
❖ Age ≥60 years
❖ Pre-existing comorbidities: Hypertension, type II diabetes mellitus, chronic kidney disease, obesity, cancers
❖ Pre-existing lung pathology: Smoking, COPD
❖ Pre-existing heart conditions: Heart failure, coronary artery disease, cardiomyopathies
❖ Pregnancy
❖ Sickle cell disease.

Environmental Factors

Transmission can occur more easily in the "Three C's":
❖ Crowded places with many people nearby, e.g., markets, shops, restaurants
❖ Close-contact settings, especially where people have conversations very near each other, e.g., restaurants
❖ Confined and enclosed spaces with poor ventilation, air conditioned rooms

The risk of COVID-19 spreading is higher in places where these "3Cs" overlap.

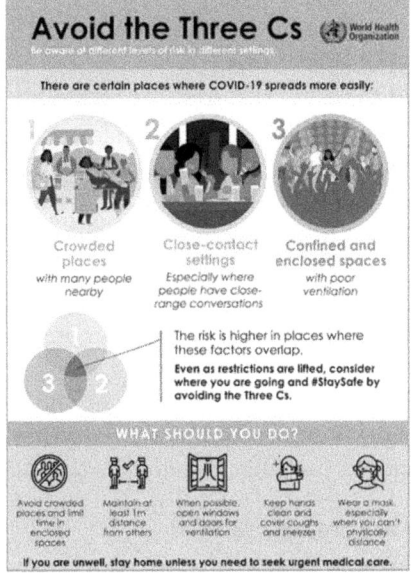

10. What are the symptoms of COVID-19?

Most common symptoms of COVID-19 (WHO):

❖ Fever
❖ Dry cough
❖ Fatigue

Less common symptoms of COVID-19:

❖ Loss of smell (anosmia)
❖ Loss of taste sensation (ageusia)
❖ Nasal congestion
❖ Conjunctivitis
❖ Sore throat
❖ Headache
❖ Muscle or joint pain
❖ Skin rashes
❖ Nausea, vomiting, diarrhea
❖ Dizziness.

11. What are the symptoms of severe COVID-19 disease?

Symptoms of severe COVID-19 disease (WHO):

❖ Shortness of breath
❖ Loss of appetite
❖ Persistent pain or pressure in the chest
❖ High grade fever (>38^{0}C/ >100.4°F)

❖ Irritability
❖ Confusion.

12. What is the case definition of a 'suspect case'?

As per WHO surveillance guidelines, a 'suspect case' is defined as:

A patient with acute respiratory illness (fever and at least one sign/symptom of respiratory disease, e.g., cough, shortness of breath), **AND** a *history of travel* to or residence in a location reporting community transmission of COVID-19 disease during the 14 days prior to symptom onset;

OR

A patient with any acute respiratory illness **AND** having been in contact with a confirmed or probable COVID-19 case in the last 14 days prior to symptom onset;

OR

A patient with severe acute respiratory illness (fever and at least one sign/symptom of respiratory disease, e.g., cough, shortness of breath; *requiring hospitalization*) **AND** in the absence of an alternative diagnosis that fully explains the clinical presentation.

13. What is the case definition of a 'probable case'?

As per WHO surveillance guidelines, a 'probable case' is defined as:
A suspect case for whom testing for the COVID-19 virus is inconclusive.

OR

A suspect case for whom testing could not be performed for any reason.

14. What is the case definition of a 'confirmed case'?

As per WHO surveillance guidelines, a 'confirmed case' is defined as:

A person with laboratory confirmation of COVID-19 infection, irrespective of clinical signs and symptoms.

15. How a confirmed COVID-19 case is assessed according to the disease severity?

According to the 'COVID-19 Clinical management' (WHO, January 2021); a confirmed COVID-19 case is assessed according to the disease severity as follows:

Severity	Clinical presentation	Clinical parameters
Mild disease	Patients with uncomplicated upper respiratory tract infection, may have mild symptoms such as fever, cough, sore throat, nasal congestion, malaise, headache	No evidence of breathlessness or hypoxia (normal saturation)
Moderate disease	Pneumonia with no signs of severe disease	Adolescent or adult with clinical signs of pneumonia (fever, cough, dyspnea, fast breathing*) and no signs of severe pneumonia, including $SpO_2 \geq 90\%$ on room air
		Child with clinical signs of non-severe pneumonia (cough or difficulty breathing + fast breathing* and/or chest indrawing) and no signs of severe pneumonia.

Contd...

Contd...

Severity	Clinical presentation	Clinical parameters
Severe disease	Severe pneumonia	Adolescent or adult with clinical signs of pneumonia (fever, cough, dyspnea, fast breathing) **plus** at least one of the following: • Respiratory rate > 30/min • Severe respiratory distress; or • SpO_2 <90% on room air. • Child with clinical signs of pneumonia (cough or difficulty in breathing) **plus** at least one of the following: • Central cyanosis or SpO_2 < 90% • Severe respiratory distress (e.g., fast breathing, grunting, very severe chest indrawing); • General danger sign: Inability to breastfeed or drink, lethargy or unconsciousness, or convulsions.
	Acute respiratory distress syndrome (ARDS)	Onset: Within 1 week of a known clinical insult (i.e., pneumonia) or new/worsening respiratory symptoms Chest imaging: Bilateral opacities Exclude cardiac failure/volume overload by doing an echocardiography Severity of ARDS in adults: | Severity	PaO_2/FiO_2 (mm Hg)
---	---
Mild ARDS:	>200 but ≤300
Moderate:	ARDS >100 but ≤200
Severe:	ARDS ≤100	 When PaO_2 is not available, SpO_2/FiO_2 ≤315 suggests ARDS.
Critical disease	Sepsis	Acute life-threatening organ dysfunction caused by a dysregulated host response to suspected or proven infection. Signs of organ dysfunction include: • Altered mental status • Difficult or fast breathing • Low oxygen saturation • Reduced urine output • Hypotension • Tachycardia • Weak pulse • Cold extremities • Skin mottling • Laboratory evidence of coagulopathy, thrombocytope-nia, acidosis, high lactate, or hyperbilirubinemia.
	Septic shock	Persistent hypotension despite volume resuscitation, requiring vasopressors
	Acute thrombosis	• Acute venous thromboembolism (e.g., deep vein thrombosis/pulmonary embolism) • Acute stroke • Acute coronary syndrome

*Definition of fast breathing:

Age group	Respiratory rate
<2 months	≥ 60/min
2-11 months	≥ 50/min
1-5 years	≥ 40/min
>5 years and adults	>30/min

16. What are the most common complications leading to death in a patient with active SARS-CoV-2 infection?

Common complications leading to death in COVID-19 include:
1. Respiratory failure
2. Acute respiratory distress syndrome (ARDS)
3. Sepsis and septic shock
4. Thromboembolism
5. Multiorgan failure.

17. What are ILI and SARI?

WHO case definition of Influenza Like Illness (ILI):

An acute respiratory infection with:
❖ Measured fever of 38^0C
❖ Cough
❖ Onset within last 10 days.

WHO case definition of Severe Acute Respiratory Infections (SARI):
An acute respiratory infection with:
❖ History of fever or measured fever of ≥38°C
❖ Cough
❖ Onset within last 10 days
❖ Requiring hospitalization.

18. Why ILI and SARI surveillance models were used in COVID-19 sentinel surveillance?

❖ Influenza and SARS-CoV-2 are two different virus causing similar type of respiratory illness
❖ Similar presentation

Symptom	COVID-19	Influenza
Fever	☑	☑
Cough	☑	☑
Fatigue	☑	☑
Shortness of breath	☑	Infrequent
Headache	Infrequent	☑
Sore throat	☑	☑
Loss of taste and smell	☑	Absent

❖ Similar case definition
❖ Similar specimen type and testing platform

❖ Already existing infrastructure
❖ To track the progress of pandemic.

19. What are the tests used to establish a diagnosis of COVID-19?

❖ ***Real time RT-PCR*** is the gold standard frontline test for diagnosis of COVID-19.
❖ Various open and closed RT-PCR platforms (Open systems RT-PCR machines, TrueNat and CBNAAT) are currently being used for COVID-19 diagnosis in India.
❖ All these platforms require specialized laboratory facilities in terms of equipment, biosafety and biosecurity.
❖ Minimum time taken for the test varies between different systems with a minimum of 2–5 hours including the time taken for sample transportation.
❖ These strict specifications limit the widespread use of the RT-PCR test.
❖ In view of this, there was urgent need of a reliable point-of-care rapid antigen detection test with good sensitivity and specificity for early detection of the disease.
❖ The rapid antigen test (RAT) which was evaluated and validated by ICMR and AIIMS, New Delhi independently was the ***Standard Q COVID-19 Ag detection*** test; it is a *rapid chromatographic immunoassay* for qualitative detection of specific antigens to SARS-CoV-2. developed by SD Biosensor, a South Korea based company, having its manufacturing unit in India.

20. Algorithm for COVID-19 test interpretation using rapid antigen point-of-care test.

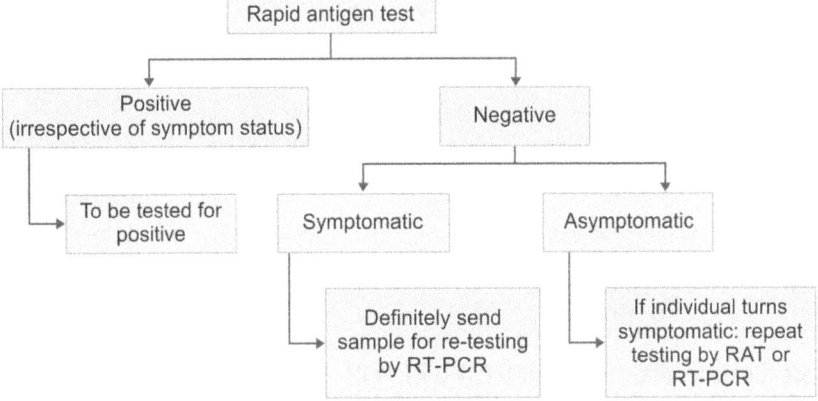

❖ ICMR recommendation on test of choice:

Situation	Test of choice
Routine surveillance in containment zones and screening at points of entry	Rapid antigen test (RAT)
Routine surveillance in non-containment areas	RT-PCR or TrueNat or CBNAAT
In hospital settings	

21. Who are to be tested for COVID-19 in a hospital setting?

❖ All patients of severe acute respiratory infection (SARI)
❖ All symptomatic (ILI symptoms) patients presenting in a healthcare setting

❖ Asymptomatic high-risk patients who are hospitalized or seeking immediate hospitalization such as immunocompromised individuals, patients diagnosed with malignant disease, transplant patients, patients with chronic comorbidities, elderly ≥ 65 years.

❖ Asymptomatic patients undergoing surgical/nonsurgical invasive procedures (not to be tested more than once a week during hospital stay)

❖ All pregnant women in/near labor who are hospitalized for delivery.

22. What are the samples used to diagnose an active COVID-19 infection?

Specimen collection details (Adapted from WHO guidelines)

Specimen	Collection material	Transport to laboratory	Storage till testing	Comment
Nasopharyngeal and oropharyngeal swab	Dacron or polyester flocked swabs	4°C	≤5 days: 4°C >5 days: -70°C	The nasopharyngeal and oropharyngeal swabs should be placed in the same tube to increase the viral load
Bronchoalveolar lavage	Sterile container	4°C	≤48 hours: 4°C >48 hours: -70°C	There might be some dilution, but still, it is a worthwhile specimen
Endotracheal aspirate, nasopharyngeal aspirate, nasal wash	Sterile container	4°C	≤48 hours: 4°C >48 hours: -70°C	-
Sputum	Sterile container	4°C	≤48 hours: 4°C >48 hours: -70°C	Ensure the sample is from lower respiratory tract
Tissue from biopsy or autopsy material	Sterile container with saline	4°C	≤24 hours: 4°C >24 hours: -70°C	Autopsy sample collection should be preferable avoided
Serum (2 samples: acute and convalescent)	Serum separator tubes (Collect 3–5 mL of whole blood in adults)	4°C	≤5 days: 4°C >5 days: -70°C	Collect paired samples: Acute: 1st week of illness Convalescent: 2–3 weeks later

23. What are the genes detected in SARS-CoV-2 RT-PCR?

❖ Initial screening RT PCR involves detection of '**E**' gene (coding for SARS-CoV-2 viral envelope)

❖ Confirmation of samples positive in screening PCR involves detection of one of the following two gene targets:
   1. **RdRp** gene (coding for SARS-CoV-2 RNA dependent RNA polymerase)
   2. **ORF** gene (coding for SARS-CoV-2 Open Reading Frame).

24. What are the precautionary measures that must be taken during sample collection?

As this is an aerosol generating procedure:
   i. Always use personal protective equipment (PPE), e.g., laboratory apron/ gown, face mask, gloves and goggles
   ii. Wipe gloves thoroughly with a disinfectant (e.g., surgical spirit) before and after taking the sample.

25. How are the samples collected to diagnose an active SARS-CoV-2 infection?

Steps to be followed for specimen collection using aseptic method [ICMR guidelines]:

NASAL SWAB COLLECTION

❖ Take a fresh sterile swab.
❖ Gently tilt the patient's head backwards and steady the chin.
❖ Insert the swab into the nostril parallel (1–2 cm) to the palate until the resistance is met at turbinate.
❖ Hold the swab in that position for few seconds and then withdraw slowly in a firmly rotating motion (5 times clockwise and 5 times anticlockwise).

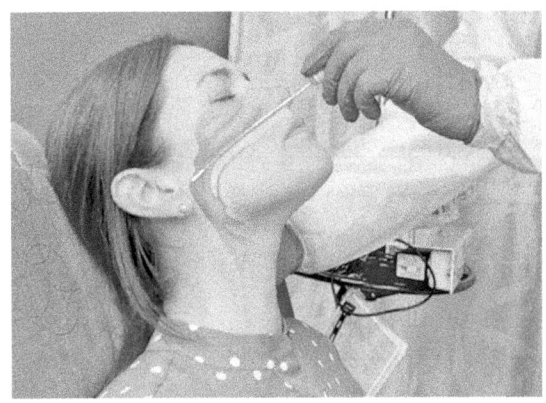

Nasal swab collection

OROPHARYNGEAL SWAB COLLECTION

❖ Gently tilt the patient's head back
❖ Steady the chin
❖ Ask the patient to open his/her mouth
❖ Use a disposable tongue depressor to hold the tongue well
❖ Insert a sterile swab
❖ Swab both the tonsils and the posterior pharynx vigorously with a rotating motion, till the patient starts to gag
❖ Remove the swab without touching the tongue
❖ The swab is then placed in the labelled tube containing viral transport medium (VTM)
❖ The applicator stick is broken off at the indicated mark (if provided) or at below the level of the tube opening
❖ Close and tightly screw cap the tube.

26. What are the guidelines followed while handing and transporting a specimen sample for diagnosis of COVID-19?

Specimen handling at collection site

❖ A unique specimen ID is written/pasted on each VTM sample by the lab technician
❖ VTM containing samples are to be kept in cool box immediately after collection
❖ VTM tube IDs are cross checked with the details in the filled sample collection form
❖ If the specimens cannot be sent to the laboratory within the specified time frame, they should be stored at or below -70°C in ultra-low freezer
❖ Repeated freezing and thawing must be avoided.

Transportation of samples from field site to testing laboratory

❖ Samples should be transported at 2–8°C within specified time frame to the testing laboratory.
❖ Samples should be kept in proper standing position in appropriate test tube rack.
❖ The VTM containing part of the tube should be in direct contact with frozen gel packs.

ICMR Specimen Referral Form for COVID-19 (SARS-CoV2)

INTRODUCTION

This form is for collection centers/laboratories to enter details of the samples being tested for COVID-19. It is mandatory to fill this form for each and every sample being tested. It is essential that the collection centers/laboratories exercise caution to ensure that correct information is captured in the form.

INSTRUCTIONS
• Inform the local/district/state health authorities, especially surveillance officer for further guidance
• Seek guidance on requirements for the clinical specimen collection and transport from nodal officer
• This form may be filled in and shared with the IDSP and forwarded to a laboratory where testing is planned
• Fields marked with asterisk (∗) are mandatory

SECTION A – PATIENT DETAILS

A.1 TEST INITIATION DETAILS

*Sample collected first time: Yes ☐   No ☐

If No, Patient ID: ....

A.2 PERSONAL DETAILS

*Patient Name: ....   Father's Name...

*Age: .... Years/Months/ Days (If age <1 yr, pls. tick months/ days checkbox)

*Gender: Male ☐ Female ☐ Transgender ☐

*Occupation: Health Care Worker☐ Police☐ Sanitation☐ Security Guards☐ Others☐

*Mobile Number: ☐☐☐☐☐☐☐☐☐☐   Mobile Number belongs to: Patient ☐ Family ☐

*Nationality: ....

*Present patient address: ....   *Downloaded Aarogya Setu App: Yes ☐ No☐

....   Pincode ....

*District ....   *State:...............................

(These fields to be filled for all patients including foreigners)

Aadhar No. (For Indians): ....

Passport No. (For Foreign Nationals): ....

*A.3 SPECIMEN INFORMATION FROM REFERRING AGENCY

*Specimen type: Throat swab ☐ Nasal swab ☐ Bronchoalveolar lavage ☐ Endotracheal aspirate ☐

Nasopharyngeal swab ☐

*Type of test: RT-PCR ☐   Rapid Antigen Test (RAT) ☐

*Name of kit used [   ]

*Collection date ☐☐ ☐☐ ☐☐☐☐

*Sample ID (Label) ....

Symptomatic ☐   Asymptomatic ☐

Contact of a lab confirmed case: Yes☐   No ☐

If, RT-PCR test, name of lab where sample is sent for testing (Drop down – list of Rt-PCR/ TrueNat/ CBNAAT labs)

* Mode of transport used to   ☐ Public – In drop down menu – Bus, Metro, Train, Cab, Auto, Ambulance
  visit testing facility
                                    ☐ Private – In drop down menu – Car, Scooty, Bike, Bicycle, Walk

                                    ☐ Not Applicable

Please Note - Hospital form is required for the patients visiting OPD, IPD and Emergency and Community form is required for patients under containment zone/Non-containment area/Point of entry/Testing on demand

*A.3.1 For Community

Sample collected from

- ☐ Containment zone
- ☐ Non-containment area
- ☐ Testing on demand
- ☐ Point of entry

Cat 1: All symptomatic (ILI symptoms) cases
Cat 2: All asymptomatic high-risk individuals (Any individual who falls under Section B2)
Cat 3: All symptomatic (ILI symptoms) individuals with history of international travel in the last 14 days
Cat 4: All individuals who wish to get themselves tested

A.3.2 For Hospital

Cat 1: All patients of severe acute respiratory infection (SARI)
Cat 2: All symptomatic (ILI symptoms) patients presenting in a healthcare setting
Cat 3: Asymptomatic high-risk patients who are hospitalized or seeking immediate hospitalization
Cat 4: Asymptomatic patients undergoing surgical/non-surgical invasive procedures (not to be tested more than once a week during hospital stay).
Cat 5: All pregnant women in/near labor who are hospitalized for delivery
Cat 6: All symptomatic neonates presenting with acute respiratory/sepsis like illness
Cat 7: Patients presenting with atypical manifestations [stroke, encephalitis, pulmonary embolism, acute coronary symptoms, Guillain–Barre syndrome, multisystem inflammatory syndrome in children (MIS-C), progressive gastrointestinal symptoms] based on the discretion of the treating physician
Cat 8: All individuals who wish to get themselves tested
*Fields marked with asterisk are mandatory to be filled
Please Note: Section B1 and B2 need to be filled for both Community and Hospital settings. Section B3 needs to be filled only for Hospital settings

SECTION B- MEDICAL INFORMATION

B.1 CLINICAL SYMPTOMS AND SIGNS

Cough	☐	Loss of taste	☐
Sore throat	☐	Diarrhea	☐
Fever	☐	Breathlessness	☐
Loss of smell	☐	Other symptoms, please specify: _____	

Date of onset of first symptom (dd/mm/yy): ☐☐ ☐☐ ☐☐☐☐

B.2 PRE-EXISTING MEDICAL CONDITIONS

Diabetes	☐	Over weight/obesity	☐
Heart disease	☐	Hypertension	☐
Chronic lung disease	☐	Cancer	☐
Chronic kidney disease	☐	Any other please specify: _____	

B.3 HOSPITALIZATION DETAILS

Hospitalized: Yes ☐   No ☐

Hospital State: .... Hospital
District: ....
Hospital Name: ....

Hospitalization Date: ☐☐ ☐☐ ☐☐☐☐
....

TEST RESULT (To be filled by COVID-19 testing lab facility)

Date of sample receipt (dd/mm/yy)	Sample accepted/ rejected	Date of testing (dd/mm/yy)	Test result (Positive/ Negative)	Repeat sample required (Yes/No)	Sign of Authority (Lab In-charge)

27. What is the current stand on re-testing for COVID-19?

As per the current ICMR guidelines:

❖ A single RT-PCR/CBNAAT/RAT positive test is to be considered confirmatory, without any repeat testing.

❖ *No re-testing is recommended prior to discharge* from a COVID-19 facility after clinical recovery, including for transfer from a COVID facility to a non-COVID facility.

❖ If symptoms develop following a negative RAT test, a repeat RAT or RT-PCR should be done.

28. What is the difference between isolation and quarantine?

Both isolation and quarantine are methods of preventing the spread of COVID-19.

❖ Quarantine is used for anyone who is a contact of someone infected with SARS-CoV-2, regardless of whether the infected person is symptomatic or not.

❖ Quarantine means that exposed person remains separated from others because he may be infected and should stay in a designated facility or at home for 14 days.

❖ Isolation is used for anyone who has been tested positive for SARS-CoV-2, regardless of whether the infected person is symptomatic or not.

❖ Being in isolation means being separated from other people, ideally in a medically facility where the diseased person can receive medical care.

❖ If isolation in a medical facility is not possible and the infected person is not at a high risk of developing severe disease, isolation can take place at home.

❖ Symptomatic COVID-19 patients should remain in isolation for at least 10 days plus an additional 3 days without symptoms.

❖ Asymptomatic COVID-19 patients should remain in isolation for 10 days from the time of being test positive.

29. What are the strategies of prevention of COVID-19?

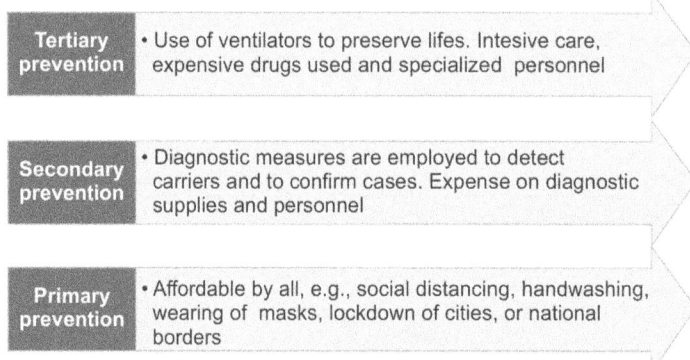

Primordial prevention: Addresses the prevention of risk factors to the onset of disease. Inculcating healthy lifestyle practices among children like hand hygiene, nutritious diet, exercise, avoiding tobacco, alcohol, drugs.

Primary prevention: Aims at avoiding the development of a disease or disability in healthy individuals.

Health Promotion

i. **P: P**ersonal hygiene.
Adopting hand washing practices using soap and water for at least 20 seconds. If not available, then hand sanitizers containing at least 70% alcohol for minimum 40 seconds may be used.

ii. **S:** Encouraging **s**ocial distancing of at least 6 feet

iii. **M:** Correct wearing of **m**asks.
   - Wearing a medical mask is one of active prevention measures that can limit the spread of certain respiratory diseases, by preventing transmission of droplets, including COVID-19 and other IPC measures to prevent human-to-human transmission of COVID-19.
   - If medical masks are worn, appropriate use and disposal are essential to ensure they are effective and to avoid any increase in transmission.
   All of the above three appropriate behaviors, when combined together, reduce the risk of acquiring the COVID-19 infection.

iv. All persons/patients need to cover their nose and mouth with a tissue or elbow when coughing or sneezing;

v. Quarantine of international travelers for the period of estimated incubation period of the COVID-19 which in this case is 14 days.

Specific Protection

A. Healthcare workers protection:
   - WHO recommend that healthcare workers should:
   - Use medical masks correctly.
   - Wear eye protection (goggles) or facial protection (face shield) to avoid contamination of mucous membranes.
   - Wear clean, non-sterile, long-sleeved gown and gloves.
   - Ensure that after patient care, appropriate doffing and disposal of all PPE and hand hygiene should be carried out.
   - A new set of PPE is needed when care is given to a different patient.
   - Equipment should be either single-use and disposable or dedicated equipment (e.g., stethoscopes, blood pressure cuffs and thermometers). If equipment needs to be shared among patients, clean and disinfect it between use for each individual patient (e.g. by using ethyl alcohol 70%).
   - Refrain from touching eyes, nose, or mouth with potentially contaminated gloved or bare hands.
   - Avoid moving and transporting patients out of their room or area unless medically necessary. Use designated portable X-ray equipment or other designated diagnostic equipment. If transport is required, use predetermined transport routes to minimize exposure for staff, other patients and visitors, and have the patient wear a medical mask.
   - Ensure that HCWs who are transporting patients perform hand hygiene and wear appropriate PPE.
   - Routinely clean and disinfect surfaces with which the patient is in contact.
   - Limit the number of HCWs, family members, and visitors who are in contact with suspected or confirmed COVID-19 patients.

B. **Airborne precautions for aerosol-generating procedures**:
Some aerosol-generating procedures, such as tracheal intubation, non-invasive ventilation, tracheostomy, cardiopulmonary resuscitation, manual ventilation before intubation, and bronchoscopy, have been associated with an increased risk of transmission of coronaviruses HCWs must ensure they perform aerosol-generating procedures by maintaining strict infection prevention and control.

C. **Immunization: COVID-19 vaccines.**

30. What are the vaccines currently being administered in India?

Two types of COVID-19 vaccines are being administered in India:
1. Covishield (made by Serum Institute of India Ltd)
2. Covaxin (made by Bharat Biotech International Ltd).

31. Who are the first beneficiaries of COVID-19 vaccines in India?

The COVID-19 vaccination drive was launched on 16th January, 2021 in India.
❖ The first group to receive COVID-19 vaccine includes healthcare and frontline workers
❖ The second group to receive COVID-19 vaccine will be persons over 50 years of age and persons under 50 years with comorbid conditions.

32. Who all should avoid getting vaccination for now?

❖ Persons with history of anaphylaxis or allergic reaction to a previous dose of COVID-19 vaccine
❖ Immediate or delayed anaphylaxis or allergic reaction to vaccines, injectable therapies, pharmaceutical products, food items, etc.
❖ Pregnant, lactating mothers and women who are not sure of their pregnancy.

33. Who all should avoid vaccination temporarily?

COVID vaccination to be deferred for 4-8 weeks after recovery in the following conditions:
❖ Persons having active symptoms of COVID-19 infection*
❖ COVID-19 patients who have been given anti-COVID-19 monoclonal antibodies or convalescent plasma
❖ Acutely unwell and hospitalized patients due to any illness.

34. Who all should take special precautions?

Vaccine should be administered with caution in persons with a history of any bleeding or coagulation disorder such as:
❖ Clotting factor deficiency
❖ Coagulopathy
❖ Platelet disorders.

---

*However, a person with a *past history* of COVID infection +/ a RT-PCR positive illness can be safely vaccinated.

35. What is the current status of COVID-19 vaccination in persons with chronic diseases or comorbidities?

Persons with the following conditions can be vaccinated:

❖ History of chronic diseases and morbidities (cardiac, neurological, pulmonary, metabolic, renal, malignancies)
❖ Immunodeficiency, HIV, patients on immunosuppression due to any condition (however, the response to the COVID-19 vaccines might be less in these individuals).

36. What are the precautionary guidelines for COVID-19 vaccination?

❖ Authorized age group: COVID-19 vaccination is indicated only for 18 years and above.
❖ Co-administration of vaccines: If required, COVID-19 vaccine and other vaccines should be separated by an interval of at least 14 days.
❖ Interchangeability of COVID-19 vaccines is not permitted: Second dose should also be of the same COVID-19 vaccine which was administered as the first dose.
❖ As with all injectable vaccines, appropriate medical treatment and supervision should always be readily available in case of an anaphylactic event following the administration of the vaccine.

COVISHIELD

Both COVISHIELD™ (manufactured by Serum Institute of India Pvt Ltd) and COVID-19 Vaccine AstraZeneca (manufactured by AstraZeneca) are ChAdOx1 nCoV-19 corona virus vaccines (recombinant).

Mechanism of action	Covishield is a monovalent vaccine composed of a single recombinant, replication-deficient chimpanzee adenovirus (ChAdOx1) vector **encoding the S glycoprotein of SARS-CoV-2**. Following administration, the S glycoprotein of SARS-CoV-2 is expressed locally stimulating neutralizing antibody and cellular immune responses.
Current trial status	The Serum Institute of India (SII) and Indian Council of Medical Research (ICMR) are jointly conducting a Phase II/III, observer-blind, randomized, controlled study to determine the safety and immunogenicity of Covishield.
Dose	One dose: 0.5 mL
Composition	One dose of Covishield contains 5×10^{10} viral particles
Storage condition	Store in a refrigerator (+2°C to +8°C) Do not freeze. Protect from light. Do not shake.
Shelf-life	6 months
Route of administration	Intramuscular (IM) injection only, preferably in the deltoid muscle
Use within	Once opened, multidose vials should be used as soon as practically possible and within 6 hours when kept between +2°C and +25°C.
Vaccination schedule	2 doses: The second dose should be administered between 4 to 6 weeks after the first dose. Protective immune response appears 4 weeks after the second dose.

Contd...

Contd...

Adverse reactions	Very common: • Headache • Nausea • Myalgia • Arthralgia • Injection site: Tenderness, pain, warmth, erythema, pruritus, swelling, bruising • Fatigue, malaise • Pyrexia, chills Common: • Injection site induration • Influenza like illness • Vomiting Uncommon: • Decreased appetite • Dizziness • Abdominal pain • Lymphadenopathy • Hyperhidrosis, pruritus, rash

COVAXIN

Covaxin, India's indigenous COVID-19 vaccine by Bharat Biotech is developed in collaboration with the Indian Council of Medical Research (ICMR) - National Institute of Virology (NIV).

Mechanism of action	Covaxin is an inactivated vaccine; containing 6 mcg of whole-virion inactivated SARS-CoV-2 antigen
Current trial status	Phase III human clinical trial ongoing
Dose	0.5 mL
Route of administration	Intramuscular (IM) injection only, preferably in the deltoid muscle
Use within	6 hours
Vaccination schedule	2 doses, 4 weeks apart
Storage condition	Store in a refrigerator (+2°C to +8°C) Do not freeze. Protect from light. Shake well before use.
Shelf-life	6 months
Adverse reactions	Injection site: • Pain, swelling, redness, itching • Stiffness in the upper arm • Weakness in injection arm • Body ache • Headache • Fever • Malaise • Weakness • Rashes • Nausea • Vomiting.

Chemoprophylaxis: Ivermectin, 12 mg on days 0, 7, 30 followed by once every month has been used in some countries like Bangladesh, India.

Secondary Prevention

    i. **Early diagnosis:** A person with COVID symptoms is advised to isolate, wear mask and immediately get tested for COVID-19.

    ii. **Treatment.**

1. What are the currently accepted treatment protocols for COVID-19 patient?

According to the 'COVID-19 Clinical Management: Living Guidance' document (Published by WHO on 25th January 2021), we will only discuss the strong recommendations as advised by WHO in brief:

Management of Mild COVID-19

❖ Patients with suspected or confirmed mild COVID-19 *should be isolated* to contain virus transmission at a designated COVID-19 health facility, community facility or at home (self-isolation).

❖ Patients with mild COVID-19 should be given symptomatic treatment such as *antipyretics* for fever and pain (preferably NSAIDs), adequate *nutrition* and appropriate *rehydration.*

❖ Counsel patients with mild COVID-19 about signs and symptoms of complications that should prompt urgent care (e.g., lightheadedness, difficulty breathing, chest pain, dehydration etc.).

❖ Routine prophylactic antibiotic therapy is discouraged in patients with mild COVID-19 as it may lead to higher bacterial resistance rates (A recent systematic review reported that only **8%** of the patients hospitalized with COVID-19 encountered bacterial or fungal coinfection during hospital admission). However some countries have used.

❖ Doxycycline 100 mg BD for 7 days, with Ivermectin 12 mg OD for 5 days, along with supportive therapy like vitamin C, Zinc, vitamin D, steam inhalation, to prevent COVID pneumonia.

❖ Monitor SPO_2 by pulse oximeter at home, and immediately report if the saturation is < 95%.

Management of Moderate COVID-19 (Pneumonia)

❖ Patients with suspected or confirmed moderate COVID-19 (pneumonia) *should be isolated* to contain virus transmission. Patients with moderate illness may not require emergency interventions or hospitalization; however, isolation is necessary for all suspect or confirmed cases.

❖ For symptomatic patients with COVID-19 and risk factors for progression to severe disease who are not hospitalized, the *use of pulse oximetry monitoring at home* as part of a package of care is recommended, including patient and provider education and appropriate follow-up.

❖ For patients with suspected or confirmed moderate COVID-19, antibiotics should not be routinely prescribed unless there is clinical suspicion of a bacterial infection.

❖ Patients with moderate COVID-19 should be closely monitored for signs or symptoms of disease progression.

Management of Severe COVID-19 (Severe Pneumonia)

❖ All areas where severe COVID-19 patients may be cared for should be equipped with pulse oximeters, functioning oxygen systems and disposable, single-use, oxygen-delivering interfaces (nasal cannula, Venturi mask and mask with reservoir bag).

❖ WHO recommends *immediate administration of supplemental oxygen therapy* to any patient with emergency signs during resuscitation to target $SpO_2 \geq 94\%$ and to any patient without emergency signs and hypoxemia to target $SpO_2 > 90\%$ or $\geq 92-95\%$ in pregnant women.

❖ Adults with emergency signs (obstructed or absent breathing, severe respiratory distress, central cyanosis, shock, coma and/or convulsions) should receive *emergency airway management* and oxygen therapy during resuscitation to target $SpO_2 \geq 94\%$.

❖ Deliver oxygen flow rates using appropriate delivery devices.

Delivery device	Oxygen flow rate
Nasal cannula	Up to 5 L/min
Venturi mask	6–10 L/min
Face mask with reservoir bag	10–15 L/min

❖ Closely monitor patients for signs of clinical deterioration, such as rapidly progressive respiratory failure and shock and respond immediately with supportive care interventions.

❖ WHO suggests awake *prone positioning* of severely ill patients hospitalized with COVID-19 requiring supplemental oxygen or noninvasive ventilation.

❖ Patients with COVID-19 should *be treated cautiously with intravenous fluids*; aggressive fluid resuscitation may worsen oxygenation, especially in settings where there is limited availability of mechanical ventilation.

❖ *WHO recommends the use of empiric antimicrobials to treat all likely pathogens for patients with suspected or confirmed severe COVID-19*, based on clinical judgment, patient host factors and local epidemiology, and this should be done as soon as possible (within 1 hour of initial assessment if possible), ideally with blood cultures obtained first. Antimicrobial therapy should be assessed daily for de-escalation.

❖ *Thromboprophylaxis*: In hospitalized patients with COVID-19, without an established indication for higher dose anticoagulation, WHO suggests administering standard thromboprophylaxis dosing of anticoagulation.

Management strategies of critical COVID-19 (ARDS, septic shock and acute thromboembolism) are out of the scope of this book because these will require in-depth understanding of Critical care Medicine.

2. What are the current stands on different therapeutics being or had been used in management of COVID-19?

By 9th February, 2021 the WHO guideline contains the following recommendations:

❖ WHO recommends against administering hydroxychloroquine for treatment of COVID-19.

❖ WHO recommends against administering Lopinavir/Ritonavir for treatment of COVID-19.

❖ In hospitalized patients with COVID-19 infection, regardless of disease severity; WHO suggests against administering Remdesivir in addition to usual care.

❖ For patients with nonsevere COVID-19-infection, WHO recommends against the administration of systemic corticosteroids.

❖ **For patients with severe or critical COVID-19-infection, WHO recommends the administration of systemic corticosteroids.**

3. What is 'Infection prevention control (IPC)'? How is it practiced in the care of COVID-19 patients?

Infection prevention control (IPC) is a critical and integral part of clinical management of COVID-19 patients and should be initiated at the point of entry of the patient to hospital (typically the Emergency Department).

At triage	• Give suspect patient a triple layer surgical mask and direct patient to separate area, an isolation room if available • Keep at least 1 meter distance between suspected patients and other patients • Instruct all patients to cover nose and mouth during coughing or sneezing with tissue or flexed elbow for others • Perform *hand hygiene* after contact with respiratory secretions.
Standard precautions	Apply standard precautions for all patients, at all times, when providing any type of patient care. Standard precautions include: • Hand hygiene • Use of personal protective equipment (PPE) in high-risk areas • Prevention of needle-stick or sharps injury • Safe waste management • Cleaning and disinfection of equipment.
Droplet precautions	• Droplet precautions prevent large droplet transmission of respiratory viruses • Use a *triple layer surgical mask* if working within 1–2 meters of the patient • When providing care in close contact with a patient with respiratory symptoms, use eye protection (face-mask or goggles), because sprays of secretions may occur.
Contact precautions	• Use *PPE* (triple layer surgical mask, eye protection, gloves and gown) when entering room and remove PPE when leaving • If an equipment (e.g., stethoscope/BP cuff/thermometer) needs to be shared among patients, clean and disinfect between each patient use • Ensure that healthcare workers refrain from touching their eyes, nose, and mouth with potentially contaminated gloved or ungloved hands • Perform hand hygiene.
Airborne precautions	• Ensure that healthcare workers performing aerosol-generating procedures (i.e., open suctioning of respiratory tract/intubation/bronchoscopy/cardiopulmonary resuscitation) use PPE, including gloves, long-sleeved gowns, eye protection, and fit-tested particulate respirators (*N95*) • Whenever possible, use adequately ventilated single rooms when performing aerosol-generating procedures, meaning *negative pressure rooms* with minimum of 12 air changes per hour.

1. What is the full form of IMCI?

Integrated management of childhood illness.

2. What is IMCI?

IMCI is an integrated approach to child health that focuses on the well-being of the whole child. It aims to reduce death, illness and disability, and to promote improved growth and development among children under 5 years of age. It includes both preventive and curative elements that are implemented by families and communities as well as by health facilities.

3. What are the components of IMCI?

The IMCI strategy includes three main components:
1. Improving case management skills of healthcare staff
2. Improving overall health systems
3. Improving family and community health practices.

4. Why is IMCI better than single-condition approaches?

Children brought for medical treatment in the developing world are often suffering from more than one condition, making a single diagnosis impossible. IMCI is an integrated strategy, which takes into account the variety of factors that put children at serious risk. It ensures the combined treatment of the major childhood illnesses, emphasizing prevention of disease through immunization and improved nutrition.

5. What are the principles of the integrated clinical case management in IMCI clinical guidelines?

A. Examining all sick children aged up to 5 years of age for general danger signs and all young infants for signs of very severe disease. These signs indicate severe illness and the need for immediate referral or admission to hospital.
B. The children and infants are then assessed for main symptoms:

In young infants (up to 2 months), the main symptoms include:
- Local bacterial infection
- Diarrhea
- Jaundice.

In older children (2 months to 5 years) the main symptoms include:
- Cough or difficulty breathing

- Diarrhea
- Fever
- Ear infection.

C. Then in addition, all sick children are routinely checked for:
  - Nutritional and immunization status
  - HIV status in high HIV settings
  - Other potential problems.

D. A combination of individual signs leads to a child's classification within one or more symptom groups rather than a diagnosis. The classification of illness is based on a color-coded triage system:
  - **"PINK"** indicates urgent hospital referral or admission
  - **"YELLOW"** indicates initiation of specific outpatient treatment
  - **"GREEN"** indicates supportive home care.

6. What are the special features of IMCI?

❖ Only a limited number of clinical signs are used, selected on the basis of their sensitivity and specificity to detect disease through classification

❖ IMCI management procedures use a limited number of essential drugs and encourage active participation of caregivers in the treatment of their children

❖ An essential component of IMCI is the counseling of caregivers regarding home care:
  - Appropriate feeding and fluids
  - When to return to the clinic immediately
  - When to return for follow-up.

Sick Young Infant Age up to 2 Months

We are discussing only two things—bacterial infection and diarrhea as they are important from examination point of view.

Bacterial Infection

Check for very severe disease and local bacterial infection

Ask:

- Is the infant having difficulty in feeding?
- Has the infant had convulsions (fits)?

Look, listen, feel:

- Count the breaths in 1 minute. Repeat the count if more than 60 breaths per minute
- Look for severe chest indrawing
- Measure axillary temperature
- Look at the umbilicus. Is it red or draining pus?
- Look for skin pustules
- Look at the young infant's movements

  If infant is sleeping, ask the mother to wake him/her
  - Does the infant move on his/her own?

  If the young infant is not moving, gently stimulate him/her
  - Does the infant not move at all?

> Young infant must be calm

Classify all young infants

Any one of the following signs:

- Not feeding well or
- Convulsions or
- Fast breathing (60 breaths per minute or more) or
- Severe chest indrawing or
- Fever (37.5°C or above) or
- Low body temperature (>35.5°C) or
- Movement only when stimulated or no movement at all

- Umbilicus red or draining pus
- Skin pustules

- None at the signs of very severe disease or local bacterial infection

Pink:
Very severe disease

Yellow:
Local bacterial infection

Green:
Severe disease or local infection unlikely

- Give the first dose of intramuscular antibiotics
- Treat to prevent low blood sugar
- Refer urgently to hospital**
- Advise mother how to keep the infant warm on the way to the hospital

- Give an appropriate oral antibiotic
- Teach the mother to treat local infections at home
- Advise mother to give home care for the young infant
- Follow-up in 2 days

- Advise mother to give home care

**These thresholds are based on axillary temperature. The thresholds for rectal temperature readings are approximately 0.5°C higher. If referral is not possible, manage the sick young infant as described in the national referral care guidelines or WHO Pocket Book for hospital care for children.

Give an appropriate oral antibiotic for local bacterial infection

❖ First-line antibiotic: _____

❖ Second-line antibiotic: _____

Age or weight	Amoxicillin Give 2 times daily for 5 days	
	Tablet 250 mg	Syrup 125 mg in 5 mL
Birth up to 1 month (4 kg)	1/4	2.5 mL
1 month up to 2 months (4–<6 kg)	1/2	5 mL

Teach the Mother to Treat Local Infections at Home

❖ Explain how the treatment is given.

❖ Watch her as she does the first treatment in the clinic.

❖ Tell her to return to the clinic if the infection worsens.

To treat skin pustules or umbilical infection	To treat thrush (ulcers or white patches in mouth)
The mother should do the treatment twice daily for 5 days:	The mother should do the treatment four times daily for 7 days:
• Wash hands	• Wash hands
• Gently wash off pus and crusts with soap and water	• Paint the mouth with half-strength gentian violet (0.25%) using a soft cloth wrapped around the finger
• Dry the area	• Wash hands
• Paint the skin or umbilicus/cord with full strength gentian violet (0.5%)	
• Wash hands	

Diarrhea

Then ask: Does the young infant have diarrhea?

If yes, look and feel:

• Look at the young infant's general condition: Infant's movements
  – Does the infant move on his/her own?
  – Does the infant not move even when stimulated but then stops?
  – Does the infant not move at all?
  – Is the infant restless and irritable?
• Look for sunken eyes
• Pinch the skin of the abdomen. Does it go back
  – Very slowly (longer than 2 seconds)?
  – Or slowly?

[box: Classify diarrhea for dehydration]

Signs	Classify as	Treatment

Two of the following signs:
• Movement only when stimulated or no movement at all
• Sunken eyes
• Skin pinch goes back very slow
	Pink:
	Severe dehydration
		• If infant has no other severe classification:
		  – Give fluid for severe dehydration (plan C)
		  OR
		  If infant also has another severe classification
		  – Refer urgently to hospital with mother giving frequent sips of ORS on the way Advise the mother to continue breastfeeding

Two of the following signs:
• Restless and irritable
• Sunken eyes
• Skin pinch goes back slowly
	Yellow:
	Some dehydration
		• Give fluid and breast milk for some dehydration (plan B)
		• *if infant has any severe classification:*
		  – Refer urgently to hospital with mother giving frequent sips of ORS on the way
		  – Advise the mother to continue breastfeeding
		• Advise mother when to return immediately
		• Follow-up in 2 days if not improving

Not enough signs to classify as some or severe dehydration	*Green:* No dehydration	• Give fluids to treat diarrhea at home and continue breastfeeding (plan A) • Advise mother when to return immediately • Follow-up in 2 days if not improving

What is diarrhea in a young infant?

A young infant has diarrhea if the stools have changed from usual pattern and are many and watery (more water than fecal matter). The normally frequent or semi-solid stools of a breastfeed baby are not diarrhea.

Plan A: Treat Diarrhea at Home

Counsel the mother on the four rules of home treatment:

1. Give extra fluid
2. Give zinc supplements (age 2 months up to 5 years)
3. Continue feeding
4. When to return.

❖ Give extra fluid (as much as the child will take):
   – **Tell the mother:**
      - Breastfeed frequently and for longer at each feed.
      - If the child is exclusively breastfed, give ORS or clean water in addition to breast milk.
   – **If the child is not exclusively breastfed, give one or more of the following:**
      - ORS solution, food-based fluids (such as soup, rice water, and yoghurt, drinks), or clean water.
   – **It is especially important to give ORS at home when:**
      - The child has been treated with Plan B or Plan C during this visit.
      - The child cannot return to a clinic if the diarrhea gets worse.
   – **Teach the mother, how to mix and give ORS. Give the mother 2 packets of ORS to use at home**
   – **Show the mother how much fluid to give in addition to the usual fluid intake:**

Up to 2 years	50–100 mL after each loose stool
2 years or more	100–200 mL after each loose stool

   Tell the mother to:
   - Give frequent small sips from a cup.
   - If the child vomits, wait 10 minutes. Then continue, but more slowly.
   - *Continue giving extra fluid until the diarrhea stops.*

❖ Give zinc (age 2 months up to 5 years)
   – **Tell the mother how much zinc to give (20 mg tab):**

2 months up to 6 months	1/2 tablet daily for 14 days
6 months or more	5 tablet daily for 14 days

   – **Show the mother how to give zinc supplements:**
      - Infants—dissolve tablet in a small amount of expressed breast milk. ORS or clean water in a cup
      - Older children—tablets can be chewed or dissolved in a small amount of water.

❖ **Continue feeding (exclusive breastfeeding if age less than 8 months)**
❖ **When to return.**

Plan B: Treat Some Dehydration with ORS

In the clinic, give recommended amount of ORS over 4 hours period

❖ **Determine the amount of ORS to give during first 4 hours:**

Weight	<6 kg	6–<10 kg	10–<12 kg	12–19 kg
Age*	Up to 4 months	4 months up to 12 months	12 months up to 2 years	2 years up to 5 years
In mL	200–450	450–800	900–960	960–1600

*Use the child's age only when you do not know the weight. The approximate amount of ORS required (in mL) can also be calculated by multiplying the child's weight (in kg) by 75.

- If the child wants more ORS than shown, give more.
- For infants under 6 months who are not breastfed, also give 100–200 mL clean water during this period and use standard ORS. This is not needed if you use new low osmolarity ORS.

❖ **Show the mother how to give ORS solution:**
- Give frequent small sips from a cup
- If the child vomits, wait for 10 minutes. Then continue, but more slowly
- Continue breastfeeding whenever the child wants.

❖ **After 4 hours:**
- Reassess the child and classify the child for dehydration
- Select the appropriate plan to continue treatment
- Begin feeding the child in clinic.

❖ **If the mother must leave before completing treatment:**
- Show her how to prepare ORS solution at home
- Show her how much ORS to give to finish 4-hour treatment at home
- Give her enough ORS packets to complete rehydration. Also give her 2 packets as recommended in Plan A
- Explain the 4 rules of home treatment:
  1. Give extra fluid
  2. Give zinc (age 2 months up to 5 years)
  3. Continue feeding (exclusive breastfeeding if age less than 6 months)
  4. When to return.

Plan C: Treat Severe Dehydration Quickly

Follow the Arrows. If Answer is 'Yes', Go Across. If 'No', Go Down

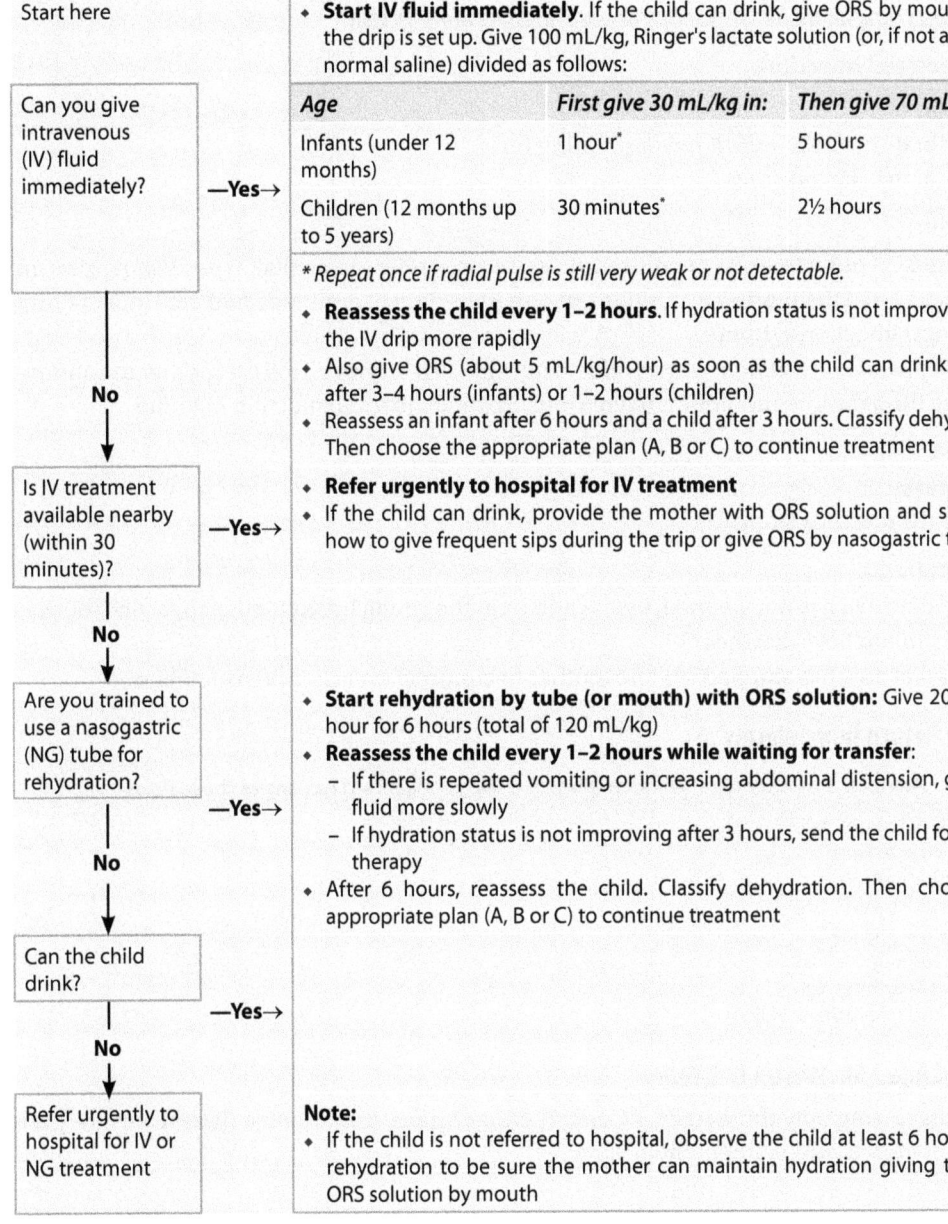

Start here	**Start IV fluid immediately**. If the child can drink, give ORS by mouth while the drip is set up. Give 100 mL/kg, Ringer's lactate solution (or, if not available, normal saline) divided as follows:		
Can you give intravenous (IV) fluid immediately? —Yes→	*Age*	*First give 30 mL/kg in:*	*Then give 70 mL/kg in:*
	Infants (under 12 months)	1 hour*	5 hours
	Children (12 months up to 5 years)	30 minutes*	2½ hours
No	** Repeat once if radial pulse is still very weak or not detectable.*		
	• **Reassess the child every 1–2 hours**. If hydration status is not improving, give the IV drip more rapidly		
	• Also give ORS (about 5 mL/kg/hour) as soon as the child can drink: Usually after 3–4 hours (infants) or 1–2 hours (children)		
	• Reassess an infant after 6 hours and a child after 3 hours. Classify dehydration. Then choose the appropriate plan (A, B or C) to continue treatment		
Is IV treatment available nearby (within 30 minutes)? —Yes→	• **Refer urgently to hospital for IV treatment**		
	• If the child can drink, provide the mother with ORS solution and show her how to give frequent sips during the trip or give ORS by nasogastric tube		
No			
Are you trained to use a nasogastric (NG) tube for rehydration? —Yes→	• **Start rehydration by tube (or mouth) with ORS solution:** Give 20 mL/kg/hour for 6 hours (total of 120 mL/kg)		
	• **Reassess the child every 1–2 hours while waiting for transfer**:		
	– If there is repeated vomiting or increasing abdominal distension, give the fluid more slowly		
	– If hydration status is not improving after 3 hours, send the child for IV therapy		
No	• After 6 hours, reassess the child. Classify dehydration. Then choose the appropriate plan (A, B or C) to continue treatment		
Can the child drink? —Yes→			
No			
Refer urgently to hospital for IV or NG treatment	**Note:**		
	• If the child is not referred to hospital, observe the child at least 6 hours after rehydration to be sure the mother can maintain hydration giving the child ORS solution by mouth		

Follow-up of bacterial infection and diarrhea.

FOLLOW-UP

Give Follow-up Care for the Young Infant

Assess every young infant for "very severe disease" during follow-up visit

Local bacterial infection

After 2 days:
- ❖ Look at the umbilicus. Is it red or draining pus?
- ❖ Look at the skin pustules.

Treatment:
- ❖ If umbilical *pus or redness remains same or is worse*, refer to hospital. If *pus and redness are improved,* tell the mother to continue giving the 5 days of antibiotic and continue treating the local infection at home
- ❖ If skin pustules are *same or worse*, refer to hospital. If it improves, tell the mother to continue giving the 5 days of antibiotic and continue treating the local infection at home.

Diarrhea
After 2 days:
Ask: Has the diarrhea stopped?

Treatment:
- ❖ If the diarrhea has not stopped, assess and treat the young infant for diarrhea. See "does in young infant have diarrhea?"
- ❖ If the diarrhea has stopped, tell the mother to continue exclusive breastfeeding.

When to Return Immediately

Advise the mother to return immediately if the young infant has any of these signs
- ◆ Breastfeeding poorly
- ◆ Reduced activity
- ◆ Becomes sicker
- ◆ Develops a fever
- ◆ Feels unusually cold
- ◆ Fast breathing
- ◆ Difficult breathing
- ◆ Palms and soles appear yellow

Sick Child Age 2 Months up to 5 Years

We are discussing only three things: General danger signs, pneumonia, diarrhea as they are important from examination point of view.

General Danger Signs

Check for general danger signs

Ask:	Look:
• Is the child able to drink or breastfeed? • Does the child vomit everything? • Has the child had convulsions?	• See if the child is lethargic or unconscious • Is the child convulsing now?

Urgent attention →

• Any general danger sign

Pink: **Very severe disease**

• Give diazepam if convulsing now
• Quickly complete the assessment
• Give any prereferral treatment immediately
• Treat to prevent low blood sugar
• Keep the child warm
• Refer urgently

A child with any general danger sign needs urgent attention; complete the assessment and any prereferral treatment immediately so referral is not delayed.

Give Diazepam to Stop Convulsions

❖ Turn the child to his/her side and clear the airway. Avoid putting things in the mouth
❖ Give 0.5 mg/kg diazepam injection solution per rectum using a small syringe without a needle (like a tuberculin syringe) or using a catheter
❖ Check for low blood sugar, then treat or prevent
❖ Give oxygen and refer
❖ If convulsions have not stopped after 10 minutes repeat diazepam dose.

Age or weight	Dose of diazepam 10 mg/2 mL
2 months up to 6 months (5–7 kg)	0.5 mL
6 months up to 12 months (7–10 kg)	1.0 mL
12 months up to 3 years (10–14 kg)	1.5 mL
3 years up to 5 years (14–19 kg)	2.0 mL

Treat the Child to Prevent Low Blood Sugar

❖ If the child is able to breastfeed:
  – Ask the mother to breastfeed the child.
❖ If the child is not able to breastfeed but is able to swallow:
  – Give expressed breast milk or a breast milk substitute
  – If neither of these is available, give sugar water
  – Give 30–50 mL of milk or sugar water* before departure.
❖ If the child is not able to swallow:
  – Give 50 mL of milk or sugar water* by nasogastric tube.
  – If no nasogastric tube available. Give 1 teaspoon of sugar moistened with 1–2 drops of water sublingually and repeat doses every 20 minutes to prevent relapse
    To make sugar water: Dissolve 4 level teaspoons of sugar (20 g) in a 200 mL cup of clean water.

Pneumonia

Then ask about main symptoms:
Does the child have cough or difficult breathing?

If yes, ask:

Look, listen, feel;

- For how long?
  - Count the breaths in 1 minute
  - Look for chest indrawing
  - Look and listen for stridor
  - Lock and listen for wheezing

Child must be calm

If wheezing with either fast breathing or chest indrawing:
Give a trial of rapid acting inhales bronchodilator for up to three times 15–20 minutes apart. Count the breaths and look for chest indrawing again, and then classify

If the child is: | **Fast breathing is:**

- 2–12 months | 50 breaths per minute or more
- 12 months–5 years | 40 breaths per minute or more

Classify cough or difficult breathing

Signs	Classify as	Treatment
• Any general danger sign or • Stridor in calm child	*Pink:* Severe pneumonia or very severe disease	• Give first dose of an appropriate antibiotic • Refer *urgently* to hospital**
• Chest indrawing or • Fast breathing	*Yellow:* Pneumonia	• Give oral amoxicillin for 5 days*** • If wheezing (or disappeared after rapidly acting bronchodilator) given an inhaled bronchodilator for 5 days**** • If chest indrawing in HIV exposed/infected give first dose of amoxicillin and refer • Soothe the throat and relieve the cough with safe remedy • If coughing for more than 14 days or recur wheeze, refer for possible TB or asthma assessment • Advise mother when to return immediately • Follow-up in 3 days
• No signs of pneumonia or very severe disease	*Green:* Cough or cold	• If wheezing (or disappeared after rapidly acting bronchodilator) give an inhaled bronchodilator for 5 days**** • Soothe the throat and relieve the cough with safe remedy • If coughing for more than 14 days or recurrent wheezing, refer for possible TB or asthma assessment • Advise mother when to return immediately • Follow-up in 5 days if not improving

If pulse oximeter is available, determine oxygen saturation and refer if <90%
** If referral is not possible, manage the child as described in the pneumonia section of the national referral guidelines or as in WHO Pocket Book for hospital care for children
*** Oral amoxicillin for 3 days could be used in patients with fast breathing but no chest indrawing in low HIV settings
**** In settings where inhaled bronchodilator is not available, oral salbutamol may be tried but not recommended for the treatment of severe acute wheeze.

Follow-up of Pneumonia

After 3 days:

Check the child for general danger signs.
Assess the child for cough or difficult breathing.
Ask:

❖ Is the child breathing slower?
❖ Is there a chest indrawing?   } See *Assess and Classify chart*
❖ Is there less fever?
❖ Is the child eating better?

Treatment:

❖ If any general danger sign or stridor, refer urgently to hospital
❖ If *chest indrawing and/or breathing rate, fever and eating are the same or worse,* refer urgently to hospital
❖ If *breathing slower, no chest indrawing, fever, and eating better,* complete the 5 days of antibiotic.

Diarrhea

Does the child have diarrhea?

It yes, ask:	Look and feel:
◆ For how long?	◆ Look at the child's general condition. Is the child:
◆ Is there blood in the stool?	– Lethargic and unconscious?
	– Restless or irritable?
	◆ Look for sunken eyes
	◆ Offer the child fluid. Is the child:
	– Not able to drink or drinking poorly?
	– Drinking eagerly, thirsty?
	◆ Pinch the skin of the abdomen. Does it go back:
	– Very slowly (longer than 2 seconds)?
	– Slowly?

For dehydration classify diarrhea

Signs	Classify as	Treatment

Two of the following signs:
◆ Lethargic or unconscious
◆ Sunken eyes
◆ Not able to drink or drinking poorly
◆ Skin pinch goes back very slowly
	Pink: Severe dehydration	◆ If child has no other severe classification:
		  – Give fluid for severe dehydration (plan C)
		    OR
		◆ If child also has another severe classification:
		  – Refer urgently to hospital with mother giving frequent sips of ORS on the way
		  – Advise the mother to continue breastfeeding
		◆ If child is 2 years or older and there is cholera in your area, give antibiotic for cholera

Two of the following signs:
◆ Restless, irritable
◆ Sunken eyes
◆ Drinks eagerly, thirsty
◆ Skin pinch goes back slowly
	Yellow: Some dehydration	◆ Give fluid, zinc supplements, and food for some dehydration (plan B)
		◆ If child also has a severe classification:
		  – Refer urgently to hospital with mother giving frequent sips of ORS on the way
		  – Advise the mother to continue breastfeeding
		◆ Advise mother when to return immediately
		◆ Follow-up in 5 days if not improving

Not enough signs to classify as some or severe dehydration	*Green:* No dehydration	◆ Give fluid, zinc supplements, and food to treat diarrhea at home (plan A) ◆ Advise mother when to return immediately ◆ Follow-up in 5 days if not improving

and if diarrhea 14 days or more

Signs	Classify as	Treatment
◆ Dehydration present	*Pink:* Severe persistent diarrhea	◆ Treat dehydration before referral unless the child has another severe classification ◆ Refer to hospital
◆ No dehydration	*Yellow:* Persistent diarrhea	◆ Advise the mother on feeding a child who has persistent diarrhea ◆ Give multivitamins and minerals (including zinc) for 14 days ◆ Follow-up in 5 days

and if blood in stool

Signs	Classify as	Treatment
◆ Blood in stool	*Yellow:* Dysentery	◆ Give ciprofloxacin for 3 days ◆ Follow-up in 3 days

Follow-up of Persistent Diarrhea

After 5 days:
Ask:
- ❖ Has the diarrhea stopped?
- ❖ How many loose stools is the child having per day?

Treatment:
- ❖ If *the diarrhea has not stopped* (child is still having 3 or more loose stools per day), do a full reassessment of the child. Treat for dehydration if present. Then refer to hospital.
- ❖ If *the diarrhea has stopped* (child having less than 3 loose stools per day), tell the mother to follow the usual feeding recommendations for the child's age.

Feeding recommendations for a child has persistent diarrhea:
- ❖ If still breastfeeding, give more frequent, longer breastfeeds, day and night.
- ❖ If taking other milk:
  - – Replace with increased breastfeeding
    OR
  - – Replace with fermented milk products, such as yoghurt
    OR
  - – Replace half the milk with nutrient-rich semisolid food.
- ❖ For other foods, follow feeding recommendations for the child's age.

Follow-up of Dysentery

After 3 days:
Assess the child for diarrhea.

Ask:
- ❖ Are there fewer stools?
- ❖ Is there less blood in the stool?
- ❖ Is there less fever?
- ❖ Is there less abdominal pain?
- ❖ Is the child eating better?

Treatment:
- ❖ If the child is *dehydrated*, then treat the dehydration
- ❖ If *number of stools, amount of blood in stools, fever, abdominal pain, or eating are worse or the same:*
  - – Change to second-line oral antibiotic recommended for dysentery in your area. Give it for 5 days. Advise the mother to return after 3 days. If you do not have the second-line antibiotic; refer to hospital.

Exceptions: If the child: • Is less than 12 months old,
OR
• Was dehydrated on the first visit,   } Refer to hospital
OR
• If he had measles within the last 3 months

❖ If *fewer stools, less blood in the stools, less fever, less abdominal pain, and eating better,* continue giving ciprofloxacin until finished.

Ensure that mother understands the oral rehydration method fully and that she also understands the need for an extra meal each day for a week.

When to Return Immediately

Advise mother to return immediately if the child has any of these signs:	
Any sick child	◆ Not able to drink or breastfeed ◆ Becomes sicker ◆ Develops a fever
If child has *cough or cold*, return if:	◆ Fast breathing ◆ Difficult breathing
If child has diarrhea, return if:	◆ Blood in stool ◆ Drinking poorly

Chapter 17

Acute Flaccid Paralysis Surveillance

DEFINITION ASSOCIATED WITH SURVEILLANCE

Surveillance

Surveillance is defined as *"the continuous scrutiny of the factors that determine the occurrence and distribution of disease and other conditions of ill health".* Surveillance is essential for effective control and prevention and includes the collection, analysis, interpretation and distribution of relevant data for action (WHO, 1981).

Types of Surveillance

1. *Passive surveillance*: Surveillance is *passive* when data/reports are sent by designated health facilities or individuals on their own periodically as a routine.
2. *Active surveillance*: Surveillance is *active* when a designated official *usually external to the health facility* visits periodically and seeks to collect data from individuals/registers/log books/medical records at a facility *to ensure that no reports/data are incomplete or missing.*

1. How surveillance can be carried out?

Surveillance can be carried out as:

❖ *Institutional surveillance*: It refers to the collection of data (actively or passively) *from pre-identified and designated fixed facilities* regardless of size.
❖ *Community based surveillance*: It refers to the collection of data *from individuals and households at the village/locality level* rather than from institutions or facilities.

2. What can you know from analyzing surveillance data?

Analysis of surveillance data helps us to know the following:

❖ Where the disease is occurring (place)?
❖ When the disease is occurring (time)?
❖ In whom the disease is occurring (person)?

DEFINITION OF AN AFP CASE

Acute flaccid paralysis (AFP) is defined as sudden onset of weakness and floppiness in any part of the body in a child <15 years of age or paralysis in a person of any age in whom polio is suspected.

BACKGROUND RATE OF AFP

❖ In other parts of the world at least one case of AFP (excluding polio) occurs annually for every 1,00,000 children less than 15 years of age. This is referred to as the "background" rate of AFP among children

❖ The nonpolio causes of AFP including (but not limited to) the following causes account for this background rate:
  – Guillain-Barré syndrome (GBS)
  – Transverse myelitis
  – Traumatic neuritis
❖ Sensitive surveillance for AFP must be able to detect a *minimum* of 1 case per 100,000 children less than 15 years of age.
❖ In India, where **the incidence of conditions such as traumatic neuritis and AFP caused by other nonpolio enteroviruses is very high,** the background nonpolio AFP rate is undoubtedly much higher than 1/1,00,000. For this reason, the operational target of nonpolio AFP case detection in India has been set to 2/1,00,000.

PURPOSE OF AFP SURVEILLANCE

❖ AFP surveillance helps to detect reliably areas where poliovirus transmission is occurring.
❖ Thus AFP surveillance helps us to identify areas of priority for focusing immunization activities.
❖ It is the most reliable tool to measure the quality and impact of polio immunization activities.
❖ *For polio free certification, it is essential to provide evidence to the certification committee of the absence of wild polio virus transmission through a functioning and sensitive surveillance system for 3 years after attaining zero polio case status.*

REASONS FOR AFP SURVEILLANCE INSTEAD OF POLIO SURVEILLANCE

❖ Polio surveillance for a case of disease in a child that "looks like polio" alone is not sufficient because **it is impossible to precisely identify all cases of paralytic polio clinically** due to confusing and ambiguous clinical signs and variable clinical knowledge and skills of doctors.
❖ To ensure that no cases of polio are missed, all cases of AFP should be reported and investigated.
❖ *If sufficient nonpolio AFP cases are being detected for investigation, it implies that the surveillance is sensitive enough to pick up polio transmission in that area if it was occurring.*

SELECTION OF AFP CASES FOR INVESTIGATION

The principle of AFP surveillance is to identify children below 15 years with the **syndrome of acute flaccid paralysis:**
❖ **Acute:** *Rapid progression or short, brief duration*
❖ **Flaccid:** *Floppy or soft and yielding to passive stretching at any time during illness*
❖ **Paralysis:** *Severe loss of motor strength*
❖ **Paresis:** *Slight loss of motor strength.*

SURVEILLANCE AT LOCAL/DISTRICT/STATE/NATIONAL LEVELS

Levels	Surveillance activities
Local level	• AFP surveillance at the local level is institution based through a comprehensive network of reporting sites which includes **reporting units and informers' unit** • They notify the DIO/SMO when they suspect an AFP case

Contd...

Contd...

Levels	Surveillance activities
District level	• *Routine activities*: The DIO/SMO reports to the state level on the **Tuesday** of each week • *Activities when AFP cases are reported*: The DIO/SMO is notified of an AFP case by a reporting unit/informers' unit/medical officer/pediatrician/other physician/nurse who sees a patient with AFP
State level	• On every **Wednesday**, the SEPIO/RC/State SMO collects the information and the linelists from all the districts in the state
National level	• At the national level, on **Thursday at** NPSU, the data from the states received in the weekly state linelist is collected, collated and compiled to prepare the national report • This is sent to the Assistant Commissioner (Immunization), Ministry of Health and Family Welfare, Government of India, New Delhi to the WHO South-East Asian Regional Office (SEARO) at New Delhi

(DIO: District Immunization Officer; SMO: Surveillance Medical Officer; SEPIO: State EPI Officer; EPI: Expanded Program of Immunization; RC: Regional Coordinator; NPSU: National Polio Surveillance Unit).

AFP surveillance at different levels is shown below:

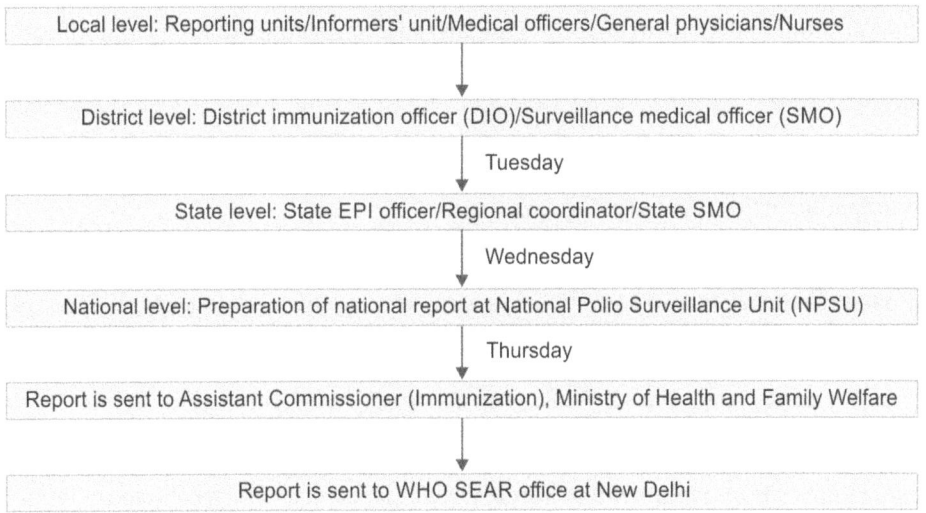

AFP surveillance at different levels

AFP SURVEILLANCE AFTER ATTAINING A ZERO POLIO STATUS

After attaining zero polio cases, it is still critical to continue active surveillance in all areas in the country to detect any wild poliovirus (WPV) case either indigenous or importation for at least 3 years after the last confirmed case. This is also a requirement for certification.

CASE NOTIFICATION

❖ *The date of notification is the date the information of the AFP case reaches the district level (DIO/SMO).*
❖ The Ministry of Health and Family Welfare, Government of India issued an official instruction in 1997 that all health facilities, clinicians and other practitioners are required to notify AFP cases immediately to the District Immunization Officer (DIO) by the fastest available means.

❖ *Immediate notification of AFP cases is essential because important activities including immediate case investigation and stool sample collection, outbreak response immunization and active searches for additional cases in the community should be ensured without delay.*

CASE VERIFICATION

❖ Once a case of AFP is reported by a physician/health unit/any other source, DIO/SMO/any other designated official must personally see the case to ascertain if the case meets the AFP case definition.
❖ If the case does not meet the case definition of AFP, DIO/SMO should discuss the findings with the RC/reporting physician/health worker and record the case as not AFP on the case investigation form.
❖ The SMO should maintain a separate file of all notified cases that he/she determined not to be AFP.

CASE INVESTIGATION

❖ Upon verification that the case meets the AFP case definition, DIO/SMO initiates the case investigation.
❖ Attempt should be made to ensure a case investigation within 48 hours of notification for all AFP cases.
❖ Any case that has had onset within 6 months of notification should be investigated.

The necessary steps in the AFP case investigation are as follows:
1. Using the case investigation form (CIF) as a guide, obtain the history and conduct a physical examination of the affected child.
2. Fill out the CIF and assign the EPID (unique case identification) number.
3. Determine carefully the travel history of the child and family 35 days prior to the onset of paralysis and *details of visitors from outside during this period to pinpoint the place of infection*, in case AFP is due to polio. The details of travel should be incorporated into the CIF. Cross notify the SMO of the concerned district where the child was probably infected to enable him to take necessary follow-up actions. Also inform state SMO/SRC/RC/NPSU.
4. *Collect two stool samples from the child at a minimum interval of 24 hours*; this is done to improve the chances for the detection of poliovirus which may be shed intermittently. *Stool cultures have the maximum probability of yielding a positive result if collected within 14 days (2 weeks) of paralysis onset*, so every effort must be made to collect specimens within this interval. The excretion of poliovirus diminishes rapidly after 14 days, but because a small proportion of cases can still excrete virus for several weeks following paralysis onset, *stool specimens should be collected from late reported cases for up to 60 days (2 months) after paralysis onset*. DIO/SMO should ensure that all reporting sites initiate stool collection for every AFP case without waiting for the case to be examined by DIO/SMO.
5. *Each specimen should be 8 g* (approximately the size of an adult thumb) and stored and transported under proper cold chain conditions.
6. If stool specimens cannot be collected within 14 days of paralysis onset, DIO/SMO should collect detailed epidemiological and clinical informations to be presented to the Expert Review Committee for classification.
7. Collect detailed information on where the patient will be located at 60 days from the time of paralysis onset as *cases with inadequate stool specimens or with vaccine virus or wild virus isolations from stool specimens will require follow-up examination between 60 and 90 days following paralysis onset*, for the determination of the presence or absence of residual weakness.

COLLECTION, TRANSPORT AND REPORTING RESULTS OF STOOL SPECIMEN

1. When to collect stool specimen from a case of AFP?

❖ *Two stool specimens must be collected from every AFP case*
❖ *Stool specimens must be collected within 14 days of onset of paralysis to maximize the chances of isolating poliovirus*
❖ *In case samples cannot be collected within 14 days, the specimens should still be collected up to 60 days of paralysis onset*
❖ The first specimen should be collected at the time of the case investigation.
❖ If the child is not able to pass stool, leave the stool collection kit and stool shipment carrier with frozen ice packs with the family so that they can collect sample from the child later
❖ The second sample should be collected at least 24 hours after the first specimen collection because virus shedding may be intermittent.

2. How to collect a stool specimen?

❖ Use a clean plastic screw cap container (it is not essential to have a sterilized container)
❖ A label with the name, identification number of the case (EPID number), specimen number and the date of collection should be pasted on the side of the container. Use a water-resistant, indelible pen to label the specimen containers
❖ If possible, collect fresh stool from the child's diapers, or get the child to defecate onto a clean paper
❖ Collect a volume of stool about the size of one adult thumb size (8 g). This amount of stool will allow additional testing, if necessary
❖ Use the spoon attached to the cap to place the specimen in the sample bottle
❖ Avoid using laxatives
❖ Do not fill the container up to the brim
❖ Do not soil the rim of the container
❖ After collection, immediately place the container in the stool shipment carrier/fridge
❖ Enema is not a preferred method for stool collection.

3. What do you mean by an "adequate stool" sample?

Two specimens collected within 14 days of paralysis onset and at least 24 hours apart; each specimen must be of adequate volume (8–10 g) and arrive at a WHO-accredited laboratory in good condition (i.e. no desiccation, no leakage, with adequate documentation and evidence that the cold chain was maintained).

Transportation of Specimens

❖ The specimens should be sent to the laboratory in "cold chain"
❖ The process of keeping the specimen in the desired temperature of 2–8°C after collection from the child to the time of reaching the laboratory is called the cold chain
❖ If there is likely to be a delay in shipment, after collection, the specimens must be placed immediately in a deep freezer or freezer compartment of a refrigerator
❖ As soon as both samples are collected, make arrangements to ship the specimens immediately
❖ Plan for the specimens to **arrive at the laboratory within 72 hours of dispatch**
❖ If this is not possible, the specimens must be frozen (at–20°C) and then shipped frozen, preferably with dry ice or with cold packs that have also been frozen at – 20°C
❖ If a cold chain is not properly maintained at all times during transport, poliovirus will not survive in the stool specimen.

Stool Collection and Handling at a Glance

Item	Details
Specimen	8 g of stools (approximately one adult "thumb-size" amount for each specimen)
Number	Two specimens taken at least 24 hours apart
When	Within 14 days of paralysis onset, and no later than 60 days following paralysis onset
Method	Preferably voided stools; by rectal tube if necessary
Temporary storage	Less than +8°C
Transportation	Less than +8°C
Label	Case identification ("EPID") number, date of specimen collection, child's name and sample number
Collection responsibility	DIO and SMO
Storage responsibility	DIO and SMO
Transportation responsibility	DIO, SMO and SEPIO

4. What is EPID number/case investigation number? What are its components?

EPID Number

❖ Every AFP case must have a unique case investigation number that is used to track the case and to link laboratory data to the case
❖ The format for the EPID number is used universally in all countries conducting AFP surveillance for polio eradication
❖ The EPID number is the basis for the case-based surveillance database of all AFP cases investigated and tracked as part of the global Polio Eradication Initiative
❖ DIO/SMO is responsible for assigning the case identification numbers.

Components of an EPID Number

The **case investigation number** (also called "EPID" number) comprises 13 alphabetic characters and digits.

Example: IND-AA-BB-##-###

Characters/digits	Meaning	Example
First 3 (IND)	3-letter country code (1st administrative level)	IND
Next 2 (AA)	2-letter state code (2nd administrative level); state where case was detected and investigated	UP
Next 3 (BBB)	3-letter district code (3rd administrative level); district where case was detected and investigated	LNO
Next 2 (##)	2 digit identification of the year of paralysis onset (according to the Gregorian calendar); Note: If a case with disease onset on 28th December 2005 is reported on 5th January 2006, it is coded 05	05
Next 3 (###)	Number of the case detected in that district in that calendar year	From 001 onwards

Example of case identification number: IND-TN-CNI-05-001.

This is a case identification number for the first case in 2005 from the district of Chennai in the state of Tamil Nadu in India.

SIXTY DAYS FOLLOW-UP EXAMINATION

❖ Sixty days follow-up is done between the 60th and 90th day in certain categories of AFP cases **to determine the presence/absence of residual paralysis.**
❖ *The presence of residual paralysis at this time is further evidence that the cause of paralysis is likely to be due to poliovirus.*
❖ The 60th day follow-up should not be done before the 60th day of onset of paralysis.

In India, the following categories should undergo 60-day follow-up:
❖ AFP cases with *inadequate stool specimen collection*
❖ AFP cases with *isolation of wild poliovirus*
❖ AFP cases with *isolation of vaccine-type (Sabin-type) poliovirus.*

During the 60-day follow-up examination, the investigator must:
❖ Verify with the family that all the information on the CIF is correct
❖ Ask if the paralysis has improved/progressed/same as before
❖ Observe how the child moves limbs or areas of the body that were paralyzed (look for areas of muscle atrophy, mid-thigh skin folds in children and if possible watch the child walk)
❖ Compare present (e.g. mid-arm/mid-thigh) circumference measurements with the measurements taken at initial case investigation to detect any wasting.
❖ Examine the tone, power and reflexes
❖ Verify sensation
❖ Even mild residual weakness is considered as residual paralysis
❖ Complete the 60-day follow-up format and send the form to NPSU according to established procedures.

OUTBREAK RESPONSE IMMUNIZATION

❖ After the AFP case investigation and stool specimen collection, outbreak response immunization (ORI) is organized in the community and performed as soon as possible
❖ Children aged 0–59 months are given one dose of bivalent oral poliovirus vaccine (bOPV) regardless of the number of doses received previously
❖ *Usually 500 children below 5 years of age from the locality/village of the AFP case are covered under ORI.*

Chapter 18

Tuberculosis and RNTCP Guidelines (2022)

TUBERCULOSIS AND GLOBAL CHALLENGES

Tuberculosis (TB) persists as a global public health problem of serious magnitude requiring urgent attention. Current global efforts to control TB have three distinct but overlapping dimensions:

 i. Humanitarian
 ii. Public health, and
iii. Economic.

BURDEN OF TUBERCULOSIS

As India is the 2nd most populous country in the world, about one-fourth of global annual TB incidence occurs in India.

MILLENNIUM DEVELOPMENT GOAL AND TUBERCULOSIS

Goal 6: "Combat HIV/AIDS, malaria and other diseases".
❖ **Target 6.C:** "To reverse the incidence of malaria and other major diseases"
 – **Indicator 6.9:** Incidence, prevalence and death rates associated with tuberculosis
 – **Indicator 6.10:** Proportion of tuberculosis cases detected and cured under directly observed treatment short course.

Components of the Stop TB Strategy, 2006

❖ Pursuing high quality DOTS expansion and enhancement
❖ Addressing TB/HIV, MDR-TB and other challenges
❖ Contributing to health system strengthening
❖ Engaging all health providers
❖ Empowering people with TB, and communities
❖ Enabling and promoting research.

Stop TB Partnership Targets

❖ **By 2005:**
- At least 70% people with sputum smear positive TB will be diagnosed
- At least 85% cured.

❖ **By 2015:**
- Global burden of TB (prevalence and death rates) will be reduced by 50% relative to 1990 levels
  - Reduce prevalence to <150 per lakh population
  - Reduce deaths to <15 per lakh population
- Number of people dying from TB in 2015 should be less than 1 million including those coinfected with HIV.

❖ **By 2050:**
- Global incidence of TB disease will be less than or equal to 1 case per million population per year.

National Strategic Plan for Tuberculosis Elimination, 2017–2025

❖ *Vision*: TB free India with zero deaths, disease and poverty due to tuberculosis
❖ *Goal*: To achieve a rapid decline in burden of TB, morbidity and mortality while working towards the elimination of TB in India by 2025.

	Baseline	Target		
Impact indicators	*2015*	*2020*	*2023*	*2025*
To reduce estimated TB Incidence rate (per 100,000)	217	142	77	44
To reduce estimated TB prevalence rate (per 100,000)	320	170	90	65
To reduce estimated mortality due to TB (per 100,000)	32	15	6	3
To achieve zero catastrophic cost for affected families due to TB	35%	0%	0%	0%

Source: RNTCP, National Strategic Plan for Tuberculosis Elimination, 2017–2025, Central TB Division, DGHS, Ministry of Health with Family Welfare, Government of India (March 2017).

REVISED NATIONAL TUBERCULOSIS CONTROL PROGRAM

Before the Revised National Tuberculosis Control Program (RNTCP) came into force the existing tuberculosis program had the following objectives:

❖ To identify and treat as large a number of TB patients as possible so that infectious cases are rendered noninfectious
❖ To reduce the magnitude of TB problem in the country to a level where it ceases to be a public health problem.

NTCP Performance and Evolution of RNTCP

❖ Despite a nationwide network of facilities, NTCP failed to yield satisfactory results. The situation did not change much
❖ The case finding efficiency was only 30 of the expected level although the mortality rate decreased to 53/10,000 population.

Implementation of RNTCP

❖ Launched in 1997 based on WHO DOTS Strategy
  – Entire country covered in March 2006 through an unprecedented rapid expansion of DOTS
❖ Implemented as 100% centrally sponsored program
  – Government of India is committed to continue the support till TB ceases to be a public health problem in the country
❖ All components of the STOP TB Strategy, 2006 are being implemented.

Program Goals of RNTCP

❖ To reduce mortality and morbidity from TB and
❖ To interrupt chain of transmission.

Objectives of RNTCP

❖ To achieve and maintain a cure rate of at least 85% among newly detected infectious (new sputum smear positive) cases.
❖ To achieve and maintain detection of at least 70% of such cases in the population.

How the Strategy Works?

❖ Augmentation of organizational support at the central and state level for meaningful coordination
❖ Increase in budgetary outlay
❖ Use of sputum microscopy as a primary method of diagnosis among self-reporting patients
❖ Standardized treatment regimens
❖ Augmentation of the peripheral level supervision through the creation of a subdistrict supervisory unit
❖ Ensuring a regular uninterrupted supply of drugs up to the most peripheral level
❖ Emphasis on training, IEC, operational research and NGO involvement in the program.

Organization and Structure of RNTCP at Different Levels

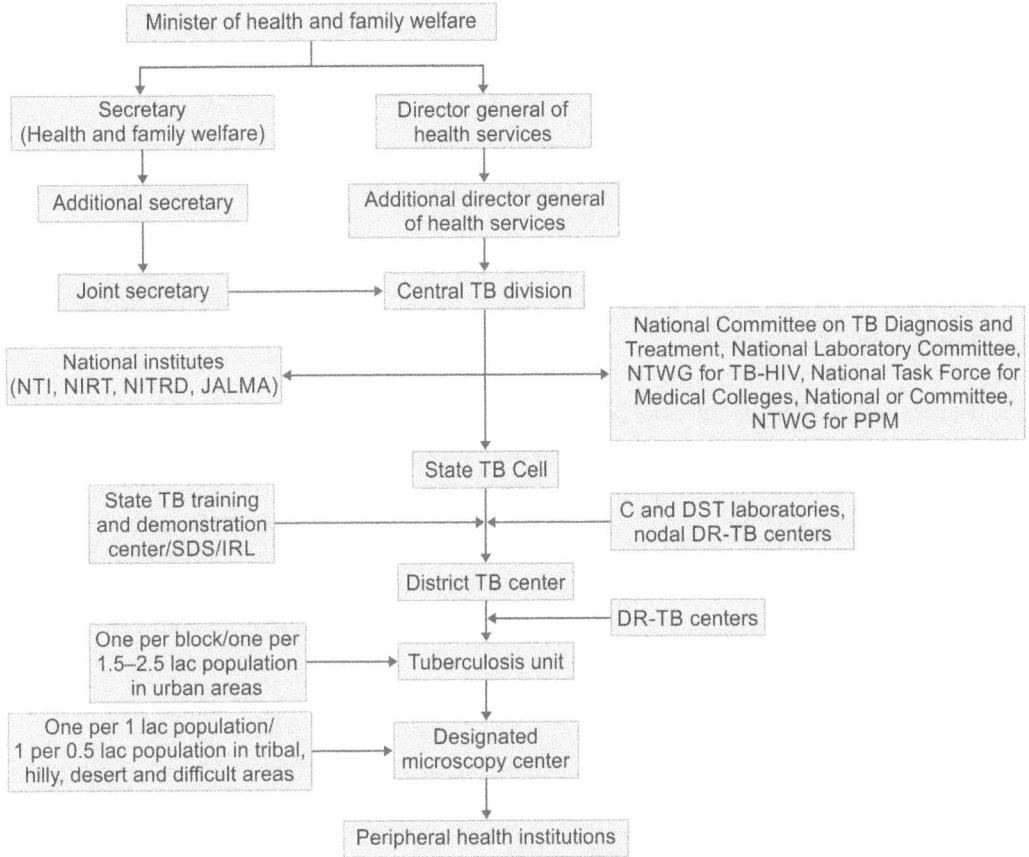

Core Elements of RNTCP

Phase I (1997–2006)

Ensure high quality DOTS expansion in the country, addressing the *five primary components of the DOTS strategy*

Components of DOTS:
 i. Political and administrative commitment
 ii. Good quality diagnosis through sputum microscopy
 iii. Directly observed treatment
 iv. Systematic monitoring and accountability
 v. Addressing stop TB strategy under RNTCP

Phase II (2006–2011)

The RNTCP phase II is envisaged to:
 i. Consolidate the achievements of phase I
 ii. Maintain its progressive trend and effect further improvement in its functioning
 iii. Achieve TB related MDG goals while retaining DOTS as its core strategy

DOTS in Context of HIV

DOTS can:
 ❖ Prolong and improve the quality of life
 ❖ Prevent emergence of MDR-TB
 ❖ Stop the spread of TB
 ❖ Reverse the trend of MDR-TB.

In the context of HIV, failure to use DOTS can result in—rapid spread of disease—tripling of cases—increased drug resistance.

Definitions Regarding Tuberculosis

Case Definitions

I. *Microbiologically confirmed TB* case refers to a presumptive TB patient with biological specimen positive for acid-fast bacilli, or positive for *Mycobacterium tuberculosis* on culture, or positive for tuberculosis through quality assured rapid diagnostic molecular test.

II. *Clinically diagnosed TB* case refers to a presumptive TB patient who is not microbiologically confirmed, but has been diagnosed with active TB by a clinician on the basis of X-ray abnormalities, histopathology or clinical signs with a decision to treat the patient with a full course of anti-TB treatment.

Classification Based on Anatomical Site of Disease

a. Pulmonary tuberculosis (PTB) refers to any microbiologically confirmed or clinically diagnosed case of TB involving the lung parenchyma or tracheobronchial tree.

b. Extrapulmonary tuberculosis (EPTB) refers to any microbiologically confirmed or clinically diagnosed case of TB involving organs other than the lungs such as pleura, lymph nodes, intestine, genitourinary tract, joint and bones, meninges of the brain, etc.

Note: A patient with both pulmonary and extrapulmonary TB should be classified as a case of PTB.

Classification Based on History of TB Treatment

a. *New case*: A TB patient who has never had treatment for TB or has taken anti-TB drugs for less than 1 month is considered as a new case.

b. *Previously treated* patients have received 1 month or more of anti-TB drugs in the past.
   - *Recurrent TB case:* A TB patient previously declared as successfully treated (cured/treatment completed) and is subsequently found to be microbiologically confirmed TB case is a recurrent TB case.
   - *Treatment after failure:* Patients are those who have previously been treated for TB and whose treatment failed at the end of their most recent course of treatment.
   - *Treatment after loss to follow-up*: A TB patient previously treated for TB for 1 month or more and was declared lost to follow-up in their most recent course of treatment and subsequently found microbiologically confirmed TB case.
   - *Other previously treated patients* are those who have previously been treated for TB but whose outcome after their most recent course of treatment is unknown or undocumented.

c. *Transferred in*: A TB patient who is received for treatment in a tuberculosis unit, after registered for treatment in another TB unit is considered as a case of transferred in.

Classification Based on Drug Resistance

a. *Monoresistance (MR)*: A TB patient whose biological specimen is resistant to one first-line anti-TB drug only.

b. *Polydrug resistance (PDR)*: A TB patient whose biological specimen is resistant to more than one first-line anti-TB drug, other than both isoniazid (INH) and rifampicin.

c. *Multidrug resistance (MDR)*: A TB patient whose biological specimen is resistant to both isoniazid and rifampicin with/without resistance to other first-line drugs based on the results from a quality assured laboratory.

Note: Patients who have any rifampicin resistance should also be managed as if they are an MDR-TB case.

d. *Extensive-drug resistance (XDR)*: A MDR-TB case whose biological specimen is additionally resistant to a fluoroquinolone (ofloxacin, levofloxacin, or moxifloxacin) and a second-line injectable anti-TB drug (kanamycin, amikacin, or capreomycin) from a quality assured laboratory.

Differences between Previous and New RNTCP Guidelines

Topics	Previous guidelines (2005)	New guidelines (2022)
Tool for case diagnosis	The main tools for diagnosis were sputum smear microscopy with ZN stain and CXR	Major importance has been given on nationally implementing molecular methods like cartridge based nucleic acid amplification test (CBNAAT) for early diagnosis
Detection of resistance	Previously detection of drug resistance was mainly culture-based (solid and liquid) and line probe assay (LPA) was available on few selected institutions	Now emphasis is given on molecular methods, diagnosis of drug resistant TB is to be done nationwide by CBNAAT/LPA; LPA is better than CBNAAT
Treatment protocol	Thrice weekly regimen. Separate tablets	Once daily regimen. Fixed dose combination (FDC)
Treatment regimen for new cases	2 (HRZE) + 4 (HR)	2 (HRZE) + 4 (HRE)
Monitoring for confirmed drug intake by patients (treatment adherence)	The principle was directly observed treatment; short-course (DOTS): • During intensive phase: Health worker watches the person swallow the drug in his presence • During continuation phase: Patient is given combipack for 1 week, the first dose of which is swallowed by the patient in the presence of health worker	Several new technologies have been implemented: • Mobile based "pill in hand" adherence monitoring tool: When patient takes a dose, a secret number appears on the strip. The patient has to make a missed call to a specified number with that digits. This will be documented by a centralized unit • Specially designed electronic pill boxes or strips with GSM connection and pressure sensor will be used by measuring the weight of remaining pills • A SMS gateway through which patient can report daily pill consumption, minor adverse effects and any need for help
Introduction of new drug through RNTCP	—	Provision to use 2 new drugs: Bedaquiline and Delamanid in drug resistant cases only if indications are met

Diagnostic Algorithm of Pulmonary TB in Adults

❖ *Presumptive pulmonary TB*: Refers to a person with any of the symptoms and signs suggestive of TB including: Cough >2 weeks, fever >2 weeks, significant weight loss, hemoptysis, any abnormality in chest radiograph

❖ Number of specimen(s) required for diagnosis of smear positive TB: 2
❖ Spot sputum specimen (Day 1)
❖ Morning sputum specimen (Day 2).

Diagnosis of TB

❖ None of the sputum smears positive: Doubtful
❖ One of the sputum smears positive: Sputum (+) pulmonary TB
❖ Both of the sputum smears positive: Sputum (+) pulmonary TB.

Grading of Smears

Examination findings	No. of fields examined	Grading	Result
No AFB in 100 oil immersion field	100	0	Negative
1–9 AFB per 100 oil immersion field	100	Scanty	Positive
10–99 AFB per 100 oil immersion field	100	1+	Positive
1–10 AFB per oil immersion field	50	2+	Positive
>10 AFB in per oil immersion field	20	3+	Positive

Diagnostic algorithm for pulmonary TB

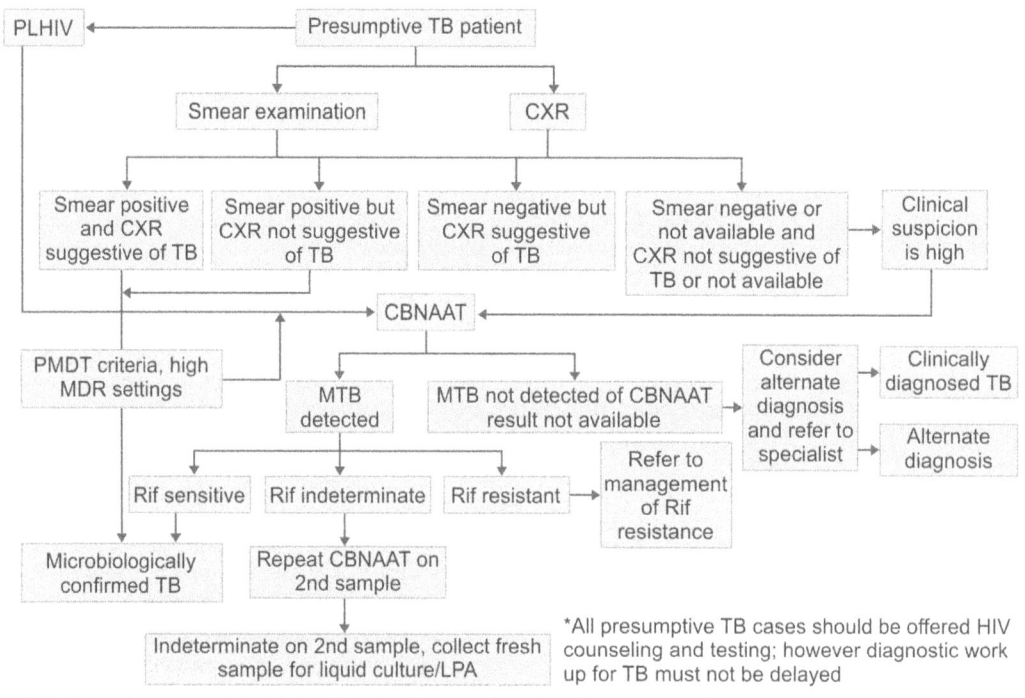

(PLHIV: People living with HIV/AIDS; CBNAAT: Cartridge based nucleic acid amplification test; LPA: Line probe assay; CXR: Chest X-ray; MTB: *Mycobacterium tuberculosis*; Rif: Rifampicin).

Programmatic Management of Drug-resistant TB (PMDT) Criteria/MDR Suspect Criteria

Criteria A	All failures of new TB cases Smear positive previously treated cases who remain smear positive at 4th month onwards All pulmonary TB cases who are contacts of known MDR TB case
Criteria B	In addition to criteria A: All smear positive previously treated pulmonary TB cases at diagnosis. Any smear positive follow-up result in new or previously treated cases
Criteria C	In addition to criteria B: All smear negative previously treated pulmonary TB cases at diagnosis HIV-TB coinfected cases at diagnosis

Diagnostic Algorithm of Pediatric Pulmonary TB

Presumptive pulmonary TB: Refers to children with persistent fever and/or cough for >2 weeks, loss of weight/no weight gain and/or history of contact with infectious TB cases.

Diagnostic algorithm for pediatric pulmonary TB

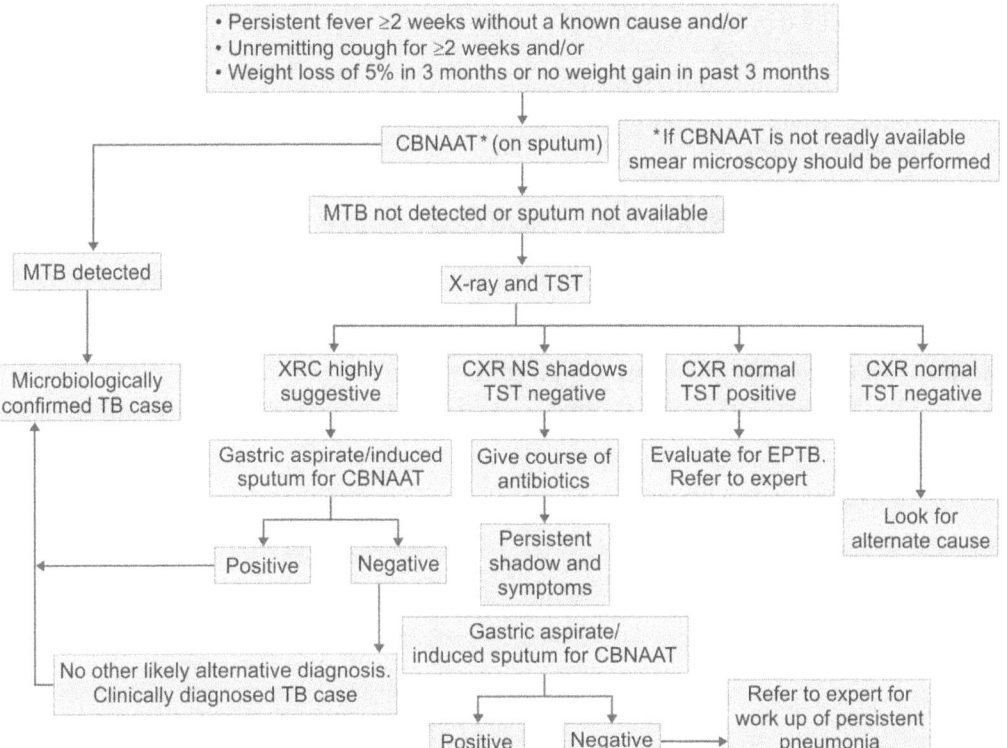

(XRC: X-ray chest; CXR: Chest X-ray; NS: Nonspecific; TST: Tuberculin skin test; EPTB: Extrapulmonary tuberculosis; CBNAAT: Cartridge based nucleic acid amplification test; TB: Tuberculosis).

XRC high suggestive means:
1. Hilar or mediastinal lymphadenopathy
2. Chronic fibrocavitatory shadows.

Special note: Antibiotics having anti-TB action (quinolones, amoxicillin/clavulanic acid, linezolid) should not be given.

Chemotherapy

Objectives

❖ To achieve a cure rate of at least 85% of all new smear positives.
❖ To achieve at least 90% treatment completion rate of all retreatment cases and sputum negative cases.

Short course chemotherapy is given in two phases:
1. Intensive phase
2. Continuation phase.

Basis of chemotherapy in tuberculosis:
❖ Continuous (daily) treatment regimens
❖ Standardized treatment regimens in two categories
❖ Regimen decided by MO on basis of:
  – Sputum smear results
  – History of previous anti-TB treatment
  – Disease classification (pulmonary/extrapulmonary)
  – Severity of illness.

DRUG SENSITIVE-TUBERCULOSIS TREATMENT AS PER NTEP (2022)

(Authors' note: This is the most recent Guideline for TB in India, so it's good to know! This complete guideline may not be required for exam, but it will be helpful for other purposes.)

Regimen for Drug Sensitive-TB Cases: 2HRZE/4HRE

This regimen is for H and R sensitive TB cases and cases where the sensitivity pattern cannot be established.

Treatment is given in two phases:

Intensive phase	Continuation phase
Consists of 8 weeks (56 doses) of Isoniazid (H), Rifampicin (R), Pyrazinamide (Z) and Ethambutol (E) given under direct observation in daily dosages as per weight band categories	Consists of 16 weeks (112 doses) of Isoniazid, Rifampicin and Ethambutol in daily dosages. • Only Pyrazinamide will be stopped in the continuation phase. The CP needs to be extended up to 24 weeks in certain forms of TB-like CNS TB, skeletal TB. • In disseminated TB or slow response treating physician may extend on case-to-case basis.

Regimen for DS-TB	IP	CP
Drugs	2HRZE	4HRE
Doses	56	112

Adult TB Treatment

Drug Dosages for First-line Anti-TB Drugs

Drugs	Doses
Isoniazid (H)	5 mg/kg daily (4 to 6 mg/kg)
Rifampicin (R)	10 mg/kg daily (8 to 12 mg/kg)
Pyrazinamide (Z)	25 mg/kg daily (20 to 30 mg/kg)
Ethambutol (E)	15 mg/kg daily (12 to 18 mg/kg)
Streptomycin (S)*	15 mg/kg daily (15 to 20 mg/kg)

*Streptomycin is administered only in certain situations, like TB meningitis or if any first line drug need to be replaced due to ADR as per weight of the patient.

Pyridoxine may be given at a dosage of 10 mg per day

Body weight category (kg)	Number of tablets (FDCs)	
	Intensive Phase (H: 75 mg; R: 150 mg; Z: 400 mg; E: 275 mg)	Continuation Phase (H: 75mg; R: 150 mg; E: 275 mg)
25–34	2	2
35–49	3	3
50–64	4	4
65–75	5	5
>75	6	6

- Fixed dose combinations (FDCs) refer to products containing two or more active ingredients in fixed doses, used for a particular indication(s).
- In NTEP, for Adults: 4-FDC (given in IP) consists of HRZE and 3-FDC (given in CP) consists of HRE.
- During treatment if weight of the patient increases by >5 kg and crosses the next weight band, then patient should be given the next higher weight band FDC drugs.

SPECIAL CONSIDERATIONS FOR DIFFERENT MANIFESTATIONS OF TUBERCULOSIS (2022)

Special Considerations for Adult TB Meningitis

❖ Intensive phase: 2 months of RHZE or RHZS
❖ Continuation phase: 3 drugs-RHE for at least 10 months*

Role of Steroids in Adult TB Meningitis

❖ Preferably Dexamethasone 0.4 mg/kg/day intravenously in 3-4 divided doses during hospital stay.
❖ If not feasible, give oral Dexamethasone 0.4 mg/kg/day in divided doses or oral Prednisolone 1 mg/kg/day in a single morning dose.
❖ Discharge on oral steroids on tapering doses for total duration of 8–12 weeks.

*Treatment duration may be increased in some cases as per the clinician decision.

❖ Regular follow up is essential every month for at least first 3 months and can be increased thereafter till treatment is stopped.
❖ Monitor liver function tests and any other features of drug toxicity.
❖ Observe for clinical improvement or any deterioration.
❖ Closely observe for development of any complications.

Special Considerations for Adult Abdominal TB

❖ Extend duration of treatment in cases of inadequate response.
❖ Refer for surgical management for complications [intestinal obstruction (due to strictures), perforation].
❖ Consider endoscopic dilatation for treatment for accessible strictures.
❖ Refer for biliary drainage in case of jaundice due to biliary obstruction (hepatobiliary obstruction/pancreatic TB).

Special Considerations for Intraocular TB

Pediatric TB Treatment

Antitubercular Treatment (ATT):
❖ 2 months of RHEZ + 7 months of RH depending on clinical response and side-effects to treatment.
❖ Add pyridoxine 10 mg/day.

Corticosteroids:
❖ Topical steroids eye drops for severe/anterior chamber inflammation.
❖ For treatment in children refer to paediatrician.
❖ Systemic corticosteroids for severe inflammation in consultation with uveitis expert.

Pediatric TB Treatment

❖ Pediatric cases are to be treated under NTEP in daily dosages as per 6 weight band categories
❖ Children and adolescents up to 18 years of age weighing less than 39 kg, are to be treated using pediatric weight bands.
❖ Those weighing more than 39 kg to be treated with adult weight bands.

Available Pediatric Dispersible FDCs and Loose Drugs

1. Dispersible FDC, flavored
❖ Rifampicin 75 mg + Isoniazid 50 mg + Pyrazinamide 150 mg
❖ Rifampicin 75 mg + Isoniazid 50 mg

2. Dispersible loose drugs
❖ Ethambutol 100 mg
❖ Isoniazid 100 mg

Drug dosages for first-line anti- TB drugs

Isoniazid (H)	7–15 mg/kg (maximum dose 300 mg/day)
Rifampicin (R)	10–20 mg/kg (maximum dose 600 mg/day)
Pyrazinamide (Z)	30–40 mg/kg (maximum 2000 mg/day)
Ethambutol (E)	15–25 mg/kg (maximum 1500 mg/day)

Weight band (kg)	Number of tablets (dispersible FDCs)			
	Intensive phase		Continuation phase	
	HRZ (50/75/150)	E (100)	HR (50/75)	E (100)
4–7	1	1	1	1
8–11	2	2	2	2
12–15	3	3	3	3
16–24	4	4	4	4
25–29	3+ 1A*	2	3+ 1A*	2
30–39	3+2A*	2	2+2A*	2

*A=Adult FDC
(HRZE = 75/150/400/275; HRE =75/150/275). It is added in higher weight band categories, i.e. > 25 kg as these children may be able to swallow tablets.
Pyridoxine may be given at a dosage of 10 mg per day

Special considerations for paediatric TB meningitis

ATT for paediatric TB meningitis
❖ HRZE and 10 HRE (in appropriate doses).

Corticosteroids
❖ Prednisolone 2 mg/kg/day for 4 weeks and then taper over 4 weeks*
❖ Slower taper needed in some patients

Special Considerations for Pediatric Abdominal TB

❖ Steroids: Not recommended
❖ Supportive treatment: Management of SAM/Malnutrition as per national guidelines
❖ Surgical treatment:
  – Acute intestinal obstruction, bowel perforation
  – Persistence of obstructive symptoms despite conservative
❖ Management and ATT. DO NOT start empirical ATT with isolated:
  – Recurrent/chronic abdominal pain without danger signs
  – Chronic diarrhea.

*Equivalent dose of another steroid formulation may be used either injectable/oral

Treatment Regimens

Basic for antitubercular drugs regimens:

Category of patient		Intensive phase*	Continuation phase**
New	New smear-positive. New smear-negative. New extrapulmonary cases	2 (HRZE)	4 (HRE)
Previously treated	Recurrent TB case. Treatment after failure. Treatment after loss to follow-up. Other previously treated patients	2 (HRZES) + 1 (HRZE)	5 (HRE)
MDR-TB cases	Resistance to (H + R ± any other first-line ATD)	6–9 months***	18 months
XDR TB cases	Resistance to H + R + fluoroquinolone (ofloxacin, levofloxacin or moxifloxacin) and a second-line injectable anti-TB drugs (kanamycin, amikacin or capreomycin)	6–12 months	18 months

* If sputum positive for AFB at end of prescribed intensive phase, extend it by 1 month.
** For patients with TB meningitis, disseminated disease and spinal TB with neurological complications continuation phase may be up to 7 months.
*** As per the new programmatic management of drug-resistant TB (PMDT) guidelines 2017, management of DRTB is completely based on drug sensitivity testing (DST). Those are complex regimens and out of the scope of undergraduates.

Schedule of Follow-up Sputum Examination

Category of the patient	Pretreatment sputum	Test at month	If result is	Then
New	+	2	–	CP: Sputum at 6 months
			+	Send LPA culture to rule out drug resistance* CP: Sputum at 6 months
	–	2	–	CP: Sputum at 6 months
			+	Send LPA culture to rule out drug resistance CP: Sputum at 6 months
Previously treated	+	3	–	CP: Sputum at 8 months
			+	Send LPA culture to rule out drug resistance CP: Sputum at 8 months

*No extension of intensive phase in daily regimen.
(LPA: Line probe assay, CP: Continuation phase).

Common Adverse Effects of First-line Anti-TB Drugs

Drug	Adverse effects
Isoniazid (H)	• Peripheral neuropathy • Skin rash • Hepatitis • Sleepiness and lethargy

(Contd...)

(Contd...)

Drug	Adverse effects
Rifampicin (R)	• GI side effects: Abdominal pain, nausea, vomiting • Hepatitis • Generalized cutaneous reactions • Idiopathic or immune thrombocytopenic purpura
Pyrazinamide (Z)	• Hyperuricemia • Hepatitis • GI side effects
Ethambutol (E)	• Retrobulbar neuritis
Streptomycin (S)	• Vestibular toxicity (nausea and vertigo) • Nephrotoxicity

Treatment in Special Situations

Hospitalization

❖ The usual mode of TB treatment is domiciliary, but in patients with pneumothorax or large accumulations of pleural fluid leading to breathlessness; massive hemoptysis, etc., the patients might need hospitalization

❖ These patients can be managed in general hospitals preferably in wards where adequate airborne infection control measures are taken to prevent the spread.

Pregnancy and Postnatal Period

❖ A successful treatment of TB is important for successful outcome of pregnancy. With the exception of streptomycin, the first-line anti-TB drugs are safe for use in pregnancy. Streptomycin is ototoxic to the fetus and should not be used during pregnancy

❖ A breastfeeding woman should receive a full course of TB treatment. Correct chemotherapy is the best way to prevent transmission of TB to baby. Breastfeeding has to be continued

❖ After ruling out active TB, the baby should be given 6 months of isoniazid preventive therapy, followed by BCG vaccination. Breastfeeding should never be discouraged.

Special Note: Isoniazid Preventive Therapy

❖ Children are more susceptible to TB infection, more likely to develop active TB disease soon after infection, and more likely to develop severe forms of disseminated TB

❖ Children <6 years of age who are close contacts of a TB patient should be evaluated for active TB by a medical officer/pediatrician. After excluding active TB he/she should be given INH preventive therapy irrespective of their BCG or nutritional status. The dose of INH for preventive therapy is 10 mg/kg body weight administered daily for a minimum period of 6 months.

TB and Contraceptive Pills Usage

❖ As rifampicin is a potent inducer of hepatic enzymes, the protective efficacy of oral contraceptive pills may be decreased

❖ Hence, women suffering from TB and using contraceptive pills should be advised to use some alternative anticontraception method

❖ Use of barrier methods (condoms/diaphragms), IUDs (CuT) or depot medroxyprogesterone (depo-provera) are recommended based on individual preference and eligibility.

Hepatic Disorders

❖ Clinical monitoring (and LFT if possible) of all patients with pre-existing liver disease should be performed during treatment
❖ If the serum ALT level is >3 times normal before the initiation of treatment, the following regimens should be considered:

Regimen containing 2 hepatotoxic drugs	9 (HRE) or 2 (HRES) + 7 (HR) or 6-9 (RZE)
Regimen containing 1 hepatotoxic drug	2 (HES) + 7 (HR)
Regimen containing no hepatotoxic drugs	18–24 (ES + 1 fluoroquinolone)

Renal Failure

❖ First-line drugs not needing renal dose adjustment: HR (Safest: Rifampicin)
❖ Second-line drugs not needing renal dose adjustment: Moxifloxacin, ethionamide, linezolid, clofazimine.

TB with HIV

Clinical staging	CD4 cell count	Timing of ART in relation to initiation of TB treatment	ART recommendations
Start ART irrespective of any clinical stage	CD4 count of any value	Start ATT first. Start ART as soon as TB treatment is tolerated (preferably between 2 weeks and 2 months)	Start ART regimen TLE for patients not on ART. First line ART for HIV-TB: Tenofovir 300 mg + lamivudine 300 mg + efavirenz 600 mg (FDC)

Rationale for ART recommendation during TB treatment: *In the absence of ART, TB therapy alone does not significantly increase the CD4 cell count.* Nor does it significantly decrease the HIV viral load. The use of highly active antiretroviral therapy (HAART) in patients with TB can lead to a sustained reduction in the HIV viral load, thus decreasing AIDS related mortality.

Treatment Outcomes for Drug-susceptible TB Patients

❖ *Cured*: Microbiologically confirmed TB patients at the beginning of treatment who was smear or culture negative at the end of the complete treatment
❖ *Treatment completed*: A TB patient who completed treatment without evidence of failure or clinical deterioration but with no record to show that the smear or culture results of biological specimen in the last month of treatment was negative, either because test was not done or result is unavailable
❖ *Treatment success*: TB patients either cured or treatment completed are accounted in treatment success
❖ *Failure*: A TB patient whose biological specimen is positive by smear or culture at the end of the treatment
❖ *Failure to respond*: A case of pediatric TB who fails to have microbiological conversion to negative status or fails to respond clinically/or deteriorates after 12 weeks of compliant intensive phase shall be deemed to have failed response provided alternative diagnoses/ reasons for nonresponse have been ruled out
❖ *Lost to follow-up*: A TB patient whose treatment was interrupted for 1 consecutive month or more

❖ *Not evaluated*: A TB patient for whom no treatment outcome is assigned. This includes former "transfer out"
❖ *Treatment regimen changed*: A TB patient who is on first line regimen and has been diagnosed as having DRTB and switched to drug resistant TB regimen prior to being declared as failed
❖ *Died*: A patient who has died during the course of anti-TB treatment.

Special Note: Bedaquiline (BDQ)

❖ Class: Bedaquiline is a new class of drug, diarylquinoline
❖ Mechanism: Bedaquiline specifically targets mycobacterial ATP synthase, an enzyme essential for the supply of energy to *Mycobacterium tuberculosis* and most other mycobacteria
❖ Salient features:
  – Strong bactericidal and sterilizing activities against *M. tuberculosis*
  – High volume of distribution with extensive tissue distribution
  – Highly bound to plasma proteins
  – Metabolized in liver
  – The drug has an extended half-life, it is present in the plasma up to 5.5 months post-stopping BDQ
  – No dosage adjustments required in patients with mild to moderate renal impairment.
❖ Specific adverse events related to BDQ:
  – AST and/or ALT elevation
  – Amylase and/or lipase elevation
  – Musculoskeletal abnormalities—myalgia
  – Gastrointestinal abnormalities—severe nausea and vomiting
  – Cardiac rhythm abnormality: QT prolongation → ventricular arrhythmia → sudden death. To monitor closely, an ECG should be obtained before initiation of therapy, then every 2 weeks for 3 months, then monthly.
❖ BDQ demonstrates no cross-resistance with existing first- and second-line anti-TB drugs and has shown significant benefits in improving the time to culture conversion in MDR-TB patients
❖ RNTCP is introducing BDQ through conditional access program at 6 sites in the country initially.

Guidelines for Use of Delamanid in the Treatment of Drug Resistant TB in India (2018)

❖ Indications:
  1. When an effective treatment regimen containing four second-line drugs in addition to pyrazinamide (Z) cannot be designed.
  2. When there is documented evidence of resistance to any FQ or second-line injectable drug in addition to MDR.
  3. When there is higher risk for poor outcomes (i.e. drug intolerance or contraindication, extensive or advanced disease).
❖ Chemical class: Nitroimidazole
❖ Mechanism of action: Bactericidal (Half-life: 36 hours)
  – By blocking the synthesis of mycolic acids (an important component of mycobacterial cell wall)
  – By poisoning them with nitric oxide (NO), which the drugs release when metabolized.
❖ Each film-coated tablet contains 50 mg delamanid
❖ Excipient: Each film-coated tablet contains 100 mg lactose (as monohydrate).

Points to be Remembered Regarding TB

❖ TB is a notifiable disease
❖ If you are not sure of individualized treatment regime, please do not start it. Instead you may register the patient under RNTCP.
❖ Do not start a fluoroquinolone to a TB suspect.
❖ Please do simple sputum microscopy for AFB smear for all TB suspects, rather than directly starting from higher investigations like CT scan.
❖ Serological TB tests are banned in India, e.g. TB IgG and TB IgM.
❖ Do not even attempt to treat drug resistant TB in the absence of requisite training. Refer to specialist/RNTCP/PMDT.
❖ "NIKSHAY", the web-based reporting for TB program has been a notable achievement initiated in 2012 and has enabled capture and transfer of individual patient data from remotest health institutions of the country.

RNTCP Treatment Card

Revised National Tuberculosis Control Program
Treatment Card

State _____ City/district _____ TB unit _____ PHI _____ TB Notification No/NIKSHAY ID _____

Name _____ Sex ☐ M ☐ F ☐ TG age: _____ Occupation: _____ Socioeconomic status: APL/BPL

Complete address: House No.: _____ Road: _____ Ward/village: _____ Town/city: _____ Taluka/mandal: _____ District: _____

State: _____ Pin Code _____ Important landmark: _____ Mobile: _____ Aadhar No.: _____ Area: Slum/Tribal/Migrant/

Refugee Name and address of Contact Person: _____ Mobile No.:

Name of treatment supporter _____ Designation _____ Mobile No.:

Initial home visit by: _____ Date: _____ Type of Treatment adherence—DOT/Family DOT/ICT supported, specify _____ / Other _____ Date

of onset of first symptom: _____ Number of healthcare providers visited before diagnosis for current episode:

Disease Classification
☐ Pulmonary
☐ Extrapulmonary
Site _____

Type of Patient
☐ New ☐ Recurrent
☐ Transfer in ☐ Treatment after failure
☐ Treatment ☐ Others, previously treated (specify) _____
After LFU

Basis of Diagnosis
☐ Microbiologically confirmed
☐ Clinical TB

Investigations (ZN/ FM/CBNAAT/Liquid C/ Solid C)	Lab	Lab No.	Test result	Sample sent to CDST (date)	DST result
Pretreatment					
End of intensive phase					
End of treatment					

Other investigations (if any) with result

History of previous ATT: _____ months of treatment _____ months since end of last episode

Source of treatment: ☐ Public ☐ Private Previous regimen: _____

HIV-related information

HIV status: ☐ Unknown ☐ Reactive ☐ NR Date _____ PID _____

CPT delivered on: (1) _____ (2) _____ (3) _____ (4) _____ (5) _____ (6) _____

Initiated on ART: ☐ No ☐ Yes Date and ART No. _____

Diabetes-related information

Diabetes status: ☐ Unknown ☐ Diabetic ☐ Non-diabetic

RBS _____ FBS _____

Initiated on ADT: ☐ No ☐ Yes Date and ADT No. _____

Other comorbidity

Details _____

Signature of MD with date _____

	<6 yr	>6 yr
No. of household contacts		
No. screened		
No. with symptoms		
No. evaluated		
No. diagnosed		
No. put on treatment		

No. of children less than 6 years given chemoprophylaxis =

Name	Wt (g)	Dose (mg)	1	2	3	4	5	6

Addiction-related information

Current tobacco user ☐ Yes ☐ NO

If yes, ☐ Smoking ☐ Smokeless Linked for cessation ☐ Yes ☐ No

If tobacco user, status of tobacco use at end of treatment ☐ Quit ☐ Not quit

History of alcohol intake ☐ Yes ☐ No

If yes, linked for deaddiction ☐ Yes ☐ No

BIBLIOGRAPHY

1. Guidelines for use of Delamanid for treatment of DR-TB in India, 2018.
2. Programmatic Management of Drug Resistant Tuberculosis (PMDT) in India; 2012.
3. Revised National Tuberculosis Control Programme DOTS-Plus Guidelines, Central TB Division, Directorate General of Health Services, Ministry of Health & Family Welfare.
4. RNTCP at a glance, Central TB Division, Directorate General of Health Services, Ministry of Health & Family Welfare.
5. TB India 2013, RNTCP annual status report Central TB Division, Directorate General of Health Services, Ministry of Health & Family Welfare.
6. Technical and Operational Guidelines for Tuberculosis Control in India; 2016.
7. The Guidelines for use of Bedaquiline in RNTCP through conditional access under the Programmatic Management of Drug Resistant Tuberculosis in India; 2016.

Chapter
19

Reproductive, Child and Adolescent Health

INTRODUCTION

❖ Mothers and children not only constitute a large group, but they are also called vulnerable or special group.
❖ They comprises 71.4% of population of the developing countries. In India, women of the child-bearing age (15–44 years) constitute 22.2% and children under 15 years of age about 35.3% of total population, together 57.7% of population consists of mothers and children.
❖ The present strategy is to provide mother and child health services as an integrated package of "essential health care" also known as *Primary Health Care.*

BASIC CONCEPT BEHIND THE SPECIAL ATTENTION OF MOTHER AND CHILD

Mother and Child—One Unit

❖ During the antenatal period the fetus is part of mother
❖ Child health is closely related to maternal health
❖ Certain diseases and conditions of the mother during pregnancy are likely to have effect upon the fetus
❖ After birth the child is dependent on mother
❖ The mother is also the first teacher of child.

Definition of Maternal and Child Health

"Maternal and child health" (MCH) refers to *the promotive, preventive, curative and rehabilitative health care for mothers and children, child health, family planning, school health, handicapped children, adolescence and health aspects of children in special setting such as day care.*

Objectives of MCH Services

❖ Reduction of maternal, perinatal, infant, and childhood mortality and morbidity
❖ Promotion of reproductive health
❖ Promotion of physical and psychological development of the adolescent within the family.

Targets of Major Policies/Projects Relevant to MCH

Indicator	Tenth Plan Goals (2002–2007)	RCH II Goals (2005–2010)	National Population Policy 2000 (by 2010)	Millennium Development Goals (by 2015)
Population growth	16.2% (2001–2011)	16.2% (2001–2011)	—	—
Infant mortality rate	45/1000	35/1000	30/1000	—
Under 5 mortality rate	—	—	—	Reduce by 2/3rd from 1990 levels
Maternal mortality ratio	200/100,000	150/100,000	100/100,000	Reduce by 3/4th from 1990 levels
Total fertility rate	2.3	2.2	2.1	—
Couple protection rate	65%	65%	Meet 100% needs	—

Components of MCH Services

Services to the mothers	Services to the children

◆ Antenatal care
◆ Intranatal care
◆ Postnatal care
◆ Other services:
  – Psychological
  – Breastfeeding
  – Family planning
  – Basic health education
	◆ Neonatal care
	◆ Continuing care of the infant
	◆ Care of the school children
	◆ Care of the children of the employed mothers
	◆ Care of the handicapped children

MCH Services Antenatal Care

The care of the women during pregnancy.

Aim

The primary aim of antenatal care is to achieve at the end of a pregnancy a healthy mother and a healthy baby.

Objectives of Antenatal Care

❖ To promote, protect and maintain the health of the mother during pregnancy.
❖ To detect "high-risk" cases and special attention.
❖ To foresee complications and prevent them.
❖ To remove anxiety and dread associated with delivery.
❖ To reduce maternal and infant mortality and morbidity.
❖ To teach the mother elements of child care, nutrition, personal hygiene and environmental sanitation.
❖ To sensitize the mother to need for family planning.
❖ To attend the under–fives accompanying the mother.

Antenatal Services Provided

Antenatal Visits

Mother should attend the antenatal clinics:
❖ Once a month during the first 7 months

❖ Twice a month, during the next month
❖ Thereafter once in a week, if everything is normal.

A minimum of three visits covering the entire period of pregnancy should be:
❖ 1st visit at 20th weeks
❖ 2nd visit at 30th weeks
❖ 3rd visit at 36th weeks.

Preventive services for mothers (before delivery):
❖ The first visit:
  – Health history
  – Physical examination
  – Laboratory examination
❖ On subsequent visits:
  – Physical examination
  – Laboratory tests
❖ Iron and folic acid supplementation
❖ Immunization against tetanus
❖ Instruction on:
  – Nutrition
  – Family planning
  – Self-care
  – Delivery and parenthood.
❖ Referral services
❖ Risk approach for high-risk cases like: elderly primi, malpresentations, antepartum hemorrhage, pre-eclampsia, anemia, twins, history of previous cesarean delivery, and general diseases like kidney disease, diabetes, tuberculosis, liver diseases, etc.
❖ Maintenance of records:
  – The antenatal care is prepared at the first examination, it includes registration number
  – Identifying data
  – Previous health history
  – Main health events.
❖ Home visits: It is the backbone of MCH services. Home visit by the health worker female or public health nurse.

Prenatal Advices

a. *Diet*: Lactation demand about 550 kcal a day.
   Weight gain during pregnancy:

Trimester	Weight gain
1st	2 kg
2nd	5 kg
3rd	5 kg
Total weight gain	**12 kg**

   b. *Personal hygiene*:
- Personal cleanliness
- Rest and sleep: 8 hours sleep and 2 hours rest
- Mild exercise
- Smoking and alcohol should be avoided
- Dental care
- Sexual intercourse: Restricted especially during last trimester.
- Drugs having serious effect on fetus (teratogenic drugs) should be avoided.

   c. *Warning signs*: Swelling of feet, fits, headache, blurred vision, bleeding or discharge per vagina.

   d. Child care special classes for mother craft consists of nutrition education, advice on hygiene and child rearing, etc.

Specific Protection

- ❖ Anemia
- ❖ Nutritional deficiencies
- ❖ Toxemias of pregnancy
- ❖ Tetanus
- ❖ Syphilis
- ❖ German measles
- ❖ Rh status
- ❖ HIV infection.

Mental Preparation

Mother craft classes at MCH centers help a great deal in achieving this objective.

Family Planning

To provide full range of family planning and contraception services.

Pediatric Component

All antenatal clinics to pay attention to the under-fives accompanying the mothers.

MCH Services for Intranatal Care

Child birth is a normal physiological process, but complications may arise, e.g. septicemia may arise result from unskilled and septic manipulations, and tetanus neonatorum (neonatal tetanus) from the use of unsterilized instruments. The emphasis on the cleanliness.

It entails:
- ❖ Clean hands and fingernails
- ❖ Clean surface for delivery
- ❖ Clean cutting and care of cord.

Aims of Intranatal Care

- ❖ Thorough asepsis.
- ❖ Delivery with minimum injury to the infant and mother

❖ Readiness to deal with complications such as prolonged labor, antepartum hemorrhage, convulsions, malpresentations, prolapse of cord, etc.
❖ Care of the baby at delivery-resuscitation, care of the cord, care of the eyes.

Intranatal Care

Domiciliary Care

Mother with normal obstetric history may be advised to have their confinement in their homes, provided the home conditions are satisfactory. In such cases the delivery may be conducted by the "health worker female or trained dai" this is known as "domiciliary midwifery service".

Advantages and disadvantages of domiciliary services:

Advantages	Disadvantages
• Mother delivers in the familiar surroundings of her home	• Mother may have less medical and nursing supervision
• Less chance of cross infection	• Mother may have less rest
• Mother is able to keep an eye upon her children and domestic affairs	• Mother resume her duties too soon
	• Diet may be neglected

Responsibilities of female health worker in domiciliary care:
She should be adequately trained to recognize the "danger signals". The danger signals are:
❖ Sluggish pains or rupture of membranes
❖ Prolapse of the cord or hand
❖ Meconium stained liquor
❖ Excessive show or bleeding during labor
❖ Late placental separation
❖ Postpartum hemorrhage or collapse
❖ Increased temperature.

Institutional Care

At about 1% of deliveries tend to be abnormal, requiring the services of a doctor institutional care is recommended for all 'high-risk' cases and where home conditions are unsuitable.

Rooming in

Keeping the baby's crib the side of the mother's bed is called "rooming-in". It also allays the fear in the mother mind that the baby is not misplaced in the central nursery.

Postnatal Care of the Mother

Postnatal care of the mother (and the newborn) after delivery is known as postnatal care.

Objectives

❖ To prevent complications of the postpartum period.
❖ To provide care for the rapid restoration of the mother to optimum health.
❖ To check adequacy of breastfeeding.
❖ To provide family planning services.
❖ To provide basic health education to mother family.

Complications of Postpartum Period

❖ Puerperal sepsis
❖ Thrombophlebitis
❖ Secondary hemorrhage
❖ Urinary tract infection and mastitis.

All these complications should be detected early to treat with prompt measure.

Restoration of Mother to Optimum Health

1. Physical examinations:
   Postnatal examinations: Soon after delivery, the health check-up must be frequent, i.e. twice a day during the first 3 days and subsequently once a day till umbilical cord drops off.

   Female health worker checks:
   – Vitals
   – Breasts
   – Progress of normal involution of uterus
   – Examines lochia for any abnormality
   – Check urine and bowels
   – Advises on perineal care.

   Further visits should be done once in 2 or 3 months during first 6 months, and after once in 2 or 3 months till the end of 1 year.
2. Laboratory investigations:
   Hb estimation: Routine Hb estimation can be done when anemia discovered, if anemia is present treatment to be continued for 1 year.
3. Nutritional advices: The nutritional needs of the mother must be adequately met.
4. Postnatal exercises: It is to bring stretched abdominal and pelvic muscle back to normal.
5. Other services:
   a. Psychological: Fear and insecurity may be eliminated by proper prenatal instruction
   b. Breastfeeding
   c. Family planning: Mother should attend postnatal contacts to adopt a suitable method for spacing the next birth
   d. Basic health education: About hygiene, feeding for mother and infant, pregnancy spacing, importance of health check-up, birth registration.

Services to the Children

1. Neonatal care:
   – Early neonatal care: The first week of life the most crucial period in the life of an infant. Objectives of early neonatal care:
     - Establish and maintenance of cardiorespiratory functions
     - Maintenance of body temperature
     - Avoidance of infection
     - Establish of satisfactory feeding regimen
     - Early detection and treatment of congenital and acquired disorders.
   – Immediate care:
     - Clearing the airway: To help to establish breathing, the airways should be cleared mucus and other secretions
     - APGAR score: It is taken 1 minute and again at 5 minutes after birth.

APGAR Score (Evaluate at 1 and 5 Minutes Postpartum)

	Sign	2	1	0
A	Activity (muscle tone)	Active	Arms and legs flexed	Absent
P	Pulse	>100 bpm	<100 bpm	Absent
G	Grimace (reflex irritability)	Sneezes, coughs, pulls away	Grimaces	No response
A	Appearance (skin color)	Normal over entire body	Normal except extremities	Cyanotic or pale all over
R	Respirations	Good, crying	Slow, irregular	Absent

Total score   = 10
Severe depression = 0–3
Mild depression   = 4–7
No depression   = 7–10

- Care of the cord: The cord should be cut and tied when it has stopped pulsating. Care must be taken to prevent tetanus of newborn by unsterilized instruments and cord ties.
- Care of the eyes: Before the eyes are open, the lid margins of the newborn should be cleaned with sterile wet swabs, one for each eye from inner to outer side.
- Care of the skin: The first bath is given with soap and warm water to remove vernix, meconium and blood clots. Some prefer to apply warm oil before the bath.
- Maintenance of body temperature: The normal body temperature of a newborn is between 36.5°–37.5°C. It is, therefore, important that immediately after birth the child is quickly dried with a clean cloth and wrapped in warm cloth and given to the mother for skin-to-skin contact and breastfeeding.
- Breastfeeding
  - Neonatal examinations
    Measuring the baby: weight, height, head circumference
  - Identification and care of "at risk" infants
  - Late neonatal care.
2. Continuing care of the infant.
3. Care of the school children
4. Care of the children of the employed mothers
5. Care of the handicapped children
6. Proper placement of the child.

REPRODUCTIVE AND CHILD HEALTH PROGRAM

Definition

Reproductive and child health approach has defined as:

"People have ability to reproduce and regulate their fertility, women are able to go through pregnancy and their birth safely, the outcome of pregnancy is successful in terms of maternal and infant survival and wellbeing and couples are able to have sexual relations free of fear of pregnancy and of contracting disease".

❖ The program was formally launched on 15 October 1997.
❖ The RCH program incorporated the earlier existing programs, i.e. National Family Welfare Program and Child Survival and Survival and Safe Motherhood Program (CSSM) and added

two more components one relating to sexually transmitted disease and the other relating to reproductive tract infections.

❖ RCH program was based on RCH approach and in management there was a paradigm shift from target-oriented to target free approach (TFA).

The **paradigm shift** can be summarized as follows:

Topic	CSSM	RCH
Goal	2 child norm	Enable clients to meet their own goal
Approach	Top → down (centralized)	Bottom → up (decentralized)
Service	Mainly family planning	Full range maternal and child health care
Quality	Compromised	High quality
Attitude to client	To motivate and give them good reasons to take a choice	To listen, assess the need of the client, inform them and advice
Monitoring	Usually targets are monitored	Some of parameter that are monitored: i. Quality of care ii. Coverage of services iii. Client satisfaction
Responsible to	To an administrative system operated by large number of officials	The client and communities

RCH Phase 1 Program Incorporated the Four Components

Family planning

Client approach to prevention health care

Child survival and safe motherhood component

Prevention/management of RTI, STDs and AIDS

Main Highlights of RCH Program

1. The program integrates *all interventions of fertility regulation, maternal and child health reproductive health for both men and women.*
2. The services to be provided are *client oriented.*
3. The program envisages *upgradation of the level of facilities for providing various interventions and quality of care.* The first referral units are being set up at sub-district level to provide comprehensive emergency obstetric and newborn care.
4. The facilities of *obstetric care, MTP and IUD insertion in the PHC level are improved. IUD insertion facilities are also available at subcenters.*
5. *Specialist facilities for STD and RTI are available in all district hospitals* and in a fair number of sub-district level hospitals.
6. The program aims at *improving the outreach of services primarily for the vulnerable population.*

Objectives of RCH Program

Immediate	Intermediate	Ultimate
To promote the health of the mothers and children to ensure safe motherhood and child survival	To reduce IMR and MMR	Population stabilization through responsible reproductive behavior

RCH Services and Major Interventions

1. *Essential obstetric care*: It aims to provide the basic maternity services to all pregnant women through:
   – Early registration of pregnancy (within 12–16 weeks)

- Provision of minimum three antenatal checkups by ANM
- Provision of safe delivery at home or institution
- Provision of three postnatal checkups to monitor the postnatal recovery and to detect complications.

2. *Emergency obstetrical care*: It is very essential to prevent maternal mortality and morbidity traditional birth attendance should be maintained in conducting the deliveries.
3. *24-hour delivery services*: At PHCs, CHCs to promote institutional deliveries, the staff should be encouraged round the clock delivery facilities at health centers.

4. *Medical termination of pregnancy through the MTP Act 1971*:
   - Aim:
     - To reduce maternal morbidity and mortality from unsafe abortions.
   - Assistance: From the central government is in the forms of training of manpower, supply of MTP equipment and provision for engaging doctors trained in MTP to visit PHCs on fixed dates to perform MTP.
5. *Control of reproductive tract infections and sexually transmitted diseases*: It has been implemented in close collaboration with National AIDS Control Organization (NACO). NACO will provide assistance for setting up RTI, STD clinics at the district level. Each district will be assisted by 2 laboratory technicians on contract basis for testing blood, urine and RTI, STI tests.
6. *The Universal Immunization Program (UIP)* became part of CSSM program in 1992 and RCH program 1997. It will continue to provide vaccines for polio, tetanus, DPT, DT, measles and tuberculosis.

7. *Essential newborn care:* The primary goal is to reduce perinatal and neonatal mortality. The main components are:
   - Resuscitation of newborn with asphyxia
   - Prevention of hypothermia
   - Prevention of infection
   - Exclusive breastfeeding and referral of sick newborn.
8. Diarrhea is one of the leading causes of child mortality.
   Oral rehydration therapy program started in 1986–1987 and is being implemented through RCH program.
   - Supplies of ORS packets to the states are being organized by central government.
   - Twice a year 150 packets of ORS are provided as part of drug kit supplied to all sub-centers in country.
   - Adequate nutritional care of the child with diarrhea and proper advice to mother on feeding are important areas.
9. *Prevention and control of vitamin A deficiency in children*: Under this program, doses of vitamin A are being given to all children under 5 years of age. The first dose (1 lakh units) is given at 9 months of age along with measles vaccination. The second dose is given along with DPT, OPV booster doses with subsequent doses (2 lakh units each) given at 6 months intervals.
10. *Acute respiratory disease control*: The standard case management of ARI and prevention of deaths due to pneumonia is now an integral part of RCH program.
    - Peripheral health workers are being trained to recognize and treat pneumonia.
    - Cotrimoxazole is being supplied to the health worker through drug kit.
11. *Prevention and control of anemia in children*: Iron deficiency anemia is widely prevalent in young children.

Under this program of control and prevention of anemia, tablets containing 2 mg of elemental iron and 0.1 mg of folic acid are provided at subcenter level.

The health workers provide 100 tablets to children clinically found to be anemic.

REPRODUCTIVE AND CHILD HEALTH PROGRAM–PHASE II

❖ *Started*: From 1st April 2005.
❖ *Focus*: To reduce maternal and child mortality and morbidity with emphasis on rural health care.
❖ Major strategies are:
  1. Essential obstetric care:
     a. Institutional delivery
     b. Skilled attendance at delivery
  2. Emergency obstetric care:
     a. First referral units
     b. PHCs and CHCs for round the clock delivery services.
  3. Strengthening referral system.
  4. Strengthening project management.
  5. Strengthening infrastructure.
  6. Capacity building.
  7. Improving referral system.
  8. Innovative schemes.

Brief discussion about the strategies:
  1. Essential obstetric care:
     a. Institutional delivery
        * 24 hours delivery centers (50% PHCs and CHCs) with emergency obstetric care and essential newborn care and basic resuscitation services round the clock
     b. Skilled attendance at delivery
        * WHO has emphasized skilled attendance at delivery to reduce maternal mortality by ANM/LVHs.
  2. Emergency obstetric care: Operationalization of FRUs and skilled attendance at birth are the activities of second phase of RCH.

     Minimum services of fully functional FRUs:
  – 24 Hours delivery services including normal and assisted deliveries.
  – Emergency obstetric care include cesarean section
  – Newborn care
  – Emergency care of sick children
  – Full range of family planning services includes laparoscopic services
  – Safe abortion services
  – Treatment of STI/RTI
  – Blood storage facility
  – Essential laboratory services
  – Referral (transport) services: There are three critical determinants of a referral facility:
     1. Availability of surgical interventions
     2. Newborn care
     3. Blood storage facility availability for 24 hours a day basis.
  – Strengthening referral system.

New initiatives:
- Training of MBBS doctors in life saving anesthetic skills for emergency obstetric care. Govt. of India is also introducing training of MBBS doctors of obstetric management skills, prepared training plan for 16 weeks in all obstetric management skills, including cesarean section operation.
- Setting up of blood storage centers at FRUs.
- Pradhan Mantri Surakshit Matritva Abhiyan (PMSMA)
- Janani Suraksha Yojana (JSY).
- Janani Shishu Suraksha Karyakaram (JSSK)
- Vandemataram scheme.
- Safe abortion services.
- Integrated Management of Childhood Illnesses.

Janani Suraksha Yojana (JSY)

It is a safe motherhood intervention under the National Rural Health Mission (NRHM).
- ❖ *Objective*:
  - Reducing maternal and neonatal mortality by promoting institutional delivery among the poor pregnant women
- ❖ *Launched on* 12th April 2005
- ❖ *Implementation:*
  - In all states and union territories with special focus on low performing states
  - The states with a low rate of institutional deliveries is classified as '*Low Performing States* (LPS)' (the states of Uttar Pradesh, Uttaranchal, Bihar, Jharkhand, Madhya Pradesh, Chhattisgarh, Assam, Rajasthan, Odisha and Jammu & Kashmir)
  - The remaining states are termed as *High Performing States* (HPS).
- ❖ *Important features of JSY*:
  - JSY is a 100% centrally sponsored scheme
  - It integrates cash assistance with delivery and post-delivery care
  - The success of the scheme would be determined by the increase in institutional delivery among the poor families.
- ❖ *Role of ASHA or other link health worker associated with JSY would be to*:
  - Identify pregnant woman as a beneficiary of the scheme and report or facilitate registration for ANC
  - Assist the pregnant woman to obtain necessary certifications wherever necessary
  - Provide and/or help the women in receiving at least three ANC checkups including TT injections, IFA tablets
  - Identify a functional government health center or an accredited private health institution for referral and delivery
  - Counsel for institutional delivery
  - Escort the beneficiary women to the predetermined health center and stay with her till the woman is discharged
  - Arrange to immunize the newborn till the age of *14 weeks*
  - Inform about the birth or death of the child or mother to the ANM/MO
  - Postnatal visit within 7 days of delivery to track mother's health after delivery and facilitate in obtaining care, wherever necessary
  - Counsel for initiation of breastfeeding to the newborn within one-hour of delivery and its continuance till 3–6 months and promote family planning.

❖ *Eligibility for cash assistance:*

LPS	All pregnant women delivering in government health centers, such as subcenters (SCs)/ primary health centers (PHCs)/community health centers (CHCs)/first referral units (FRUs)/ general wards of district or state hospitals or accredited private institutions
HPS	All BPL/scheduled caste/scheduled tribe (SC/ST) women delivering in a government health center, such as SC/PHC/CHC/FRU/general wards of district or state hospital or accredited private institutions

❖ *Scale of cash assistance for institutional delivery:*
  - Rural areas:

Category	Mother's package (in ₹)	ASHA's package* (in ₹)	Total package (in ₹)
LPS	1,400	600	2,000
HPS	700	600	1,300

  - Urban areas:

Category	Mother's package (in ₹)	ASHA's package** (in ₹)	Total package (in ₹)
LPS	1,000	400	1,400
HPS	600	400	1000

* ASHA package of ₹ 600 in rural areas include ₹ 300 for ANC component and ₹ 300 for facilitating institutional delivery.
** ASHA package of ₹ 400 in urban areas include ₹ 200 for ANC component and ₹ 200 for facilitating institutional delivery.
Note: In addition to institutional delivery benefit, BPL pregnant women who prefer to deliver at home are entitled to a cash assistance of ₹ 500 per delivery under the JSY.
[*Reference:* Annual Report on (RMNCH + A) Program (2014–2015), Chapter 4, Ministry of Health and Family Welfare]

While mother will receive her entitled cash, the scheme does not provide for ASHA package for such pregnant women choosing to deliver in an accredited private institution.

❖ *Limitations of cash assistance for institutional delivery :*
  - LPS: All births, delivered in a health center—government or accredited private health institutions
  - HPS: Up to 2 live births.
❖ *Payment of cash assistance:* As the cash assistance to the mother is mainly to meet the cost of delivery, it should be paid effectively at the institution itself
❖ *ASHA package in rural areas:* Includes the following three components:
  1. *Cash assistance for referral transport:* To go to the nearest health center for delivery. The state will determine the amount of assistance (should not below ₹ 250/- per delivery) depending on the topography and the infrastructure available in their state.
  2. *Cash incentive to ASHA:* This should not be below ₹ 200/- per delivery in lieu of her work relating to facilitating institutional delivery.
     (Generally, ASHA should get this money after her postnatal visit to the beneficiary and after the child has been immunized for BCG.)
  3. *Transactional cost (Balance out of ₹ 600/-)* is to be paid to ASHA in lieu of her stay with the pregnant woman in the health center for delivery to meet her cost of boarding and lodging, etc. Therefore, this payment should be made at the hospital/heath institution itself.

❖ *Other cash assistance*:
  – JSK subsidizes cost of cesarean sections and for management of obstetric complications, up to ₹ 1500/- delivery to Govt. institutions where Govt. specialists are not in positions.
  – In LPS and HPS 19+ BPL woman gets ₹ 500/- delivery up to 2 live births.
❖ *Monitoring of JSY*:
  – Monthly meeting of all ASHAs/health workers working under an ANM should be held by the ANM
  – Monthly reports and annual reports also need to be submitted to the department in a format decided by the government for the effective monitoring at the government level.

Janani-Shishu Suraksha Karyakram (JSSK)

Introduction

❖ To complement JSY, Government of India launched Janani Shishu Suraksha Karyakaram (JSSK) on 1st June 2011, to eliminate out of pocket expenditure for pregnant women and sick newborns and infants on drugs, diet, diagnostics, user charges, referral transport, etc.
❖ The scheme entitles all pregnant women delivering in public health institutions to absolutely free and no expense delivery including cesarean section
❖ This initiative also provides for free transport from home to institution, between facilities in case of a referral and drop back home.

Services and Facilities under JSSK

Services/facilities	For pregnant women	For sick newborn till 30 days after birth
Free and zero expense delivery and cesarean section	√	—
Free diet during stay in the health institutions	Up to 3 days for normal delivery and 7 days for cesarean section	—
Free drugs and consumables	√	√
Free essential diagnostics	√	√
Free provision of blood	√	√
Free transport	√	√
Exemption from all kinds of user charges	√	√

Vandemataram Scheme

This is a voluntary scheme wherein any Obstetrician and Gynecologist speciality, maternity home, nursing home, lady doctor, MBBS doctor can volunteer themselves for providing safe motherhood services.
❖ The enrolled doctors will display "Vandemataram logo" at their clinic.
❖ Iron and folic acid tablets, oral pills, TT injections, etc. will be provided by the respective district medical officers to the Vandemataram doctors clinics for free distribution to beneficiaries.
❖ Safe abortion services:
  – Medical method
    - Termination of early pregnancy (49 days) using 2 drugs:
      * Mifeprestone followed by misoprostol
  – Manual vacuum aspiration
    - Safe and simple technique for termination of pregnancy

- Can be used at PHC or comparable facility
- FOGSI, WHO and State Govt. are coordinating the project.

Referral Transport

Key issues: Roads, transportation, RCH I funds poorly utilized, community participation lacking.

Under consideration:
- ❖ Place funds in cooperation with AWW/ANM under JSY
- ❖ Develop community mechanisms
- ❖ Provide outsource ambulance services at PHCs, CHCs, and FRUs.

Reproductive, Maternal, Newborn, Child and Adolescent Health (RMNCH+A) Strategy, 2013

Introduction

- ❖ In February 2013, the Government of India held its own historic Summit on the Call to Action for Child Survival, where it launched "A Strategic Approach to Reproductive, Maternal, Newborn, Child, and Adolescent Health (RMNCH+A) in India." Since that time, RMNCH+A has become the heart of the Government of India's flagship public health program, National Rural Health Mission (NRHM)
- ❖ The RMNCH+A strategy is based on provision of comprehensive care through the 5 pillars of reproductive, maternal, neonatal, child and adolescent health
- ❖ The "plus" within the strategy focuses on including adolescence for the first time as a distinct life stage.

Objectives

The 12th Five Year Plan has defined the national health outcomes and the three goals that are relevant to RMNCH+A strategic approach as follows:
1. Reduction of infant mortality rate (IMR) to 25 per 1,000 live births by 2017
2. Reduction in maternal mortality ratio (MMR) to 100 per 100,000 live births by 2017
3. Reduction in total fertility rate (TFR) to 2.1 by 2017.

Strategic RMNCH+A Interventions Across Life Stages

Life stage	Priority interventions under RMNCH+A strategy
Pregnancy and childbirth	• Delivery of antenatal care package and tracking of high-risk pregnancies • Skilled obstetric care • Immediate essential newborn care and resuscitation • Emergency obstetric and newborn care • Postpartum care for mother and newborn • Postpartum IUCD and sterilization • Implementation of PCPNDT Act
Newborn and childcare	• Home-based newborn care and prompt referral • Facility-based care of the sick newborn • Integrated management of common childhood illnesses (diarrhea, pneumonia and malaria) • Child nutrition and essential micronutrients supplementation • Immunization • Early detection and management of defects at birth, deficiencies, diseases and disability in children (0–18 years)

Contd...

Contd...

Life stage	Priority interventions under RMNCH+A strategy
Adolescent	• Adolescent nutrition; iron and folic acid supplementation • Facility-based adolescent reproductive and sexual health services [through adolescent friendly health clinics (AFHC)] • Information and counseling on adolescent sexual reproductive health and other health issues • Menstrual hygiene • Preventive health checkups
Through the reproductive years	• Community-based promotion and delivery of contraceptives • Promotion of spacing methods (interval IUCD) • Sterilization services (vasectomies and tubectomies) • Comprehensive abortion care (includes MTP Act) • Prevention and management of sexually transmitted and reproductive infections (STI/RTI)

Pradhan Mantri Surakshit Matritva Abhiyan (PMSMA)

Introduction

❖ The Pradhan Mantri Surakshit Matritva Abhiyan (PMSMA) is being introduced to ensure quality antenatal to over 3 crore pregnant women in the country

❖ Under the campaign, a minimum package of antenatal care services would be provided to the beneficiaries on the 9th day of every month at the Pradhan Mantri Surakshit Matritva Clinics to ensure that every pregnant woman receives at least one checkup in the 2nd and 3rd trimester of pregnancy

❖ If the 9th day of the month is a Sunday/a holiday, then the clinic should be organized on the next working day.

Target Beneficiaries:

The program aims to reach out to all pregnant women who are in the 2nd and 3rd trimesters of pregnancy.

Packages of Services

❖ Routine antenatal check up

❖ Diagnostic services

❖ Identification and management of high-risk pregnancy

❖ Counseling on nutrition, family planning, birth preparedness, newborn and postnatal care.

Movement of Beneficiaries in PMSMA Clinics

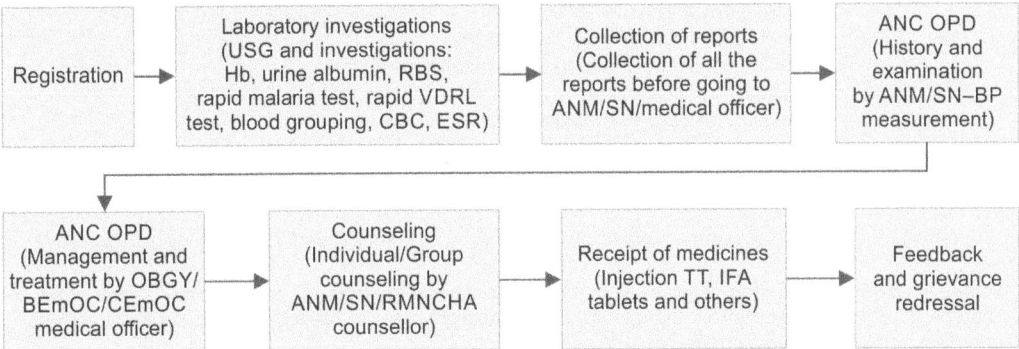

Source: PMSMA Guidelines (Maternal Health Division Ministry of Health & Family Welfare), Dated 18.4.2016.

ADOLESCENT HEALTH

Rashtriya Kishor Swasthya Karyakram (RKSK)

Introduction

❖ Adolescent health component includes the:
  – Adolescent Reproductive and Sexual Health (ARSH) program
  – Menstrual Hygiene Scheme (MHS)
  – Weekly Iron and Folic Acid Supplementation (WIFS) program components
❖ The newly launched Rashtriya Kishor Swasthya Karyakram (RKSK) subsumes these components into a comprehensive program
❖ RKSK is underpinned by evidence that adolescence is the most important stage of the life cycle for health interventions
❖ RKSK is a paradigm shift from the existing clinic-based services to promotion and prevention and reaching adolescents in their own environment, such as in schools and communities.

The objectives and functions of each component of RKSK are as follows:

Adolescent Reproductive and Sexual Health (ARSH) Program

Introduction

ARSH focuses on reorganizing the existing public health system in order to meet health service needs of adolescents through provision of promotive, preventive and curative services at designated Adolescent Friendly Health Clinics (AFHC) across level of care.

Package of AFHC Services

Information	• IEC and IPC for nutrition, sex and reproductive health, mental health, gender-based violence, noncommunicable disease, substance misuse
Commodities	• IFA/albendazole tablets • Sanitary napkin • Contraceptives (condoms, OCP, ECP) • Other medicines (e.g. paracetamol, anti-spasmodic and first aid) • Pregnancy testing kits
Services	• BMI screening • Hb testing • RTI/STI management • ANC for pregnant adolescents • Counseling* • Management of menstrual problems • Management of iron deficiency anemia • Screening for diabetes and hypertension • Management of common adolescent health problems • HIV testing and counseling • Management of physical violence and sexual abuse • Linkages with de-addiction centers and referrals • Treatment by specialists • Referral services

(IEC: Information, education and communication; IPC: Interpersonal communication; ECP: Emergency contraceptive pills).

* Counseling is given on nutrition, puberty-related concerns, premarital counseling, sexual problems, contraceptive, abortion, RTI/STI, substance abuse, learning problems, stress, depression, suicidal tendency, violence, sexual abuse, other mental health issues, health lifestyle, risky behavior.

Menstrual Hygiene Scheme (MHS)

Introduction

❖ The scheme for Promotion of Menstrual Hygiene has been initiated for rural adolescent girls in the age group of 10–19 years.
❖ This program aims at that girls in rural areas have adequate knowledge and information about menstrual hygiene and have access to high quality sanitary napkins along with safe disposal mechanisms.

Key activities under the scheme include:

❖ Community-based health education and outreach in the target population to promote menstrual health
❖ Ensuring regular availability of sanitary napkins to the adolescents (Central supply: 'Free-days')
❖ Sourcing and procurement of sanitary napkins
❖ Storage and distribution of sanitary napkins to the adolescent girls
❖ Training of ASHA and nodal teachers in menstrual health
❖ Safe disposal of sanitary napkins.

Weekly Iron and Folic Acid Supplementation (WIFS) Program

❖ The Ministry of Health and Family Welfare has rolled out the Weekly Iron and Folic Acid Supplementation (WIFS) program in 2012–2013 to meet the challenge of high prevalence and incidence of iron deficiency anemia amongst adolescent girls and boys.
❖ WIFS program includes:
  – Weekly supervised administration of iron and folic acid supplements (containing 100 mg elemental iron and 500 µg folic acid) to in-school adolescent girls and boys and out-of-school adolescent girls
  – Screening of target groups for moderate/severe anemia and referral to nearest centers
  – Biannual de-worming (400 mg, 6 months apart)
  – Information and counseling for improving dietary intake and for taking actions for prevention of intestinal worm infestation.

Guidelines on Consumption of WIFS Tablets

❖ Adolescents will be advised to take iron-folic acid tablets after meals (approximately one hour) to prevent side effects such as nausea
❖ Adolescent girls or boys who complain of side effects will be advised to take the IFA supplements after dinner and before retiring to sleep
❖ Increase intake of foods rich in vitamin C such as lemon, amla, etc. will help to absorb iron from the vegetarian Indian diet. Use of iron vessels for cooking will also be encouraged
❖ Drinking of tea or coffee within an hour of consuming main meals will be discouraged
❖ Adolescent boys and girls will be motivated to follow correct hygiene practices and the habit of using footwear to prevent worm infestation.

Diagnosis and Treatment for Malaria
(According to New NVBDCP Operational Guidelines, 2022)

INTRODUCTION

National Framework for Malaria Elimination in India 2016–2030 (Launched in February, 2016)

Vision:
Eliminate malaria nationally and contribute to improve health, quality of life and alleviation of poverty.

Goals:
❖ Eliminate malaria (zero indigenous cases) throughout the entire country by 2030
❖ Maintain malaria-free status in areas where malaria transmission has been interrupted and prevent re-introduction of malaria.

Salient Points Under Diagnosis of Malaria

❖ A confirmed malaria case is one in which the parasite has been detected by a diagnostic test, i.e. microscopy, rapid diagnostic test (RDT) or molecular diagnostic tests
❖ *Microscopy is the gold standard for malaria diagnosis.* Availability of quality microscopy for malaria diagnosis is mandatory at all PHCs and above levels
❖ *Quality assured antigen detecting bivalent RDTs* are recommended for use under National Vector Borne Diseases Control Program (NVBDCP)
❖ If there is a high clinical suspicion of malaria (intermittent fever with rigors and sweating in a high-endemic area) in a RDT negative patient when no other cause can be found, the RDT should be repeated after about 24 hours and all efforts made to obtain the microscopy result rapidly
❖ *Special note:* Antigens can persist for up to 4 weeks after clearance of parasitemia resulting in false positive test results. If a patient, who has been treated, is febrile within 1 month after the treatment and the RDT is positive, the malaria diagnosis should be confirmed by microscopy before treatment is started.

Case Management

Objectives of case management of malaria are:
- ❖ Ensure radical, clinical and parasitological cure to malaria cases
- ❖ Prevent severe malaria and deaths due to malaria
- ❖ Reduce malaria transmission and
- ❖ Prevent relapses of *P. vivax* malaria.

All fever cases diagnosed as malaria by either rapid diagnostic test or microscopy should be promptly given effective treatment. The medicine chosen will depend upon whether the patient has vivax malaria/falciparum malaria diagnosed by blood tests.

Diagnosis and Treatment Protocol For Malaria

Where microscopy result is available within 24 hours

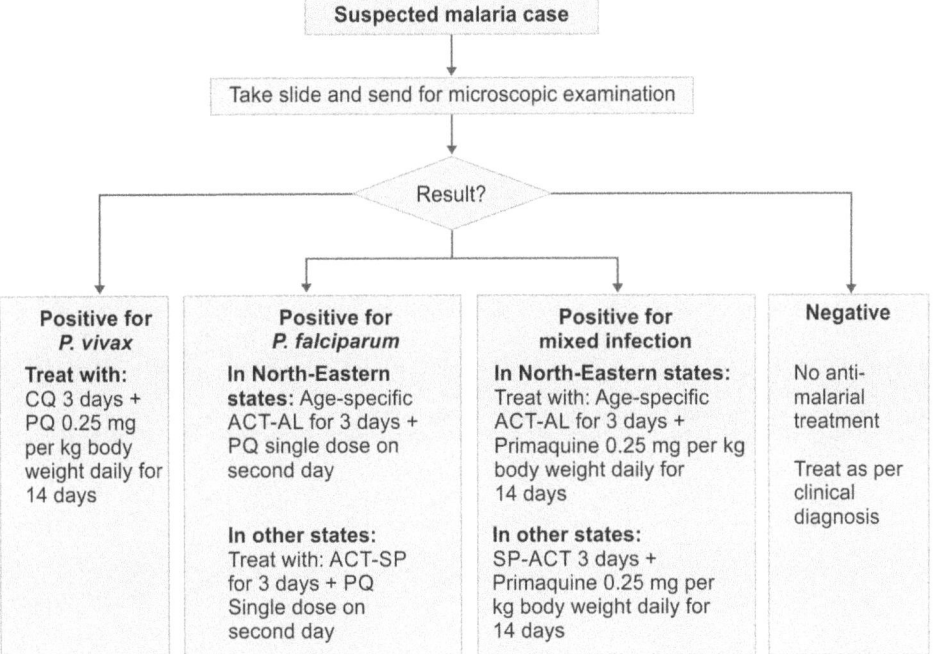

[ACT-AL: Artemisinin-based Combination Therapy-Artemether-Lumefantrine; ACT-SP: Artemisinin-based Combination Therapy (Artesunate+Sulfadoxine-Pyrimethamine); CQ: Chloroquine; PQ: Primaquine]

Where microscopy result is not available within 24 hours and monovalent RDT is used

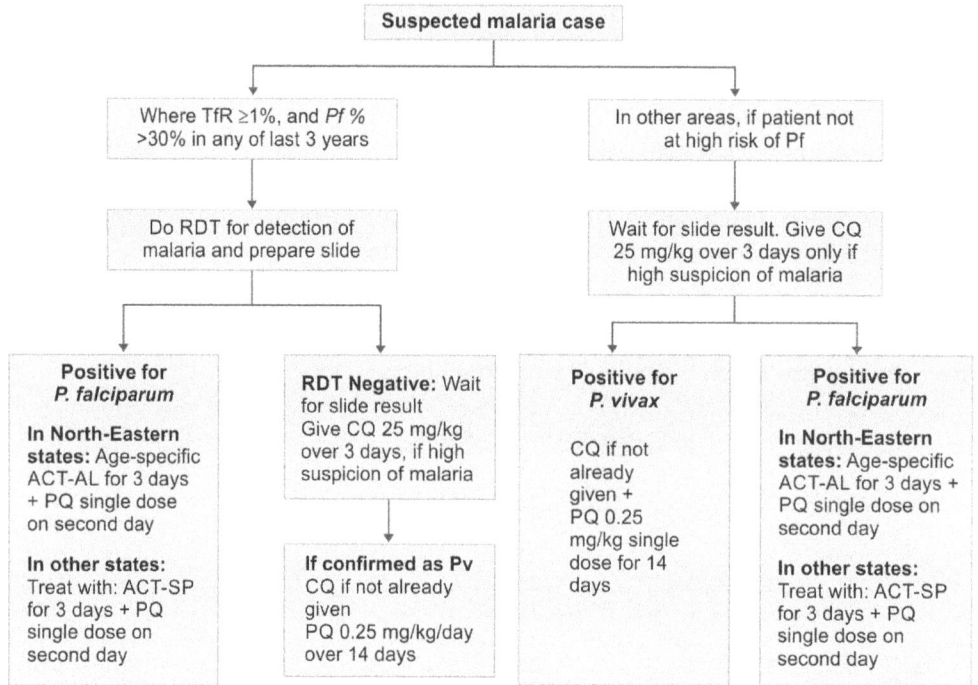

(TfR: test falciparum rate; ACT-AL: Artemisinin-based Combination Therapy-Artemether-Lumefantrine; ACT-SP: Artemisinin-based Combination Therapy (Artesunate+Sulfadoxine-Pyrimethamine); CQ: Chloroquine; PQ: Primaquine)

Note:
• If a patient has severe symptoms at any stage, then immediately refer to a nearest PHC or other health facility with indoor patient management or a registered medical doctor.
• PQ is contraindicated in pregnancy and in children under 1 year (infant).

Where microscopy result is not available within 24 hours and bivalent RDT is used

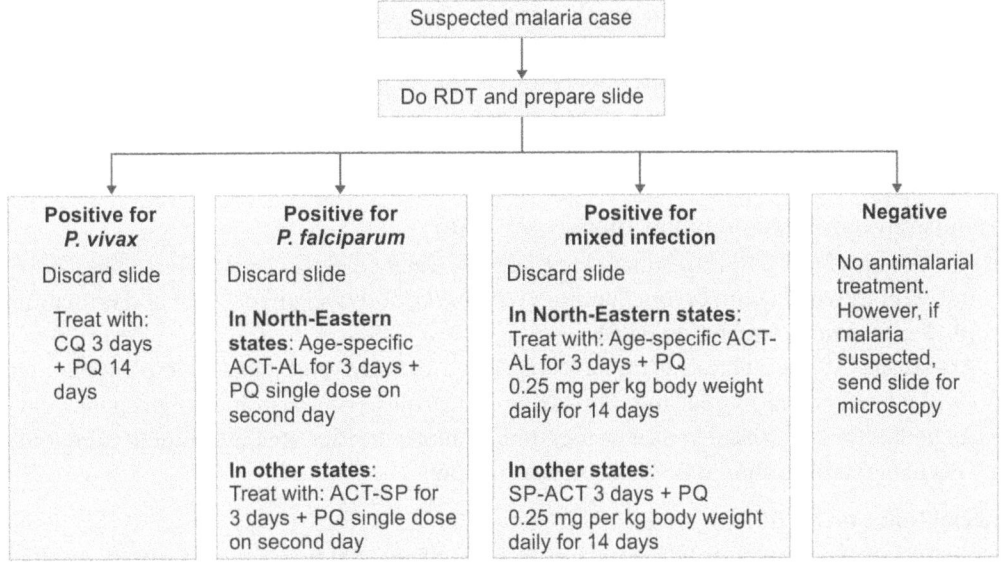

(ACT-AL: Artemisinin-based Combination Therapy-Artemether-Lumefantrine; ACT-SP: Artemisinin-based Combination Therapy (Artesunate+Sulfadoxine-Pyrimethamine); CQ: Chloroquine; PQ: Primaquine)

Note:
• If a patient has severe symptoms at any stage, then immediately refer to a nearest PHC or other health facility with indoor patient management or a registered medical doctor.
• PQ is contraindicated in pregnancy and in children under 1 year (infant).

TREATMENT OF *P. VIVAX* MALARIA

Diagnosis of *P. vivax* malaria may be made by the use of RDT (Bivalent) or microscopic examination of the blood smear. On confirmation following treatment is to be given:

Drug Schedule for Treatment of *P. vivax* Malaria

1. *Chloroquine*: 25 mg/kg body weight divided over 3 days:
   – 10 mg/kg on day 1
   – 10 mg/kg on day 2 and
   – 5 mg/kg on day 3.
2. *Primaquine*: 0.25 mg/kg body weight daily for 14 days.

Special Notes on Use of Primaquine
❖ Primaquine is contraindicated in:
   – Infants
   – Pregnant women
   – Individuals with G6PD deficiency (Special care to be taken in patients with anemia).
   – The 14-days regimen of primaquine should be given under supervision. The patient should be followed up to ensure compliance to 14 day treatment with primaquine.
   – Patients given primaquine must be instructed to stop primaquine if they develop high coloration of urine or blue coloration of lips and report immediately.

TREATMENT OF *P. FALCIPARUM* MALARIA

Diagnosis of *P. falciparum* malaria may be made by the use of RDT (monovalent or bivalent) or microscopic examination of the blood smear. It is imperative to start the treatment for falciparum malaria immediately on diagnosis. The treatment for falciparum malaria is as follows:

Drug Schedule for Treatment of Uncomplicated *P. falciparum* Malaria

In other States

Artemisinin-based Combination Therapy (ACT-SP)

❖ The dosage of ACT-SP is artesunate 4 mg/kg body weight daily for 3 days plus sulfadoxine (25 mg/kg body weight) and pyrimethamine (1.25 mg/kg body weight) on day 1 and Primaquine (0.75 mg/kg body weight) on day 2

❖ Artesunate (AS), available as 50 mg tablets are given for 3 days, and sulfadoxine-pyrimethamine (S-P) tablets, containing 500 mg sulfadoxine and 25 mg pyrimethamine are given for 1 day

❖ All tablets for a day should be taken together, swallowed with water. In addition, primaquine (PQ Large) tablets should be given on the 2nd day.

Special Notes on ACT-SP

❖ SP is not to be given to children below 5 months of age and they should be treated with an alternate ACT

❖ Primaquine and ACT-SP are not to given to pregnant women and they should be treated with an suitable alternate ACT

❖ Sulfadoxine in ACT-SP can, in rare cases, cause serious cutaneous or mucocutaneous eruptions and/or agranulocytosis. Any patient with such reactions developing within a month after taking ACT-SP should be considered *allergic to sulfonamides* and not be given sulfonamides again

❖ As there is a risk of the parasite developing artemisinin resistance, oral monotherapy with artemisinin derivatives should not be given under any circumstance for uncomplicated malaria. Therefore, the Drug Controller General (India) has issued instructions to the state drug controllers to not issue any new license for oral artemisinin derived monotherapies and for licenses granted earlier to be withdrawn

❖ Treatment failures with ACT are very rare and in most cases, failure to respond to treatment is due to inadequate patient compliance. However, any ACT treatment failure should be treated with quinine plus tetracycline/doxycycline/clindamycin for 7 days.

In North-Eastern States (NE States)

Due to signs of *P. falciparum* developing resistance to ACT-SP in some areas in the NE States, Artemether-lumefantrine (ACT-AL) has been introduced as the ACT combination to be used for treatment of *P. falciparum* cases in NE States under the national drug policy.

1. *ACT-AL*: Coformulated tablet of: Artemether (20 mg)—Lumefantrine (120 mg) for 3 days
2. *Primaquine*: 0.75 mg/kg body weight on day 2.

Special Notes on ACT-AL

❖ Primaquine is given in a single dose of 0.75 mg/kg body weight on day 2 for its gametocytocidal properties

❖ ACT-AL is not to be used in women in 1st trimester of pregnancy.

TREATMENT OF UNCOMPLICATED *P. FALCIPARUM* CASES IN PREGNANCY

Points of Concern

❖ Malaria in pregnancy, especially malaria due to *P. falciparum*, is a serious condition as there is reduction of hemoglobin with each bout of fever rapidly leading to severe anemia

❖ There is a high risk of abortion with malaria in early pregnancy and increased chances of stillbirth, intrauterine growth retardation and low birth weight with malaria later in the pregnancy.

Therefore, every effort should be made in pregnant women to diagnose and treat malaria at the earliest.

Treatment in First Trimester

Quinine salt 10 mg/kg 3 times daily for 7 days.

Note: Quinine may induce hypoglycemia; pregnant women should not start taking quinine on an empty stomach and should eat regularly, while on quinine treatment.

Second and Third Trimester

Area-specific ACT as per dosage schedule:
❖ ACT-AL in North-Eastern States
❖ Any ACT combination other than ACT-SP in other states.

MIXED INFECTIONS

Treatment of *P. vivax* + *P. falciparum* Cases

All mixed infections should be treated with full course of ACT and Primaquine 0.25 mg per kg body weight daily for 14 days.

In North-Eastern States: Treat with: Age-specific ACT-AL for 3 days + Primaquine 0.25 mg per kg body weight daily for 14 days.

In Other States: ACT-SP 3 days + Primaquine 0.25 mg per kg body weight daily for 14 days.

Treatment of *P. ovale* + *P. malariae* Cases

In India, these species are very rarely found in few places. *P. ovale* should be treated as *P. vivax* and *P. malariae* should be treated as *P. falciparum*.

Note:
All cases of mixed infection are to be treated as Pf as per the drug policy applicable in the area plus primaquine for 14 days.

Use of Paracetamol

Paracetamol tablets are available as part of the ASHA kit also in the health facilities. Paracetamol usually brings down fever from any cause within half an hour. However, paracetamol does not cure the disease that is causing the fever. So, its effect does not last long. The fever remains low for about 4–6 hours, and then the fever can rise again. Paracetamol can be safely given at any age and even during pregnancy, in the dose shown in the dosage chart. In this dose, it can be given 3-4 times a day if needed. If the fever is not very high, and the patient is able to tolerate the fever, there is no need to give paracetamol.

Dosage Chart for Use of Paracetamol

Age	No. of tablets of paracetamol (500 mg tablets)
Less than 1 year	¼
1–4 years	½
5–8 years	¾
9–14 years	1
15 years or more	1 or 2

SEVERE AND COMPLICATED MALARIA

A case of uncomplicated malaria usually presents with fever, rigors, headache, bodyache, fatigue, anorexia and nausea.

Serious complications can arise in *P. falciparum* infection and rarely in *P. vivax*. They may sometimes develop suddenly over a span of time as short as 12-24 hours and may lead to death, if not treated promptly and adequately.

Definition: Severe falciparum malaria is defined as one or more of the following, occurring in the absence of an identified alternative cause and in the presence of *P. falciparum* asexual parasitemia:

❖ Impaired consciousness
❖ Prostration (generalized weakness)
❖ Multiple convulsions
❖ Acidosis
❖ Hypoglycemia
❖ Severe anemia
❖ Renal impairment
❖ Jaundice
❖ Pulmonary edema
❖ Significant bleeding
❖ Shock
❖ Hyperparasitemia.

Chemotherapy of Severe and Complicated Malaria

Initial parenteral treatment for at least 48 hours: choose 1 of following 4 options:	Follow-up treatment, when patient can take oral medication following parenteral treatment:
Quinine: 20 mg quinine salt/kg body weight on admission (IV infusion or divided IM injection)	Quinine: 10 mg/kg 3 times a day
	With
Followed by maintenance dose of, 10 mg/kg 8 hourly;	Doxycycline 100 mg once a day or
Infusion rate should not exceed 5 mg/kg per hour.	Clindamycin in pregnant women and children under
Loading dose of 20 mg/kg should not be given, if the patient has already received quinine	8 years of age to complete 7 days of treatment

Contd...

Contd...

Initial parenteral treatment for at least 48 hours: choose 1 of following 4 options:	Follow-up treatment, when patient can take oral medication following parenteral treatment:
Artesunate: 2.4 mg/kg IV or IM given on admission (time=0), then at 12 h and 24 h, then once a day Or Artemether: 3.2 mg/kg bw IM given on admission then 1.6 mg/kg per day Or Arteether: 150 mg daily IM for 3 days in adults only (not recommended for children)	Full oral course of area-specific ACT: In North-Eastern states: Age-specific ACT-AL for 3 days + PQ Single dose on second day In other states: Treat with: ACT-SP for 3 days + PQ single dose on second day

Note: The parenteral treatment in severe malaria cases should be given for minimum of 24 hours once started (irrespective of the patient's ability to tolerate oral medication earlier than 24 hours).

After parenteral artemisinin therapy, patients will receive a full course of area-specific oral ACT for 3 days. Those patients who received parenteral quinine therapy should receive any one of the below:

Oral quinine 10 mg/kg 3 times a day for 7 days (including the days when parenteral quinine was administered) + Doxycycline 3 mg/kg once a day
Clindamycin 10 mg/kg 12-hourly for 7 days or area-specific ACT as described (doxycycline is contraindicated in pregnant women and children under 8 years of age)

CHEMOPROPHYLAXIS

Chemoprophylaxis should be administered only in selective grips in high *P. falciparum* endemic areas. Use of personal protection measures including Insecticide-Treated Bed Nets (ITNs)/Long-Lasting Insecticidal Nets (LLINs) should be encouraged for pregnant women and other vulnerable population including travelers for longer stay. However, for longer stay of military and para-military forces in high *P. falciparum* endemic areas, the practice of chemoprophylaxis should be followed wherever appropriate, e.g. troops on night patrol duty and decisions of their Medical Administrative Authority should be followed.

SHORT-TERM CHEMOPROPHYLAXIS (UP TO 6 WEEKS)

Doxycycline

100 mg once daily for adults and 1.5 mg/kg once daily for children.

The drug should be:
- Started 2 days before travel and
- Continued for 4 weeks after leaving the malarious area.

Note: It is not recommended for pregnant women and children less than 8 years.

CHEMOPROPHYLAXIS FOR LONGER STAY (MORE THAN 6 WEEKS)

Mefloquine

250 mg weekly for adults and should be administered:
- Two weeks before entering the high-risk area

❖ Continued during the stay
❖ Till 4 weeks after leaving the area.

Note: Mefloquine is contraindicated in individuals with history of convulsions, neuropsychiatric problems and cardiac conditions. Therefore, necessary precautions should be taken and all should undergo through this before prescription of the drug.

INTEGRATED VECTOR MANAGEMENT

Definition

Integrated vector management (IVM) is defined by WHO as a rational decision making process for the optimal use of resources for vector control. It entails use of a range of biological, chemical and physical interventions of proven efficacy, separately or in combination, in order to implement cost-effective control and reduce reliance on any single intervention.

Vector Control and Personal Protection Measures

Adult mosquito control	Indoor residual spray (IRS)
Personal protection and adult mosquito control	Bed nets: Long-lasting insecticide treated nets (LLIN) Insecticide-treated bed nets (ITN)
Larval control	Source reduction and chemical, biological and environmental measures

Principles

The prioritization for implementation of vector control measures in India is broadly based on the API (annual parasitic incidence) of the area. Stratification for IVM activities is required to be done up to subcenter level which is the unit for IVM.

$$API = \frac{\text{Total no. of positive for parasite in a year}}{\text{Total population}} \times 1000$$

Category-wise Vector Control Measures

API of area	Major activities according to API
<1	• Vector control by minor engineering measures like desilting, removal of weeds and cleaning of canals and irrigation channels, control by use of larvicides and environmental management
1–2	• Vector control by source reduction and biological control. The LLIN shall be distributed in the areas having API>1 in identified districts based on priority and availability of resources (LLIN)
2–5	• Vector control by distribution of LLIN if acceptability of IRS is low • For areas which can be supervised and accessible, quality IRS for selective vector control based on epidemiological impact of earlier vector control measures, if needed; these areas can also be provided with LLINs

>5	• For areas having seasonal transmission (less than 5 months in a year):
	  – 1 round of IRS with DDT before start of transmission
	  – Focal spray in and around 50 houses of positive cases
	  – Priority distribution of LLINs
	• Areas with perennial transmission (>5 months in a year):
	  – 2 rounds of IRS with DDT and 3 rounds with malathion
	  – Priority distribution of LLINs as per the guidelines
	  – Vector bionomics studies for future change of strategy

Source: Operational Manual for Integrated Vector Management in India, Ministry of Health & Family Welfare, Government of India (March 2016).

Biomedical Waste Management

BIOMEDICAL WASTE (MANAGEMENT AND HANDLING) RULES (2016)

Major Differences Between BMW Rules of 1998 and 2016

Points	1998	2016
• Authorization	• Only occupiers with more than 1,000 beds were required to obtain authorization	• Every occupier generating biomedical waste including health camp or Ayush infrastructures are required to obtain authorization
• Operator duties	• Absent	• Duties of the operator listed
• Categories	• Biomedical wastes were divided into 10 categories	• Biomedical wastes are divided into 4 categories
• Rules restricted to:	• In healthcare establishments with >1,000 beds only	• Treatment and disposal of biomedical waste made mandatory for all health-care establishments
• Annual report	• No format for annual report	• A format for annual report has been introduced with new rules
• Schedule	• I, II, III, IV, V	• I, II, III, IV

Introduction

Biomedical waste (BMW) management and handling is under the Ministry of Environment and Forests and Climate Change, Government of India.

- **BMW rules are not applicable to:**
  1. Radioactive waste
  2. Lead and batteries
  3. Hazardous waste
  4. Electronic waste (e-waste)
  5. Hazardous microorganisms.
- Immunize health workers handling biomedical wastes with hepatitis and tetanus vaccine.
- **Contents of BMW rules 2016:**
  1. Schedules 1–4
  2. Forms 1–5
  3. Rules 1–18.

- **Categories under BMW rules 2016:**
  1. Yellow
  2. Red
  3. White
  4. Blue.

Category	Type of waste	Discarding mechanism
Blue	**Glassware** **Metallic body implants:** Medicine vials and ampoules	• Disinfection (by soaking the washed glass waste after cleaning with detergent and sodium hypochlorite treatment) or • Autoclaving or • Microwaving or • Hydroclaving and then sent for recycling
White (translucent)	**Waste sharps:** including metals Needles, syringes with fixed needles, needles from needle tip cutter or burner, scalpels, blades	Autoclaving/dry heat sterilization → shredding/ mutilation/encapsulation → sent for final disposal to iron foundries or sanitary landfill or designated concrete waste sharp pit
Red	**Contaminated waste (recyclable):** Tubing, bottles, intravenous tubes and sets, catheters, urine bags, syringes (without needles and fixed needle syringes) and vaccutainers with their needles cut and gloves	• Autoclaving or microwaving/hydroclaving → shredding/mutilation or • Combination of sterilization and shredding
Yellow	a. **Human anatomical waste:** Human tissues, organs, body parts and fetus below the viability period	
	b. **Animal anatomical waste:** Experimental animal carcasses, body parts, organs, tissues, including the waste generated from animals used in experiments	Deep burial*
	c. **Soiled waste:** Items contaminated with blood, body fluids like dressings, plaster casts, cotton swabs and bags containing residual or discarded blood and blood components	Incineration or plasma pyrolysis
	d. **Expired or discarded medicines**	Encapsulation
	e. **Chemical waste:** Chemicals used in production of biological and used or discarded disinfectants	Incineration/plasma pyrolysis/encapsulation

Contd...

* Disposal by deep burial is permitted only in rural or remote areas where there is no access to common biomedical waste treatment facility.

Contd...

Category	Type of waste	Discarding mechanism
f	**Chemical liquid waste:** Silver X-ray film developing liquid, discarded formalin, infected secretions, aspirated body fluids, liquid from laboratories	Pretreatment before mixing with other wastewater
g.	**Discarded linen, mattresses, beddings contaminated with blood or body fluid**	Nonchlorinated chemical disinfection → Incineration/plasma pyrolysis
h.	**Microbiology, biotechnology and other clinical laboratory waste:** Blood bags, vaccines, culture	Nonchlorinated chemical disinfection → Incineration

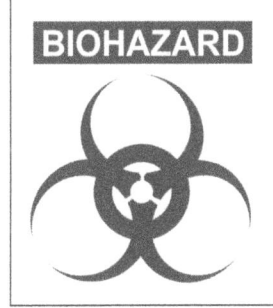

Cytotoxic hazard symbol

Handle with care   Handle with care

Label for biomedical waste containers or bags

New Requirements/Recommendations as Stated in BMW Amendment Rules, 2018

1. Pretreatment of laboratory waste, microbiology waste, blood samples by autoclave before giving to disposal*
2. Phase out chlorinated bags, gloves, blood bags
3. Training of healthcare workers about handling of biomedical waste*
4. Immunization of healthcare workers for hepatitis B and tetanus*
5. Barcode system for bags or containers containing biomedical waste
6. Health checkup of healthcare workers during induction and annually thereafter*
7. Maintain and update biomedical waste management register and monthly report on website
8. Major accidents to be reported along with annual report
9. Maintain records of autoclaving, microwaving, etc. for a period of 5 years*
10. Annual reporting on website
11. Setup BMW management committee, and meetings to be done biannually.*

*Effective immediately.

Chapter 22

Incubation and Isolation Period of Some Important Diseases

INCUBATION PERIOD

Definition

Incubation period is defined as "the time interval between invasion by an infectious agent and appearance of the first sign or symptom of the disease in question."

Significance

During the incubation period, the infectious agent undergoes multiplication in the host. When a sufficient density of the disease agent is built up in the host, the health equilibrium is disturbed and the disease becomes overt.

Diseases	Causative organism	Incubation period
Respiratory infections		
Smallpox	Variola virus	7–14 days
Chickenpox	Human herpes virus 3	14–16 days
Measles	RNA paramyxovirus	10–14 days
Rubella	RNA togavirus	14–21 days
Mumps	RNA myxovirus	14–21 days
Influenza	Orthomyxovirus	18–72 hours
Diphtheria	Corynebacterium diphtheriae	2–6 days
Whooping cough	Bordetella pertussis	7–14 days
Meningococcal meningitis	Neisseria meningitidis	3–4 days
Tuberculosis	Mycobacterium tuberculosis	Variable
Intestinal infections		
Polio	Poliovirus	7–14 days
Hepatitis A	Enterovirus 72	15–45 days
Hepatitis B	Hepadnavirus	45–180 days
Hepatitis C	Hepacivirus	30–120 days
Hepatitis D	Deltavirus	30–90 days
Hepatitis E	Calcivirus	21–45 days
Cholera	Vibrio cholerae	1–2 days

Contd...

Contd...

Diseases	Causative organism	Incubation period
Typhoid fever	*Salmonella typhi*	10–14 days
Staphylococcal food poisoning	*Staphylococcus aureus*	1–6 hours
Ascariasis	*Ascaris lumbricoides*	2 months
Hookworm	*Ancylostoma duodenale*	5 weeks to 9 months
Arthropod borne infections		
Dengue	*Arbovirus*	3–10 days
Malaria	*Plasmodium vivax*	8–17 days
	P. falciparum	9–14 days
	P. malariae	18–40 days
	P. ovale	16–18 days
Lymphatic filariasis	*Wuchereria bancrofti*	8–16 months
Zoonoses		
Rabies	*Lyssavirus type 1*	3–8 weeks
Yellow fever	*Flavivirus*	2–6 days
Japanese encephalitis	*Flavivirus*	5–15 days
Chikungunya fever	*Chikungunyavirus*	4–7 days
Bubonic/septicemic plague	*Yersinia pestis*	2–7 days
Pneumonic plague	*Yersinia pestis*	1–3 days
Taeniasis	*Taenia solium/Taenia saginata*	8–14 weeks
Kala-azar	*Leishmania donovani*	1–4 months
Surface infections		
Tetanus	*Clostridium tetani*	6–10 days
AIDS	*HIV*	Months to years
Leprosy	*Mycobacterium leprae*	5–20 years

Isolation Period

Definition

Isolation is defined as "separation for the period of communicability of infected persons or animals from others in such places and under such conditions, as to prevent or limit the direct or indirect transmission of the infectious agent from those infected to those who are susceptible, or who may spread the agent to others."

Significance

The purpose of isolation is to protect the community by preventing transfer of infection from the reservoir to the possible susceptible hosts.

Disease	Duration of isolation
Chickenpox	Until all the lesions crusted usually about 6 days after onset of rash
Measles	From the onset of catarrhal stage through 3rd day of rash
Cholera, diphtheria	3 days after antibiotics started until 48 hours of antibiotics/negative cultures after treatment
Shigellosis, salmonellosis	Until 3 consecutive negative stool cultures
Hepatitis A	3 weeks
Influenza	3 days after onset
Polio	2 weeks in adult, 6 weeks in pediatric age group
Confirmed TB	Until 3 weeks of effective chemotherapy
Herpes zoster	6 days after onset of rash
Mumps	Until swelling subsides
Pertussis	4 weeks/until paroxysms cease
Meningococcal meningitis, streptococcal pharyngitis	Until the first 6 hours of effective antibiotic therapy are completed

National Health Policy and Elimination of Some Diseases

NATIONAL HEALTH GOALS FOR COMMUNICABLE AND NONCOMMUNICABLE DISEASES UNDER 12TH FIVE-YEAR PLAN OF NATIONAL HEALTH MISSION (2012–2017)

1. Reduce maternal mortality ratio (MMR) to 1/1,000 live births
2. Reduce infant mortality rate (IMR) to 25/1,000 live births
3. Reduce total fertility rate (TFR) to 2.1
4. Prevention and reduction of anemia in women aged 15–49 years
5. Prevent and reduce mortality and morbidity from communicable, noncommunicable; injuries and emerging diseases
6. Reduce household out-of-pocket expenditure on total healthcare expenditure
7. Reduce annual incidence and mortality from tuberculosis by half
8. Reduce prevalence of leprosy to <1/10,000 population and incidence to zero in all districts
9. Annual malaria incidence to be <1/1,000
10. Less than 1% microfilaria prevalence in all districts
11. Kala-azar elimination by 2015, <1 case per 10,000 population in all blocks.

SMALLPOX ERADICATION

❖ Last indigenous case in India: 17th May, 1975.
❖ Last known case in India: 24th May, 1975 (imported from Bangladesh).
❖ Last case of smallpox in the world: 26th October, 1977 (Somalia).
❖ India declared smallpox free: April, 1977.
❖ WHO declared global eradication of smallpox: 8th May, 1980.

POLIOMYELITIS ERADICATION

❖ Last recorded wild case of poliovirus:
   – Type 2 → 1999
   – Type 3 → 11th November 2012.
❖ All reported cases since 11th November 2012 have been of type 1.
❖ Last case of polio due to wild poliovirus in India was detected on 13th January 2011 in Howrah District of West Bengal.
❖ WHO certified entire South East Asia Region (including India) as "polio free" on 27th March, 2014.
❖ Now only three countries, i.e. Pakistan, Nigeria and Afghanistan are endemic for wild poliovirus.

INDIA HAS ELIMINATED FOLLOWING DISEASES

Eliminated diseases from India:
1. Guinea worm/Dracunculiasis (Feb, 2000)*
2. Leprosy (December, 2005)
3. Yaws (September, 2006)
4. Maternal neonatal tetanus (on 14th July, 2016).

*In 2016 only 2 cases of Guinea worm were detected in Chad. It is the second human disease to be in line to be eradicated after smallpox.

Disease	Elimination level/ criteria	
Leprosy	<1/10,000 population	
Neonatal tetanus	<0.1/1000 live births TT2 coverage >90% Attended deliveries >75%	
Polio	Certification of polio eradication is conducted on a regional basis. Each region can consider certification only when all countries in the area demonstrate the absence of wild poliovirus transmission for at least three consecutive years in the presence of certification standard surveillance	
TB (WHO and Stop TB strategy)	<1 case per million population (to eliminate TB as a public health problem)	
Criteria for tracking progress towards IDD elimination	*Indicator*	*Goal*
	Proportionate with enlarged thyroid age (6–12 years)	<5%
	Urinary iodine excretion <100 µg/L	<50%
	Urinary iodine excretion <20 µg/L	<20%
	Proportionate of houses consuming adequately iodized salt	>90%

Current Public Health-related Statistics and Recent Updates

Authors' Note

In this chapter, we have discussed the latest health-related statistics from the most reliable sources. We have put our best efforts to give you the most updated information. If anyhow, the numerical values of health indicators or targets given in other chapters of this book differs from this chapter; please confirm the data from this chapter only.

SOCIOECONOMIC INDICATORS

Human Development Index (HDI)

Rank	Country	HDI value	Category
1	Norway	0.957	Very high development
131	India	0.645	Medium development
189	Niger	0.394	Low development

Source: Human Development Report 2020 (United Nations Development Programme)

GROSS DOMESTIC PRODUCTS (GDP)

Definition

According to **Organization for Economic Cooperation and Development (OECD)**: Gross domestic products (GDP) is "An aggregate measure of production equal to the sum of the gross values added of all resident institutional units engaged in production (plus any taxes, and minus any subsidies, on products not included in the value of their outputs)."

For India:

GDP: 2.87 trillions of US $

Rank: 5

Source: World Bank and International Monetary Fund (IMF) Report.

BELOW POVERTY LINE (BPL)

Definition

Internationally, an income of less than $1.90 per day per head of purchasing power parity is defined as extreme poverty.

By this estimate, *about 21.2% of Indians are extremely poor.*

Income-based poverty lines consider the bare minimum income to provide basic food requirements.

It does not account for other essentials such as health care and education.

Source: "Poverty and Equity—India" The World Bank (2012).

NATIONAL SOCIODEMOGRAPHIC GOALS OF NPP, 2000 (ACHIEVED BY 2010)

1. Address the unmet needs for basic reproductive and child health services, supplies and infrastructure.
2. Make school education up to age 14 free and compulsory, and reduce drop outs at primary and secondary school levels to below 20% for both boys and girls.
3. Reduce infant mortality rate (IMR) to below 30 per 1000 live births.
4. Reduce maternal mortality ratio (MMR) to below 100 per 100,000 live births.
5. Achieve universal immunization of children against all vaccine preventable diseases.
6. Promote delayed marriage for girls, not earlier than age 18 and preferably after 20 years of age.
7. Achieve 80% institutional deliveries and 100% deliveries by trained persons.
8. Achieve universal access to information/counseling, and services for fertility regulation and contraception with a wide basket of choices.
9. Achieve 100% registration of births, deaths, marriage and pregnancy.
10. Contain the spread of acquired immunodeficiency syndrome (AIDS), and promote greater integration between the management of reproductive tract infections (RTIs) and sexually transmitted infections (STIs) and the National AIDS Control Organisation.
11. Prevent and control communicable diseases.
12. Integrate Indian Systems of Medicine (ISM) in the provision of reproductive and child health services, and in reaching out to households.
13. Promote vigorously the small family norm to achieve replacement levels of total fertility rate (TFR).
14. Bring about convergence in implementation of related social sector programs so that family welfare becomes a people centered program.

SUSTAINABLE DEVELOPMENTAL GOALS

Officially known as *"Transforming our world: The 2030 Agenda for Sustainable Development".*

It is a set of 17 aspirational "Global Goals" with 169 targets between them.

Difference with Millennium Development Goals

Millennium development goals (MDGs) was outdated in the year 2015. MDG dealt only with developing countries. In contrast sustainable development goals (SDGs) deal with all countries and has a wider perspective.

1. **No poverty:** End poverty in all its forms everywhere.
2. **Zero hunger:** End hunger, achieve food security and improved nutrition and promote sustainable agriculture.

3. **Good health and well-being:** Ensure healthy lives and promote well-being for all at all age.
4. **Quality education:** Ensure inclusive and equitable quality education and promote lifelong learning opportunities for all.
5. **Gender equality:** Achieve gender equality and empower all women and girls.
6. **Clean water and sanitation:** Ensure availability and sustainable management of water and sanitation for all.
7. **Affordable and clean energy:** Ensure access to affordable, reliable, sustainable and modern energy for all.
8. **Decent work and economic growth:** Promote sustained, inclusive and sustainable economic growth, full and productive employment and decent work for all.
9. **Industry, innovation and infrastructure:** Build resilient infrastructure, promote inclusive and sustainable industrialization and foster innovation.
10. **Reduced inequalities:** Reduce income inequality within and among countries.
11. **Sustainable cities and communities:** Make cities and human settlements inclusive, safe, resilient and sustainable.
12. **Responsible consumption and production:** Ensure sustainable consumption and production patterns.
13. **Climate action:** Take urgent action to combat climate change and its impacts by regulating emissions and promoting developments in renewable energy.
14. **Life below water:** Conserve and sustainably use the oceans, seas and marine resources for sustainable development.
15. **Life on land:** Protect, restore and promote sustainable use of terrestrial ecosystems, sustainably manage forests, combat desertification, and halt and reverse land degradation and halt biodiversity loss.
16. **Peace, justice and strong institutions:** Promote peaceful and inclusive societies for sustainable development, provide access to justice for all and build effective, accountable and inclusive institutions at all level.
17. **Partnerships for the goals.**

Remember 5 'P's in SDGs:
1. People
2. Planet
3. Prosperity
4. Peace
5. Partnership.

HEALTH-RELATED GOALS

By 2030, targets are:
- Global MMR <70/1 lakh live births
- Neonatal mortality rate <12/100 live births
- Under 5 mortality rate <25 live births
- Reduce by 33% premature mortality from noncommunicable diseases (NCDs)
- About 50% reduction in global deaths injuries from road traffic accidents (RTAs).

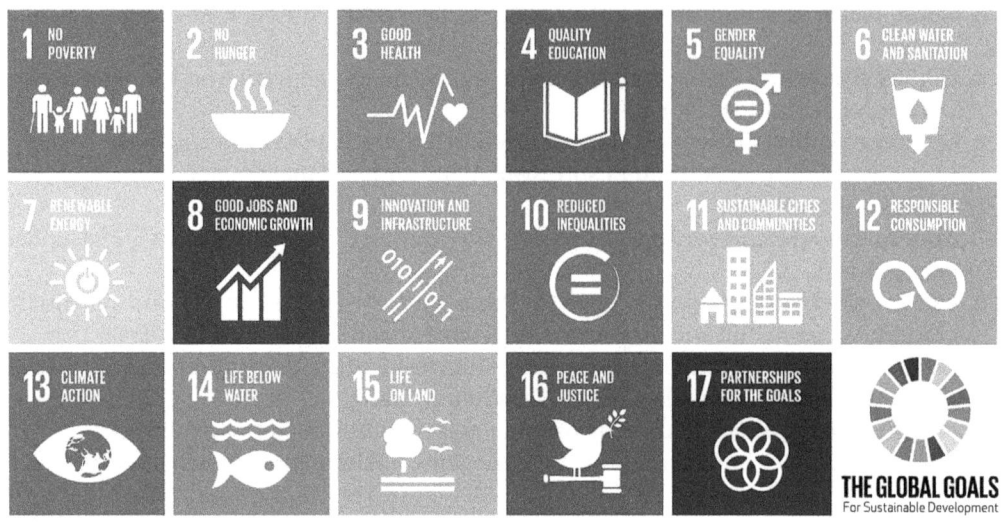

New Targets under Financial Budget in India (2017–2018)

	Disease	*Year*
Elimination	Filariasis	2017
	Kala-azar	2017
	Leprosy	2018
	Measles	2020
	Tuberculosis	2025
Reduction	Infant mortality rate to 28	2025
	Maternal mortality rate to 100	2018–2020

GLOBAL STRATEGY FOR WOMEN'S, CHILDREN'S AND ADOLESCENT'S HEALTH (2016–2030)

Vision

By 2030, a world in which every woman, child and adolescent in every setting realizes their rights to physical and mental health and well-being, has social and economic opportunities and is able to participate fully in shaping prosperous and sustainable societies.

Objectives and Targets Aligned with Sociodemographic Goals

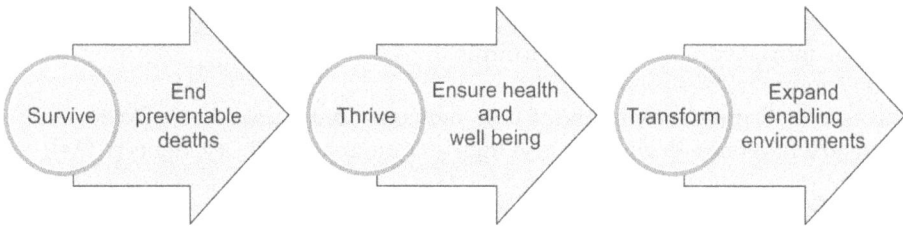

RECENT HEALTH-RELATED STATISTICS

Population	
Global	World population reached 7.67 billion (2019)
India	1,366 million
Sex ratio	
At birth	900
Adult	940 (Census)
	919 (NFHS 4)
Population density	464 persons/sq. km

Important statistics
Source: NITI Aayog (2018)

Infant mortality rate (IMR): 34 per 1,000 livebirths

Birth rate: 20.4%

Crude death rate (CDR): 6.4%

Immunization coverage: 62%

Life expectancy at birth: 67.9 years

Sex ratio at birth: 900 females/1000 males

Total fertility rate (TFR): 2.3

Maternal mortality rate (MMR): 130 per 100,000 live births

RECENT UPDATES REGARDING INFECTIOUS DISEASES

Recent Updates Regarding HIV (2022)

Revised guidelines on initiation of anti-retroviral therapy (updated on 2022):

As per revised guidelines, it has been decided to **treat all people living with HIV (PLHIV) with antiretroviral therapy (ART)** *regardless of CD4 count, clinical stage, age or population.*

A. Patients who are in pre-ART care should undergo a fresh CD4 count, if it is more than 3 months old and baseline investigations before ART initiation as per revised criteria.

B. Adequate counseling and preparedness needs to be ensured before ART initiation in all PLHIV.

C. Particularly for these with higher CD4 count as they are likely to be asymptomatic and more likely to default.

D. The guidelines remains same for what regimens to start:
   – The basic principle for first-line ART for treatment-naive adult and adolescent patients is to use a triple drug combination from two different classes of ARVS.
   – The first-line ART essentially comprises of a nucleotide/nucleoside reverse transcriptase inhibitor (NRTI) backbone, preferably non-thymidine **(Tenofovir Plus Lamivudine) and one integrase strand transfer inhibitor (INSTI) preferably Dolutegravir (DTG).**
   – In consideration of the WHO guidelines and based on recommendations of NACO Technical Resource Group, it has been decided to include Dolutegravir-containing regimens as the preferred first-line treatment for HIV-positive adults, adolescents and

children (weighing more than 20 kg/age more than 6 years) under the NACP since July 2020.
- Based on the evidence supporting better efficacy and fewer side effects, the preferred first-line ART regimen for all People Living with HIV (PLHIV) with age >10 years and weight >30 kg is as follows:
  - Tenofovir (TDF 300 mg) + Lamivudine (3TC 300 mg) + Dolutegravir (DTG 50 mg) Regimen (TLD) as FDC in a single pill once a day fat a fixed time every day as per patient's convenience.
- This regimen has the advantage of harmonization in the treatment of all adults, adolescents, pregnant women including those with HIV-1, HIV-2, HIV-1 and 2, women exposed to single dose Nevirapine in the past and those co-infected with TB or hepatitis.
- It is a simple, potent and well-tolerated regimen that offers the advantage of a decentralized service delivery and monitoring. It also simplifies the supply chain and minimizes monitoring requirements.

GENERAL GUIDANCE

❖ A single pill of TLD should be taken preferably at bedtime, and instances where additional dose of DTG is indicated should be taken preferably in the morning.
❖ Patients with severe diabetes and hypertension should be monitored more closely for Tenofovir toxicity. Patients starting on DTG should be monitored for blood glucose (six monthly) and weight gain (on monthly visits). Appropriate physical activity should be advised to prevent weight gain.

Pediatric Antiretroviral Regimens

❖ *The choice of drugs depends on the child's age and body weight. Abacavir* (ABC) is the preferred NRTI for initiation in children less than 10 years of age and body weight of less than 30 kg at present.
❖ For all children above 10 years and above 30 kg body weight, Tenofovir (TDF) is the preferred drug for initiation. This is the simplest, most potent and least toxic regimen that offers.
❖ The advantage of a decentralized service delivery and monitoring as it harmonizes with adult ART regimen. It also simplifies the supply chain and minimizes the monitoring requirements.
❖ Lopinavir/Ritonaviris recommended as the preferred third drug in all children less than 6 years of age and less than 20 kg body weight till the availability of pediatric formulations of Dolutegravir under the national programme. For children older than 6 years of age and body weight of more than 20 kg, DTG is recommended as the preferred third drug.

Recent WHO Target for HIV

90–90–90 target

By 2020
- 90% of all people living with HIV will have been diagnosed
- 90% of all people with HIV diagnosed HIV infection will receive ART
- 90% of all people on ART will have viral suppression

Special Notes

❖ WHO certifies India to have eliminated Yaws and Maternal Neonatal Tetanus (on 14th July 2016)

❖ India is the first country to eliminate Yaws under 2012 neglected tropical disease.

Recent Treatment Protocol of Leishmaniasis

❖ Drug of choice: Liposomal amphotericin B given IV
❖ Alternative: Miltefosine (oral)
❖ Sodium stibogluconate is *No Longer Used.*

Polio Eradication and Endgame Strategic Plan (2013–2018)

Introduction: The Polio Eradication and Endgame Strategic Plan (2013–2018) represents a major milestone in polio eradication and describes specific steps to take to successfully achieve eradication.

The plan was developed by the Global Polio Eradication Initiative (GPEI) in consultation with national health authorities, global health initiatives, scientific experts, donors and other stakeholders, in response to a directive of the World Health Assembly.

Objectives are as follows:

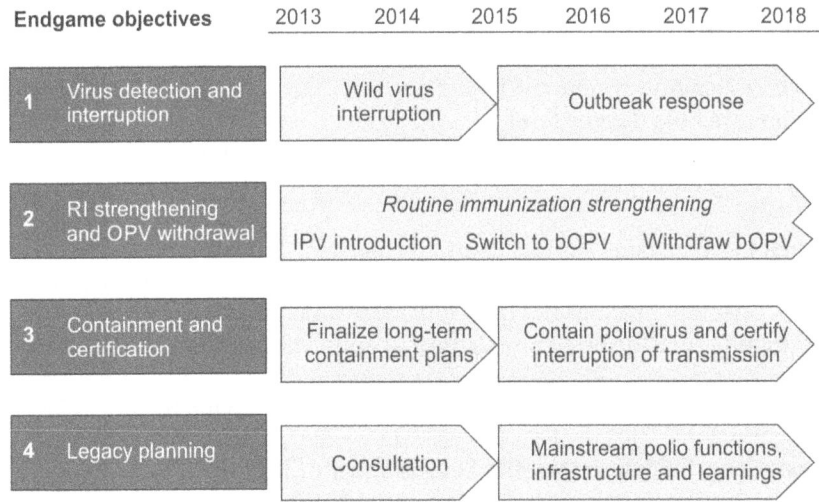

(RI: Routine immunization; OPV: Oral polio vaccine; IPV: Inactivated polio vaccine; bOPV: Bivalent oral polio vaccine)

Global Health Sector Strategy on Viral Hepatitis (2016–2021)

Vision	• A world where viral hepatitis transmission is halted and everyone living with hepatitis has access to safe, affordable and effective care and treatment
Goal	• Eliminate viral hepatitis as a major public health threat
Global targets	• Reduce new cases of chronic HBV and HCV infections by 90% by 2030 • Reduce deaths due to viral hepatitis by 65% by 2030
Preventive interventions	• Three doses of HBV vaccine for infants • Prevention of PTCT of HBV • Blood safety and injection safety • Harm reduction for drug users
Treatment interventions	• Diagnosis of HBV and HCV • Treatment of HBV and HCV

(HBV: Hepatitis B virus; HCV: Hepatitis C virus; PTCT: Plasma thromboplastin component test)

National Framework for Malaria Elimination in India (2016–2030)

Goals

❖ Eliminate malaria (zero indigenous cases) throughout the entire country 2030
❖ Maintain malaria-free status in areas where malaria transmission has been interrupted and prevent reintroduction.

Zika Virus Update

❖ Zika virus (ZIKV) is a member of the virus family *Flaviviridae*.
❖ Spread: It spreads by daytime-active *Aedes* mosquitoes, such as *A. aegypti* and *A. albopictus.*

Zika Fever

❖ Zika fever (also known as Zika virus disease) is an illness caused by the Zika virus.
❖ Symptoms:
  – Most cases have no symptoms (80% of persons), but when present they are usually mild and can resemble dengue fever.
  – Symptoms may include fever, red eyes, joint pain, headache, and a maculopapular rash.
  – Symptoms generally last <7 days. It has not caused any reported deaths during the initial infection.
  – Pregnant women can be infected at any trimester.
  – Infection during pregnancy causes microcephaly and other brain malformations in some babies. Infection in adults has been linked to Guillain–Barré syndrome (GBS).
❖ Vaccine: In June 2016 the FDA granted the first approval for a human clinical trial for a Zika vaccine
❖ Treatment: Supportive care is recommend. No specific antiviral treatment for Zika virus.

National Operational Guidelines: Measles Rubella Vaccine (2017)

❖ In September 2013, India resolved to eliminate measles and control rubella/congenital rubella syndrome (CRS) by 2020
❖ Accordingly, MHFW is introducing rubella vaccine in its UIP as measles-rubella (MR) vaccine

❖ The vaccine will be introduced as MR Campaign, targeting children from 9 months to 15 years, in a phased manner over 2–3 years, followed by inclusion of the vaccine in routine immunization (RI)

❖ *This is the 1st time rubella vaccine is introduced in India* and will replace measles with MR vaccine.

RECENT UPDATES REGARDING NONCOMMUNICABLE DISEASES

❖ *25 by 25:* Bring 25% reduction in premature deaths by NCDs by 2025
❖ *Cancer:*
  – Strikes more women in India, but kills more men
  – **Onco-collect**: A software to see how a patient react to a drug and how they fare long time.
❖ *Diabetes mellitus:*
  – Burden of diabetes mellitus in India: 72.96 million (for year 2017)
  – Prevalence: 11.8% of adult population
  – Government of India has launched **M-diabetes**: Mobile health initiative for prevention and care of diabetes.
❖ *Depression:*
  – Leading cause of disability worldwide
  – Prevalence in India: 4% (as per WHO)
  – Campaign slogan for depression is "**Let's talk**".

Mental Health Bill (2017)	
◆ Recent modification to "Right-based approach" from "Assurance-based approach"	
◆ Components are as follows:	
Rights of mentally ill	Advance directive
Mental health authorities	Decriminalizing suicide, prohibiting electroconvulsive therapy

JUVENILE JUSTICE ACT, 2015

❖ Effective from 15th January 2016
❖ Replaces existing Indian Juvenile Delinquency Law, Juvenile Justice Act (2000)
❖ Juveniles in conflict with law in age group of 16–18 years, if involved in heinous crimes, can be tried as adults.

RECENT UPDATES REGARDING BLINDNESS AND VISUAL IMPAIRMENT

❖ The nomenclature of the scheme "National Program for Control of Blindness" has been changed to "National Program for Control of Blindness and Visual Impairment"
❖ Updated WHO definition of blindness: *Presenting distance visual acuity less than 3/60 (20/400) in better eye and limitation of field of vision to be less than 10 degrees from center of fixation*
❖ Updated WHO definition of visual impairment: *Presenting distance visual acuity less than 6/18 and better than or equal to 3/60 in the better eye.*

RECENT MORTALITY STATISTICS

❖ Overall (According to Indian Statistics):
  – Most common cause: Cardiovascular disease (ischemic heart disease—15.7% of deaths)
  – Respiratory disease (COPD—10% of deaths)
  – Cerebrovascular accidents
  – Lower respiratory tract infection
  – Diarrhea
  – Tuberculosis
  – Chronic kidney disease
  – Neonatal preterm birth-related problems
  – Road traffic accident.
❖ Adult young men: Most commonly die due to road traffic accident
❖ Adult young female: Most commonly die due to suicide (most common method hanging).

RECENT UPDATES IN NUTRITION

Healthy Diet

Definition of healthy diet in adult (as per WHO recommendation 2015):

❖ Fruits, vegetables, legumes (e.g., lentils, beans), nuts and whole grains (e.g., unprocessed maize, millet, oats, wheat, brown rice).
❖ At least 400 g (5 portions) of fruits and vegetables a day. Potatoes, sweet potatoes, cassava and other starchy roots are not classified as fruits or vegetables.
❖ Less than 10% of total energy intake from free sugars which is equivalent to 50 g (or around 12 level teaspoons) for a person of healthy body weight consuming approximately 2000 calories per day, but ideally less than 5% of total energy intake for additional health benefits. Most free sugars are added to foods or drinks by the manufacturer, cook or consumer, and can also be found in sugars naturally present in honey, syrups, fruit juices and fruit juice concentrates.
❖ Less than 30% of total energy intake from fats.
  Unsaturated fats (e.g., found in fish, avocado, nuts, sunflower, canola and olive oils) are preferable to saturated fats (e.g., found in fatty meat, butter, palm and coconut oil, cream, cheese, ghee and lard). Industrial trans fats (found in processed food, fast food, snack food, fried food, frozen pizza, pies, cookies, margarines and spreads) are not part of a healthy diet.
❖ Less than 5 g of salt (equivalent to approximately 1 teaspoon) per day and use iodized salt.

Definition of healthy diet for infants and young children (as per WHO recommendation 2015):

In the first 2 years of a child's life, optimal nutrition fosters healthy growth and improves cognitive development. It also reduces the risk of becoming overweight or obese and developing NCDs later in life.

Advice on a healthy diet for infants and children is similar to that for adults, but the following elements are also important:

❖ Infants should be breastfed exclusively during the first 6 months of life.
❖ Infants should be breastfed continuously until 2 years of age and beyond.
❖ From 6 months of age, breast milk should be complemented with a variety of adequate, safe and nutrient dense complementary foods. Salt and sugars should not be added to complementary foods.

FAMILY PLANNING RELATED UPDATES

The National Family Planning Programme introduced three new methods to expand contraceptive choices:

Injectable contraceptive (DMPA)	3 monthly DMPA under Antara Programme
Chhaya/Saheli	Centchroman once a week nonhormonal pill
Progesterone only pill	For lactating mothers

MISCELLANEOUS RECENT UPDATES

Antibiotic resistance red line:
- ❖ To curb antibiotic resistance
- ❖ Cannot be obtained without prescription.

Environmental friendly activities undertaken by Government of India:
- ❖ Plastic bags <50 microns is banned (earlier 40)
- ❖ Swachh Bharat Abhiyan.

SWACHH BHARAT ABHIYAN

Introduction

Swachh Bharat Abhiyan was announced by honorable Prime Minister of India on Indian Independence Day and launched on 2 October 2014, 145th birth anniversary of Mahatma Gandhi. The Government of India has aimed to make India a clean India by 2nd of October 2019 (means 150th birth anniversary of the Mahatma Gandhi) through this campaign.

Goal

To achieve "Swachh Bharat" by 2019.

Aim

- ❖ Stamp out open defecation system
- ❖ Eliminate manual scavenging
- ❖ Convert insanitary toilets into clean flush toilets
- ❖ Strengthen the sanitation system in urban and rural areas
- ❖ Motivate and spread cleanliness awareness among people.

Activities

Swachh Bharat Mission (Urban)

- ❖ Under the programme, community toilets will be built in residential areas where it is difficult to construct individual household toilets.
- ❖ Public toilets will also be constructed in designated locations such as tourist places, markets, bus stations, railway stations, etc.
- ❖ The program will be implemented over a five-year period and will include:
  - – Solid waste management
  - – Construction of individual household toilets

- Construction of community toilets
- Public awareness campaigns.

Swachh Bharat Mission (Gramin)

This programme includes:

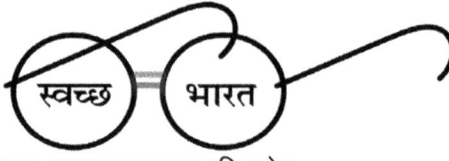

- ❖ Construction of individual household toilets
- ❖ To provide water availability for storing, hand-washing and cleaning of toilets
- ❖ To convert waste into wealth in rural India in the forms of bio-fertilizer and different forms of energy
- ❖ To motivate Communities and Panchayati Raj Institutions to adopt sustainable sanitation practices and facilities through awareness creation and health education.

Kayakalp Programme

- ❖ Part of Swachh Bharat Abhiyan
- ❖ Encouraging sanitation at public health facilities in country.

Performances

As of January 2021: Total sanitation coverage throughout India has raised to 99.95% from 38.70% in October 2014.

AYUSHMAN BHARAT

Ayushman Bharat, a flagship scheme of Government of India, was launched as recommended by the National Health Policy 2017, to achieve the vision of Universal Health Coverage (UHC). This initiative has been designed to meet Sustainable Development Goals (SDGs) and its underlining commitment, which is to "*leave no one behind*".

Ayushman Bharat is an attempt to move from sectoral and segmented approach of health service delivery to a comprehensive *need-based health care service*. This scheme aims to undertake path breaking interventions to holistically address the healthcare system (covering prevention, promotion and ambulatory care) at the primary, secondary and tertiary level. Ayushman Bharat adopts a continuum of care approach, comprising of two inter-related components, which are:

- ❖ Health and Wellness Centers (HWCs)
- ❖ Pradhan Mantri Jan Arogya Yojana (PM-JAY)

Health and Wellness Centers (HWCs)

In February 2018, the Government of India announced the creation of 1,50,000 Health and Wellness Centers (HWCs) by transforming the existing subcenters and primary health centers. These centers are to deliver **Comprehensive Primary Health Care (CPHC)** bringing healthcare closer to the homes of people. They cover both, maternal and child health services and noncommunicable diseases, including **free essential drugs and diagnostic services**.

Health and Wellness Centers are envisaged to deliver an expanded range of services to address the primary healthcare needs of the entire population in their area, expanding access, universality and equity close to the community. The emphasis of health promotion and prevention is designed to bring focus on keeping people healthy by engaging and empowering individuals and communities to choose healthy behaviors and make changes that reduce the risk of developing chronic diseases and morbidities.

Pradhan Mantri Jan Arogya Yojana (PM-JAY)

The second component under Ayushman Bharat is the Pradhan Mantri Jan Arogya Yojna or PM-JAY as it is popularly known. This scheme was launched on 23rd September, 2018 in Ranchi, Jharkhand by the Hon'ble Prime Minister of India.

Ayushman Bharat PM-JAY is the largest health assurance scheme in the world which aims at providing a health cover of ₹ 5 lakhs per family per year for secondary and tertiary care hospitalization to over 10.74 crores poor and vulnerable families (approximately 50 crore beneficiaries) that form the bottom 40% of the Indian population. The households included are based on the deprivation and occupational criteria of Socio-Economic Caste Census 2011 (SECC 2011) for rural and urban areas respectively. PM-JAY is fully funded by the Government and cost of implementation is shared between the Central and State Governments.

Key Features and Benefits of PM-JAY

❖ PM-JAY is the world's largest health insurance/assurance scheme fully financed by the government.
❖ It provides a cover of ₹ **5 lakhs per family per year** for secondary and tertiary care hospitalization across public and private empaneled hospitals in India.
❖ Over **10.74 crore** poor and vulnerable entitled families (approximately 50 crore beneficiaries) are eligible for these benefits.
❖ PM-JAY provides **cashless access to healthcare services** for the beneficiary at the hospital.
❖ It covers **up to 3 days of prehospitalization and 15 days posthospitalization expenses** such as diagnostics and medicines.
❖ There is no restriction on the family size, age or gender.
❖ All pre-existing conditions are covered from day one. This means that any eligible person suffering from any medical condition before being covered by PM-JAY will now be able to get treatment for all those medical conditions as well under this scheme right from the day they are enrolled.
❖ Benefits of the scheme are portable across the country, i.e., a beneficiary can visit any empaneled public or private hospital in India to avail cashless treatment.
❖ Services include approximately 1,393 procedures covering all the costs related to treatment, including but not limited to drugs, supplies, diagnostic services, physician's fees, room charges, surgeon charges, OT and ICU charges, etc.:
  – Medical examination, treatment and consultation
  – Prehospitalization
  – Medicine and medical consumables
  – Nonintensive and intensive care services
  – Diagnostic and laboratory investigations
  – Medical implantation services (where necessary)
  – Accommodation benefits
  – Food services
  – Complications arising during treatment
  – Posthospitalization follow-up care up to 15 days
❖ Public hospitals are reimbursed for the healthcare services at par with the private hospitals.

Special Notes

A. Water availability:
   - 7.6% crore in India deprived of safe drinking water (5% of Indian population)
   - Highest in the world.
B. Cigarette package warning:
   - From 1st April 2016 India made 85% on both sides of cigarette packet mandatory for tobacco products
   - WHO has now advised for plain packaging of tobacco from 31st May
   - Tobacco is responsible for 40–50% of cancers.

Other Important Updates

❖ From 1st April 2017 India will move Bharat Stage IV emission norm fuels.
❖ Yellow fever vaccine validity now life long
❖ Government has linked aadhar to school mid-day meals
❖ 90% of India has a 12 digit identity (**Aadhar card**)
❖ United funds for subcenter increased to INR 20,000 per month
❖ **NeHA**: Stands for *"National e-health Authority"*
   It is used for digitization of health information
❖ No liquor shops will be in 500 meters from highway.

IMPORTANT PUBLIC HEALTH DAYS

Month	Date	Day
January	Last Sunday	World Leprosy Eradication Day
February	4	World Cancer Day
	10	National Deworming Day
March	16	Measles Immunization Day
	24	World TB Day
April	25	World Malaria Day
	Last week (24th–30th)	World Immunization Week
May	16th (Recent update)	National Dengue Day
	28th	International Women's Health Day/International Menstrual Hygiene Day
	31st	World No Tobacco Day
June	5th	World Environment Day
	21st (Recent update)	International Day of Yoga
July	1st	National Doctors Day
August	1st–7th	World Breastfeeding Week
October	Whole month	Breast Cancer Awareness Month
	10th	World Mental Health Day
	24th	World Polio Day
November	10th	World Immunization Day
December	1st	World AIDS Day

Drug of Choice for Some Important Communicable Diseases

Disease/condition	Drug of choice
First line therapy for visceral leishmaniasis/ kala-azar	Liposomal amphotericin B
River blindness (onchocerciasis)	Ivermectin
Scabies (also children and pregnant women)	5% permethrin single overnight application
Uncomplicated gonococcal infection	Single dose ceftriaxone IM (or) oral cefixime + single dose azithromycin/doxycycline
Lymphogranuloma venereum (LGV)	Doxycycline
Donovanosis	Azithromycin
Syphilis	Benzathine penicillin G
Neurosyphilis	Aqueous penicillin G
Congenital syphilis	Penicillin G
Meningococcal meningitis cases and carriers	Injection ceftriaxone
Cholera in adult	Doxycycline
Cholera in children	Azithromycin
Cholera in pregnancy	Azithromycin
Cholera in doxycycline resistant area	Ciprofloxacin
Cholera chemoprophylaxis	Tetracycline
Plague	Streptomycin
Plague chemoprophylaxis	Tetracycline
Whooping cough chemoprophylaxis	Erythromycin
Leptospirosis Anthrax Actinomycosis Trench bite Rat bite fever	Penicillin
Leptospirosis	Doxycycline
Neurocysticercosis	Albendazole
Pneumonia	Cotrimoxazole

Contd...

Contd...

Disease/condition	Drug of choice
Epidemic typhus	
Endemic typhus	Tetracycline
Q fever	
Trachoma	Azithromycin
Brucellosis	Doxycycline + Streptomycin
Pertussis	Erythromycin
Typhoid in pregnancy	Ceftriaxone
Severe/complicated malaria (also in pregnancy)	Injectable artesunate
Malaria in pregnancy	Chloroquine
Prevention of HIV transmission from mother to child	Nevirapine in low risk infants and Zidovudine + Nevirapine in high risk infants
Treatment of newborn when mother has active TB and taking ATT	BCG + INH for 6 weeks + breastfeeding
Prophylaxis of diphtheria contacts	Erythromycin

Most common neonatal disease screened	Congenital hypothyroidism
Most common opportunistic infection in AIDS in India	Tuberculosis
Most common opportunistic infection in AIDS in world	Bacterial pneumonia
Most common parasitic infection in AIDS	*Cryptosporidium parvum*
Most common cancer seen in AIDS	Lymphoma (MC: Diffuse large B cell lymphoma)
Most common cause of meningitis in AIDS patient	*Cryptococcus*
Most common cancer in Indian males	Cancer of lip and oral cavity
Most common cancer in Indian females	Breast cancer
Most common cause of death among Indian geriatrics above 70 years of age	Cardiovascular disease
Most common disorder in post disaster phase	Gastroenteritis
Most common mental disorder causing DALY loss	Unipolar depression
Most common psychiatric disorder in India/world	Major depression
Most common age group of major depression	Middle-aged females
Most common gram-positive organism causing meningitis	*Streptococcus pneumoniae*
Most common gram-negative organism causing meningitis	*Neisseria meningitidis*
Most common source of meningococcal meningitis	Carrier
Most common hepatitis virus transmitted perinatally	HBV
Most common time of perinatal transmission of HBV	Time of delivery
Most common virus associated with transfusion hepatitis	HCV
Most common organ affected in visceral leishmaniasis	Spleen
Most common STD worldwide	Genital herpes (HSV2)
Most common organism causing STD in India	*Chlamydia trachomatis*
Most common virus causing diarrhea in infants	Rotavirus
Most common chronic occupational lung disease in world	Silicosis
Most common age group of rheumatic fever	5–15 years
Most common complication of pregnancy in India	Anemia
Most common complication of IUCD	IUD expulsion
Most common cause of failure of vasectomy	Mistaken identification of vas deferens
Most common cause of chronic hepatitis/cirrhosis	Hepatitis B

Contd...

Contd...

Most common cause of fulminant hepatitis in pregnancy	Hepatitis E
Most common cause of hepatic encephalopathy in pregnancy	
Most common cause of infant mortality in world	Prematurity
Most common cause of infant mortality in India	Low birth weight and prematurity
Most common cause of early neonatal mortality in India	Preterm birth
Most common cause of late neonatal mortality in India	Infections
Most common cause of under 5 mortality in India	Pneumonia
Most common cause of traveller's diarrhea in infants	Enterotoxigenic *E. coli* (ETEC)
Most common cause of heart disease in 5–30 years age group globally	Rheumatic fever
Most common complication of chicken pox in children	Secondary bacterial infection
Most common complication of measles in children	Otitis media
Most common presentation of polio	Subacute/inapparent infection
Most common site of scabies	Interdigital space and anterior wrist
Most common site of oral cancer worldwide	Lateral border of tongue
Most common site of oral cancer in India	Alveobuccal complex

Index

A

Aadhar card 606
Abdominal pain 402
Abdominal tenderness 98
Abortion 385, 450
  incomplete 187
  mid-trimester 187
  safe 88, 569
  spontaneous 197, 299
  unsafe 109, 449
Accident 120, 290, 449, 450
Accredited Social Health Activist 86
  scheme 86, 253
  worker
    responsibilities of 86, 253
    role of 86, 253
Acculturation 202
  barriers of 203
  effects of 203
Acellular pertussis DPT vaccine 357
Acids 154
Acne, mild to moderate 397
Acquired immunodeficiency syndrome 104, 272, 286, 589
  control 287
Actinomycosis 607
Acute flaccid paralysis 533
  background rate of 533
  selection of 534
  surveillance 533, 535
    purpose of 534
    reasons for 534
  syndrome of 534
Acute infection 112
Acute respiratory disease
  control 567
  syndrome 503, 504
Acute respiratory infection 106, 107
AD syringe 375
Additional manpower resources 107, 110, 113, 117, 121, 129

Adenomyosis 398
Adequate stool sample 537
Adjuvant therapy 392
Administration, signs of 36, 164, 351
Adolescent Friendly Health Clinics services, package of 181, 574
Adolescent health 574
  care 88
  program 180
Adolescent Reproductive and Sexual Health Program 181, 574
Adult literacy 199
Adverse events following immunization 346
  cause-specific categorization of 346
  monitoring, importance of 348
  surveillance 349
Aedes aegypti 285
  index 285
Aerosol-generating procedures, airborne precautions for 512
African tick paralysis 330
African trypanosomiasis 177, 178
Age-sex pyramid 183, 184
  use of 184
Age-specific death rate 441
Age-specific fertility rate 58
Ageusia 501
Air pollution
  index 205
  indicators of 205, 206
Albendazole 219, 607
Alcohol 35, 179
  consumption 203
  control of 42
Alcoholism 102, 158, 311
Alkalis 154
All India Blind Relief Society 251
All India Women's Conference 251
Allergic disease, severe 402
Aluminium phosphate 355

Alum-precipitated toxoid 356
Alveobuccal complex 610
Ambulatory care 115
Amenorrhea 398
Amniotomy 187
Amoebiasis 218, 219
Amphixenosis 175
Amphotericin B 33
Amplifier host 278
Anaerobic biofilters 209
Analytical epidemiology 327
Anaphylaxis 347
Anatomy, father of 1
Ancylostoma duodenale 589
Anemia 83, 101, 109, 135, 136, 311, 393, 397, 420, 449, 450, 451, 609
  severe 112, 188
Anemia Mukt Bharat campaign 200
Anesthesia 188, 294, 479
Anganwadi worker 87, 93, 106, 109, 113, 117, 125, 129, 133, 141, 144, 323
Angular stomatitis 127
Animal anatomical waste 586
Ankle edema 139
Annual parasite incidence 284
Anopheles mosquito 2
Anorexia 98, 372
Anosmia 501
Antenatal care, objectives of 560
Antenatal check-up 254, 291
Antenatal factors 67
Antenatal services 560
Antenatal visits 560
Anterior wrist 610
Anthrax 1, 175, 607
Anthropometric examination 74
Anthropozoonosis 175
Antibiotics 357
Antibodies 340
Antilarval measures 97, 99
Antirabies vaccine, intradermal regimes of 286

Antiretroviral therapy 597
Antitubercular treatment 550
Anxiety 63, 120, 217
Apgar score 565
Apneic spells 487
Appetite, loss of 501
Appropriate technology 85, 249
Aqueous penicillin G 607
Argemone oil, detection of 72
Artemisinin-based combination
    therapy 580
Artesunate, injectable 608
Arthralgia 28, 29
Arthropod borne infections 589
Ascariasis 589
Ascaris lumbricoides 589
Asherman's syndrome 392
Asthma 83, 311, 451
Atherosclerosis 194
Autism 275
Autoimmune response 411
Autoimmunity 2
Auxiliary nurse midwife 93, 106,
    109, 113, 117, 121, 125, 129,
    133, 137, 141, 144, 491
Awareness programme 108
Axillary temperature 484
AYUSH 251
Ayushman Bharat 604, 605
Azithromycin 476, 478, 607, 608

B

Baby-friendly hospital
    initiative 189
Bacillary dysentery 218, 219
Bacillus anthracis 175
Bacillus Calmette-Guérin 349, 354
    osteitis 347
    vaccination 354
    vaccine 162, 351-353
Backache, lower 476, 478
Backwardness 203
Bacterial infection 520, , 521
    secondary 610
Bacterial pneumonia 609
Bacteriological examination 38
Bacteriological index 39
Bacteriology, father of 1
Balanced diet 438
    essential components of 302
Bar diagram 460, 462
Barrier
    methods 385, 494
    types of 243

Basal body temperature 405
    method 385
Basic sanitation 128
Battered baby syndrome 193, 438
Bedaquiline 555
Behavioral disease 271
Behavioral therapy 314
Below poverty line 593
Beneficiaries, movement of 573
Benzathine penicillin G 607
Berksonian bias 10
Betel quid 42
BG Prasad scale, modified 467
Bharadwaj scale 467
Bharat Sevak Samaj 250
Bhore committee 247
    report 248
Bioactive intrauterine
    devices 390
Biochemical tests 76
Biohazard symbol 492
Biological pond 221
Biological transmission 168
Biology, father of 1
Biomedical waste 439, 585
    color coding of 307
    containers, label for 587
    improper handling of 308
    management 585
    rules 585
        contents of 585
    tracking, importance of 224
    types of 225
Biotechnology 587
Biphasic pill 396
Birth 63, 291
    asphyxia 487
    control
        method 381
        role in 405
    injury 106
    rate 58
    registration 314
    spacing 115, 135
    weight 186, 496
Bitot's spot 127, 372
Bivalent oral polio vaccine 599
Bladder 83, 311
Bleeding 401, 493
    disturbances 398
Blindness 52, 234, 601
    causes of 52
    controlling of 52, 53
    major causes of 52
    under national programme for
        control of blindness 52

Block medical officer of health 20,
    93, 106, 108, 109, 113, 117,
    121, 125, 129, 133, 137, 141,
    144
    duties of 90, 96 105, 108, 112, 116,
        124, 127, 132, 135, 140, 144
    functions of 90, 91, 95
    role of 120, 136
    writing duties of 92
Block primary health nurse 93,
    106, 109, 113, 117, 121, 125,
    129, 133, 137, 141, 144
Block sanitary inspector 93, 106,
    109, 113, 117, 121, 125, 129,
    133, 137, 141, 144
Blood
    cells, cancers of 83
    clotting 398
    disorder 311
    groups, distribution of 463
    pressure 43, 216, 473
        classification of 435
    smear 101
    tests 103
    transfusion 188, 294
Blueberry muffin spots 274
Body
    mass index 178, 290
    parts of 37
Bone marrow aspiration 101
Bordetella pertussis 588
Bore hole latrine 210
Borrelia burgdorferi 175
Borrelia duttoni 330
Botany, father of 1
Brain-tissue vaccines 172
Break point chlorination 305
    achievement of 207, 305, 306
Breast
    cancer 398, 450, 609
        awareness month 606
    carcinoma promoting factor 455
    disorders, benign 397
    milk 471
    tenderness 398, 402
    tumor 455
Breastfeeding 416, 493
    benefits of 188
    position 471
    promotion of 47
    types of 471
Breath, shortness of 501
Broken
    bones 193
    family 64, 102
Brucellosis 197, 608

Bruises 193
Bubonic plague 589
Bulbar polio 27
Bulbospinal polio 27
Burning sensation 477
Burns 193

C

Cafeteria choice 383
    principle of 383
Calcivirus 588
Calculate maternal mortality ratio
    449, 450, 451
Calendar method 407
Calorie 201
Cancer 194, 234, 289
    breast 398
    danger signs of 41, 180
    genitals 398
    lip 609
    oral cavity 609
Capitulum 330
Carbohydrate deficiency 155
Carbon monoxide 206
Carcinogenesis 398
Cardiac abnormalities 398
Cardiac failure 73
Cardiovascular disease 398, 602,
    609
CARE India 255
Carriers
    importance of 162
    types of 161
Cartridge based nucleic acid
    amplification test 546, 547
Case control 7, 8
    study 8, 10, 265, 328
        advantages of 10, 11
        disadvantages of 10, 11
Case fatality rate 6, 158, 159, 442
Case finding methods 21
Cash assistance, payment of 570
Cataract 52, 275
Category-wise vector control
    measures 584
Cefixime 219, 476, 478
Ceftriaxone 219, 607, 608
Cellular fragment vaccine 345
Census 436, 472
Centchroman 402
Central Government Health
    Scheme 252
Central Maternity Benefit Act 79

Central Social Welfare Board 250
Cerebral palsy 275, 453
Cerebral thrombosis 398
Cerebrovascular accidents 602
Cervical cancer 398
Cervical hyperplasia 402
Cervical motion tenderness 478
Cervical mucus method 385, 406
Cervical tears, repair of 187
Cesarean section 187
Chagas disease 176, 177
Chemical
    hazards 229
    liquid waste 587
    methods 384, 388
    reactions 221
    waste 225, 586
Chemoprophylaxis 20, 514, 583
    short-term 583
Chemotherapy 2, 280, 548, 582
Chest
    pressure in 501
    X-ray 546, 547
Chickenpox 1, 274, 443, 588, 590,
    610
Chikungunya 283
    fever 589
    virus 589
Child death rate 447
Child health 559
    care 88
Child labor 468
Child mortality rates 446
Child nutrition 257
Child survival and safe
    motherhood 339, 371
    program 64
Child's growth curve, direction of
    192, 297
Childhood illnesses, integrated
    management of 569
Chills 28
Chlamydia 274, 475
    trachomatis 609
Chlorination 206, 208, 305
    phases of 207
Chlorine 304, 305
    action of 206
    dose 207
    residuals 207
Chloroquine 254, 291, 608
Cholera 120, 218, 219, 234, 449,
    588, 590, 607
    chemoprophylaxis 607
    vibrio 2

Cholestatic jaundice 398
Christian missionaries 321
Chromosomal abnormality 112,
    195
Chronic noncommunicable
    disease, epidemiology of
    41, 288
Ciprofloxacin 219, 607
Cirrhosis 609
Citizens forum 321
Classroom hunger 72, 202
Clinical laboratory waste 587
Clinical trial, heart of 263
Clofazimine 21, 22, 171, 480
Clostridium tetani 589
Cluster sample 240
CO poisoning 229
Cognitive-behavioral therapy 314
Cohort studies 7, 8, 328
Cold
    box 379
    chain 375
    shock 228
    storage 492
    water hazards 228
Coliform organisms 306
Colitis 64
Colorectal cancer 398
Combined methods 384, 388
Combined oral contraceptive pills,
    adverse effects of 398
Combined pill 385, 401
Combined vaccine 344, 345
Common cold 161
Common homemade oral
    rehydration salt 170
Common peroneal nerve 480
Communicable diseases 433, 607
    epidemiology of 17, 168, 269
    prevention of 190
Communication 83, 130, 181, 241,
    316, 574
    barriers of 242
    channels of 241, 242
    types of channels of 242
Community 74, 265
    diagnosis 148, 324, 325, 431
    health
        care of 84, 249, 320
        center 54, 451
    intervention 29
    medicine 259, 431, 609
    members, importance of 227
    need assessment 88
    oriented activities 23

participation 84, 249
treatment 431
Complicated malaria 582, 608
    chemotherapy of 582
Comprehensive primary health
    care 604
Comprehensive village health
    plan, development of 254
Condom 56, 59, 254, 291, 383-386,
    417
    non-contraceptive use of 387
    promotion 104
    proper use of 386
    types of 387
Confusion 502
Congenital anomalies 106, 274
Congenital defects 234
Congenital rubella syndrome 600
Conjunctival xerosis 371, 372
Conjunctivitis 481, 501
Constructional strategies 54
Consumption unit 468
Contagious disease 432
Contaminated waste 586
Contamination 431
Continuous data 473
Continuous water supply 470
Contraception 88, 232, 381
    methods of 55, 384, 406
Contraceptive
    benefits 397
    choices 603
    methods 383, 493, 414
        advantages of 58, 59, 417
        choice of 59
        disadvantages of 58, 59,
            417
        evaluation of 414
    pills
        benefits of 397
        usage 553
Contractures, prevention of 24
Control epidemic dropsy 72
Control measures,
        implementation of 94, 96,
            97, 99, 101, 103, 105, 131
Conventional contraceptives 383,
    385
Conventional vasectomy 410
Convulsions 45, 46, 527
Cord, condition of 106
Corneal blindness 52
Corneal ulcer 372, 481
Corneal xerosis 372

Corticosteroids 550
    therapy 374
Corynebacterium diphtheriae 588
Cost-benefit analysis 338
Cost-effective analysis 338
Cotrimoxazole 607
Cough 504
Couple protection rate 59, 132,
    382, 383, 493
Covaxin 514
COVID-19 499, 500, 502, 504, 505,
    510
    care of 517
    diagnosis of 505, 507
    disease, severe 516
    infection, diagnose active 506
    management of 516
    mild 515
    moderate 515
    prevention of 510
    sentinel surveillance 504
    symptoms of 501
    test 505
    treatment protocols for 515
    vaccination
        current status of 513
        precautionary guidelines
            for 513
    vaccines 512
        first beneficiaries of 512
Covishield 513
CoVs
    genre of 499
    structure of 499
    types of 499
Cowpox 342
Coxsackie virus 274
Crime 204
Criticism 152
Cross infection 327
Cross-sectional study 265, 328
Croup 481
Crude birth rate 444, 447
Crude death rate 5, 441
Cryptococcus 609
Cryptosporidium parvum 609
Curve, direction of 192, 297
Custodial separation 385
Cystic fibrosis 232, 313

D

Danger signs 41, 180

Danida 321
Dapsone 21, 22, 171, 480
Data 473
    analysis 13, 31, 91, 92, 124
    collection 92, 124, 148
        methods of 149
        procedure of 474
        tools of 149
Dawson's disease 481
Dawson's encephalitis 481
Day carriers 379
Death 63, 106, 228, 291
Deep well 336, 337
Deformities, prevention of 24
Dehydration 49, 524
    mild 219
    severe 219, 525
Delamanid, use of 555
Delayed immunization 373
Delayed motor milestones
    196, 299
Delivery device 516
Delivery services 187, 293
Deltavirus 588
Demographic cycle 183
Demography 55, 182, 291, 436
Dengue 29, 97, 177, 178, 190, 283,
    589
    clinical presentation of 99
Depo medroxy progesterone
    acetate 57
Depot formulations 60, 385, 403,
    418
Depression 120, 194
Dermatitis 311
Descriptive epidemiology 327
Determinants, assessment of 95-
    97, 102
Diabetes 194
    epidemiology 288
    mellitus 178, 188, 44, 288,
        398
        diagnostic criteria of 44, 45
        management of 44, 45
        risk factors of 178
Diagnostic test 16, 336
Dial thermometer 491
Diaphragm 59, 384, 385, 387, 417
Diarrhea 73, 106, 218, 254, 291,
    426, 443, 501, 518, 519, 522,
    523, 530, 531, 602
    management of 282
    persistent 531
    treatment for 281, 424

Diazepam 46, 527
Diet survey 76
  methods of 76
Dietary fiber 179, 302
Dietary goals 438
Dietary intake, assessment of 76
Different biomedical waste
  disposal of 225
  treatment of 225
Diffuse large B cell lymphoma 609
Diloxanide furoate 219
Diphtheria 197, 217, 349, 588, 590
  contacts, prophylaxis of 608
  immunization, types of 356
  pertussis and tetanus vaccine
    355, 356
  tetanus vaccine 357
  toxoid 355
Dipylidium caninum 175
Directly Observed Treatment,
  Short-course 279
  components of 543
Disability 23, 326, 430
  adjusted life year 152, 429
  limitation 22, 24, 27
  prevention of 23
Disaster 439
  cycle, phases in 226
  management 225, 309, 439
  preparedness 226, 227, 439
    implementation strategy of
    228
    WHO strategy for 227
  vaccination in 229
Discarded medicines 586
Disease
  anatomical site of 433, 544
  biological transmission of 168
  carrier state of 262
  chronic 513
  control 325, 429
  elimination 325, 430
  eradication 325, 430
  germ theory of 1
  iceberg concept of 155
  natural history of 156, 157, 429
  prevalence 21
  routes of transmission of 214
  screening for 15, 266
  severe 503
  specific death rate 6
Disinfection, process of 206
Dispersion 315

Disposable delivery kit 254, 291,
  422, 323
  supply of 119
District Blindness Control
  Society 54
District immunization officer 535
Dizziness 225, 402, 501
DNA vaccination 345
Domestic violence 451
Domiciliary care 563
Donovanosis 607
Dorsal shield 330
Doxycycline 477, 478, 583, 607,
  608
Drain 213
Drinking water 208
Drowning 228
Drug
  abuse 203, 204
  addiction 158
    treatment of 314
  dosages 549
  resistance 434, 544
  schedule 579, 580
Drug-sensitive-tuberculosis
  treatment 548
Drug-resistant tuberculosis
  programmatic management of
    547
  treatment of 555
Drug-susceptible tuberculosis 554
Dry skin 372
Drying process 296
Dug well latrine 210, 211
Dust 205
Dye 83
Dysentery 120, 262
  follow-up of 531
Dysmenorrhea 397, 476, 478
Dyspareunia 476, 478
Dyspnea 73
Dysuria 476, 478

E

Ear infection 519
Early neonatal mortality rate 444
Eclampsia 187, 449, 450, 451
Ecological factors, evaluation
  of 15
Ectopic pregnancy 397, 416, 493
Edema 127
Education 4, 130, 181, 257, 574
Educational qualifications 467

Egg
  allergies 341
  protein 303
Electrocution 228
Electrolytes 283
Electronic vaccine intelligence
  network 351
Eligible couple 382, 493
Embryology, father of 1
Emergency
  care 190
  contraception 400
    aims of 400
  contraceptive pills 181, 574
  obstetric care 65
Emotional immaturity 102
Emphysema 194
Employees State Insurance Act
  79, 80
  corporation 80
  hospitals 54
Encephalitis 365
Encephalopathy 347, 357
Endemic cretinism 196, 299
Endemic typhus 608
Endometrial cancer 398
  risk of 392
Endometriosis 398
Enteroviruses 274, 588
Entomological factors, evaluation
  of 31
Environment 77, 205, 303
Environmental sanitation 199
Enzyme-linked immunosorbent
  assay 481
Enzymes 155
EPID number 538
  components of 538
Epidemic 11, 159
  confirmation of existence of
    13, 30, 92
  curve 160
    application of 160
  frequency 30
  investigation of 11, 13
  types of 11, 160
  typhus 175, 608
Epidemiological methods
  7, 261
Epidemiological studies 7, 8
  classification of 7
  types of 262
Epidemiological triad 154, 429

Epidemiology 7, 158, 431
  father of 1
  principle of 7, 261
Epilepsy 398
Epithelium, hyperkeratinization
    of 372
Ergonomics 81, 231
  objectives of 231
Erythromycin 607, 608
Erythroplakia 42
Essential newborn care 567
Essential obstetric care 65
Ethambutol 549
Exclusive breastfeeding 471
Experimental vaccine 344
Expired medicines 586
Explosive outbreaks 278
Extrapulmonary tuberculosis 434,
    547
Extrinsic incubation period 329
Eye
  health 53
    services 190
  pallor of 139
  problems 275

F

Face-to-face communication 242
Facilitating healthy growth 72, 202
Factories Act 230
Factors influencing acculturation
    202
Family 62, 464
  and Child Welfare 257
  classification of 61
  cycle
    phases of 465
    stages of 60, 62, 465
  functions of 465
  head of 466
  member, chronic illness of 203
  Pension Scheme 79
  physician 147
    functions of 147
    role of 147
  planning 55, 88, 115, 291, 381,
      382, 436, 493
    advices 55, 415, 416, 493,
        494
    Association of India 250
    concept 339
    methods 494
    mode of intervention of 384
    recent updates in 385

related updates 603
scopes of 381
services, benefits of 384
unmet need of 184, 384
role of 60, 62
structure of 464
types of 60, 61, 464
welfare
  concept 339, 382
  services awareness 88
Fasciola
  hepatica 175
  infestation 175
Fast breathing 504
Fat 155
Fatigue 101, 229, 402, 501
Febrile seizures 347
Fecal contamination 306
Fecal disease transmission, routes
    of 210
Fecal-borne diseases, breaking
    transmission cycle of 303
Feeding
  difficulties 487
  recommendations 531
Female condom 384-387
Female sterilization 55, 60, 385,
    411, 419
Fertile period 407
Fertility
  indicators 58, 442
  return of 407
Fetus 340
Fever 101, 254, 274, 291, 354, 476,
    478, 501, 504, 519
  acute onset of 98
  hemorrhagic 330
  high grade 501
  treatment depots 173
Fibroadenoma 397
Fibrocystic disease 397
Field cancerization 43
Filariasis 278
First aid 190
  services 254, 291
First pregnancy, age of 115
First trimester, treatment in 581
First true epidemiologist,
    father of 1
First-line anti-tuberculosis
    drugs 549
  common adverse effects of 552
Fish tape worm 218
Fixing priorities 94, 107, 110, 114,
    130, 134, 138, 246

Flash method 197
Flavivirus 589
Flood 120
  health hazards of 228
Fluorescent leprosy antibody
    absorption test 40
Fluorine 300
Fluorosis, types of 300
Fly hazards 191
Folic acid 107, 420
Folk media 242
Follicular hyperkeratosis 372
Food
  adulteration 331
  enrichment 438
  fortification 331, 438
  hygiene 438
  intoxicants, types of 72
  poisoning 228
  safety 438
Forceps delivery 188, 453
Ford foundation 321
Formal education 257
Fostering social equality 72, 202
Fractured bones 193
Frequency distribution 459
  table 462
Frequency histogram 459
Frequency polygon 459, 560
Friction 155
Front load refrigerators 378
Frustration 217
Fulminant hepatitis 610
Funeral expenses 81

G

G6PD deficiency 232, 313
Gallbladder disease 398
Gambling 204
Gas hazards 228
Gastroenteritis 609
Gastrointestinal tract 372
Gender equity 72, 202
General danger signs 527
  check for 527
General fertility rate 58, 444
General marital fertility rate 58
Generation time 329
Genetic 232, 313
  abnormalities 195
  counseling 232, 313
    significance of 232, 313
  diseases 313

Genital
  herpes 609
  swelling 475
  ulcer 103, 475, 477
  wart 475
Genotoxic waste 224, 225
Geriatric
  population, health problems of 194
  preventive medicine in 64, 185, 292
Germ theory 1
Gestational age, small for 274
Giardiasis 218
Glaucoma 52, 73, 194, 275
Global Health Sector Strategy on Viral Hepatitis 600
Global Polio Eradication Initiative 599
Global Strategy for Women's, Children's and Adolescent's Health 596
Goals 338
  partnerships for 595
GOBI-FFF campaign 257
Goiter 196, 298, 299
Gonorrhea 262, 475
Good clinical trial, criteria for 263
Government health services, facilitation of utilization of 254
Gram stain 476
Greater auricular nerve 37
Grit 205
Gross domestic products 593
Gross reproduction rate 58
Group 243
  discussion 316, 318, 338
  model of 243
  matching 10
Growth
  chart 296, 495, 495, 497
    role of 296
  curve, direction of 497
  monitoring 123, 198, 296, 332
  retardation 372
Guillain-Barré syndrome 274, 347, 365
Guineaworm 218
Gynecology, preventive medicine in 437

H

Haemophilus influenzae 358
Hand pump 213
Handicap 326, 430
Handicapped children, education of 191
Hantavirus pulmonary syndrome 175
Hard physical labor 112
Hard tick 330
Hazards 224, 439
Headache 28, 29, 225, 398, 402, 501
Health 67, 77, 195, 205, 232, 257, 258, 295, 303, 313, 428
  and disease, concept of 3, 149, 258, 428
  and Wellness Centers 604
  appraisal 189
  assistant 121, 137
  care 84, 249, 320, 323
    planning 245
    waste 223
    workers 165, 511
  check-up 198
  determinants of 3, 4
  education 24, 135, 143, 191, 219, 289, 316-318, 336, 440
    communication for 83, 241, 316
  facility 187
  hazards 120, 228
  indicators of 4, 5
  information
    and basic biomedical statistics 83, 233, 314
    source of 233
  intersectoral action for 440
  mortality indicators of 5
  operational definition of 428
  planning
    and management 84, 245, 318
    steps of 245
  Programs in India 45, 180, 290
  promotion 511
  propaganda 317, 336
  related goals 595
  situation, analysis of 246
  statistics 440
Healthy diet 195, 602

Hearing
  defects 196, 299
  impairment 275
Heart
  disease 450, 610
  rate 216
Height 75, 127
Hemoglobinopathies 195
Hemolytic disease 106
Hemophilia 232, 313
Hemorrhage 109
  antepartum 449
  intraventricular 487
Hemorrhagic manifestations 28, 29
Henderson scale 467
Hepacivirus 588
Hepatic disorders 554
Hepatic encephalopathy 610
Hepatitis 229, 349
  A 120, 218, 588, 590
  B 262, 349, 588, 609
    birth dose of 369
    vaccine 164, 165, 368-370
    virus 345, 369
  C 456, 588
  chronic 609
  D 588
  E 120, 218, 588, 610
Hepatocellular adenoma 398
Hepatosplenomegaly 275
Herd immunity 341
  determinants of 341
Herpes zoster 590
High fever 28
High-temperature, short-time continuous method 197
Hind Kusht Nivaran Sangh 250
Hindu Ood of medicine, father of 1
Hirsutism 397
Histamine test 39
Holder method 197
Holligsheed scale 467
Homeopathy 2
  father of 1
Hookworm 589
  infection 219
  infestation 266
Hormonal contraceptives 60, 418
Hormonal methods 385, 395
Hormone 155
  replacement therapy 392
Hospital medicine 325

Hospital records 315
Hospital waste management 78, 223, 307, 439
Hospitalization 553
Host 431
  factors 32, 100
  types of 431
Housing 306, 468, 469
  standards 128
Human anatomical waste 586
Human development index 149-151, 429, 593
Human diploid cells 171
Human herpes virus 588
Human immunodeficiency virus 271, 286, 435, 554, 589, 597
  control 287
  pretest counseling of 272
  symptomatic 374
  transmission 287
    prevention of 608
Human rabies immunoglobulin 36
Hydatid disease 218
Hygiene 431
Hyperbilirubinemia 487
Hyperglycemia 398
Hyperlipidemia, congenital 398
Hypertension 63, 83, 288, 311, 398
  guidelines 43
  modifiable risk factors for 179
Hypertensive disorders, severe 187
Hyperventilation mediated reactions 348
Hypogammaglobulinemia 164
Hypoglycemia 487
Hypopigmented patches 37, 479
Hyporesponsive episode 347
Hypothermia 487
Hypothesis
  formulation of 15, 31, 91
  testing of 15, 91
Hypothyroid cretinism 196, 299
Hypothyroidism 196, 299
  congenital 609
Hypotonic episode 347

I

Iatrogenic infection 265
Ice lined refrigerator 376, 377
Ice pack 379, 490
Iceberg disease 288
  submerged part of 260

Iceberg phenomenon 156
  significance of 156, 260
Illiteracy 112
Illness 63
Immune disorder 341
Immunity 32, 188, 341, 356
  active 340
  cross 327
  herd 341
  passive 340
  types of 367
Immunization 89, 123, 198, 254, 291, 340, 342, 359, 362, 492, 512
  anxiety-related reaction 346, 348
  error-related reaction 346, 347
  expanded program of 535
Immunological test 40
Immunology, father of 1
Immunoprophylaxis 20
Immunosuppression 374
Impaired glucose tolerance 45
Impaired memory 194
Impairment 326, 430
Implementation strategy 228
Inactivated polio vaccine 351, 362, 599
Inapparent infection 610
Incidence 278, 335
Incubation period 329, 433, 588
Indian Council for Child Welfare 250
Indian Medical Association 251, 321
Indian Medicine, father of 1
Indian Red Cross Society 250, 254
Indian Surgery and Plastic Surgery, father of 1
Industrial accidents 312
Infant mortality 445
  rate 104, 444
Infections 109, 188, 224, 431, 487, 610
  chain of transmission of 265
  prevention control 517
  types of 224
Infectious disease 432, 597
Infectious waste 225
Infective dermatosis 164
Infestation 431
Influenza 217, 234, 504, 588, 590
Information 130, 181, 574
  education and communication activities 131
  campaign 139
  types of 149

Inguinal swelling 103
Injectable contraceptives under national program, recent updates in 403
Injury 63, 120, 367
Insecticide treated nets 29
Institutional care 563
Institutional delivery 65, 292
Integrase strand transfer inhibitor 597
Integrated Child Development Scheme 68, 197
  growth chart, interpretation of 191, 296
  scheme 87, 198
Integrated child development services 85
Integrated clinical case management, principle of 518
Integrated Counseling and Testing Center
  functions of 174
  location of 174
  target group of 174
Integrated disease surveillance projects 88
Integrated Management of Childhood Illness 518
  classification placement 48, 50
  clinical guidelines 518
  components of 518
  features of 519
  guidelines 518
Integrated vector management 176, 584
  goal of 176
  key elements of 176
Intensified national iron plus initiative 69, 199, 200
Interdigital space 610
Internal injuries 193
International Day of Yoga 606
International Ergonomics Association 439
International Health 89
  Organizations 254
International Menstrual Hygiene Day 606
International travelers 165
International Women's Health Day 606
Interpersonal communication 181, 242, 317, 574

Interpretation 151, 191, 241, 296
Intersectoral coordination 84, 91, 249, 251, 440
place of 252
Interval procedure 412
Intervention, modes of 24
Intestinal infections 588
Intracranial pressure 216
Intradermal schedule 172
Intramuscular regimes 286
Intramuscular schedules 172
Intranatal care 563
aims of 562
Intranatal factors 67
Intraocular tuberculosis 550
Intrauterine contraceptive devices 57
complications of 609
Intrauterine death 197, 299
Intrauterine device 60, 385, 389, 417
classification of 390
insertion of 391
non-contraceptive benefits of 392
types of 390
Intrauterine infection 112
Intravenous rehydration 219
Intrinsic educational value 72, 202
Intrinsic incubation period 329
Iodine deficiency disorder
public health significance of 298
spectrum of 196
Iodized salt, use of 70
Ion absorption, physiological basis of 424
Iron 107, 420
deficiency anemia 397
tablets 420
Irritability 194, 217, 502
Ischemic heart disease 602
Isolation 327, 510
duration of 590
period 588, 589
Isoniazid 549
preventive therapy 553
Ivermectin 607

J

Janani Shishu Suraksha Karyakaram 569, 571
Janani Suraksha Yojana 569
Japanese encephalitis 278, 589
incidence of 278

Jaundice 416, 494, 518
cholestatic 398
recent history of 402
Joint family 61, 465
advantages of 465
disadvantages of 465
Joint pain 501
Junior red cross 322
Juvenile delinquency 193, 437
prevention of 193
Juvenile Justice Act 601

K

Kala-azar 3, 100, 176, 177, 589
control of 31
elimination 33, 101
epidemiology of 31
first line therapy for 607
resurgence of 31, 34
Kangaroo mother care 115, 185
benefits of 186
eligibility criteria for 186
initiation of 186
stopping of 186
Kangaroo nutrition 186
Kayakalp programme 604
Keratomalacia 372
Kidney
disease 311
chronic 602
problems 83
Killed polio vaccine, injectable 362
Killed vaccine 343, 344
Koch's phenomenon 2
Koch's postulate 2
Kulshrestha scale 467
Kuppuswami scale, modified 467
Kwashiorkor 331

L

Laboratory tests 76
Lactational amenorrhea 189
method 406, 419
Laparotomy 187
Late neonatal mortality rate 444
Lateral popliteal nerve 37
Lead 83
time 167, 267, 432
concept of 167
Legal restriction 73
Leishmania donovani 589

Leishmaniasis
cutaneous 177
treatment protocol of 599
Lepromin test 40
Leprosy 19, 234, 276, 435, 589
case detection campaign 21
diagnosis of 37
diagnostic protocol of 20
management of 21, 41, 171
multidrug therapy for 21, 170, 171
treatment of 276
Leptospirosis 607
Lethal disease 269
Levonorgestrel 401
intrauterine devices 391
Life expectancy 5, 436
Life index, physical quality of 149, 150
Life table method 414
Lifestyle modifications, role of 45
Line probe assay 546
Lions clubs 321
Liposomal amphotericin B 33, 101, 607
Lips, pallor of 139
Liquid vaccine 351
Listeriosis 197
Literate 467
Live attenuated vaccine 342, 343, 344, 351
Live births, total number of 449
Liver
disease 311, 398
disorders 398
Living, level of 149
Local bacterial infection 518
Longitudinal studies 328
Long-term health benefits 189
Long-term program 248
Loose stool 47
Louse borne typhus 234
Low birth weight 106, 112, 437, 610
babies 112
proportion of 112
Low blood sugar 46, 527
Low couple protection rate 132
Low osmolarity ORS 282
Low socioeconomic status 112
Lower abdominal pain 103, 475, 476, 478
Lower respiratory tract infection 602

Lung
  active tuberculosis of 311
  disease, chronic 83, 311
Lyme disease 175
Lymph nodes, enlarged 477
Lymphadenitis, suppurative 347
Lymphatic filariasis 176-178, 589
Lymphogranuloma venereum 607
Lymphoma 609
Lyssavirus 589

M

Major depression 609
Major policies, targets of 560
Malaria 2, 96, 112, 172, 173, 175-
    178, 234, 262, 450, 589, 608
  active surveillance 172, 173
    components of 173
  control, setbacks of 285
  diagnosis for 576, 577
  salient points under diagnosis
    of 576
  severe 582, 608
  surveillance, objectives of 172
  treatment for 576, 577
Male condom 384-386
Male pill 403
Male sterilization 56, 60, 385, 409,
    418
Male vasectomy 56, 60, 418
Malformations, congenital 195
Malignant ovarian disease 397
Malnutrition 73, 106
  large number of 67
Manpower 113
  training 71, 201
Manual management 188, 294
Marasmus 331
Marital disharmony 203
Marriage
  age of 115
  pattern of 464
  sanction of 464
Mass
  communication 71, 201, 242
  media 119, 315
  strategy 288
Maternal and child health services
    562
  antenatal care 560
  components of 560
  objectives of 559
Maternal death 292, 450, 451
  causes of 292

Maternal diabetes 179
Maternal health 559
Maternal mortality
  rate 108, 293
  ratio 449, 450, 451
Maternity benefit 81
Mathematical representation 454
Maturation pond 221
Measles 229, 277, 342, 349, 588,
    590, 610
  elimination campaign,
    strategies of 169
  immunization day 606
  infection 270, 301
  rubella vaccine 600
  vaccination strategy, recent
    updates in 170
  vaccine 364-366
Mebendazole 219
Medical
  benefit 79, 80
  care 79, 320
  facilities provision 253
  management 187
  nutrition therapy 44, 45
  research team 455
  statistics 457
  Termination of pregnancy
    Act 403
    Rules 404
  treatment 314
Medicated intrauterine devices
    390
Medicine 1, 77, 202
  father of 1
Mefloquine 583
Meningococcal meningitis 229,
    588, 590, 607, 609
Menorrhagia 393
Menstrual hygiene scheme
    181, 575
Menstrual irregularities 476
Menstruation 397
Mental
  and emotional instability 203
  deficiency 299
  deficit 196
  disorders 217
  health 188, 190, 314
    Bill 601
  preparation 562
  retardation 275
  stress 229
Metabolic acidosis 487
Metabolic disorders 195
Metronidazole 219, 477, 478

Microbiology 587
  and Protozoology, father of 1
Microorganisms 154
Mid-arm circumference 75, 127
Mid-day meal 303, 457
  scheme 71, 201
    new guidelines for 202
    rationale of 71, 202
Migraine 398
Milk 303
  pasteurization of 197
Millennium development goals
    153, 540, 594
Miltefosine 33
Mini-lap operation 385
Minimeasles 365
Miscarriage 197, 299
Missed pills 397, 400
Mission Indradhanush 349
Mixed vaccine 345
Model 154, 209, 243
Modern physiology and
    experimental medicine,
    father of 1
Modern surgery, father of 1
Molds 229
Monitoring 430
  and evaluation 111, 115, 123,
    132, 135
  and surveillance 71, 140, 201
Monophasic pill 396
Morbidity 442
Morphological index 39
Mortality rates 441, 442
Mosquito
  bite 278
  breeding habits of 284
  types of 284
Mucosal ulcers 101
Multibacillary leprosy 20
Multidimensional family therapy
    314
Multidrug therapy 21, 38, 170
Multidrug-resistant tuberculosis
    280
Multiload 375 394
Multiorgan failure 504
Multiphase sample 239
Multiphasic screening 167
Multiple gestation 112
Multiple pregnancy 112
Multipurpose worker 93, 106, 109,
    113, 117, 125, 129, 133, 141,
    144
Mumps 342, 588, 590

Muscle
  pain 501
  wasting 127
  weakness 196, 299
Muscular dystrophy 232, 313
Myalgia 28, 29
Mycobacterium
  leprae 589
  tuberculosis 433, 546, 588
Myocardial infarction 234

N

Narrow birth space 112
Nasal congestion 501
Nasal smear 39
Nasal swab collection 507
Nasopharyngeal disease,
  moderate 482
National AIDS Control
  Programme 88
National Dengue Day 606
National Deworming Day 606
National Doctors Day 606
National Family Planning
  Programme 603
National Framework for Malaria
  Elimination in India 576,
  600
National Health Goals for
  Communicable and
  Noncommunicable
  Diseases 591
National Health Mission 591
National Health Policy 591
National Health Programmes 88
National Immunization Schedule
  349
National Iodine Deficiency
  Disorder Control
  Programme 70, 85, 200
National Leprosy Eradication
  Programme 21, 88
  guidelines 171
National Malaria Eradication
  Programme 34
National Operational Guidelines
  600
National Polio Surveillance Unit
  535
National Program for Control of
  Blindness 52, 88, 371
  and visual impairment 601
  structural organization of 54

National Program for Prevention
  and Control of Cancer,
  Diabetes, Cardiovascular
  Diseases and Stroke 88
National Program for Prevention
  of Nutritional Blindness 69,
  199, 371
National Rural Health Mission
  371
National Strategic Plan for
  Tuberculosis Elimination
  541
National Tuberculosis Control
  Programme performance
  542
National Vector Borne Disease
  Control Programme 29, 88
Natural family planning methods
  385, 405
Nausea 401, 501
Negative predictive value 433, 454
Neisseria meningitidis 588, 609
Neonatal deaths 448
  causes of 106
Neonatal health 89
Neonatal mortality 445
  rate 444
Neonatal preterm birth-related
  problems 602
Neonatal tetanus 116, 485
  prevention of 118, 323
Nephritis 83, 311
Nerve
  deafness 194
  thickening 479
Net reproduction rate 58, 383, 436
Neurocysticercosis 607
Neurological cretinism 196, 299
Neurological effects 196, 299
Neurosyphilis 607
Nevirapine 608
New Integrated Child
  Development Scheme
  growth chart 333
Night blindness 371, 372
Nitric acid test 72
Nitrogen dioxide 206
No scalpel vasectomy 385, 410
No touch insertion technique 394
Noise
  pollution
    effects of 215
    hazards of 214
    source of 215
Nomenclature 342

Nonchemical vector control
  methods 177
Noncommunicable disease 290,
  435, 601
  epidemiology of 178
  prevention of 288
Non-contraceptive benefits 392,
  397
Nonformal preschool education
  198
Nongonococcal urethritis 475
Non-medicated intrauterine
  devices 390
Norplant 385
Nuclear family 61, 465
  advantages of 465
  disadvantages of 465
Nucleoside reverse transcriptase
  inhibitor 597
Nutrition 67, 195, 257, 295, 438
  and Health Education 198
  recent updates in 602
  value 201
Nutritional anemia 135, 420
  causes of 135, 136
Nutritional programs 67
  overview of 68
Nutritional services 190
Nutritional status 484
  assessment of 74
Nutritional surveillance 74, 332,
  438
Nutritional survey 74

O

Obesity 178, 179
  childhood 188
  measure of 290
Objectives 113, 117, 124, 338, 596
Observation 247
Obstetrics, preventive medicine in
  64, 185, 292, 437
Obstructed labor 109, 449, 450,
  451
Occupation 4, 32
Occupational diseases 230
  prevention of 310
Occupational health 78, 230, 310,
  439
Ofloxacin 219
Old Integrated Child Development
  Scheme growth chart 333
Onchocerciasis 177, 607

One-way communication 316
Open vial policy 380
Open wounds 229
Optic atrophy 275
Oral antibiotic 521
Oral cancer 610
    epidemiology of 41, 42
    prevention of 42
Oral cefixime 607
Oral contraceptive pill 57, 179, 494
Oral pill 254, 291, 385, 395
Oral polio vaccine 24, 273, 359,
    363, 599
    administration 360
Oral rehydration salt 107, 281,
    322-425
    administration 424
        physiological basis of 423
    components of 423
    mechanism of action of 424,
    425
Oral rehydration therapy 219
Organization, cornerstone of 227
Oropharyngeal swab collection
    507
Orthomyxovirus 588
Osmolar concentration 423
Osteopenia 398
Osteoporosis 194, 398
OT test 208, 306
OTA test 208, 306
Otitis media 481, 610
Outbreak response immunization
    539
Ovarian cancer 397
Ovarian cysts 397
Ovarian disease, benign 397
Overcrowding 217, 468
Overweight 290
Oxidation pond 220
    advantages of 222
Oxygen flow rate 516
Ozone 206

P

Pallor 127, 130
Panel discussion 244, 318, 338
    formats of 244
    procedure of 244
Paper chromatography test 72
Paracetamol, use of 581, 582
Parapet wall 212
Paratyphoid fever 218
Partography 188
Parvovirus B19 274

Passive immunization 365, 369
Pasteurization 197, 334, 438
    methods of 197
Pathology, father of 1
Paucibacillary leprosy 20
Pearl index 414
Pediatric
    antiretroviral regimens 598
    component 562
    preventive medicine in 64, 185,
    292, 437
    pulmonary tuberculosis 547
    tuberculosis treatment 550
Pelvic inflammatory disease 397,
    493
Penicillin 607
    G 607
Pentavalent vaccine 351, 358, 359
Peptic ulcer 63, 311
Performances 604
Perinatal mortality rate 446, 447
Periodic examination 310, 334
Periodic fluctuations 9
Periodic mass screening 261
Peripheral nerve involvement
    170, 276
Permanent disablement
    benefit 81
Permethrin single overnight
    application 607
Persistent diarrhea 531
    follow-up of 531
Persistent pain 501
Personal prophylaxis 34, 102
Personality formation 63
Pertussis 342, 590, 608
    killed acellular bacilli 355
Petechial rash 274
Pharmaceutical waste 224, 225
Phenomena after vaccination
    163, 352
Phlebotomus argentipes 32
Physical
    examination 37
    injuries 228
    methods 384
    rehabilitation 81
Pie chart 460, 461, 463
Pie diagram 463
Placenta 63
    condition of 106
    manual removal of 188
Placental abnormalities 112
Placental insufficiency 112
Plague 234, 281, 607
    chemoprophylaxis 607

Plan vaccination schedule 492
Planning 245
    cycle 245
Plasma insulin 398
Plasmodium
    falciparum malaria, treatment
        of 580, 581
    ovale, treatment of 581
    vivax 589
        malaria, treatment of 579,
        581
Platform 212
Plot weight 497
Pneumococcal conjugate vaccine
    351
Pneumoconiosis 78, 311, 439
    types of 78
Pneumonia 50, 481, 515, 528, 607,
    610
    follow-up of 529
    severe 503, 515
Pneumonic plague 589
Poisons 154
Policy decisions 65
Polio 229, 234, 349, 588, 590
    eradication 273
        and endgame strategic plan
        599
    certification of 273
    surveillance 534
    vaccine 362
        father of 1
        injectable 24, 25, 363
        types of 362
Poliomyelitis 24, 218, 274
    eradication 591
Poliovirus 588
Polycystic ovarian disease 397,
    402
Polyunsaturated fatty acid 178
Pomeroy technique 312
Poor feeding 274
Poor nutritional habits 158
Poor personal hygiene 158
Poor sanitation 158
Population 473
    groups 286
    movement 32
    pyramid 183, 330
Positive predictive value 266, 433,
    454, 457
Postcoital contraception 400
Postcoital pill 385, 400
Post-conceptional methods 385
Posterior capsular
    opacification 52

Posterior segment disorder 52
Posterior tibial nerve 480
Postexposure passive
immunization 36
Postexposure prophylaxis 35, 172,
285
Postexposure vaccination 36
Postnatal care 563
Postnatal check-up 254
Postnatal factors 67
Postnatal mortality 445
rates 444
Postnatal period 553
Post-neonatal
deaths 446
mortality rate 444
Postpartum hemorrhage 449-
451
Postpartum period, complications
of 564
Post-traumatic stress disorder 120
Postvaccination encephalitis 347
Postvasectomy pain syndrome 411
Poverty 203
Povidone iodine 35
Pradhan Mantri Jan Arogya Yojana
605
benefits of 605
Pradhan Mantri Surakshit Matritva
Abhiyan 569, 573
Prasad scale 467
Precancerous lesions 311
treatment of 43
Predictive values 266
Preg-color test 476
Pregnancy 187, 340, 375, 404, 493,
553, 581, 607, 608
complications of 609
termination of 232
toxemias in 109, 112
typhoid in 608
Premature babies 374
Prematurity 610
retinopathy of 487
Prenatal advices 561
Prenatal Diagnostic Techniques
(Regulation and Prevention
of Misuse) (PNDT) Act 195
Prepathogenesis phase 156
Preplacement examination 311,
334
Pressure 155
Preterm birth 610
Prevalence 335
criteria 372
Prevalent disease 269

Prevention
level of 19, 24
types of 157
Preventive medicine 64, 185, 292,
431, 437
Preventive strategies 73
under national program 47
Primaquine, use of 579
Primary health care 249, 252, 254,
321, 320, 440
delivery of 85
elements of 249
functions of 87
principle of 84, 249
Primary health center 54
Primary prevention 19, 42, 510
Primordial prevention 510
Procaine penicillin G 482
Professional bodies 251
Progestasert 391
Progesterone only
injectables 385, 403
pill 385, 399
Progressive neurological disease
374
Proportional mortality rate
limitation of 6
use of 6
Prostitution 102, 204
Protein 155, 201
energy malnutrition 67
Pseudomeasles 365
Psychiatric disorders, stress-
related 348
Psychoanalysis, father of 1
Psychological benefits 72, 202
Public health 341, 431
days 606
issue 288
father of 1
Puerperal sepsis 449, 450
Puffy face 139
Pulmonary tuberculosis 433, 442,
545, 546
period prevalence of 442
Pulse immunization 362
Pulse polio 433
immunization 362
Purified chick embryo cell rabies
vaccine 171
Purified toxoid aluminium
hydroxide 356
phosphate 356
Purified vero cell rabies vaccine
171

Pyrazinamide 549
Pyridoxine 549

Q
Q fever 608
Quality of life 149
measurement of 149
Quantitative data 473
Quarantine 327, 510

R
Rabies 1, 234, 589
immunoglobulin
administration 35
postexposure prophylaxis of
172, 285
vaccination
indication for 171
schedule for 172
vaccine 171
administration sites 36
types of 171
Radial nerve, dorsal branch of 37
Radiation 154
Radioactive substances 83
Radioactive waste 224, 225
Ramp method 216
Random blood glucose 456
Random sampling 236
Randomization 263
role of 263
Rapid antigen point-of-care
test 505
Rapid sand filter 337
Rash 28, 29
Rashtriya Kishor Swasthya
Karyakram 180, 574
Rat bite fever 607
RCA latrine 211, 212
Real time RT-PCR 505
Recombinant vector 345
Record-keeping, importance
of 309
Recurrent respiratory tract
infections 372
Red blood cell count 473
Referral services 198, 254, 294
Referral transport 572
Refractive error 52
Rehabilitation 23, 24, 27, 259, 314,
430
aim of 314
community-based 23
types of 259

Relapsing fever 234
Renal failure 554
Report writing 31
Reporting 143
Reproductive and child health 339, 371
    program 64, 565, 566, 568
        objectives of 566
        strategies of 64
        services 566
Reproductive problems 372
Reproductive tract
    anomaly 493
    infection 493
        control of 567
    malignant growth in 493
Reproductive, Maternal, Neonatal, and Child Health guidelines 412
Resource 95
    analysis 93
    assessment of 129, 246
    mobilization of 94, 122, 131
Respiratory disease 602
Respiratory distress 487
Respiratory failure 504
Respiratory infections 588
Respiratory rate 50, 484
Respiratory tract 372
    infections 120
Retinopathy 275
Retro-orbital pain 28, 29
Retrospective genetic counseling 232
Revised Integrated Child Development Scheme
    growth chart 297
Revised National Tuberculosis Control Program 88, 541
    core elements of 543
    guidelines 540
    implementation of 542
    objectives of 542
    organization of 543
    program goals of 542
    structure of 543
    treatment card 557
Rheumatic fever 610
Rheumatism 64
Rhythm method 385
Rickettsia prowazekii 175
Rifampicin 21, 22, 171, 480, 546, 549
Ringworm 175
River blindness 607
RNA
    myxovirus 588

paramyxovirus 588
togavirus 588
Road traffic accident 140, 451, 602
Rockefeller foundation 321
Rocky mountain spotted fever 330
Rotary clubs 321
Rotavirus 218, 609
    vaccine 350
Rough skin 372
Roundworm 218
Routine immunization 273, 599
Rubella 588
    congenital 234
Ruptured uterus 450
    repair of 187
Rural housing standards 470

S

Safe abortion service 88, 569
Safe drinking water 199
Safe period 385
    method 60, 418
Salmonella typhi 589
Salmonellosis 175, 234, 590
Salt intake 179
Samples
    collection 506
    separation of 239
    transportation of 507
Sampling 235, 474
    importance of 236
    techniques, types of 236
Sandfly control 34, 102
Sanitary land fill 216
Sanitary latrine 209, 210, 468
    criteria for 210
    types of 210
Sanitary well 212, 213
Sanitation 257
    barrier 213, 218, 303
    measures 34, 102
    promotion of 88
SARS-CoV-2 499, 504, 506
    communicability of 500
    induced pneumonia, pathogenesis of 500
    infection 499, 504, 507
    transmission of 499
Saturated fat 179
Scabies 607, 610
Scar 354
Scheme, components of 253
Schistosomiasis 177, 218
School
    dropout 468

health
    records 191
    services 88, 189
    participation 202
Scoring system 466
Scrape method 38
Screening 15, 16, 167, 267, 432
    test 16, 269, 336, 455
        criteria for 16
        sensitivity of 457
Scrotal swelling 103, 475
Scutum 330
Second trimester 581
Secondary prevention 20, 24, 26
Sedentary
    lifestyle 178
    obese 43
Seizures 347, 399
Selection bias 10
Senile cataract 194
Sensation, loss of 479
Sensitivity 267, 432, 433, 454
Sentinel surveillance 157, 261
Sepsis 503, 504
    severe 187
Septic shock 503, 504
Septicemia 188
Septicemic plague 589
Serology 101
Services, packages of 573
Severe COVID-19
    disease, symptoms of 501
    infection 516
    management of 515
Severe malaria 582, 608
    chemotherapy of 582
Sewage 439
Sex
    ratio 436
    separation 217, 469
    specific death rate 441
Sex-linked disorders 195
Sexual abuse 193
Sexual dimorphism 330
Sexual disharmony 102
Sexuality and gender information 135
Sexually transmitted diseases 102, 567
    syndromic management of 269
Sexually transmitted infections 102
Shallow well 336, 337
Shigellosis 590
Shock, hemorrhagic 187

Short-term fluctuations 9
  types of 9
Short-time control measures 33
Sickle cell disease 232, 313
Sickness
  absenteeism 312
  benefit 80, 81
Significance 148, 248
Silica 83
Silicosis 609
Simple formulas 433
Simple random sampling 237
Single dose
  azithromycin 607
  ceftriaxone 607
Situation analysis 92, 120, 124,
    127, 132, 136
Sixty days follow-up examination
    539
Skilled worker 467
Skin 311
  disease 83, 120
  fold thickness 75, 127
  lesion 170, 276
  light yellow appearance of 139
  rashes 501
  smear 38, 170, 276
Sleep, lack of 217
Sleeping sickness 177, 178
Slide positivity rate 284
Slow epidemic 13
Slow sand filter 337
  mechanism of 220
Small family norm 58, 135, 382
Smallpox 342, 588
  eradication 277, 591
  vaccine 2
Smears, grading of 546
Smell, loss of 501
Smoking 158, 203
Soakage
  pit 208, 209
    model of 209
  trench 209
Social
  and economic rehabilitation
    23
  assistance 335
  development 294
  medicine 147, 148, 324, 431
  problems 466
  sciences 77, 202
  security 79, 204, 335
  stigma 102
  welfare officer 93, 106, 109,
    113, 117, 121, 125, 129, 133,
    137, 141, 144

Socialization 63
Socialized medicine 324
Society 204
Socioeconomic
  indicators 593
  scales 467
  status 32, 466
Sodium
  balance, maintenance of 423
  intake 179
Soft tick 330
Solid organ transplantation 165
Sore throat 501
Spacing methods 384
Spastic diplegia 196, 299
Spastic quadriplegia 196, 299
Special senses, failure of 194
Specific death rate 4, 442
Specific protection 20, 24, 290,
    511, 562
Specificity 433, 454
Specimen 420
  handling 507
  transportation of 537
Speech defects 196, 299
Spermicidal foams 384
Spermicidal jelly 384
Spermicides 59, 417
Spinal polio 26
Spontaneous recanalization 411
Squint 197, 299
Srivastava scale 467
Standard days method 408
Standard deviation 315
Standard Q COVID-19 AG
    detection test 505
Staphylococcal food
    poisoning 589
Staphylococcus aureus 589
State blindness control society 54
Stem thermometer 491
Sterilization 232, 334, 387, 422
  methods 408
Steroids, role of 549
Stillbirths 451
Stool
  collection 538
  specimen 537
    collection of 537
    reporting results of 537
    transport of 537
Stop tuberculosis strategy,
    components of 540
Stratified random sampling 238,
    239
Strengthening referral system 66
Streptococcal pharyngitis 590

Streptococcus pneumoniae 609
Streptomycin 549, 607, 608
Stress 179
Stroke 234
Study
  design 473
  population 473
  type 473
  unit of 8
Subacute infection 610
Subacute sclerosing
    panencephalitis 365
Subnormal intelligence 196
Subunit vaccine 344
Suicidal deaths 450
Suicide 194, 451
Sulfur dioxide 205, 206
Supervisory functions 90
Supplementary feeding 47
Supplementary nutrition 69, 198,
    199, 254, 338
Surface infections 589
Surveillance 264, 274, 533, 534
Surveillance medical officer 535
Surveillance, types of 533
Survival rate 159
Sustainable developmental
    goals 594
Swachh Bharat Mission 89, 603
  gramin 604
  urban 603
Sweating 216
Symptothermal method 408, 385
Synechiolysis 392
Syphilis 274, 607
Syphilis, congenital 607
Systematic random sample 237,
    238
Systemic corticosteroids 516

T

Taenia saginata 589
Taenia solium 589
Taeniasis 589
Tamoxifen 392
Tapeworm infestation 175
Target couples 382
Taste sensation, loss of 501
Teaching, tool for 296
Teenage pregnancy 112
Temperature 154
Temporary disablement benefit 81
Tenesmus 478
Tenofovir 598
  plus lamivudine 597

Tension 63
Terminal methods 385, 408
Tertiary prevention 24, 27
Tetanus 106, 229, 277, 349, 589
    toxoid 107, 355, 366, 367
        administration of 119
        immunization 198
Tetracycline 219, 607, 608
Thalassemia 232, 313
Therapeutic nutrition 338
Thimerosal 355
Third trimester 581
Threadworm 218
Three generation family 61
Thrombocytopenia 347, 365
Thromboembolism 398, 504
Thrombosis, acute 503
Tick typhus 330
Tincture iodine 35
Tobacco 154
    consumption, control of 42
Tolerable level 215
Tongue
    lateral border of 610
    pallor of 139
Total births 451
Total fertility rate 58, 383
Toxemia 109, 112
Toxic shock syndrome 365, 388
Toxins 274
Toxoid 344
    antitoxin flocculus 356
Toxoplasma gondii 175
Toxoplasmosis 175
Trachoma 608
Trained birth attendant 116, 323
Transactional cost 570
Transfusion hepatitis 609
Transmission, mode of 32, 100, 218
Transport host 432
Transverse myelitis 274
Trauma 154
Traumatic neuritis 274
Traveller's diarrhea 610
Trench bite 607
Trench method 216
Triage 225, 309, 439
    phases of 226, 309
    system 225, 309
    types of 226, 309
Trichomoniasis 475
Triphasic pill 396
Tubectomy 55, 187
Tuberculin 2
    skin test 547

Tuberculosis 197, 217, 234, 442, 481, 540, 544, 547, 553, 554, 588, 602, 609
    abdominal 550, 551
    Association of India 250
    burden of 540
    case fatality rate for 442
    childhood 349
    diagnosis of 279, 546
    different manifestations of 549
    meningitis 549, 551
    mortality rates for 442
    treatment 434, 544, 549
Tuberculous bacilli 2
Tularemia 330
Tumors 274
Two-way communication 316
Typhoid 120, 161, 218
    fever 197, 219, 262, 589
    transmission of 283

U

Udai Pareek scale 467
Ulnar nerve 37
Ultra-high temperature
    continuous method 197
Uncomplicated gonococcal
    infection 607
Uncomplicated Plasmodium
    falciparum, treatment of 580, 581
Under five mortality rate 294, 446, 447
Underweight 290
UNICEF 89, 256, 321
    role of 89
Unipolar depression 609
Universal Immunization
    Program 567
    recent updates on 350
    vaccines 490
Unsafe drug use behavior 271
Unsafe sexual behavior 271
Unskilled worker 467
Upper respiratory tract
    infections 9
Urban basic services 257
Urethral discharge 103, 475
Urinary tract 372
Urine examination 476
Urine tests 103
Uterine bleeding, abnormal 398
Uterine synechiae 392

V

Vaccination 24, 229, 341, 342, 512
    age for 163, 352
    maximum age of 372
Vaccine 342, 347, 490
    arrangement of 377, 490
    associated paralytic
        poliomyelitis 25, 347, 361
    carrier 379
    derived polioviruses 25
    efficacy 368
    heat sensitivity of 165
    nature of 355, 362
    placement of 378
    product-related reaction 346
    quality defect-related
        reaction 346
    storage of 376
    vial 490
    vial monitor 374
Vacuum extraction 188
Vaginal bleeding, irregular 478
Vaginal discharge 103, 475, 476, 478
Vaginal rings 385
Vaginal sponge 384, 385, 388
Vaginal tears, repair of 187
Vagrancy 204
Vandemataram Scheme 569, 571
Variola virus 588
Vasectomy 187, 385
    complications of 411
    failure of 411, 609
    features of 409
Vasovagal mediated
    reactions 348
Vector borne diseases 229
Vector control methods,
    summary of 176
Venous thrombosis 398
Ventilation 468, 469
Vibrio cholerae 588
Violence 204, 217
Viral encephalitis 330
Viral infections 274
Virology, father of 1
Virulence 342
Visceral leishmaniasis 176, 177, 609
    first line therapy for 607
Vision 596
Visual impairment 601
Vital layer 219, 306

Vitamin
 A 350, 370, 373
  daily intake of 371
  deficiency 69, 371, 567
  prophylaxis 123
  source of 371
  strength of 371
  supplementation 47, 270, 301
Vocational rehabilitation 81
Voluntary health agencies 250
Voluntary muscle testing 23
Vomiting 45, 225, 401, 501

W

Waist circumference 178
Waist hip ratio 178
Waste
 sharps 586
 types of 586
Water
 absorption of 283
 bodies 208
 chlorination of 206, 208
 disinfection of 305
 purification of 304, 306
 quality monitoring 88
 supply 128, 257
Water-borne disease 218, 219, 228
 classification of 218
 control of 218
 prevention of 218
 signs of 218
Weekly iron and folic acid supplementation
 program 182, 575
 tablets, consumption of 182, 575

Weight 74, 114, 127
 gain 178, 398
 loss 101
 normal 290
Weil's disease 218
Well disinfection 222
 steps of 222
Wet smear 476
WHO recommended
 policy 164, 353
 strain 162
WHO, functions of 89
Whooping cough 161, 349, 588
 chemoprophylaxis 607
Wildlife 229
Women's Empowerment Programs 199
Word, derivation of 231
Work, types of 231
Workers
 health of 230
 preplacement examination of 311
 safety of 230
 welfare 230
Workmen's Compensation Act 79
World AIDS Day 606
World Bank 321
World Breastfeeding Week 606
World Cancer Day 606
World Environment Day 606
World Immunization Day 606
World Immunization Week 606
World Leprosy Eradication Day 606
World Malaria Day 606
World Mental Health Day 606
World No Tobacco Day 606

World Polio Day 606
World TB Day 606
Wound, local treatment of 35, 285
Writing up formulated plan 94, 107, 110, 114, 122, 126, 134, 138, 142, 145, 246
Wuchereria bancrofti 589

X

Xerophthalmia 371, 372
X-ray 83
 chest 547

Y

Yellow fever 175, 229, 234, 275, 589
Yersinia pestis 175, 589

Z

Zika fever 600
 update 600
Zinc
 mechanism of action of 426
 therapy 282, 426
Zooanthroponosis 175
Zoology, father of 1
Zoonoses 175, 589
 control of 176
 types of 175
Zoonotic diseases, spectrum of 175

EU GSPR Authorised Reprsentative
Logos Europe, 9 rue Nicolas Poussin
1700, La Rochelle, France
Phone: +33 (0) 6 67 93 73 78
E-mail: contact@logoseurope.eu

www.ingramcontent.com/pod-product-compliance
Ingram Content Group UK Ltd.
Pitfield, Milton Keynes, MK11 3LW, UK
UKHW051420270526

12721UKWH00014B/1133

9 789354 653407